OPTIMUM VITAMIN NUTRITION

for More Sustainable Poultry Farming

OPTIMUM VITAMIN NUTRITION

for More Sustainable Poultry Farming

E.O. Oviedo-Rondon, A.C. Barroeta, R. Cepero Briz, G. Litta, and J.M. Hernandez

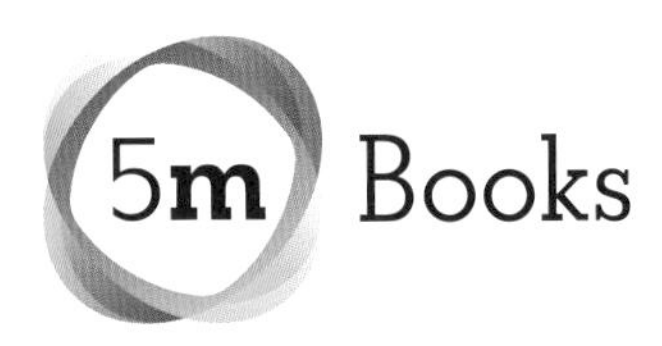

First published 2023

DSM Nutritional Products Ltd
Animal Nutrition & Health
PO Box 2676
4002 Basel, Switzerland
Phone: +41 61 815 8888
Fax: +41 61 815 8270
www.dsmnutritionalproducts.com

Published by
5M Books Ltd,
Lings, Great Easton,
Essex CM6 2HH, UK,
Tel: +44 (0)330 1333 580
www.5mbooks.com

Follow us on
Twitter @5m_Books
Instagram 5m_books
Facebook @5mBooks
LinkedIn @5mbooks

A Catalogue record for this book is available from the British Library

ISBN 9781789182248
eISBN 9781789182323
DOI 10.52517/9781789182323

Book layout by Cheshire Typesetting Ltd, Cuddington, Cheshire
Printed by Bell & Bain Ltd, Glasgow
Photos by the authors unless otherwise indicated

CONTENTS

Authors and acknowledgements vi
List of abbreviations vii

Chapter 1 Contribution of vitamin nutrition to a more sustainable farming 1
Chapter 2 A brief history of vitamins 21
Chapter 3 Introduction to vitamins 29
Chapter 4 Vitamin description 48
Chapter 5 Optimum vitamin nutrition in poultry breeders 151
Chapter 6 Optimum vitamin nutrition in broilers and turkeys 199
Chapter 7 Optimum vitamin nutrition in laying hens 279

Bibliography 329
Index 421

Authors and acknowledgements

E.O. Oviedo-Rondon
Prestage Department of Poultry Science, North Carolina State University

A.C. Barroeta
Animal Nutrition and Welfare Service, Department of Animal and Food Science, Universitat Autònoma de Barcelona, Bellaterra, Spain

R. Cepero Briz
Department of Animal Production and Food Science, Faculty of Veterinary Science, University of Zaragoza, Spain

G. Litta and J.M.Hernandez
DSM Nutritional Products, Animal Nutrition and Health

The authors are grateful to Dr. Lina Maria Peñuela, Dr. Paula Lozano Cruz, Dr. Jhon Nicolás Mejía and Dr. Valmiro Aragão Neto, who supported the work of Dr. Edgar O. Oviedo-Rondon at North Carolina State University; to Dr. G. Gonzales, Dr. J. Sanz, Dr. R. Davin, Dr. M. D. Baucells and Dr. A. Blanco Perez who supported the work of Dr. Ana Barroeta and Dr. Ricardo Cepero Briz; and to Dr. C. Lozano, Dr. F. Nell, and Dr. B. Shi from DSM Nutritional Products.

Abbreviations

ACP	acyl groups carrier protein
ACTH	adrenocorticotropic hormone
ADP	adenosine diphosphate
ALH	amplitude of lateral head
aP	available phosphorus
ARC	Agriculture Research Council
ASA	acetylsalicylic acid
ATP	adenosine triphosphate
BBS	black bone syndrome
BV	both vitamins (liposoluble and water-soluble)
BW	body weight
CaBP	calcium-binding protein
CDP	cytidine diphosphocholine
CNS	central nervous system
CoA	coenzyme A
CRALBP	cellular retinaldehyde binding protein
DBP	(vitamin) D-binding protein
DBS	dried blood spots
DEX	dexamethasone
DHA	docosahexaenoic acid
DOI	day of injection
DSID	dietary supplement ingredient database
EL	effective layer
ELISA	enzyme-linked immunosorbent assay
ETKA	erythrocyte transketolase activity
FA	folic acid
FAD	flavin adenine dinucleotide
FCR	feed conversion ratio
FDA	Food and Drug Administration
FEDNA	Fundación Española para el Desarrollo de la Nutrición Animal (Spanish Foundation for the Development of Animal Nutrition)
FGF23	fibroblast growth factor 23
FLKS	fatty liver and kidney syndrome
FMN	flavin mono-nucleotide
FPD	foot pad dermatitis
FSH	follicle-stimulating hormone
GABA	gamma-aminobutyric acid
GHG	greenhouse gas
GHR	growth hormone receptor
HB	hock burn

HC	haptocorrin
HDL	high-density lipoprotein
HDP	hen day production
HPLC	high-performance liquid chromatography
IgA	immunoglobulin A
IgG	immunoglobulin G
INRAE	Institut National de Recherche Agronomique et l'Environnement (National Institute for Agricultural Research and Environment)
IU	international unit
LDL	low-density lipoprotein
LH	luteinizing hormone
LHR	luteinizing hormone receptor
LPS	lipopolysaccharide
LV	liposoluble vitamins
MDA	malondialdehyde
ML	mammillary layer
MNB	menadione nicotinamide bisulfite
MTHFR	N10-methylene-tetrahydrofolate reductase
MV	medullary cavity volume
NAD	nicotinamide adenine dinucleotide (oxidized form)
NADH	nicotinamide adenine dinucleotide (reduced form)
NADP	nicotinamide adenine dinucleotide phosphate (oxidized form)
NADPH	nicotinamide adenine dinucleotide phosphate (reduced form)
NRC	National Research Council
OVN	Optimum Vitamin Nutrition
PABA	para-aminobenzoic acid
PAF	platelet-activating factor
PC	pyruvate carboxylase
PL	pyridoxal
PLP	pyridoxal-5'-phosphate
PM	pectoralis major
PMP	pyridoxamine-5'-phosphate
PN	pyridoxol or pyridoxine
PNG	pyridoxine-5'-beta-D-glucoside
PNP	pyridoxine-5'-phosphate
PSE	pale, soft, and exudative
PTH	parathyroid hormone
PUFA	polyunsaturated fatty acids
RAR	retinoic acid receptors
RBP	retinol-binding protein
RDA	recommended daily allowances
RIA	radioimmunoassays
ROS	reactive oxygen species
RXR	retinoid X receptor
SC	satellite cells
SD	standard deviation
SM	shell membrane
SRBC	sheep red blood cells

TBARS	thiobarbituric acid reactive substances
TC	transcobalamin
TCA	tricarboxylic acid
TD	tibial dyschondroplasia
THF	tetrahydrofolate
TMP	thiamine monophosphate
TPP	thiamine pyrophosphate
TPV	total pore volume
TTP	thiamine triphosphate
USP	United States Pharmacopeia
UV	ultraviolet
VBP	vitamin D-binding protein
VDR	vitamin D receptor
VLDL	very-low-density lipoprotein
WS	white striping
WV	water-soluble vitamins

Chapter 1

Contribution of vitamin nutrition to a more sustainable farming

ADDRESSING THE CHALLENGES OF TODAY AND TOMORROW

Today, well into the 21st century, the crucial issues relating to food production are changing. Key concepts such as productivity and efficiency continue to be of vital importance. Still, more and more, the emphasis is on the significance of terms such as sustainability, animal health and welfare, food quality from animal origin, and food waste.

Everything indicates that continuous development in the field of animal nutrition is becoming essential to meet current and future challenges. Challenges such as replacing antibiotics and coccidiostats, combatting higher incidences of more aggressive animal diseases, and responding to a growing focus on more sustainable farming, in which our industry has a critical role to play in shaping a better world in line with the Sustainable Development Goals of the United Nations. Specifically, our industry needs to:

- produce cost-effective animal protein production – for all
- provide high-quality food and feed – for a better life for all
- develop proper livelihoods – for 30% of the world population working today in agriculture
- treat animals well until the end of their life – all of them
- eliminate the negative impact of food production – on us and the environment.

In parallel, as a player who aspires to be a leader in climate action, it is important for the feed industry to lead by example, constantly seeking to reduce the carbon emissions and the environmental footprint of products and processes. That means closely managing absolute greenhouse gas (GHG) emissions and energy efficiency. A growing number of companies are setting long-term goals, validated by the Science Based Targets initiative (SBTi) aligned with the Paris Climate Agreement (COP 21) of 2015, to reach net-zero emissions before 2050. These are ambitious and long-term challenges in which the optimal use of vitamins in animal nutrition should be part of the solution.

COMMITMENT TO SUSTAINABILITY

Providing the right levels of high-quality and sustainably produced vitamins to feed mills, integrators, and farmers will help them improve animal health, well-being, and performance, while also protecting the environment, succeeding in a dynamic and ever-changing global market, and enhancing both profits and environmental sustainability.

Optimizing the performance and improving the sustainability of feed additives and premixes plays an important role in reducing the environmental burden of animal protein production.

Excipients such as rice hulls and calcium carbonate can make up to 50% of a premix composition, but little can be done to reduce their carbon footprint further. The critical products with the potential to contribute to carbon footprint and environmental impact reductions in premixes are the nutritional supplements such as vitamins.

Reducing the impact of vitamins and other feed additive operations might enable feed mills and farmers to become more sustainable, reduce their risk profile, and potentially benefit from the value created from future carbon tax savings (Figure 1.1).

Carbon pricing – whether implemented as a tax or cap and trade system – seeks to reduce GHG emissions by putting a direct financial liability on industries and activities that are large GHG emitters. It is a policy intervention to encourage the reduction of harmful activities.

The sustainability of mainstream animal production is increasingly questioned as demand rises. International bodies agree that animal protein production is one of the activities that need to reduce carbon emissions if we want to solve the climate crisis. Reductions in the impact of agricultural and animal production processes can be supported by greater use of sustainably produced nutritional solutions.

Additionally, governments may seek to impose low-carbon product standards, further environmental regulation, or tax schemes, on animal protein production or products as an incentive to reduce emissions and steer consumer consumption. The groundwork for these interventions is already being laid. In Germany, value-added tax increases on meat and dairy products are being proposed. The New Zealand government has agreed to include farm-level emissions in its Emissions Trading Scheme by 2025, and the Dutch government has committed to studying 'fair meat prices' ahead of fiscal reforms in 2022.

The agricultural and animal protein products supply chain prepare to minimize the risks posed by these changes or face severe financial penalties. The only way to do this is to significantly reduce animal production's impact on the climate and the environment. Equally, redesigning existing incentive systems (i.e. subsidies) and scaling up high-quality voluntary carbon credit systems to directly reward emission reductions can significantly accelerate the transition.

This transition to a lower-carbon future for animal proteins can be facilitated by supplying nutritional ingredients, such as vitamins, with industry-leading performance to improve the efficiency of animal production systems while reducing the carbon footprint of these feed additives and those within which they are utilized (Figure 1.2).

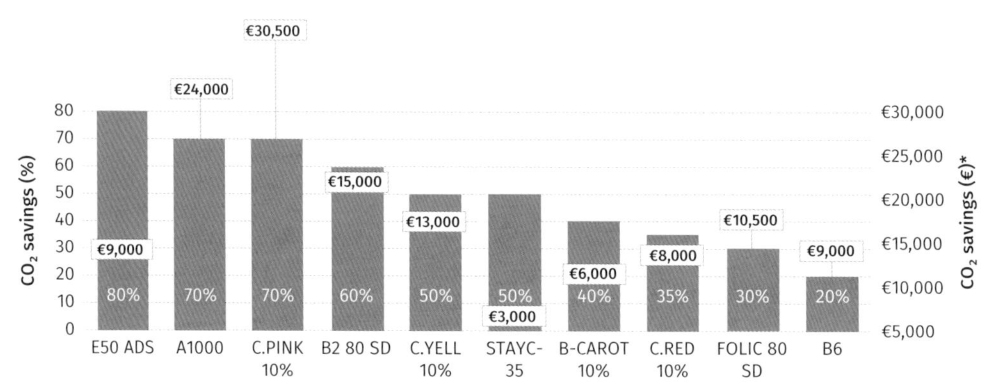

Figure 1.1 Carbon dioxide savings and potential value (carbon tax) per 10 t of feed additive: DSM product vs. the main alternative (source: DSM Animal Nutrition and Health, unpublished)

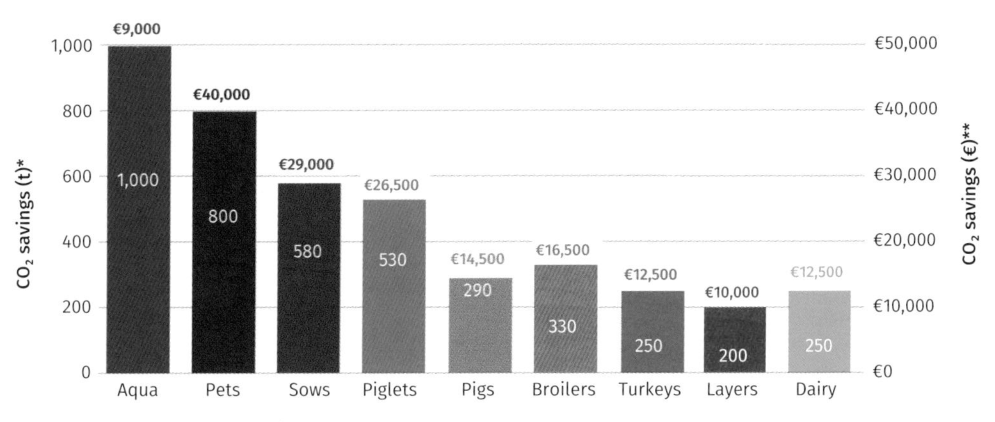

Figure 1.2 Carbon dioxide savings and potential value (carbon tax) of a more sustainable vitamin source for 100,000 t of feed produced (source: DSM Animal Nutrition and Health, unpublished)

UPDATING THE NUTRITIONAL STANDARDS OF VITAMINS IN A CONSTANTLY EVOLVING WORLD

Vitamins play a decisive role in both human and animal nutrition. As organic catalysts present in small quantities in most foods, they are essential for the normal functioning of metabolic and physiological processes such as growth, development, health, and reproduction. The requirements for vitamins in animals are dynamic: they vary according to new genotypes, levels of yield, and production systems. Vitamin functions and requirements are becoming increasingly well known.

The concept of OVN Optimum Vitamin Nutrition® for animals is essential today. Its objective is to develop a new standard for vitamin supplementation in feed in order to improve animal health status and resilience to diseases and environmental stress, which will translate into better animal productivity and homogeneity. Moreover, the quality of food produced by those animals can be enhanced, improving human health and reducing food waste. The latter is critical in a global society in which, unfortunately, many people still do not have access to the correct quantity and quality of food.

When we talk about optimum vitamin supplementation in the diet of animals, we refer to the provision of vitamin levels both over and above the established minimum requirements for avoiding deficiencies and adapted to the specific conditions of each animal species to achieve the objectives mentioned above.

Historically, the objective of the vitamin recommendations provided by various international scientific organs – such as the National Research Council (NRC USA), the Agriculture Research Council (ARC UK), and the National Research Institute for Agriculture, Food and Environment (Institut National de Recherche Agronomique et l'Environnement, INRAE, France) – was preventing nutritional shortages or deficiencies. Some of the studies on which they are based are over 40 years old. We all know that the livestock industry today has not much in common with the industry as it was at that time. Figure 1.3 shows that broiler body weight and feed conversion ratio (FCR) have improved up to 30% in the last 20 years, mainly due to genetic improvements.

Therefore, it is logical to infer that nutrition programs for farm animals must be adjusted, including vitamin supplementation, consistently with improved animal management techniques and genetic make-up. The case of vitamin D (Figure 1.4) illustrates how an improved broiler FCR requires adjustment of vitamin levels:

- as 170 g less feed is needed to reach 2.3 kg body weight (–5%) when comparing 2017 to 2021 Ross 308 genetics
- then vitamin D_3 level in feed (International Unit (IU)/kg) should be increased by 5% to keep the same vitamin D_3 intake by the bird.

Likewise, in recent times there have been important legislative changes around the world which limit the use of compounds such as antibiotics and growth promoters, substances that until recently had formed a regular part of animals' diets and the animal trials on which vitamins requirements were based.

At the same time, many countries are developing new rules on animal welfare which, in the short to medium terms, will entail less "intensiveness" in the livestock industry, aiming to improve the animals' health and well-being. Meanwhile, our farmers need to be competitive

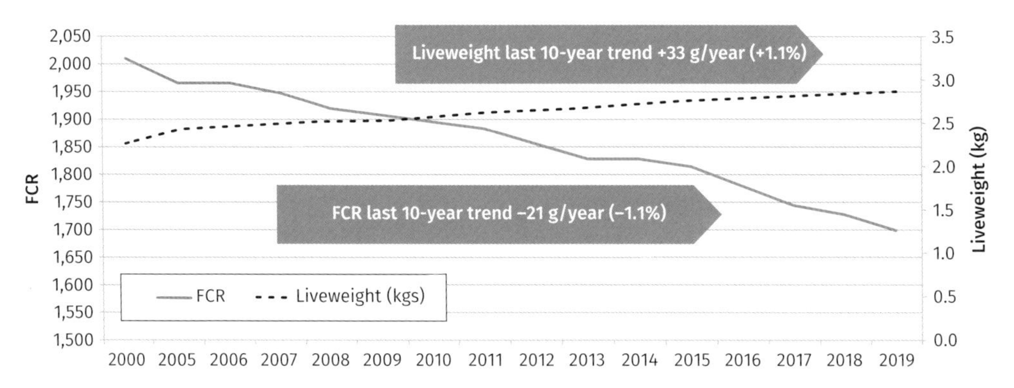

Figure 1.3 Genetic improvement in broilers: long-term field trend for liveweight and FCR (source: National Chicken Council, USA, 2022)

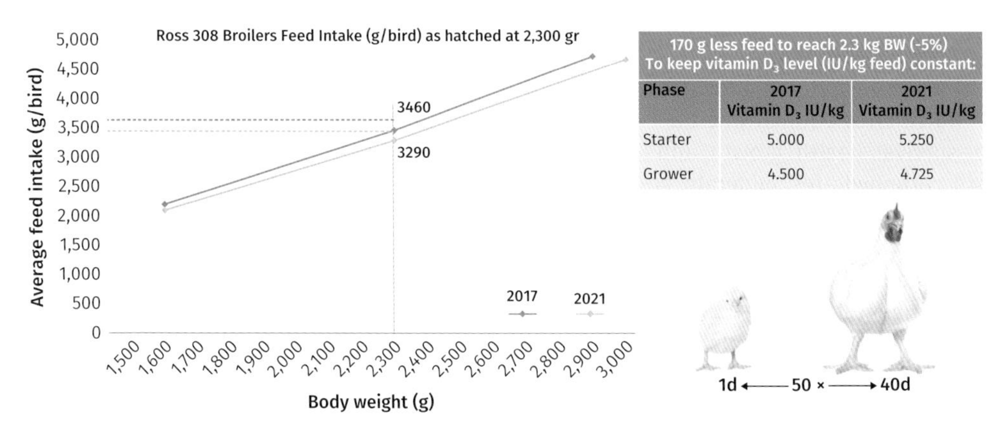

170 g less feed to reach 2.3 kg BW (-5%) To keep vitamin D_3 level (IU/kg feed) constant:		
Phase	2017 Vitamin D_3 IU/kg	2021 Vitamin D_3 IU/kg
Starter	5.000	5.250
Grower	4.500	4.725

Figure 1.4 Impact of broiler genetic progress on net vitamin intake (source: elaboration by DSM Animal Nutrition and Health, unpublished, based on Aviagen and Ross 308 Performance objectives)

enough regarding livestock productivity (weight gain, FCR, the final weight of the animal, mortality, etc.) to survive strong international competition where free trade is a tangible reality.

From the nutritional point of view, in these fast-changing circumstances, so different from those we have become accustomed to in recent years, it is essential to re-evaluate the vitamin requirements of animals with the aim of safely and efficiently producing healthy and nourishing food that meets consumer expectations, always under sustainable farming practices.

VITAMINS: ESSENTIAL MICRONUTRIENTS IN THE ANIMAL ORGANISM

Vitamins are unique and crucial nutrients in the diet of people and animals. They are important elements in the organism's vital functions: maintenance, growth, development, health, and reproduction. They also combine 2 characteristics.

- The daily requirement for each of the vitamins is very small, an aspect in which they differ from macronutrients such as carbohydrates, fats, and proteins.
- Vitamins are organic compounds, unlike other essential nutrients such as minerals (iron, iodine, zinc, etc.).

The discovery of vitamins and their function in preventing the classical deficiency diseases are milestones that stand among the most important achievements of the last century. Vitamins are particularly important because they allow optimum metabolism of other nutrients in the animal diet. In general, humans and animals need to derive them from their diet as they cannot produce the appropriate quantities by themselves. Vitamins are present in more than 30 reactions of the cellular metabolism and play, particularly in combination, a critical role in the Krebs or citric acid cycle (Figure 1.5).

Vitamins may only represent less than 1% of the cost of animal feed, but they are present in 100% of metabolic functions. This fact gives them the status of micronutrients of macro importance. Vitamins are found in minimal quantities in most feedstuffs. Their absence from the diet gives rise to specific deficiency diseases because of their significance for the normal functioning of the metabolism.

While the need to provide additional vitamins in feed is unquestioned, the levels of supplementation needed to achieve an optimum economic return in field conditions are open to debate. As a general rule, the optimum economic supplementation level is that which achieves the best index of growth, feed conversion, health status – including the immunocompetence – and which, in addition, provides the reserves appropriate for the organism.

Nutrition is optimal when an animal efficiently utilizes the nutrients provided in the feed for survival, health, growth, and reproduction. Although all the nutrients, including proteins, fats, carbohydrates, minerals, and water, are essential for carrying out these vital functions, vitamins play a key role in basic functions, such as an appropriate immune response in animals.

As mentioned already, several factors – e.g., increased productivity driven by genetic improvement, intensive farming, and higher susceptibility to diseases – give rise to a growing vulnerability to vitamin deficiencies and a yield below the optimum. A great majority of nutritionists and investigators recognize that the minimum vitamin requirements needed to prevent clinical deficiency symptoms may not be sufficient to achieve an optimum state of health and yield. In Chapter 4 we will review the multiple metabolic functions specific to each of the vitamins in greater depth.

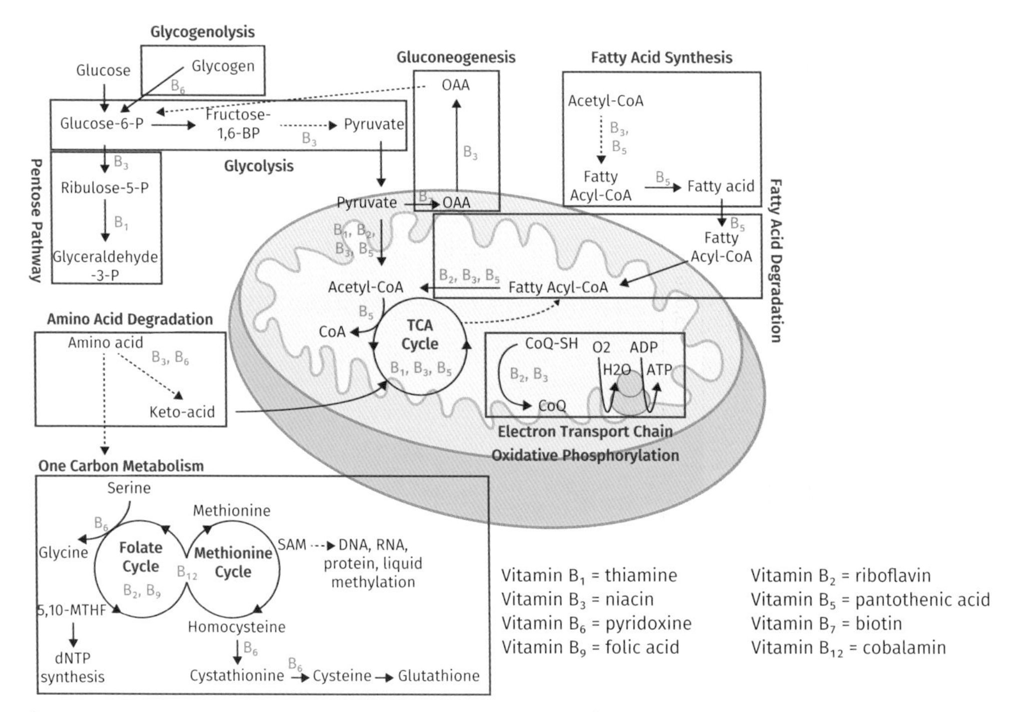

Figure 1.5 Metabolic functions and interactions of B vitamins (source: Godoy-Parejo *et al.*, 2020)

VITAMIN LEVELS IN ANIMAL DIET: THE NUTRITIONIST'S GREAT UNKNOWN QUANTITY

Establishing the vitamin supplementation level is something all nutritionists should concern themselves with. Economic cost and benefit must be a fundamental reason for revising and determining vitamin supplements in feed. The cost of supplementing feed with essential vitamins must be assessed considering the risk of suffering losses from deficiency symptoms and productive yields below the optimum. The great challenge for nutritionists is choosing a particular level from the numerous recommended tables.

There are currently various sets of recommendations for vitamin levels in feed available from industries in the animal feed sector, research institutes, animal genetics companies, and vitamin manufacturers themselves (Figure 1.6). In turn, fundamental differences can be seen in how the studies have been produced.

The ARC in the UK and the NRC in the USA periodically publish nutritional recommendations for different species, which generally constitute reference sources of limited value from the viewpoint of commercial feed formulation. The recommendations are based on establishment of the vitamin levels necessary to prevent clinical deficiency symptoms. NRC recommendations, for example, are revisions usually carried out based on studies done in experimental conditions that are perfectly controlled and therefore far removed from commercial conditions. For instance, they do not account for the stress factor, a frequent part of livestock rearing, which stress can drastically influence nutritional needs. For example, Liu *et al.* (2022) studied the effect of a coccidiosis vaccine challenge, a stress factor, on broilers fed OVN™ to simulate challenging practical farm conditions (Figures 1.7 and 1.8).

Female parent stock nutrient specifications 5-stage rearing program

		Starter 1	Starter 2	Grower	Developer	Pre-Breeder	Breeder 1	Breeder 2	Breeder 3
Added vitamins per kg	Unit	0–21 days	22–42 days	43–105 days	106–140 days	141 days to 5% production	>5% production to 224 days	225 – 350 days	After 351 days
Vitamin A	IU	13,000					15,000		
Vitamin D_3	IU	4,000					5,000		
Vitamin E	IU	100					130		
Vitamin K (menadione)	mg	6					9		
Thiamine (B_1)	mg	5					6		
Riboflavin (B_2)	mg	15					20		
Niacin	mg	50					70		
Pantothenic acid	mg	20					25		
Pyridoxine	mg	5					8		
Biotin	mg	0.3					0.6		
Folic acid	mg	3					5		
Vitamin B_{12}	mg	0.05					0.07		

Figure 1.6 Nutrition specifications for Ross 308 FF parent stock (source: Aviagen 2022)

The coccidiosis challenge resulted in higher intestinal lesion scores (1.8 *vs.* 0.8), especially for scores 2 and 3 when compared to the control, and significantly lower plasma absorption of vitamin A (–25%), vitamin E (–70%), and vitamin D_3 (–35%). Broilers in the coccidiosis challenge treatment (T2) achieved poorer weight gain and feed conversions *than*

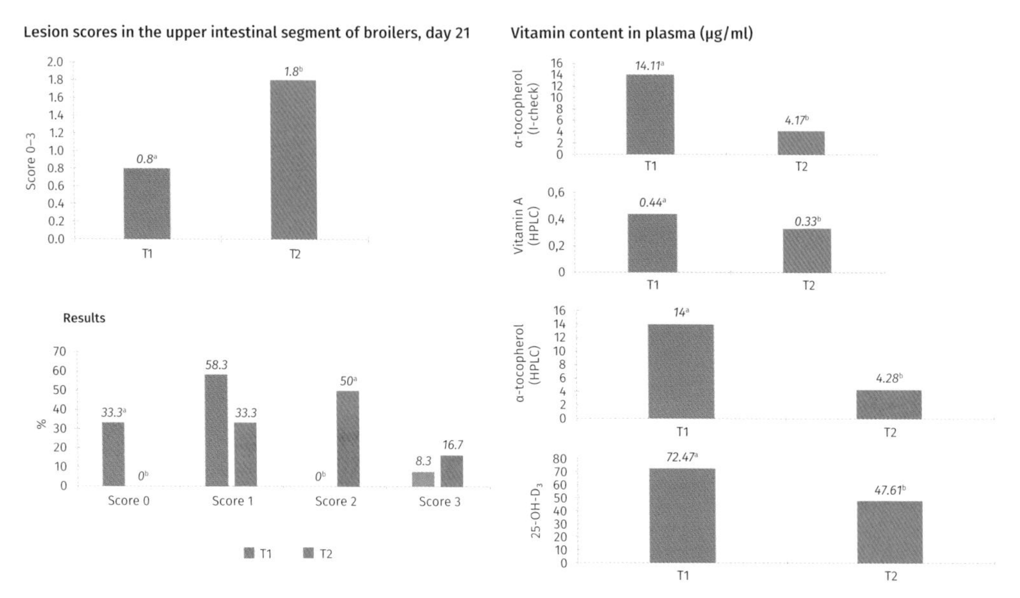

Figure 1.7 Effect of coccidiosis vaccine challenge on intestinal lesion score and plasma vitamin level of 21-day broilers fed with an OVN® diet (source: Liu *et al.*, 2022) ([a,b] $P < 0.05$)

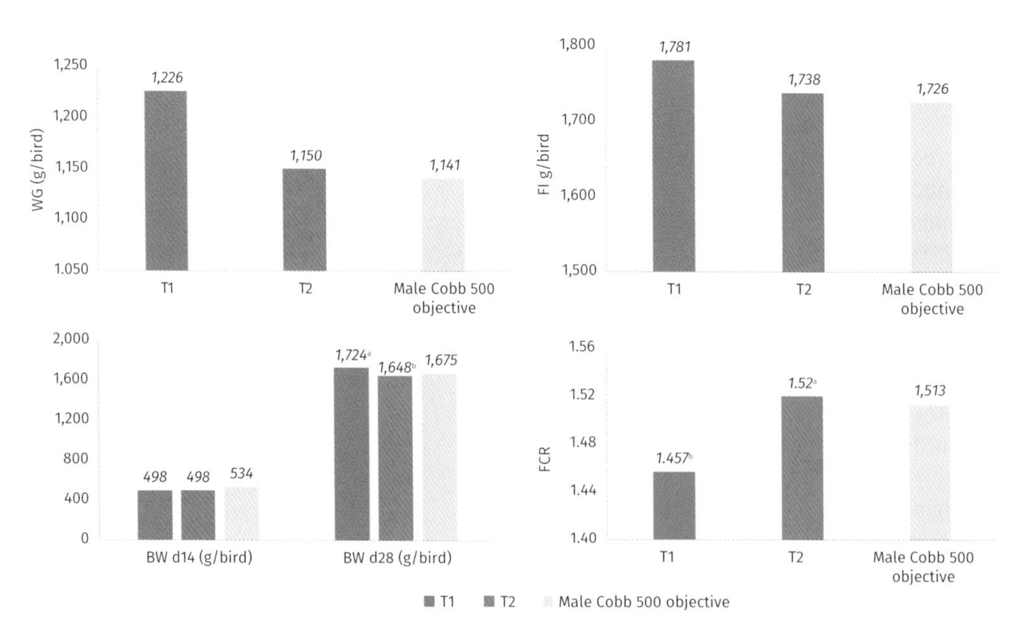

Figure 1.8 Effect of coccidiosis vaccine challenge on growth performance of 21-day broilers fed with an OVN™ diet (source: Liu *et al.*, 2022) ([a,b] $P < 0.05$)

non-challenged birds (T1), similar to Cobb 500 objective. The non-challenged OVN™ diet (T1) birds performed better than Cobb 500 objectives.

To make more efficient use of the NRC's vitamin recommendations, it is advisable to take into account the following considerations.

1. The indicated levels have been established to prevent deficiencies in the animal.
2. They do not include any kind of safety margin to prevent loss of vitamin activity stemming from usual feed storage conditions or feed processing. In other words, the recommended NRC levels must be those present in the animal's feed and when the animal is eating it.
3. They do not include safety margins for the eventuality that the animals are subjected to some sort of stress or subclinical disease.
4. They do not consider possible adverse environmental conditions, such as high temperatures, which may reduce the animal's food consumption.
5. In most cases, they are not specific to the new animal genotypes that are now being produced to optimize livestock farming.

Nutritionists usually consider stress and other economically important variables in their formulations. There is a great disparity between the levels of supplementation prescribed by the industry and those indicated by both NRC and ARC. While the industry continues to adjust vitamin supplementation in feed to achieve an optimum yield and state of health in the animal, the NRC has introduced only a few minor changes for most animal species in the last few decades. Moreover, the previous edition of the nutritional recommendations for poultry is dated 1994. Logically, the vitamin needs established nearly 3 decades ago do not apply to today's animals. Most nutritionists agree on this aspect, and supplements of many vitamins are given at levels 5 or 10 times higher than those recommended by the NRC. The greatest differences are in the vitamins A, D_3, E, B_{12}, riboflavin, pantothenic acid, and folic acid, while variations are lower with K_3, niacin, and B_6.

BIOAVAILABILITY OF VITAMINS IN ANIMALS

Many feed materials used in animal nutrition contain variable quantities of vitamins. The amounts of vitamins available in the feed are limited by the nutritional requirements of these materials: hence, the vitamin levels in the diet obtained from feedstuffs tend to vary considerably. The overall content is low, and their presence in the feed does not guarantee their bioavailability or that the animal will indeed benefit from them.

It is well accepted that vitamin levels in feedstuffs vary significantly from one geographical region to another as well as depending on the time of harvesting and the climatic conditions at each harvest. Long storage periods and the use of preservatives, fungicides, etc., negatively affect the vitamin content. Some of the factors which most adversely affect the level of vitamins in the ingredients of feed are:

- origin of the harvest
- use of fertilizers
- genetic modifications, which increase productive yield
- climate
- agricultural practices, such as crop rotation
- harvesting conditions

- storage conditions and the use of preservatives
- bioavailability.

The real content of vitamins in feed is determined by complex chemical and microbiological analysis methods carried out in authorized laboratories, which provide the real value at a given time for a certain sample or batch of the respective ingredient. But given the great number of factors that affect the stability of vitamins (temperature, humidity, light, etc.), it would be necessary to undertake costly systematic analyses of the principal feed materials to be able to use those values reliably in the formulation – at minimum cost – of the feed, with the constant adaptation of the values to avoid possible variations of the desired level.

In many cases, vitamins derived from the feedstuffs are present in compound forms that are not bioavailable, hence, not available to be absorbed and participate in the animal's physiological and metabolic processes.

In commercial vitamin preparations, various substances protect them from harm during feed production processes and from aggressive environmental agents during storage. Therefore, it is essential to consider the bioavailability of these substances when determining the vitamin content of any feed ingredient. Figure 1.9 shows the commercial form of vitamin A – A 1000 prod. Z – is not bioavailable as the other 2 preparations.

In contrast, in nature, both in vegetable and animal products, substances can effectively destroy the vitamin activity or limit their bioavailability. These antinutritional agents can also be released by certain types of bacteria or fungi – e.g., mycotoxins – as by-products of their metabolic activity, as well as being present in the normal environment of the production facilities. Their most frequent mechanism of action consists of deactivating the free form of the vitamin or preventing its absorption.

The addition of fats and oils as an energy source is common practice in the manufacture of feed. Attention should be paid to the total content of unsaturated fatty acids since they increase the likelihood that the oils and fats will become rancid. This would affect the absorption of fat-soluble vitamins such as A, E and D. Likewise, oxidation of the fats would also contribute to biotin deactivation.

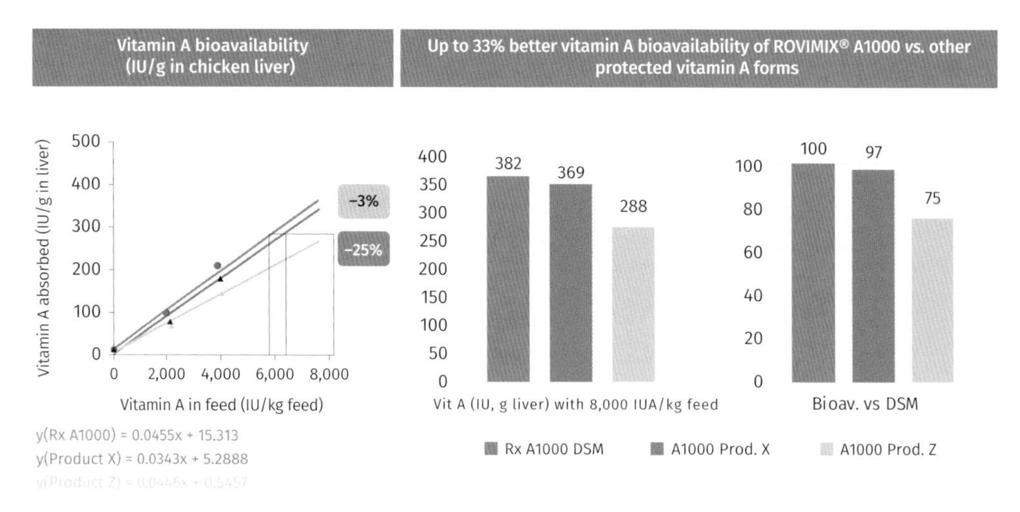

Figure 1.9 Impact of different commercial forms of ethoxyquin-free vitamin A on vitamin A bioavailability in broilers (source: Ludwig-Maximilian University, Munich, unpublished)

STABILITY OF VITAMINS IN ANIMAL FEED

Diverse factors can affect the stability of substances as volatile as vitamins, whether in their pure commercial form, in vitamin-mineral premixes, or after the manufacture of compound feed and its subsequent storage. Some of these factors are connected with the catalytic activity of the molecules themselves, the handling of commercial forms and their premixes, the characteristics of the blend, the presence of various antagonistic substances, and the storage conditions.

The vitamins present in primary materials are very susceptible to the adverse conditions mentioned above, and a heavy loss of vitamin activity is a common occurrence in these macro-ingredients. In contrast, the highest-quality commercial forms of vitamins are produced from industrial processes, which stabilize and protect the molecules of active substance during manufacture and storage, both in premixes and the feed.

Since African swine fever became a pandemic in China, the Chinese feed mills implemented specific thermal processing to inactivate the virus. Yang *et al.* (2020) carried out a trial to measure vitamin stability. They concluded that most B complex vitamins have great stability in feed processing, but the stability of fat-soluble vitamins was negatively affected by feed processing. In addition, microencapsulated vitamins had greater stability compared to non-microencapsulated vitamins. Based on these results, decreasing the strength of feed processing and choice of suitable forms of the vitamin could be recommended in feed production.

Recent data from a European premix company shows large differences in vitamin A stability in pelleted feed at 90°C with 30, 60, or 120 seconds of holding time (up to 50%) when comparing 3 different vitamin A product forms (Figure 1.10).

However, it must again be emphasized that the stabilization of the vitamins must not compromise their bioavailability in the animal. Different methods are used to stabilize vitamins.

- **Use of antioxidants** – Antioxidants are included in the formulation of commercial vitamin products to prevent fat-soluble vitamins' oxidation and prolong these compounds' shelf life. In general, those commercial forms with an appropriate quantity of antioxidant

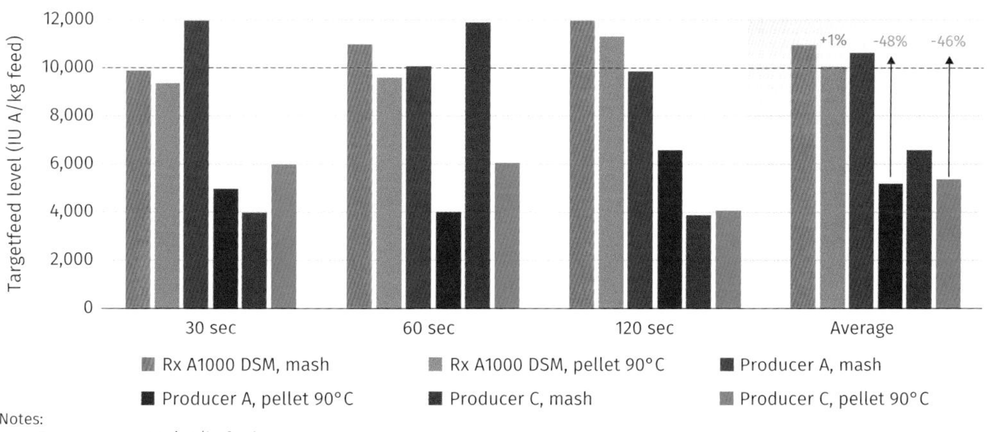

Notes:
- Target = 10,000 IU vit A/kg feed
- Premixes produced by large EU premixer with 3 different vitamin A products
- Feed corn/wheat/soy produced by Kolding Tech. Institute, Denmark
- Vitamin analyses carried out by LUFA Kiel lab, Germany (method REG(EC) 152/2009, IV, A)

Figure 1.10 Vitamin A stability in a 90°C pelleted feed at 30, 60, and 120 seconds holding time (source: elaboration by DSM Animal Nutrition and Health based on data from a European premix company, 2020 unpublished)

substances have a longer effective shelf life. This period, during which vitamin content is guaranteed, will depend to a great extent on storage conditions. The ban of ethoxyquin in the EU and some other countries has put additional pressure on vitamin, premix, and feed manufacturers to adapt their product formulation technologies and sources to guarantee the right content of the active substance in the products they market.
- **Mechanical methods** – The process, in this case, covers the active substance with a stabilizing coat. This covering protects the vitamin molecule inside it from the adverse effect of aggressive external agents, such as the presence of oxygen, ultraviolet radiation, sunlight, humidity, different temperatures, etc. (Figure 1.11).

On a practical level, this method has proved highly effective in protecting these substances and, depending on their characteristics, can be combined with a process of spray drying, which provides a large number of active particles (all with the active form of the vitamin), which facilitates a subsequent homogenous mixture in the animal's food. This is particularly relevant for vitamins like biotin or B_{12} added into feed at very low levels (Figure 1.12).

At all events, the factors mentioned above affect different vitamins in different ways.

- Vitamins A, D, and carotenoids:
  - are prone to oxidation when exposed to air
  - are sensitive to oxidizing agents
  - isomerize in acid pH
  - are sensitive to prolonged heat
  - are sensitive to the catalytic effect of minerals.
- Vitamin E:
  - is prone to oxidation in the presence of air
  - is sensitive to alkaline mediums
  - the ester is relatively more stable.

Additive	Temperature	Oxygen	Humidity	Light
Vitamin A	++	++	+	++
Vitamin D	+	++	+	+
$25OHD_3$ (calcifediol)	++	++	+	+
Vitamin E	0	+	0	+
Vitamin K_3	+	+	++	0
Vitamin B_1	+	+	+	0
Vitamin B_2	0	0	+	+
Vitamin B_6	++	0	+	+
Pantothenic acid	+	0	+	0
Nicotinates	0	0	0	0
Biotin	+	0	0	0
Folic acid	++	0	+	++
Vitamin C	++	++	++	0

++ Marked effect
+ Moderate effect
0 No effect

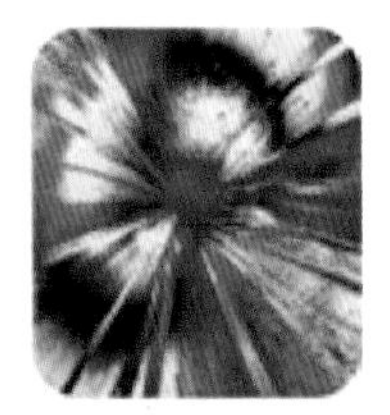

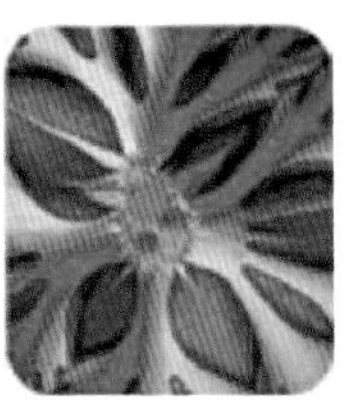

Figure 1.11 External factors influencing the stability of non-formulated vitamins (source: DSM Animal Nutrition and Health, DSM Product Forms. Quality feed ingredients for more sustainable farming, 2022)

Physical characteristics	DSM ROVIMIX® Biotin 2% SD	DSM ROVIMIX® Biotin HP 10% SD	Biotin 2% Triturate A
Soluble in water	yes	yes	no
Flowability (sec-100g)	medium	medium	low flow, tapping required
Average practical size (µm)	66	73	296
Mixability in feed, CV %	6%	5.7%	10.8%
Total particles per g product	>21 mio	>20 mio	>10 mio
Active particles per g product	100%	100%	2% (98% carrier)
Active Biotin particles per animal/day @ 0.2 mg biotin/Kg feed @ 10 g feed/day/chick	2000	400	20

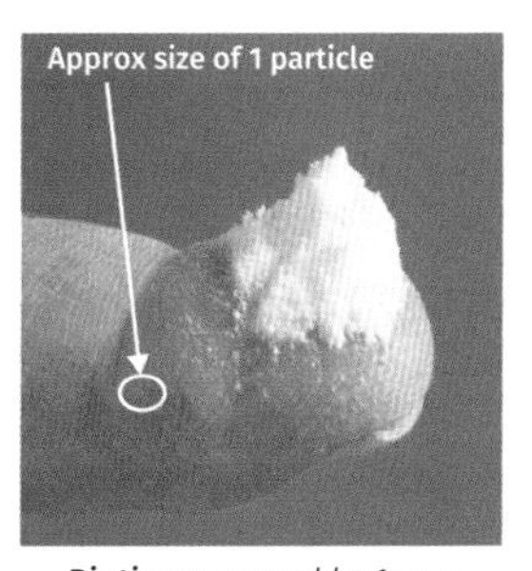

Biotin** consumed by **1 sow** **(or 20 birds,** or **1 dog** or **4 salmon) per year

Figure 1.12 Confrontation of physical characteristics of biotin spray-dried form against biotin triturate (source: DSM Animal Nutrition and Health, unpublished)

- Vitamin K:
  - is sensitive to heat
  - is prone to oxidation in the presence of oxygen.
- Vitamin B_1 (thiamine):
  - is stable with low pH, loss of activity when pH of the medium increases
  - is sensitive to the presence of oxygen and other oxidizing agents in neutral or alkaline solutions
  - splits on reacting with sulfites, with immediate separation at pH 6
  - is sensitive to metallic ions, such as copper
  - the thiaminases present in some animal and vegetable products are known antagonists of this vitamin.
- Vitamin B_2 (riboflavin):
  - is sensitive to light, especially in alkaline solutions
  - is stable in acid and neutral mediums
  - is unstable in alkaline solutions
  - is sensitive to reducing agents.
- Vitamin B_6 (pyridoxine):
  - is sensitive to light
  - is relatively stable in acid solutions and dry mixes.
- Vitamin B_{12} (cyanocobalamin):
  - has little stability in alkaline or slightly acid mediums
  - is sensitive to oxidizing reactions and reducing agents
  - the metabolites of ascorbic acid, thiamine, and nicotinamide accelerate this vitamin's decomposition
  - is sensitive to light in very dilute solutions.
- Niacin (vitamin B_3):
  - is relatively stable under practical conditions.

- Pantothenic acid (vitamin B_5):
  - has little stability in alkaline or acid mediums
  - is very hygroscopic, especially in its dl-calcium pantothenate form
  - decomposes through hydrolysis, especially at low and high pH values.
- Biotin (vitamin B_7):
  - is stable in air, acids, and at neutral pH
  - is slightly unstable in alkaline solutions.
- Folic acid (vitamin B_9):
  - has little stability in acid solutions below pH 5
  - is sensitive to oxidizing reactions and reducing agents
  - decomposes in sunlight
  - Has little stability in hygroscopic environments and the presence of minerals.
- Vitamin C:
  - is sensitive to radiation
  - oxidizes rapidly in all types of solution
  - is catalyzed by metallic ions, such as copper and iron
  - degrades rapidly at high temperatures.

OPTIMUM VITAMIN NUTRITION IN PRACTICE

The objective of OVN™ is to supplement the diet of animals with the amounts of each vitamin considered most appropriate (the optimum) to optimize the state of health and the productivity of farm animals while guaranteeing the efficiency (desired effect at minimum cost) of the recommended levels.

As already said, the levels of supplementation required for OVN™ are generally higher than those necessary to prevent clinical deficiency symptoms. These optimum supplementation levels should likewise compensate for the stress factors affecting the animal and its diet, thus guaranteeing these factors do not limit the animal's yield and health.

The following describes the concept of a *cost-effective window* for vitamin supplementation. This level must satisfy but not exceed the aim of achieving a state of optimum health and productivity. Below are some definitions of terms applicable to the OVN™ concept (Figure 1.13).

1. **Average animal response** refers to productivity results – FCR, growth rate, reproductive status, level of immunity, the animal's health status, etc. – as a consequence of the ingestion of vitamins.
2. **Total vitamin intake** describes the total level of vitamins in the diet, feedstuff's bioavailable quantity, and supplementation.
3. **Deficient** or **minimum vitamin intake** refers to the vitamin level that puts the animal in danger of showing clinical deficiency symptoms and metabolic disorders and in which the level of vitamins falls short of the NRC supplementation level.
4. **A suboptimum intake** prevents the appearance of clinical deficiency symptoms. Its supplementation levels comply with or exceed the NRC's guidelines but are inadequate to permit an optimum state of health and productivity.
5. **An optimum intake** compensates for the negative factors which influence an animal's yield and therefore contributes to achieving an optimum state of well-being, health, and productivity.
6. **Special applications** are above optimum intake levels of vitamin supplementation for optimizing certain attributes such as immunity, meat quality, bone health, etc., or are directly

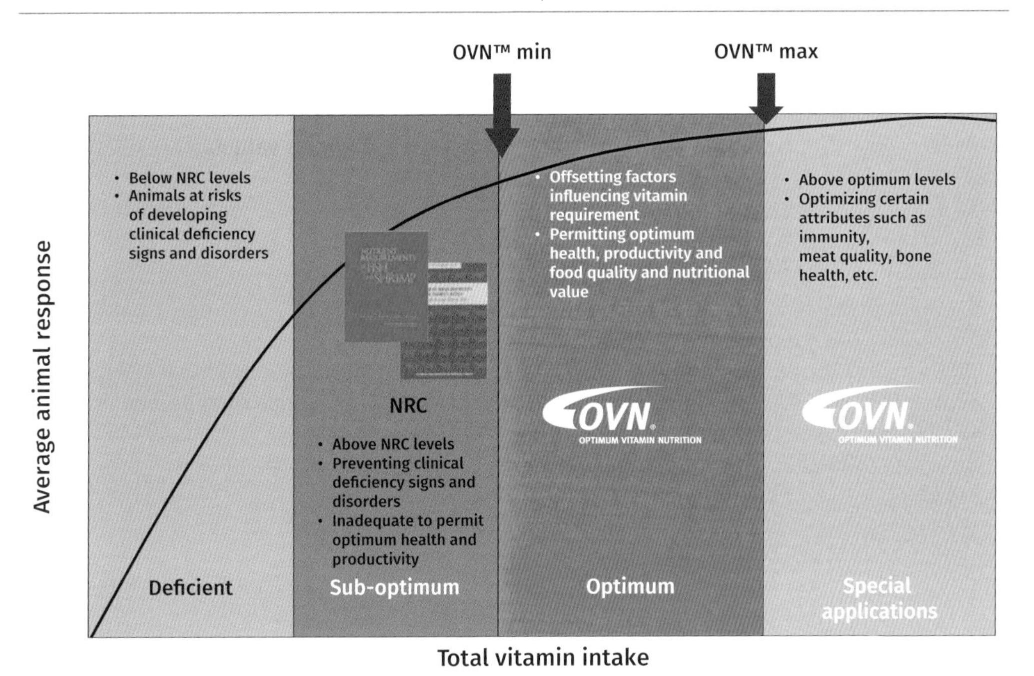

Figure 1.13 The OVN Optimum Vitamin Nutrition® concept (source: DSM, 2022)

used to produce vitamin-enriched meat or eggs. Concerning the safety of vitamins, only very large quantities (between 10 and 100 times the levels used in practice) of some vitamins such as A and D_3 in feed might occasionally cause some sort of disorder in animals. There is a growing demand for food with a greater added value, such as vitamin-rich eggs, meat, or milk, the occasional consumption of which contributes to a balanced human diet. This would necessitate such a higher vitamin content in the feed.

In summary, we can say that implementing a nutritional program with the most appropriate levels of all the vitamins in an animal's diet aims to offer the following benefits to the food chain.

1 **Optimum health and welfare** of animals are a prerequisite for producing safe and healthy meat.
2 **Optimum productivity**, given better sanitary conditions and greater efficiency in animal farming within parameters such as FCR, final weight, weight gain, mortality, etc.
3 **Optimum food quality** offered to consumers provides them with whole food with balanced nutrient content.

1. Optimizing animal health and welfare

It is common knowledge that there is a close relationship between nutrition, health, and well-being. Improving the health and well-being of an animal nowadays constitutes a crucial aspect in the production of any food type of animal origin, so one essential objective regarding nutrition and management programs would be limiting the incidence of diseases and their debilitating effect on animals. Supplementing an animal's diet with optimum quantities of vitamins at times of greatest vulnerability to infection reduces the risk of contracting a disease.

Health and immunity

Vitamins, in sufficient quantities, play a fundamental role in the capacity of an animal's organism to develop an effective immune response to disease. Since the onset of an illness cannot be predicted, the immune system must be prepared to act before the disease attacks the organism.

Various studies have demonstrated a close relationship between low levels of vitamin E in the tissues and a decrease in immunocompetence (the immune system's response) long before any clinical signs of disease appear. Vitamins E and C are powerful antioxidants that protect cells from free radicals and other types of by-products harmful to an animal's metabolism.

The same studies proved that high levels of vitamin E in feed during the first 3 weeks produced:

- an improvement in the immune response to infection and vaccination
- improvement in batches affected by subclinical infections
- fewer relapses due to secondary infections.

Reproduction

When breeding animals were fed diets rich in vitamin E during their periods of growth and production, the results were:

- improved response in the production of antibodies during vaccination
- a clear association between high levels of vitamin E in the liver and improved viability of newborn animals.

It is thus more effective to increase levels during embryogenesis when the immune system is developing at a greater rate.

Welfare

Infections cause pain and suffering in animals. In general, farmers, rearing businesses, and other people involved in their care have the greatest interest in their animals and will assume responsibility for ensuring satisfactory standards of well-being.

In the food sector, too, there are ever more retailers, wholesale distributors, and even fast-food chains which have incorporated animal welfare standards in their best practices, aiming to give animals a healthy life that will contribute to guaranteeing more nutritious food to their consumers. Optimum vitamin supplementation in an animal's diet will contribute to improving its welfare because:

- optimum vitamin levels contribute to improving the metabolism, nutrition, and well-being of the bird
- improving immunity increases resistance to diseases
- some vitamins, such as biotin, contribute to reducing the incidence of digital dermatitis, thus preventing certain types of lameness, while others, such as vitamin C, alleviate the negative effects of stress on health, and others like 25OHD_3, a more active D_3 metabolite, will improve bone health, reducing lameness and other painful skeletal issues.

2. Optimizing productivity

In animals, advances have been achieved over decades through natural genetic selection, accelerating growth rates, and favoring certain genotypes to increase meat production. These have changed broilers' nutritional requirements because of feed use improvements.

Recent data have demonstrated that animals grow faster under experimental and commercial conditions when the supplementation of vitamins in the diet is increased according to their requirements. From the economic viewpoint, the improvement in productive yield after optimizing the supply of vitamins in the feed gave rise to a significantly better cost-to-benefit ratio, in turn recompensing the farmer.

In commercial conditions, stress represents a serious threat to achieving optimum yield. It reduces feed intake, increasing the vitamin concentration needed to satisfy an animal's needs. Besides, stress alters the animal's metabolic needs, turning a nutritionally balanced meal into a diet with possible nutritional deficiencies. For example, recent investigations indicate that an appropriate supplement of vitamin C can alleviate the harmful effects of the stress caused by heat on the quality of semen, thus satisfying the nutritional requirements of roosters in such demanding conditions. Various recently published North American studies in growing birds suggest that a diet with high levels of B group vitamins can improve the yield and productivity of broilers. In turkeys, many studies show that high levels of biotin can improve feed utilization and live weight gain while also reducing mortality. Likewise, various tests on increasing absorbable biotin in wheat-based diets showed improved live weight and feed utilization in broilers.

Likewise, in breeding birds, it has been shown that high vitamin levels are vital for the production of viable chicks, since during its development, the embryo is very sensitive not only to changes in its environment but also to insufficient supplies of the majority of vitamins, and embryonic mortality and malformations are some of the main symptoms of deficiency in one or several vitamins.

In recent years various tests, both experimental and in the field, have been carried out to evaluate the potential synergistic effect on the principal productive parameters of feeding animals with an OVN™ level compared with the average level used by the industry. Some of these results in poultry farming show how diets with an optimum vitamin level increased the final weight of chickens by 2.7% (Figure 1.14), with a considerable economic benefit.

3. Optimizing the quality of food for the consumer

Meat is an essential source of protein in the human diet. Likewise, a gradual and continuous increase in demand for processed meat products can be observed. This fact should be considered when defining the nutritional strategy that should be developed in animal diets. Lipid oxidation constitutes a problem for the conservation of meat since it can give rise to undesirable smells and flavors associated with rancidification, a fact of major relevance in processed meat particularly susceptible to this oxidation process.

Feeding animals a diet rich in unsaturated vegetable fats can considerably increase levels of monounsaturated and polyunsaturated fatty acids in meat. There exist a series of polyunsaturated fatty acids that react with molecular oxygen until they are finally degraded to undesirable compounds with short chains, which cause the meat's organoleptic characteristics to deteriorate and, consequently, reduce acceptance of the meat by the consumer. Animals fed on diets with high levels of vitamin E can counteract this effect and so improve the final quality of the meat:

- by protecting the meat's lipids from oxidation and reducing the formation of undesirable smells and flavors
- by reducing the loss of exudates and improving the texture of the meat.

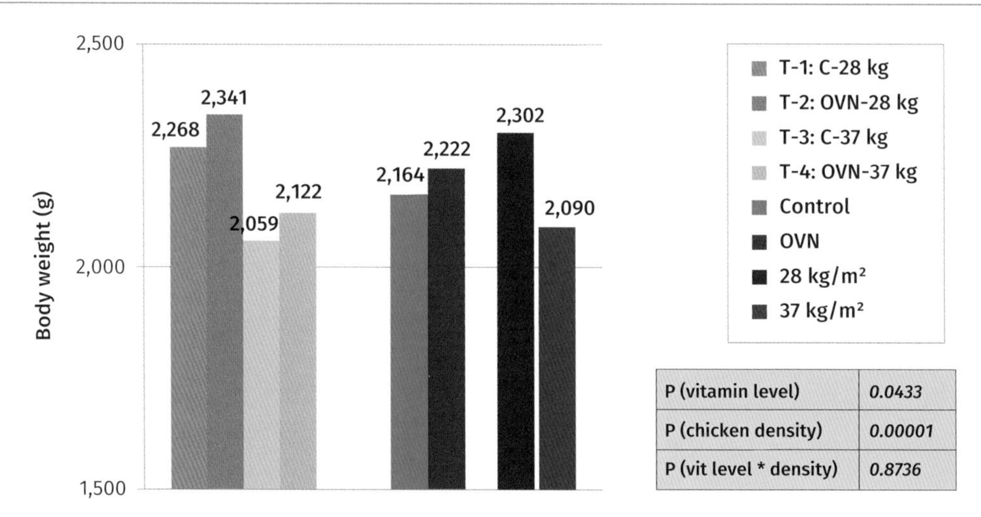

Figure 1.14 Body weight of 40-day broilers with 2 animal densities (28 kg/m^2 and 37 kg/m^2) and fed with vitamins at industry practice level against OVN™ levels (source: Pérez-Vendrell *et al.*, 2002)

Concerning other food of animal origin, levels of some vitamins present in meat have a direct relationship to the vitamin levels in the diet of the chicken. Pérez-Vendrell *et al.* (2002) showed that breasts of 40-day chickens fed a diet with an optimum level of vitamins contained a higher quantity of some nutrients such as vitamins E, B_1, and pantothenic acid, having, therefore, a better nutritional value (Figures 1.15, 1.16 and 1.17).

OPTIMUM VITAMIN NUTRITION: A DYNAMIC PROCESS IN CONSTANT EVOLUTION

Optimum vitamin supplementation in an animal's diet, over and above the established minimum needs and adapted to the specific conditions of each animal species, will permit an improvement in the state of health and welfare of the animal, thus optimizing its productive potential at the same time as facilitating the production of high-quality food, which is nutritionally balanced.

These optimum levels are based on many studies carried out at university and industrial centers, on the requirements published by different associations and principal animal genetic producers and vitamin manufacturers, and on the continuous experience of the worldwide agricultural industry. These optimum levels guarantee farmers minimum impact of negative nutritional factors, such as variability in the natural content of feed ingredients, the existence of antinutritional factors, and different levels of stress.

Although the vitamin recommendations for feed also attempt to compensate for the majority of the factors mentioned that influence an animal's vitamin needs, in extreme conditions where the processing of premix or feed is very aggressive (e.g., the inclusion of trace minerals or choline chloride, the use of feed expanders or extruded feed) supplementary quantities of some vitamins may be necessary. The negative effect on the stability of vitamins can be reduced by using high-quality commercial vitamin forms where their covering and the bioavailability of the active substance they contain are key elements to be taken into account. And all this is considering the environmental impact of how vitamins are manufactured.

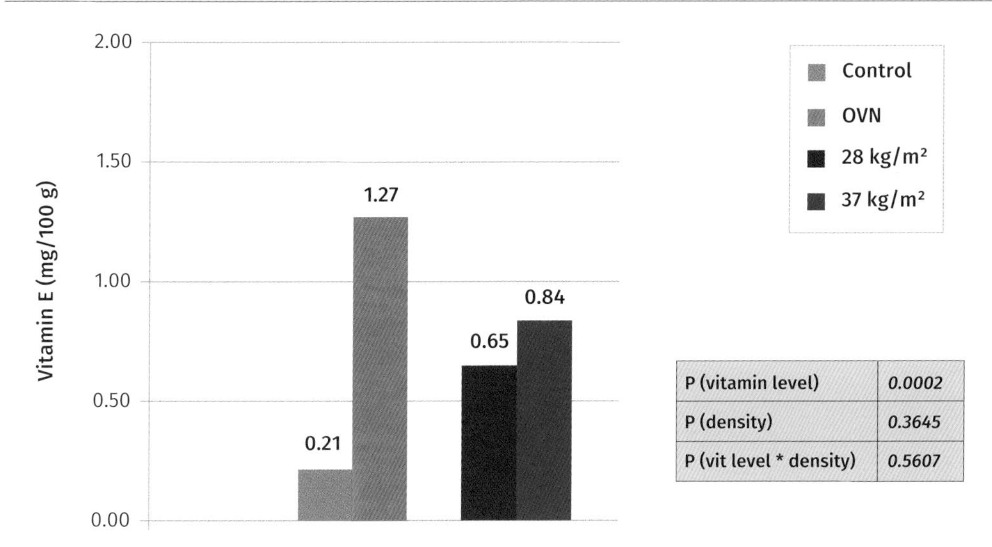

P (vitamin level)	*0.0002*
P (density)	*0.3645*
P (vit level * density)	*0.5607*

Figure 1.15 Vitamin E content in the breast of 40-days broilers with 2 animal densities (28 kg/m^2 and 37 kg/m^2) and fed with vitamins at industry practice level against OVN™ levels (source: Pérez-Vendrell *et al.*, 2002)

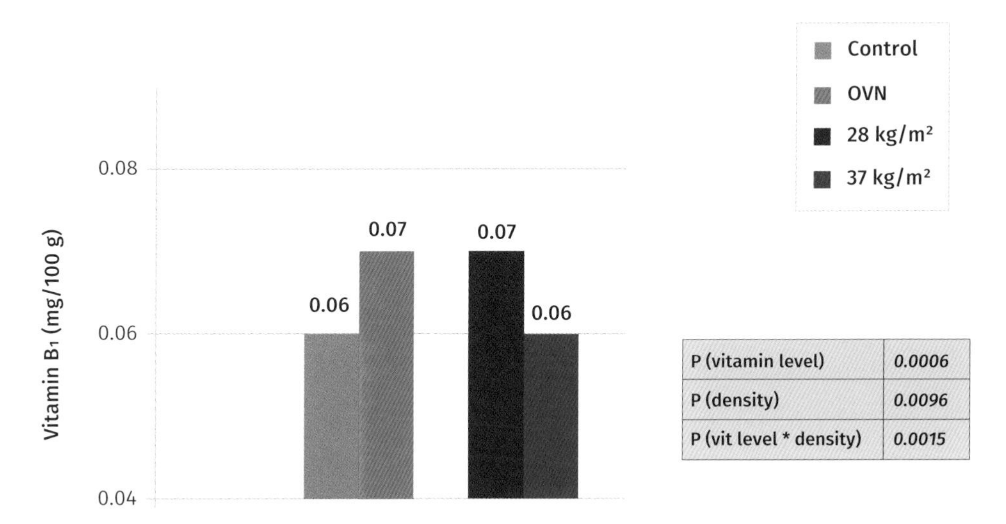

P (vitamin level)	*0.0006*
P (density)	*0.0096*
P (vit level * density)	*0.0015*

Figure 1.16 Vitamin B_1 content in the breast of 40-days broilers with 2 animal densities (28 kg/m^2 and 37 kg/m^2) and fed with vitamins at industry practice level against OVN™ levels (source: Pérez-Vendrell *et al.*, 2002)

In Chapters 4, 5, and 6 of this book, many international publications on the impact of vitamins in poultry nutrition are reviewed. These studies have endeavored to emphasize the beneficial effects that optimum vitamin levels have on an animal, both on the level of health and welfare and concerning productivity. The chapters also identify aspects on which there is currently insufficient information available, intending to address these gaps in future research and editions of this book.

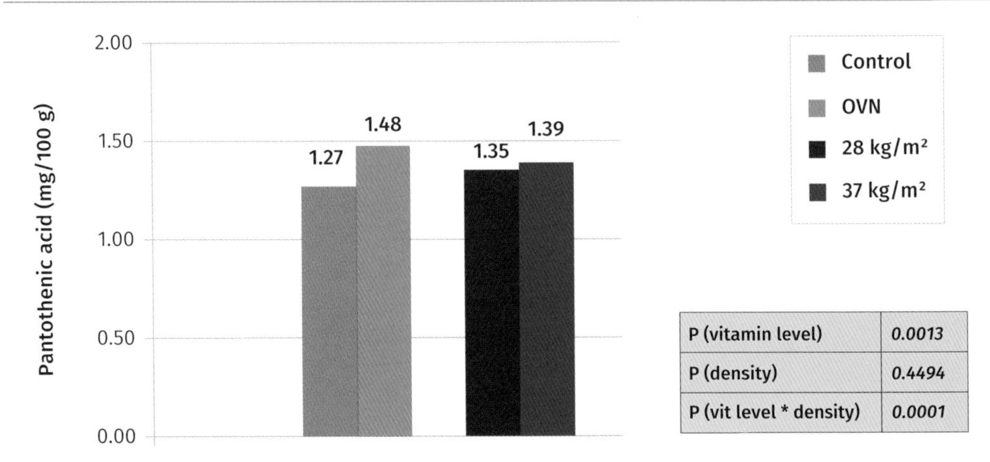

Figure 1.17 Pantothenic acid content in the breast of 40-days broilers with 2 animal densities (28 kg/m^2 and 37 kg/m^2) and fed with vitamins at industry practice level against OVN™ levels (source: Pérez-Vendrell *et al.*, 2002)

Given that animal farming is a dynamic process levels of vitamin supplementation need to be reassessed more frequently – this is a change demanded, in the majority of cases, by society, for economic reasons related to the productivity of animals and by farming systems.

The concept of OVN™ always considers the costs of vitamin supplementation in an animal's diet (in many cases, less than 1% of the cost of feed, even less if we consider the impact on meat production cost) against the risk of suffering losses through vitamin deficiencies and through working with yield indices below the optimum.

Nutritionists who follow the recommended guidelines based on the OVN™ concept ensure that vitamins enable the development of an animal's genetic potential and contribute to a more sustainable animal farming.

Chapter 2

A brief history of vitamins

Vitamins were mostly discovered in the 20th century and were once regarded as "unknown growth factors" (Eggersdorfer *et al.*, 2012). The first phase of developing the concept of vitamins began many centuries ago and gradually led to the recognition that night blindness, xerophthalmia, scurvy, beriberi, and rickets are dietary diseases. These diseases had long plagued humankind and were mentioned in the earliest written records. Records of medical science from antiquity attest that researchers had already linked certain foods and diseases or infirmities, postulating that food constituents played a causal or a preventive role. These are considered the nebulous beginnings of essential nutrients (Eggersdorfer *et al.*, 2012).

Beriberi is probably the earliest documented deficiency disorder being recognized in China as early as 2697 BC. By 1500 BC, scurvy, night blindness, and xerophthalmia were described in Egyptian writings. Two books of the Bible contain accounts that point to vitamin A deficiency (McDowell, 2006). Jeremiah 14:6 states: "and the asses did stand in high places, their eyes did fail because there was no grass." In addition, the Bible mentions that fish bile was used to cure a blind man named Tobias.

In 400 BC, the Greek physician Hippocrates, known as the Father of Medicine, reported using raw ox liver dipped in honey to prevent night blindness. He also described soldiers afflicted with scurvy. Scurvy took a heavy toll on the Crusades of the Middles Ages because the soldiers traveled far from home, and their diet was deficient in vitamin C. During the long sea voyages between 1492 and 1600, scurvy posed a serious threat to the health of sailors and undermined world exploration. For example, while sailing worldwide, Magellan lost 80% of his crew to the disease. Vasco de Gama, another great explorer, lost 60% of his 160-man crew while mapping the coast of Africa. In 1536, during Jacques Cartier's expedition to Canada, 107 out of 110 men became sick with scurvy. However, the journey was saved when the Indians shared their knowledge of the curative value of pine needles and bark. In 1593, British Admiral Richard Hawkins wrote: "I have seen some 10,000 seamen die of scurvy; some sailors tried treating themselves by trimming the rotting, putrid black flesh from their gums and washing their teeth in urine."

In 1747, James Lind, a British naval surgeon, carried out the first controlled clinical experiment aboard a ship to find a cure for scurvy. Twelve patients with scurvy were divided into 6 treatment groups. Two sailors received a dietary supplement of oranges and lemons, while the other treatment groups were given nutmeg, garlic, vinegar, cider, and seawater, respectively. The 2 men who had received the citrus fruit were cured of scurvy. Where did Lind get the idea that scurvy was related to nutrition? He had been told a story of an English sailor with scurvy who was left to die on a lonely island with no food. Feeling hungry, the man nibbled a few blades of beach grass. The next day, he felt stronger and ate some more grass. After a few weeks on this "diet," he was completely well.

In the second half of the 19th century, it was another disease that killed thousands of sailors in the Japanese navy. In 1880, the Japanese navy recorded almost 5,000 deaths from beriberi in 3 years. Patients with beriberi became weak and eventually partially paralyzed, lost weight, and died. Doctors tried to find the germ that was causing beriberi. Finally, they listened to Japanese naval surgeon Kamekiro Takaki, who believed the sailors' diet was causing beriberi. Takaki noted a 60% incidence of beriberi on a ship returning from a 1-year voyage during which the sailors' diet had been mostly polished rice and some fish. He sent out a second ship under the same conditions but substituted barley, meat, milk, and fresh vegetables for some of the rice. The dietary change eliminated beriberi, but Takaki incorrectly concluded that the additional protein prevented the beriberi. Regardless, the Japanese knew they could avoid beriberi by not relying on polished rice as the only dietary staple.

Before the beginning of the 20th century, there was a growing body of evidence that nutritional factors, later known as vitamins, were implicated in certain diseases. Louis Pasteur was the chief opponent of the "vitamin theory," which held that certain illnesses resulted from a shortage of specific nutrients in foods. Pasteur believed there were only 3 classes of organic nutrients: carbohydrates, fats, and proteins. His research showed that microorganisms caused disease and made scientists with medical training reluctant to believe the vitamin theory. It has been said that the immensely successful "germ theory" of disease, coupled with toxin theory and the successful use of antisepsis and vaccination, convinced scientists of the day that only a positive agent could cause disease (Guggenheim, 1995). Until the mid-1930s, most US doctors still believed that pellagra was an infectious disease (McDowell, 2006).

VITAMIN THEORY TAKES SHAPE

Beginning in the mid-1850s, German scientists were recognized as leaders in the field of nutrition. In the late 1800s, Professor C. von Bunge, who worked at the German university in Dorpat, Estonia, and then at Basel, Switzerland, had some graduate students conduct experiments with purified diets for small animals (Wolf and Carpenter, 1997). In 1881, N. Lunin, a Russian student studying in von Bunge's laboratory, observed that some mice died after 16 to 36 days when fed a diet composed solely of purified fat, protein, carbohydrate, salts, and water. Lunin suggested that natural foods such as milk contain small quantities of "unknown substances essential to life."

Many great scientific advances have come about due to chance observations made by men and women of inspiration. In 1896, Dutch physician and bacteriologist Christiaan Eijkman made a historic finding concerning a cure for beriberi. Eijkman was researching in Indonesia to identify the causal pathogen of beriberi. He astutely observed that a polyneuritis condition in chickens produced clinical signs similar to those in humans with beriberi. This chance discovery was made when a new head cook at the hospital discontinued the supply of "military" rice (polished rice), and the chickens fed the wholegrain "civilian" rice recovered from the polyneuritis. After extensive experimentation, Eijkman proved that both polyneuritis and beriberi were caused by eating polished white rice. Both afflictions could be prevented or cured when the outer portions of the rice grain (e.g., rice bran) were consumed. Thus, Eijkman became the first to produce a vitamin deficiency disease in an experimental animal. He also noted that prisoners with beriberi eating polished rice tended to get well when fed a less milled product. In 1901, Grijns, one of Eijkman's colleagues in Indonesia, was the first to come up with a correct interpretation of the connection between the excessive consumption of polished rice and the etiology of beriberi. He concluded that rice contained "an essential nutrient" found in the grain's outer layers.

In 1902, a Norwegian scientist named Holst conducted some experiments on "ship-beriberi" (scurvy) using poultry, but the experiments failed. In 1907, Holst and Frolich produced experimental scurvy in guinea pigs. Later it was learned that poultry could synthesize vitamin C while guinea pigs could not.

In 1906, Frederick Hopkins, working with rats in England, reported that "no animal can live upon a mixture of pure protein, fat, and carbohydrate and even when the necessary inorganic material is supplied, the animal cannot flourish." Hopkins found that small amounts of milk added to purified diets allowed rats to live and thrive. He suggested that unknown nutrients were essential for animal life, calling them "accessory food factors." Hopkins' experiments were like those of Lunin; however, they were more in depth. He played an important role by recording his views in memorable terms that received wide recognition (McCollum, 1957). Hopkins also expressed that various disorders were caused by diets deficient in unidentified nutrients (e.g., scurvy and rickets). He was responsible for opening a new field of discovery that largely depended on experimental rats.

In 1907, Elmer McCollum (Figure 2.1) arrived in Wisconsin to work on a project to determine why cows fed wheat or oats (versus yellow corn) gave birth to blind or dead calves. The answer was found to be that wheat and oats lacked the vitamin A precursor carotene. Between 1913 and 1915, McCollum and Davis discovered 2 growth factors for rats, "fat-soluble A" and "water-soluble B." By 1922, McCollum had identified vitamin D as a substance independent of vitamin A. He bubbled oxygen through cod liver oil to destroy its vitamin A; the treated oil remained effective against rickets but not against xeropthalmia. Thus, "fat-soluble vitamin A" had to be 2 vitamins, not just one (DeLuca, 2014).

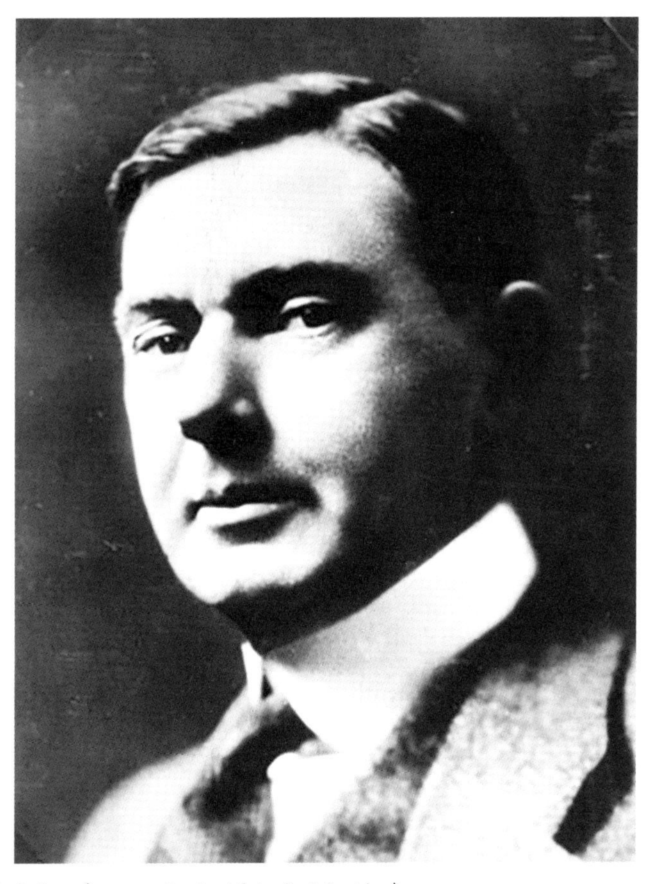

Figure 2.1 Elmer McCollum (source: Roche Historical Archive)

In 1912, Casimir Funk (Figure 2.2), a Polish biochemist working at the Lister Institute in London, proposed the "vitamin theory" (Funk and Dubin, 1922). He had reviewed the literature and made the important conclusion that beriberi could be prevented or cured by a protective factor present in natural food, which he successfully isolated from rice by-products. What he had isolated was named "beriberi vitamin" in 1912. This term "vitamin" denoted that the substance was vital to life and chemically an amine (vital + amine). In 1912, Funk proposed the theory that other "deficiency diseases" in addition to beriberi were caused by a lack of these essential substances, namely scurvy, rickets, sprue, and pellagra. He was the first to suggest that pellagra was a nutrient deficiency disease.

In 1923, Evans and Bishop discovered that vitamin E deficiency caused reproductive failure in rats. Steenbock (1924) showed that irradiation of foods as well as animals with ultraviolet light produced vitamin D. In 1928, Szent-Györgyi isolated hexuronic acid (later renamed "ascorbic acid") from foods such as orange juice. One year later, Moore proved that the animal body converts carotene to vitamin A. This experiment involved feeding 1 group of rats carotene and finding higher levels of vitamin A in their livers compared to controls. By 1928, Joseph Goldberger and Conrad Elvehjem had shown that vitamin B was more than one substance. After the "vitamin" was heated, it was no longer effective in preventing beriberi (B_1), but it was still good for rat growth (B_2). The 1930s and 1940s were the golden age of vitamin research.

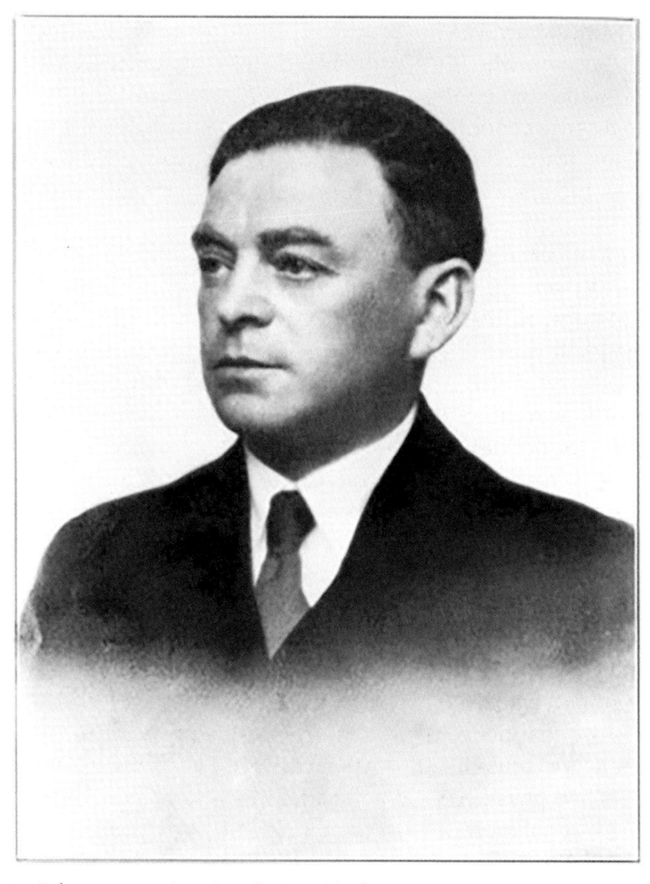

Figure 2.2 Casimir Funk (source: Roche Historical Archive)

During this period, the traditional approach was to (1) study the effects of a deficient diet, (2) find a food source that prevents the deficiency, and (3) gradually concentrate the nutrient (vitamin) in a food and test potency. Laboratory animals were used in these procedures.

Henrick Dam of Denmark discovered vitamin K in 1929 when he noted hemorrhages in chicks fed a fat-free diet. Ironically 1 year earlier, Herman Almquist, working in the United States, had discovered both forms of the vitamin (K_1 and K_2) in studies with chicks. Unfortunately, university administrators delayed the review of his paper, and when it was finally submitted to the journal *Science*, it was rejected. Therefore, only Henrick Dam received a Nobel prize for discovering vitamin K.

Vitamin B_{12} was the last traditional vitamin to be identified, in 1948. Shortly after that, it was discovered that cobalt was an essential component of the vitamin. Simple monogastric animals were found to require the vitamin, whereas ruminants and other species with large microbial populations (e.g., horses) require dietary cobalt rather than vitamin B_{12}.

Compared with the situation for night blindness, xeropthalmia, beriberi, scurvy, and rickets, there were no records from the ancient past of the disease of pellagra. The disease was caused by niacin deficiency in humans, a problem prevalent mainly in cultures where corn (maize) was a key dietary staple (Harris, 1919). Columbus took corn to Spain from America. Pellagra was not recognized until 1735, when Gaspar Casal, physician to King Philip V of Spain, identified it among peasants in northern Spain. The local people called it "mal de la rosa," and Casal associated the disease with poverty and spoiled corn. The popularity of corn spread eastward from Spain to southern France, Italy, Russia, and Egypt, and so did pellagra. James Woods Babcock of Columbia, South Carolina, who identified pellagra in the United States by establishing a link with the disease in Italy, studied the case records of the South Carolina State Hospital and concluded that the disease condition had occurred there as early as 1828. Most cases occurred in low-income groups, whose diet was limited to inexpensive foodstuffs. Diets characteristically associated with the disease were the 3 Ms, specifically meal (corn), meat (backfat), and molasses.

The word pellagra means rough skin, which relates to dermatitis. Other descriptive names for the condition were "mal de sol" (illness of the sun) and "corn bread fever." In the early 1900s in the United States, particularly in the South, it was common for 20,000 deaths to occur annually from pellagra. It was estimated that there were at least 35 cases of the disease for every death due to pellagra. Even as late as 1941, 5 years after the cause of pellagra was known, 2,000 deaths were still attributed to the disease. The clinical signs and mortality associated with pellagra are the 4 Ds: dermatitis (of areas exposed to the sun), diarrhea, dementia (mental problems), and death. Several mental institutions in the United States, Europe, and Egypt were primarily devoted to caring for pellagra sufferers or pellagrins.

In 1914, Joseph Goldberger, a bacteriologist with the US Public Health Service, was assigned to identify the cause of pellagra. His studies observed that the disease was associated with poor diet and poverty and that well-fed persons did not contract the disease (Carpenter, 1981). The therapeutic value of good diets was demonstrated in orphanages, prisons, and mental institutions in South Carolina, Georgia, and Mississippi. Goldberger, his wife, and 14 volunteers constituted a "filth squad" who ingested and injected various biological materials and excreta from pellagrins to prove that pellagra was not an infectious disease. These extreme measures did not result in pellagra, thus demonstrating the non-infectious nature of the disease. At the time, researchers and physicians did not want to believe that pellagra resulted from poor nutrition. They sought to link it to an infection in keeping with the popular "germ theory" of diseases (McDowell, 2006). An important step toward isolating the preventive factor for pellagra involved the discovery of a suitable laboratory animal for testing its potency in various concentrated preparations. It was found that a pellagra-like disease (black tongue) could be produced in dogs. Elvehjem and his colleagues (2002) isolated nicotinamide from the liver and identified it as the factor that could cure black tongue in dogs. Reports of niacin's dramatic therapeutic effects in human pellagra cases quickly followed from several clinics.

In 1824, James Scarth Combe first discovered fatal anemia (pernicious anemia) and suggested it was linked to a digestive disorder. George R. Minot and William Murphy reported in 1926 that large amounts of the raw liver would alleviate the symptoms of pernicious anemia. In 1948, E. L. Rickes and his colleagues in the United States and E. Lester Smith in England isolated vitamin B_{12} and identified it as the anti-pernicious anemia factor (McDowell, 2006). Much earlier, in 1929, W. B. Castle had shown that pernicious anemia resulted from the interaction between a dietary factor (extrinsic) and a mucoprotein substance produced by the stomach (intrinsic factor). Castle used an unusual but effective method to relieve the symptoms of pernicious anemia patients. He ate some beef, and after allowing enough time for the meat to mix with gastric juices, he regurgitated the food and mixed his vomit with the patients' food. With this treatment, the patients recovered because they received both the extrinsic (vitamin B_{12}) and intrinsic (a mucoprotein) factors from Castle's incompletely digested beef meal.

The importance of vitamins was well accepted in the first 3 decades of the 20th century. Table 2.1 provides an overview of the chronological evolution of the discovery, isolation, and assignment of the chemical structure and first production of the individual vitamins. The development of synthetic production of vitamins started in 1933 with ascorbic acid/vitamin C from Merck (Cebion®), which was isolated from plant leaves. However, the first industrial-scale chemical production of vitamin C was achieved by F. Hoffmann-La Roche in 1934 based on a combined fermentation and chemical process developed by Tadeus Reichstein. These scientific innovations were recognized with 12 Nobel Prizes and 20 laureates (Table 2.2). A complete description of the history of discovery, first syntheses, and current industrial processes used for producing each vitamin was described by Eggersdorfer *et al.* (2012) and McDowell (2013).

Table 2.1 Discovery, isolation, structural elucidation, and synthesis of vitamins (source: Eggersdorfer *et al.*, 2012)

Vitamin	Discovery	Isolation	Structural elucidation	First synthesis
Vitamin A	1916	1931	1931	1947
Vitamin D	1918	1932	1936	1959
Vitamin E	1922	1936	1938	1938
Vitamin B_1	1912	1926	1936	1936
Vitamin B_2	1920	1933	1935	1935
Niacin	1936	1936	1937	1994
Pantothenic acid	1931	1938	1940	1940
Vitamin B_6	1934	1938	1938	1939
Biotin	1931	1935	1942	1943
Folic acid	1941	1941	1946	1946
Vitamin B_{12}	1926	1948	1956	1972
Vitamin C	1912	1928	1933	1933

Table 2.2 Nobel prizes for vitamin research (source: Eggersdorfer *et al.*, 2012)

Year	Recipient	Field	Citation
1928	Adolf Windaus	Chemistry	Research into the constitution of steroids and connection with vitamins
1929	Christiaan Eijkman	Medicine, Physiology	Discovery of antineuritic vitamins
	Sir Frederick G. Hopkins	Medicine, Physiology	Discovery of growth-stimulating vitamin
1934	George R. Minot, William P. Murphy, George H. Whipple	Medicine, Physiology	Discoveries concerning liver therapy against anemias
1937	Sir Walter N. Haworth	Chemistry	Research into the constitution of carbohydrates and vitamin C
	Paul Karrer	Chemistry	Research into the constitution of carotenoids, flavins, and vitamins A and B_2
	Albert Szent-Györgyi	Medicine, Physiology	Discoveries in connection with biological combustion processes, with special reference to vitamin C and catalysis of fumaric acid
1938	Richard Kuhn	Chemistry	Work on carotenoids and vitamins
1943	Carl Peter Henrik Dam	Medicine, Physiology	Discovery of vitamin K
	Edward A. Doisy	Medicine, Physiology	Discovery of chemical nature of vitamin K
1953	Fritz A. Lipmann	Medicine, Physiology	Discovery of coenzyme A and its importance for intermediary metabolism
1964	Konrad E. Bloch, Feodor Lynen	Medicine, Physiology	Discoveries concerning mechanism and regulation of cholesterol and fatty acid metabolism
	Dorothy C. Hodgkin	Chemistry	Structural determination of vitamin B_{12}
1967	Ragnar A. Granit	Medicine, Physiology	Research which illuminated electrical properties of vision by studying wavelength discrimination by eye
	Halden K. Hartine	Medicine, Physiology	Research on mechanisms of sight
	George Wald	Medicine, Physiology	Research on chemical processes that allow pigments in the eye retina to convert light into vision

Vitamins became available in the following years through chemical synthesis, fermentation, or extraction from natural materials (Table 2.1). From 1930 to 1950, there was mainly small-scale production in several countries to reach local markets, but, as demand grew, larger plants became more common from 1950 to 1970. Still, it was not until 1987 that all the vitamins were accessible by industrial processes. Nowadays, chemical synthesis is still the dominant method of industrial production.

The large companies Hoffmann-La Roche (Figure 2.3) and BASF were market leaders, but numerous European and Japanese pharmaceutical companies produced and sold vitamins.

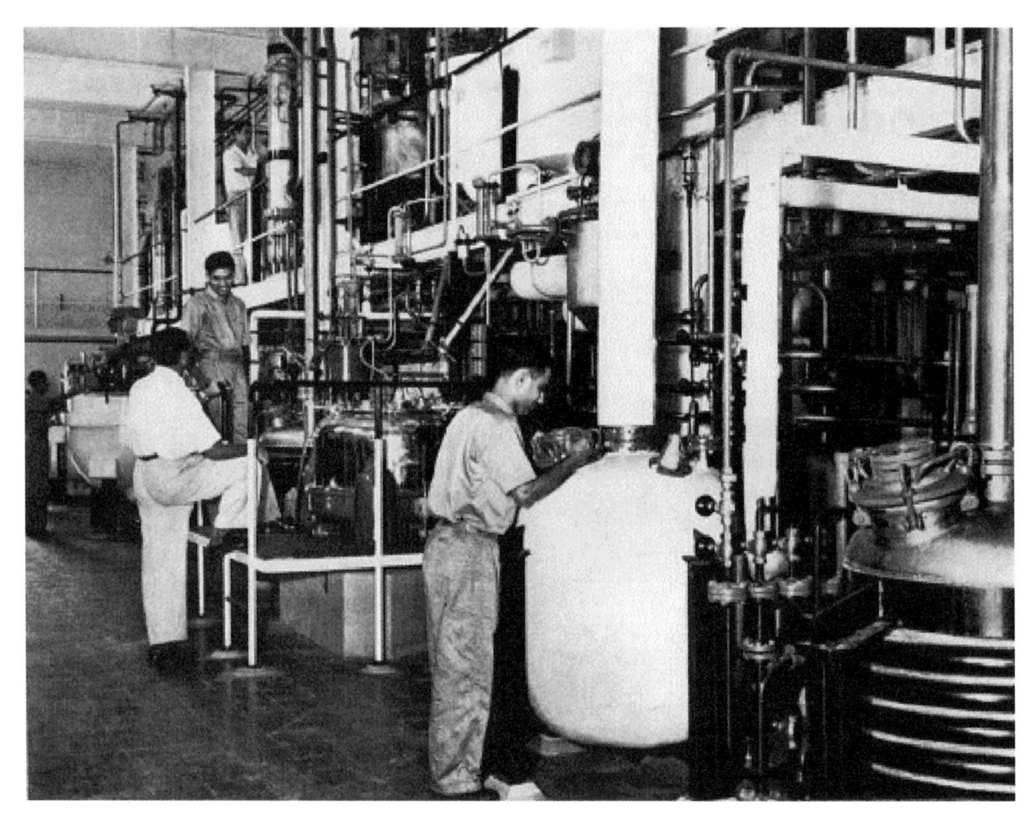

Figure 2.3 Early production of vitamin A at Roche Nutley, USA (source: Roche Historical Archive).

Between 1970 and 1990, production plants became even bigger and with global reach, and since 2000 China has become a larger producer. Fermentation technology started to gain importance, especially for vitamin B_{12} and B_2. New technologies have been emerging in the past 10 years, such as the overexpression of vitamins in plants by either using traditional breeding or genetically modified plants (Eggersdorfer *et al.*, 2012).

Chapter 3

Introduction to vitamins

VITAMIN DEFINITION AND CLASSIFICATION

A vitamin is an organic substance that is:

- a component of a natural compound but distinct from other nutrients such as carbohydrates, fats, proteins, minerals, and water
- present in most foods in a minute amount
- essential for normal metabolism in physiological functions such as growth, development, maintenance, and reproduction
- a cause of a specific deficiency disease or syndrome if absent from the diet or if improperly absorbed or utilized
- not (with very few exceptions) synthesized by the host to meet physiological demands and therefore must be obtained from the diet.

Vitamins are differentiated from the trace elements, also present in the diet in small quantities, by their organic nature. Some vitamins deviate from the preceding definition in that they do not always need to be constituents of food (McDowell, 2000a). For example, companion animals and farm livestock but not fish can synthesize vitamin C (ascorbic acid). Nevertheless, a deficiency has been reported in some species that synthesize vitamin C, and supplementation with this vitamin has been shown to have value for certain disease conditions, support stress conditions, restore productivity, or maximize performance.

Likewise, for most species, niacin can be synthesized from the amino acid tryptophan (but not by the cat or the fish species studied to date) and choline from the amino acid methionine. Nevertheless, dietary supplementation with both niacin and choline is necessary for animal farming. Finally, vitamin D can also be synthesized in the skin under UV light stimulation. Still, the diets of all animals are supplemented with this vitamin to provide the required quantity primarily for proper bone development.

The quantities of vitamins required are very small, but they are essential for tissue integrity, normal development of organic functions, and health maintenance. Their physiological and metabolic roles vary and are of great importance. They are involved in many biochemical reactions and participate in the metabolism of the nutrients derived from the digestion of carbohydrates, lipids, and proteins.

A single vitamin may have several different functions, and many interactions between them are known. Classically, vitamins have been divided into 2 groups based on their solubilities in fat solvents or water. Fat-soluble vitamins include A, D, E, and K, while B complex vitamins and vitamin C are water soluble.

Fat-soluble vitamins are found in feedstuffs in association with lipids. The fat-soluble vitamins are absorbed along with dietary fats, apparently by mechanisms like those involved in fat absorption. The 13 recognized vitamins with main functions and deficiency symptoms are listed in Table 3.1.

Conditions favorable to fat absorption, such as adequate bile flow and good micelle formation, also favor absorption of the fat-soluble vitamins (Scott *et al.*, 1982; McDowell, 2000a). Water-soluble vitamins are not associated with fats, and alterations in fat absorption do not affect their absorption. The fat-soluble vitamins A and D and, to a lesser extent, E are generally stored in appreciable amounts in the animal body. Water-soluble vitamins are not stored, and excesses are rapidly excreted, except for vitamin B_{12} and perhaps biotin.

Table 3.1 Main functions of vitamins and symptoms of deficiency in poultry (source: DSM Animal Nutrition and Health, unpublished)

Vitamin	Main functions	Deficiency symptoms
Vitamin A	• Essential for growth, health (immunity), reproduction (steroid synthesis), vision, development and integrity of skin, epithelia and mucosa	• Blindness or night-blindness (xeropthalmia) • Loss of appetite, poor absorption of nutrients, impaired growth and, in severe cases, death • Decreased egg production and hatchability • Reduced immune response and increased risk of infections (respiratory and intestinal) • Keratinization of epithelial tissues
Vitamin D_3	• Homeostasis of calcium and phosphorus (intestine, bones and kidney) • Regulation of bones calcification and eggshell formation • Modulation of the immune system • Muscular cell growth	• Rickets, osteomalacia and bone disorders • Lower eggshell quality (more cracked eggs) • Reduced hatchability • Reduced growth rate • Muscular weakness
$25OHD_3$	• Major serum metabolite of vitamin D_3 • More efficient absorption in the intestine • Faster response for calcium homeostasis • More efficient modulation of the immune system and muscular cells than vitamin D_3	• Rickets, osteomalacia and bone disorders • Lower eggshell quality (more cracked eggs) • Reduced hatchability • Reduced growth rate • Muscular weakness
Vitamin E	• Most powerful fat-soluble antioxidant • Immune system modulation • Tissue protection • Fertility • Meat quality	• Muscular dystrophy and myopathy • Reduced immune response • Encephalomalacia ("crazy chick disease") • Reduced fertility and hatchability • Meat quality defects: drip-loss, off-flavors
Vitamin K_3	• Blood clotting and coagulation • Coenzyme in metabolic process related to bone mineralization (Ca binding proteins) and protein formation	• Increased clotting time • Hemorrhages • Anemia • Bone disorders • Rough plumage

Table 3.1 (continued)

Vitamin	Main functions	Deficiency symptoms
Vitamin B_1	• Coenzyme in several enzymatic reactions • Carbohydrate metabolism (conversion of glucose into energy) • Involved in ATP, DNA and RNA production • Synthesis of acetylcholine, essential in transmission of nervous impulses	• Loss of appetite up to anorexia • Reduced growth rate • Neuropathies (polyneuritis with neck twisting) • General muscle weakness, poor leg coordination • Embryo mortality • Fatty degeneration and necrosis of heath fibers (cardiac failure) • Mucosal inflammation
Vitamin B_2	• Fat and protein metabolism • Flavin coenzyme (FMN and FAD) synthesis, essentials for energy production (respiratory chain) • Involved in synthesis of steroids, red blood cells and glycogen • Integrity of mucosal membranes and antioxidant system within cells	• Reduced feed intake and growth • Reduced absorption of zinc, iron and calcium • Inflammation of the mucous membranes of the digestive tract • Peripheral neuropathy, "curled toe paralysis", chickens walking on their hocks • Reduced egg production • Increased embryo mortality and reduced hatchability
Vitamin B_6	• Coenzyme in amino acid, fat and carbohydrate metabolism • Essential for DNA and RNA synthesis • Involved in the synthesis of niacin from tryptophan	• Reduced growth rate, lesser feed intake and protein retention • Dermatitis, rough and deficient plumage • Inflamed edema of the eyelids • Disorders of blood parameters, anemia and ascites • Muscular convulsions followed by paralysis • Reduced hatchability
Vitamin B_{12}	• Synthesis of red blood cells and growth • Involved in methionine metabolism • Coenzyme in nucleic acids (DNA and RNA) and protein metabolism • Metabolism of fats and carbohydrates	• Anemia • Reduced growth rate and lower feed conversion • Defective feathering, poor plumage • Leg weakness, perosis • Gizzard erosion • Reduced hatchability and higher embryo mortality
Niacin or Vitamin B_3	• Coenzyme (active forms NAD and NADP) in amino acid, fat and carbohydrate metabolism • Required for optimum tissue integrity, particularly for the skin, the gastrointestinal tract and the nervous system	• Nervous system disorders • Inflammation and ulcers of mucous membranes • Reduced growth and feed efficiency • Lameness in young birds • Reduced feathering • Reduced egg production and hatchability
Biotin or Vitamin B_7	• Coenzyme in protein, fat and carbohydrate metabolism • Normal blood glucose level • Synthesis of fatty acids, nucleic acids (DNA and RNA) and proteins (keratin)	• Fertility disorders • Rough and brittle feathers, poor plumage • Dermatitis of foot pads • Deformation of the beak • Fatty liver and kidney syndrome (FLKS)

Table 3.1 (continued)

Vitamin	Main functions	Deficiency symptoms
d-Pantothenic acid or Vitamin B_5	• Present in Coenzyme A (CoA) and Acyl Carrier Protein (ACP) involved in carbohydrate, fat and protein metabolism • Biosynthesis of long-chain fatty acids, phospholipids and steroid hormones	• Functional disorders of nervous system • Rough feathering and depigmentation • Crusts at the corner of the beak, exudates on eyelids • Fatty degeneration of the liver • Reduced antibody formation • Reduced growth and laying performance • Reduced hatchability and increased embryo mortality
Folic acid or Vitamin B_9	• Coenzyme in the synthesis of nucleic acids (DNA and RNA) and proteins (methyl groups) • Stimulates hematopoietic system • With vitamin B_{12} it converts homocysteine into methionine	• Megaloblastic (macrocytic) anemia • Skin damages, rough plumage and feather depigmentation • Cervical paralysis, leg weakness, perosis • Reduced laying performance and hatchability • Increased embryo mortality
Vitamin C	• Intracellular (water-soluble) antioxidant • Immune system modulation: stimulation of phagocytosis • Egg shell membrane formation • Formation of collagen, connective tissues, cartilage and bones • Synthesis of corticosteroids and steroid metabolism • Conversion of vitamin D_3 to its active form $1{,}25(OH)_2D_3$	• Lower resistance to stress (e.g., low/high temperatures) • Weakness and fatigue • Reduced immune response • Hemorrhages of the skin, muscles and adipose tissues • Reproductive failures
Choline	• Membrane structural component (phosphatidylcholine) • Fat transport and metabolism in the liver • Support nervous system function (acetylcholine) • Source of methyl donors for methionine regeneration from homocysteine	• Fatty liver • Reduced growth rate

Table 3.2 lists the solubility characteristics of 16 vitamins classified as either fat or water soluble. Although metabolically essential, not all these vitamins would be dietary essentials for all species.

Vitamins can seldom be regarded as nutrients in isolation because they display a wide variety of interactions with each other and other nutrients (Bains, 1999). For example, the fat-soluble vitamins compete for intestinal absorption, with the result that an excess of one may cause deficiencies in the others. The vitamins of the B group are regulators of intermediary metabolism. Some of the metabolic processes are interdependent: for example, choline, B_{12}, and folic acid interact in the methyl groups' metabolism, so a lack of one of them increases the requirement for the others. The same thing happens between B_{12} and pantothenic acid. It may also occur that an excess of 1 vitamin induces a deficiency of others. Thus, biotin status deteriorates if the diet is supplemented with high levels of choline and other vitamins of the B group. High choline levels may similarly affect other vitamins during feed storage.

Vitamins are also known to interact in diverse ways with other nutrients, such as amino acids. For example, there is notable genetic variability in birds' capacity to synthesize nicotinic acid from tryptophan, so their requirements differ between strains. Both methionine and choline can be a source of methyl groups, which are needed to synthesize both, and this relationship is of commercial importance because supplementation entails economic cost. Biotin, folic acid, and B_6 play a part in metabolic interconversions of amino acids, so their requirement increases if protein levels are high. The same applies to those vitamins involved in the metabolism of carbohydrates (biotin, B_1), the requirements for which are higher with low-fat diets. Finally, there are also interactions between minerals and vitamins. The best-documented example is that between selenium and vitamin E. All these aspects will be treated more in detail in Chapter 4.

These interactions make it somewhat difficult to estimate the requirements for each vitamin precisely, and it is probably more appropriate to focus on the problem generally. Whitehead (1987) gives a clear explanation of the situation. The classic evaluation of the dose–response curve, so widely used to estimate the requirements of other nutrients, is not an appropriate technique in the case of vitamins, as their cost is generally low concerning the value of the response value and the potential consequences of inadequate levels. For these reasons, the usual practice is to define vitamin requirements by considering the maximum response obtained with the chosen evaluation criteria, traditionally weight gain or growth and FCR. However, growth is not a specific response: it may be affected by other factors associated with the feed (palatability, particle size, levels of other nutrients, etc.). This issue may explain the great variability in response levels between studies on a particular vitamin, even if they are almost concurrent. According to Whitehead (1987), it would not be possible to establish precise mathematical relationships regarding vitamin requirements until all their interactions are known in detail, taking at the same time into account many factors like various diet types and changes in physical composition.

VITAMIN CONVERSION FACTORS

In May 2016, the US Food and Drug Administration (FDA) announced regulations that require amendments to the existing supplement facts label, which uses units and conversions based on the 1968 Recommended Daily Allowances (RDA). The new regulations became mandatory in 2019/20 (Table 3.3). The changes that will affect the application of Dietary Supplement Ingredient Database (DSID) results are the changes in the units used to declare vitamins and minerals on supplement labels. The FDA permits manufacturers to include the amounts of nutrients in the old units in parentheses adjacent to the quantities in the new units.

VITAMINS IN FEEDSTUFFS

The vitamin content of feedstuffs is highly variable, and current values have not been completely evaluated recently. There are severe limitations in relying on average tabular values of vitamins in feedstuffs. As an example, the vitamin E content of 42 varieties of corn varied from 11.1 to 36.4 mg/kg, a 3.3-fold difference (McDowell and Ward, 2008; Chen *et al.*, 2019; Combs and McClung, 2022).

Table 3.2 Vitamin solubility characteristics (source: DSM Animal Nutrition and Health, unpublished; solubility characteristics from *United States Pharmacopeia*, 1980)

	Molecular weight	Water	Glycerol	Alcohol	Propylene glycol	Ethyl acetate	Ethanol
Vitamin A (retinol)	286.44						
Vitamin D_3	384.62						
Vitamin E (tocopherol)	430.69						
Vitamin K_1	450.68						
Vitamin K_2	580.9						
Vitamin K_3	17.21						
Vitamin B_1 (thiamine)	337.28						
Vitamin B_2 (riboflavin)	376.36						
Niacin	123.11						
Pantothenic acid (vitamin B_5)	219.23						
Vitamin B_6 (pyridoxine hydrochloride)	205.64						
Biotin (vitamin B_7)	244.31						
Folic acid (vitamin B_9)	441.4						
Vitamin B_{12} (cyanocobalamin)	1355.42						
Choline	121.18						
Vitamin C (ascorbic acid)	176.12						

Insoluble | Practically Insoluble | Slightly soluble

Methanol	Chloroform	Fats-oils	Organic solvents	Ether	Benzene	Acetone	Comments
							Freely soluble in dioxane and glacial acetic acid; moderately soluble in amyl alcohol
							Practically insoluble in butanol; Relatively soluble in acetic acid, phenol, pyridine, and solutions of alkali hydroxides and carbonates

Soluble

Not mentioned

Table 3.3 Vitamin conversion factors (source: DSM Animal Nutrition and Health, unpublished)

Vitamin (active substance)	Unit	Conversion factor active substance form to vitamin form	Product form
Vitamin A (retinol)	IU	1 IU Vitamin A = 0.344 µg Vitamin A acetate (retinyl acetate)	ROVIMIX® A 1000
			ROVIMIX® A 500 WS
			ROVIMIX® A Palmitate 1.6
			ROVIMIX® AD3 1000/200
Vitamin D_3 (cholecalciferol)	IU	1 IU Vitamin D_3 = 0.025 µg Vitamin D_3	ROVIMIX® D3-500
			ROVIMIX® AD3 1000/200
$25OHD_3$ (25 hydroxy-cholecalciferol)	mg	1 µg $25OHD_3$ = 40 IU Vitamin D_3	ROVIMIX® Hy•D 1.25%
Vitamin E (tocopherol)	mg	1 mg Vitamin E = 1 IU Vitamin E = 1 mg all-rac-α-tocopheryl acetate	ROVIMIX® E-50 Adsorbate
			ROVIMIX® E 50 SD
Vitamin K_3 (menadione)	mg	1 mg of Vitamin K_3 = 2 mg of Menadione Sodium Bisulfite (MSB)	K_3 MSB
		1 mg of Vitamin K_3 = 2.3 mg of Menadione Nicotinamide Bisulfite (MNB)	ROVIMIX® K_3 MNB
Vitamin B_1 (thiamine)	mg	1 mg of Vitamin B_1 = 1.088 mg of Thiamine mononitrate	ROVIMIX® B_1
Vitamin B_2 (riboflavin)	mg		ROVIMIX® B2 80-SD
Vitamin B_6 (pyridoxine)	mg	1 mg Vitamin B_6 = 1.215 mg Pyridoxine hydrochloride	ROVIMIX® B_6
Vitamin B_{12} (cyanocobalamin)	mg		Vitamin B_{12} 1% Feed Grade
			ROVIMIX® B_{12}
Vitamin B_3 (Niacin; nicotinic acid and nicotinamide)	mg	1 mg Nicotinic acid = 1 mg Niacin	ROVIMIX® Niacin
		1 mg Nicotinamide (or Niacinamide) = 1 mg Niacin	ROVIMIX® Niacinamide
Vitamin B_7 (d-Biotin)	mg	1 mg of Biotin = 1 mg D-Biotin	ROVIMIX® Biotin ROVIMIX® Biotin HP
Vitamin B_5 (d-Pantothenic acid)	mg	1 mg d-Pantothenic acid = 1.087 mg Calcium d-pantothenate or 2.174 mg Calcium dl-pantothenate	ROVIMIX® Calpan
Vitamin B_9 (Folic acid)	mg		ROVIMIX® Folic 80 SD

Content (min.)	Formulation technology	Application*
1,000,000 IU/g	Beadlet	M, P, EXP, EXT
500,000 IU/g	Spray-dried powder, water dispersible	MR/W
1,600,000 IU/g	Oily liquid, may crystalize on storage	Oily solution
Vitamin A 1,000,000 IU/g Vitamin D_3 200,000 IU/g	Beadlet	M, P, EXP, EXT
500,000 IU/g	Spray-dried powder, water dispersible	M, P, EXP, EXT, MR/W
Vitamin A 1,000,000 IU/g Vitamin D_3 200,000 IU/g	Beadlet	M, P, EXP, EXT
1.25% 25OHD_3 (12.5 g/kg)	Spray-dried powder, water dispersible	M, P, EXP, EXT, W
50% (500 g/kg)	Adsorbate on silicic acid	M, P, EXP, EXT
50% (500 g/kg)	Spray-dried powder, water dispersible	M, P, EXP, EXT, MR/W
Menadione: 51.5% (515 g/kg)	Fine crystalline powder	M, P, EXP, EXT, MR/W
Menadione: 43% (430 g/kg) Nicotinamide: 30.5% (305 g/kg)	Fine crystalline powder	M, P, EXP, EXT
98% (980 g/kg)	Fine crystalline powder	M, P, EXP, EXT
80% (800 g/kg)	Spray-dried powder	M, P, EXP, EXT, MR/W
99% (990 g/kg)	Fine crystalline powder	M, P, EXP, EXT, MR/W
1% (10 g/kg)	Fine powder	M, P, EXP, EXT
1% Feed Grade 1% (10 g/kg)	Spray-dried powder	M, P, EXP, EXT
99.5% (995 g/kg)	Fine crystalline powder	M, P, EXP, EXT
99.5% (995 g/kg)	Fine crystalline powder	M, P, EXP, EXT, MR/W
2% (20 g/kg) 10% (100 g/kg)	Spray-dried powder, water dispersible	M, P, EXP, EXT, MR/W
98% Calcium d-pantothenate (980 g/kg) Calcium 8.2 – 8.6% (82 – 86 g/kg)	Spray-dried powder, water dispersible	M, P, EXP, EXT, MR/W
80% (800 g/kg)	Spray-dried powder, water dispersible	M, P, EXP, EXT, MR/W

Table 3.3 (continued)

Vitamin (active substance)	Unit	Conversion factor active substance form to vitamin form	Product form
Vitamin C	mg	1 mg Vitamin C = 1 mg L-Ascorbic acid	STAY-C® 35
			STAY-C® 50
			ROVIMIX® C-EC
			Ascorbic acid
β-Carotene	mg		ROVIMIX® β-Carotene 10%
			ROVIMIX® β-Carotene 10% P
Astaxanthin	IU		CAROPHYLL® Pink 10%-CWS
			CAROPHYLL® Pink

* M: Mash; P: Pellet; EXP: Expansion; EXT: Extrusion; MR/W: Milk replacer/Water
For more information about further DSM products and product forms please ask your local DSM representative

As a reference, the average vitamin levels in some common feed ingredients are presented in Table 3.4 (Chen *et al.*, 2019). Other sources of information (Combs and McClung, 2022) still rely on data published by Scott *et al.* (1982a,b).

Generally, these average values are based on a limited number of assays published more than 50–70 years ago and were not adjusted for bioavailability and variations of vitamin levels within ingredients. Therefore, they may not reflect the changes in genetic characteristics, handling, and storage of crops, cropping practices, and processing of feedstuffs over the years. Changing processing methods can greatly alter vitamin feed levels. For example, with changes in sugar technology, literature values for pantothenic acid content of beet molasses have decreased from 50 to 110 mg/kg in the 1950s to about 1–4 mg/kg (Palagina *et al.*, 1990). Likewise, heat treatments in feed processing like pelleting and extrusion improve nutrient digestibility, reduce antinutritional factors, and eventually control *Salmonella* and other pathogens, resulting in greater vitamin destruction (Gadient, 1986; Svihus and Zimonja, 2011; Yang *et al.*, 2020). In addition, values for some vitamins were not determined by current, more precise assay procedures. Additional information on the limitations of using average values of vitamins in feedstuffs when formulating animal rations have been reported (Kurnick *et al.*, 1972).

Vitamin levels from simple rations of feedstuff are generally lower than in complex rations. The currently used diets (e.g., corn-soybean meal) for animals exclude or contain lower amounts of the more costly vitamin-rich ingredients. The vitamin fortification levels in these simpler diets should be increased to "fill in the gaps" resulting from the reduced amounts of vitamins supplied by feedstuffs.

Since ingredient changes are frequent and unpredictable in computerized best-cost diet formulation, the low levels of vitamins likely to be supplied by feedstuffs should be disregarded and adequate dietary vitamin fortification provided.

Vitamins, as pure substances, are almost all sensitive to various physical stress factors. Table 3.5 provides a simple qualitative overview of the sensitivity of each vitamin to

Content (min.)	Formulation technology	Application*
35% of total phosphorylated ascorbic acid activity (350 g/kg)	Spray-dried powder	M, P, EXP, EXT
50% of total phosphorylated sodium salt ascorbic acid activity (500 g/kg)	Spray-dried powder	M, P, EXP, EXT, MR/W
97.5% (975 g/kg)	Ethyl-cellulose coated powder	M, P, MR/W
99 – 100% (990 – 1000 g/kg)	Crystalline powder	MR/W
10% (100 g/kg)	Beadlet	M, P, EXP, EXT
10% (100 g/kg)	Cross linked beadlet	M, P, EXP, EXT
10% astaxanthin	Beadlet (Cold Water Soluble)	M, P, EXP, EXT, W
8% astaxanthin	Beadlet	M, P, EXP, EXT

these factors. This explains the importance, for industrial application, of properly formulating each vitamin to make it more stable and ensuring that the calculated amount per kilogram of feed is really reaching the animal.

FACTORS AFFECTING VITAMIN REQUIREMENTS AND UTILIZATION

1. Physiological make-up, genetics, and production function

Vitamin requirements of animals and humans depend greatly on their physiological make-up related to the traits developed by decades of genetic selection, age, health, and nutritional status and function (such as producing meat, milk, eggs, hair or wool, or carrying a fetus) (Roche, 1979). For example, breeder hens have higher vitamin requirements for optimum hatchability since vitamin requirements for egg production are generally less than for egg hatchability. Higher levels of vitamins A, D_3, and E are needed in breeder hen diets than in feeds for rapidly growing broilers.

Selection for a faster growth rate may allow animals to reach much higher weights at much younger ages with less feed consumption. This rapid growth may influence birds' ability to develop their skeleton accordingly (Williams *et al.*, 2000a,b).

Dudley-Cash (1994) concludes that since genetic potential has improved FCR by 0.8% yearly and most of the NRC vitamin requirement data are 45–65 years old, vitamin requirements determined several decades ago may not apply to today's poultry. Leeson (2007) reached basically the same conclusion: for layers, the estimate is around a 1% yearly decline in vitamin intake per egg produced, while for meat birds, there has been a 0.6–0.8% yearly decline per kilogram body gain.

Leg problems still observed in commercial strains of broilers and broiler breeders can be corrected partly by higher levels of biotin, folacin, niacin, and choline, and more available vitamin D (Roche, 1979). Vitamins C and E can also mitigate the severity of myopathies observed in broilers (Wang *et al.*, 2020a,b).

Table 3.4 Vitamin concentrations of feedstuffs, mean (SD) (source: adapted from Chen *et al.*, 2019)

	Vitamins, mg/kg – mean (standard deviation)								
Feed ingredients	β-carotene	Vitamin E	Vitamin B_6	Folic acid	Niacin	Pantothenic acid	Vitamin B_2 (riboflavin)	Vitamin B_1 (thiamine)	Choline
Corn	1.62 (0.44)	18.67 (9.48)	3.05 (1.19)	0.08 (0.07)	3.68 (1.73)	3.98 (1.20)	1.30 (0.20)	0.61 (0.17)	292.82 (80.55)
Corn DDGS	2.16 (0.58)	39.24 (9.97)	0.99 (0.47)	0.57 (0.31)	23.23 (13.13)	15.55 (3.02)	3.73 (0.66)	2.14 (0.54)	337.36 (173.38)
Corn germ meal	0.36 (0.09)	19.31 (5.89)	4.44 (1.80)	0.72 (0.49)	29.42 (5.73)	5.35 (2.98)	3.95 (2.28)	4.14 (2.34)	818.00 (513.98)
Corn gluten meal	11.10 (4.05)	7.00 (1.51)	2.13 (0.93)	0.02 (0.02)	36.46 (5.90)	3.93 (2.06)	0.72 (0.36)	0.37 (0.13)	80.04 (13.16)
Corn gluten feed	0.56 (0.11)	9.89 (2.62)	4.15 (1.01)	1.30 (0.46)	52.65 (11.94)	12.56 (3.14)	1.89 (0.80)	5.11 (1.04)	1525.18 (242.75)
Wheat	–	7.27 (1.73)	2.23 (1.33)	0.40 (0.18)	32.86 (8.63)	7.36 (3.60)	0.57 (0.19)	2.12 (1.09)	234.29 (81.65)
Wheat bran	–	19.79 (5.86)	6.52 (1.19)	0.40 (0.18)	102.53 (14.81)	12.35 (4.02)	0.96 (0.26)	2.52 (0.58)	931.59 (121.89)
Wheat shorts	–	9.03 (4.28)	3.93 (1.23)	0.62 (0.27)	4.54 (1.31)	8.18 (0.96)	1.18 (0.12)	3.69 (1.26)	830.48 (226.78)
Soybean meal	–	2.42 (0.85)	6.43 (1.07)	0.51 (0.11)	62.03 (6.21)	3.63 (0.85)	1.77 (0.37)	9.13 (1.51)	1686.54 (144.07)
Rapeseed meal	–	8.66 (2.40)	3.46 (1.80)	0.65 (0.47)	72.82 (10.53)	6.73 (2.75)	1.53 (0.41)	2.14 (0.90)	2276.32 (193.22)
Peanut meal	–	0.67 (0.27)	5.44 (1.11)	104.96 (13.40)	104.96 (14.07)	18.27 (3.46)	1.65 (0.41)	4.22 (1.47)	1527.60 (130.54)
Cottonseed meal	–	10.57 (7.83)	6.30 (1.64)	9.15 (1.87)	9.15 (1.87)	6.75 (1.92)	2.19 (0.32)	1.63 (0.48)	1546.24 (272.49)
Sunflower seed meal	–	1.04 (0.30)	7.57 (0.49)	183.91 (14.60)	183.91 (14.60)	27.25 (1.52)	3.65 (0.16)	1.78 (0.34)	399.96 (69.15)

2. Confined production versus access to pasture

The complete confinement of poultry has been common for many decades, and consequently, vitamin nutrition has played an important role in the success of poultry production. The new trends are to give access to pasture in free-range systems. Since young, lush, green grasses or legumes are good vitamin sources, these production systems could provide significant quantities of most vitamins. More available vitamins A and E are present in pastures and green forages, which contain ample amounts of β-carotene, α-tocopherol, and flavonoids, compared to levels found in grains, which are lower in bioavailability. The outdoor system has been proven to improve polyunsaturated omega-3 and the ratio between omega-6 and omega-3 fatty acids (Dal Bosco *et al.*, 2016). However, negative effects on oxidative stability have been observed.

Consequently, free-range poultry could also benefit from vitamin supplementation. The effect of foraging in birds is complex, depending on the balance between anti- and pro-oxidant compounds and on the kinetic activity of the animal, which drives oxidation (Sossidou *et al.*, 2011). Oxidation may be low with grass intake because green forage has high levels of tocopherols, tocotrienols, carotenoids, vitamin C, and polyphenols (Mugnai *et al.*, 2014). The current poultry rearing systems do not emphasize outdoor grazing areas for poultry (Horsted *et al.*, 2007); however, studies on crop content indicate that slow-growing poultry strains have a large intake of pasture and other accessible foods (Mwalusanya *et al.*, 2002; Dal Bosco *et al.*, 2014). Therefore, it is crucial to assess the intake and the nutritional relevance of pasture, the ability to transfer the compounds mentioned above into poultry products, and the development of suitable feed for free-range birds (Dal Bosco *et al.*, 2016).

Table 3.5 Sensitivity of vitamins to physical stress factors (source: DSM Animal Nutrition and Health, unpublished)

Additive	Temperature	Oxygen	Humidity	Light
Vitamin A				
Vitamin D				
25OHD$_3$ (calcifediol)				
Vitamin E				
Vitamin K$_3$				
Vitamin B$_1$				
Vitamin B$_2$				
Vitamin B$_6$				
Vitamin B$_{12}$				
Pantothenic acid				
Nicotinates				
Biotin				
Folic acid				
Vitamin C				
Carotenoids				

Marked effect   Moderate effect   No effect

3. Antioxidants and immunological role of vitamins

Immunological response and disease conditions are intimately related to the requirements for certain vitamins (Surai *et al.*, 2016; Surai *et al.*, 2019). Disease conditions influence the antioxidant vitamins (vitamin E, vitamin C, and β-carotene). These nutrients play important roles in animal health by inactivating harmful free radicals from various stressors produced through normal cellular activity. Free radicals can be extremely damaging to biological systems (Surai *et al.*, 2016; Mishra and Jha, 2019). Free radicals, including hydroxy, hypochlorite, peroxy, alkoxy, superoxide, hydrogen peroxide, and singlet oxygen, are generated by autoxidation, radiation or some oxidases, dehydrogenases, and peroxidases. Also, phagocytic granulocytes undergo respiratory bursts to produce oxygen radicals to destroy pathogens. However, these oxidative products can, in turn, damage healthy cells if they are not eliminated. Antioxidants stabilize these highly reactive free radicals, maintaining cells' structural and functional integrity (Chew, 1995; McDowell, 2006). Therefore, antioxidants are very important to poultry's immune defense and health (Surai *et al.*, 2016; Mishra and Jha, 2019; Surai *et al.*, 2019).

Tissue defense mechanisms against free-radical damage generally include vitamin C, vitamin E, and β-carotene as the major vitamin antioxidant sources. In addition, several metalloenzymes, which include glutathione peroxidase (selenium), catalase (iron), and superoxide dismutase (copper, zinc, and manganese), are also critical in protecting the internal cellular constituents from oxidative damage. These nutrients' dietary and tissue balance is important in protecting tissues against free-radical damage (Surai *et al.*, 2016; Mishra and Jha, 2019; Surai *et al.*, 2019; Combs and McClung, 2022).

Both *in vitro* and *in vivo* studies show that the antioxidant vitamins generally enhance cellular and noncellular immunity. The antioxidant function of these vitamins could, at least in part, enhance immunity by maintaining the function and structural integrity of important immune cells. A compromised immune system will reduce animal production efficiency through increased susceptibility to disease, leading to animal morbidity and mortality.

Vitamin C is the most important antioxidant in extracellular fluids. It can protect biomembranes against lipid peroxidation damage by eliminating peroxyl radicals in the aqueous phase before the latter can initiate peroxidation (Frei *et al.*, 1989; Ahmadu *et al.*, 2016). In data from rats, vitamin C was required for an adequate immune response in limiting lung pathology after influenza virus infection (Li *et al.*, 2006). One of the protective effects of vitamin C may partly be mediated through its ability to reduce circulating glucocorticoids (Degkwitz, 1987; Ahmadu *et al.*, 2016). In addition, ascorbate can regenerate the reduced form of α-tocopherol, perhaps accounting for the observed sparing effect of these vitamins (Jacob, 1995; Tanaka *et al.*, 1997). In the process of sparing fatty acid oxidation, tocopherol is oxidized to the tocopheryl free-radical. Ascorbic acid can donate an electron to the tocopheryl free-radical, regenerating the reduced antioxidant form of tocopherol (Ahmadu *et al.*, 2016; Min *et al.*, 2018).

Vitamin C and E supplementation resulted in a 78% decrease in the susceptibility of lipoproteins to mononuclear cell-mediated oxidation (Rifici and Khachadurian, 1993). As an effective scavenger of reactive oxygen species, ascorbic acid minimizes the oxidative stress associated with activated phagocytic leukocytes' respiratory burst, thereby controlling the inflammation and tissue damage associated with immune responses (Chien *et al.*, 2004). Ascorbic acid is very high in phagocytic cells, with these cells using free radicals and other highly reactive oxygen-containing molecules to help kill pathogens that invade the body. However, these reactive species may damage cells and tissues in the process. Ascorbic acid helps to protect these cells from oxidative damage (Min *et al.*, 2018; Combs and McClung, 2022).

Vitamin A strongly influences the immunological response, although it has less antioxidant potential than β-carotene. Animals deficient in vitamin A will show increased frequency and severity of bacterial, protozoal, and viral infections and other disease conditions. As a function of vitamin A, part of the disease resistance is related to maintaining mucous membranes and normal adrenal gland functioning which produces the corticosteroids needed to combat disease. An animal's ability to resist illness depends on a responsive immune system, and a vitamin A deficiency causes a reduced immune response (Combs and McClung, 2022).

Vitamin A deficiency affects immune functions, particularly the antibody response to T-cell-dependent antigens (Ross, 1992). The RAR-alpha mRNA expression and antigen-specific proliferative response of T-lymphocytes are influenced by vitamin A status *in vivo* and directly modulated by retinoic acid (Halevy *et al.*, 1994). Vitamin A deficiency affects several cells of the immune system. Repletion with retinoic acid effectively re-establishes the number of circulating lymphocytes (Zhao and Ross, 1995) and even can have transgenerational effects on the progeny when supplemented with hens (Lin *et al.*, 2002).

A diminished primary antibody response could also increase the severity and duration of an episode of infection. In contrast, a diminished secondary reaction could increase the risk of developing a second disease episode. Vitamin A deficiency causes decreases in phagocytic activity in macrophages and neutrophils. The secretory immunoglobulin A (IgA) system is an important first line of defense against infections of mucosal surfaces (McGhee *et al.*, 1992). Several studies in animal models have shown that the intestinal IgA response is impaired by vitamin A deficiency (Davis and Sell, 1989; Wiedermann *et al.*, 1993; Stephensen *et al.*, 1996).

An optimal vitamin A range enhances vitamin A responses because both deficient and excessive levels suppress immune function. In many experiments with laboratory and domestic animals, the effects of both clinical and subclinical deficiencies of vitamin A on the production of antibodies and the resistance of different tissues to microbial infection or parasitic infestation have frequently been demonstrated (Kelley and Easter, 1987). Supplemental vitamin A improved the health of animals infected with roundworms and hens infected with *Capillaria* (Herrick, 1972).

A combination of vitamin A (15,000 IU/kg) and vitamin E (250 mg/kg) was more effective than either vitamin alone in reducing heat stress-related (32°C) decreases in broiler performance (Sahin *et al.*, 2001). High environmental temperature harms laying performance and can impede disease resistance (Lin *et al.*, 2006). Vitamin A supplementation at high levels (2–3 times the NRC requirement) to commercial layer hens under heat stress was beneficial to laying performance and immune function (Lin *et al.*, 2002). Hens suffering heat stress immediately after Newcastle disease vaccination need higher dietary vitamin A intake to obtain the maximal level of antibody production (Davis and Sell, 1989). Vitamin A could alleviate the oxidative injuries induced by heat exposure and immune challenge (Lin *et al.*, 2002).

Vitamin A-deficient chicks showed rapid loss of lymphocytes, and deficient rats showed atrophy of the thymus and spleen and reduced response to diphtheria and tetanus toxoids (Krishnan *et al.*, 1974). Mortality from fowl typhoid (*Salmonella gallinarum*) was decreased in chicks fed vitamin A levels greater than the normal levels in high-protein diets. Chicks' serum antibody levels were increased two- to fivefold by high dietary vitamin A concentrations. The immune response from the introduced Newcastle disease virus was higher for broiler chicks receiving a 2,500 IU/kg diet of vitamin A than controls and the best for those receiving 20,000 IU/kg (Serman and Mazija, 1985).

Animal studies indicate that certain carotenoids like canthaxanthin with antioxidant capacities, but without vitamin A activity, can enhance many aspects of immune functions and can act directly as antimutagens and anticarcinogens. They can protect against radiation damage and block photosensitizers' damaging effects. Also, carotenoids can directly affect gene expression, and this mechanism may enable carotenoids to modulate the interaction between B-cells and T-cells, thus regulating humoral and cell-mediated immunity (Koutsos, 2003). A lack of carotenoids was reported to increase parameters of systemic inflammation in growing chicks (Koutsos *et al.*, 2006).

Vitamin E is perhaps the most studied nutrient related to the immune response (Meydani and Han, 2006). Evidence accumulated over the years and in many species indicates that vitamin E is an essential nutrient for the normal function of the immune system. Furthermore, studies suggest that the beneficial effects of certain nutrients, such as vitamin E, on reducing disease risk can affect the immune response. Deficiency in vitamin E impairs B- and T-cell-mediated immunity. Vitamin E partially reduces prostaglandin synthesis and prevents the oxidation of polyunsaturated fatty acids (PUFAs) in cell membranes (Shanker, 2006).

Considerable attention is presently being directed to vitamin E and selenium's role in protecting leukocytes and macrophages during phagocytosis, the mechanism whereby animals immunologically kill invading bacteria. Both vitamin E and selenium may help these cells survive the toxic products produced to effectively kill ingested bacteria (Badwey and Karnovsky, 1980).

Macrophages and neutrophils from vitamin E-deficient animals have decreased phagocytic activity (Burkholder and Swecker, 1990). Large doses of vitamin E protected chicks and poults against *Escherichia coli* with increased phagocytosis and antibody production (Tengerdy and Brown, 1977). Vitamin E supplementation in feed at levels of 150–300 mg/kg decreased chick mortality due to *E. coli* challenge from 40%, in the birds not supplemented with vitamin E, to 5% in supplemented birds (Tengerdy and Nockels, 1975). Chicks fed vitamin E at a 100 mg/kg diet had increased weight gains and reduced mortality during the coccidiosis challenge (Colnago *et al.*, 1984). Heat stress severely reduced broilers' growth performance and immune response, whereas the immune response of broilers was improved by vitamin E (Niu *et al.*, 2009). Broiler chicks fed 80 mg vitamin E/kg had increased innate and humoral immune response against coccidiosis vaccine and an *Eimeria* (protozoan parasites) challenge (Perez-Carbajal *et al.*, 2010).

Since vitamin E acts as a tissue antioxidant and aids in quenching free radicals produced in the body, any infection or other stress factor may exacerbate depletion of the limited vitamin E stores from various tissues. Regarding immunocompetency, dietary requirements may be adequate for normal growth and production; however, higher levels have improved cellular and humoral immune status. The former 2 responses are generally used as criteria for determining the requirements of a nutrient. There is an increase in glucocorticoids, epinephrine, eicosanoids, and phagocytic activity during stress and disease. Eicosanoid and corticoid synthesis and phagocytic respiratory bursts are prominent producers of free radicals that challenge the antioxidant systems. Vitamin E has been implicated in stimulating serum antibody synthesis, particularly IgG antibodies (Tengerdy, 1980). The productive effects of vitamin E on animal health may reduce immunosuppressive glucocorticoids (Golub and Gershwin, 1985). Vitamin E also most likely has an immuno-enhancing impact by altering arachidonic acid metabolism and subsequent prostaglandin synthesis, thromboxanes, and leukotrienes. Under stress conditions, increased levels of these compounds by endogenous synthesis or exogenous entry may adversely affect immune cell function (Hadden, 1987). These results suggest that the criteria for establishing requirements based on overt deficiencies or growth do not consider optimal health.

4. Stress, disease, or adverse environmental conditions

Intensified production increases stress and subclinical disease level conditions because of higher densities of animals in confined areas. Stress and disease conditions in animals may increase the basic requirement for certain vitamins. Several studies indicated that nutrient levels adequate for growth, feed efficiency, gestation, and lactation might not be sufficient for normal immunity and maximizing the animal's resistance to disease (Cunha, 1985; Nockels, 1988; Ward, 1993).

The adverse effect of environmental stress on a chicken's health, welfare, and performance cannot be overemphasized. Environmental stressors can cause an upsurge in stress hormone secretion, which negatively affects growth and leads to mortality in severe cases. However, effective management techniques are key to raising healthy chickens and profit maximization in the poultry industry. To enhance chickens' adaptability under stress conditions, it is essential to understand the functions of different vitamins and the appropriate dosage in chicken diets to alleviate stress. The synergistic effects of various vitamins and minerals could promote growth performance and reduce environmental stress in chickens (Akinyemi and Adewole, 2021).

Diseases or parasites affecting the gastrointestinal tract will reduce the intestinal absorption of vitamins from dietary sources and those synthesized by microorganisms. If they cause diarrhea or vomiting, they will decrease intestinal absorption and increase vitamin needs. Vitamin A deficiency is often seen in heavily parasitized animals that supposedly receive an adequate amount of the vitamin (McDowell, 2004).

Any disease that includes bleeding of the intestinal wall increases both vitamin loss and vitamin requirements for tissue regeneration. Likewise, a condition that causes a loss in appetite and feed intake increase the need for vitamins per unit of feed consumed to meet daily body needs. Diseases that adversely affect the integrity of the intestinal wall may interfere with vitamin A conversion from carotene and increase the animal's vitamin A needs. Cunha (1987) suggested that the transformation of vitamin D to its functional forms in the liver and kidney would be affected by diseases of these organs.

Mycotoxins are known to cause a digestive disturbance, such as vomiting and diarrhea, as well as internal bleeding, and interfere with the absorption of dietary vitamins A, D, E, and K. In broiler chickens, moldy corn containing mycotoxins have been associated with deficiencies of vitamin D (rickets) and vitamin E (encephalomalacia) even though these vitamins were supplemented at levels regarded as satisfactory.

A disorder dubbed "spiking syndrome" in broilers caused a sharp rise in mortality at about 14 days of age. Some nutritionists feel this problem may be associated with *Fusarium* mycotoxins, although the exact cause is unclear. Increased levels of thiamine reduce the rate of mortality, and it is suggested that when either corn quality is poor or mycotoxin levels and mold counts are high, thiamine should be increased by 1.11 to 1.65 mg/kg in the starter feed (Gadient, 1986).

Mortality from fowl typhoid (*Salmonella gallinarum*) was reduced in chicks fed vitamin levels greater than normal (Hill *et al.*, 1961). Vitamin E supplementation at a high level decreased chick mortality due to *E. coli* challenge from 40 to 5% (Tengerdy and Nockels, 1975). Scott *et al.* (1982) concluded that coccidiosis produces triple stress on vitamin K requirements as follows: (1) coccidiosis reduces feed intake, thereby reducing vitamin K intake; (2) coccidiosis injures the intestinal tract and reduces the absorption of the vitamin; and (3) sulfaquinoxaline treatment and other coccidiostats causes an increased requirement for vitamin K.

Egg shell quality can be severely depressed by various stresses, including disturbance and heat stress. Vitamin C has been found to promote vitamin D metabolism and is also known to counter the effects of multiple stresses. Heat stress depresses a range of egg production and quality characteristics. Ascorbic acid supplementation has improved these traits (Cheng *et al.*, 1990). Ascorbic acid can also alleviate nutritional stress. Balnave *et al.* (1991) showed that the poor shell quality of hens given saline drinking water could be overcome by adding ascorbic acid to the water (1 g/l).

Although vitamin C is commonly associated with alleviating the effects of heat stress in laying hens, recent work has demonstrated that vitamin E can also play an important role. Depression in egg production in laying hens brought about by heat stress can be partially prevented by dietary supplementation with vitamin E (Utomo *et al.*, 1994). Vitamin E enhances the immune status of layers during heat stress and potentially during other stress periods, such as transport, vaccination, and molt (Scheideler, 1998). There was a positive correlation between enhanced immunity and a positive effect on production parameters such as egg production and egg mass during stress in layers.

Developing new techniques to cope with heat stress, which adversely influences the performance and meat quality during the rearing period, is a main aim of the poultry industry. To enhance chickens' tolerance to high temperatures, understanding the functions of different supplementations and manipulating diets seem promising methods to quickly reduce the adverse effects of heat stress.

The synergistic effects of selenium and vitamins E and C, employing multiple mechanisms, enhance growth performance in broiler chickens challenged with acute heat stress. Emerging literature reveals that selenium and vitamins E and C interact closely to protect proteins and lipids from oxidative damage. Combining them can be considered an important solution to cope with heat stress. Meanwhile, selenium is involved in the glutathione pathway, which is part of the ascorbate cycle (Shakeri *et al.*, 2020).

Ward (1993) fed vitamins at 5 levels to 9,600 broilers over 42 days to compare the potential effects of stress conditions on vitamin requirements. The 5 levels were: NRC; low 25% industry (Ward, 1993); average industry; high 25% industry and high 25% + 25%. Birds were subjected to 3 stress levels (minimum, moderate, and relatively high) based on different levels of coccidia, *E. coli*, placement density, and nutritional plane. The results showed that bird performance declined as the degree of stress increased. Furthermore, although the highest level of vitamins did not completely overcome the detrimental effect of stress, the higher levels did improve performance over the lower levels.

5. Vitamin antagonists

Vitamin antagonists (anti-metabolites) interfere with the activity of various vitamins. Oldfield (1987) summarized the action of antagonists, which:

- could cleave the vitamin molecule and render it inactive, as occurs with thiaminase, found in raw fish and some feedstuffs, and thiamine (pyrithiamine is another thiamine antagonist)
- could bind with the metabolite, with similar results, as happens between avidin, found in raw egg white, and streptavidin, from *Streptomyces* mold and biotin
- could, because of structural similarity, occupy reaction sites and thereby deny them to the vitamin, as with dicumarol, found in certain plants, and vitamin K
- inactivate, through rancid fats, biotin and destroy vitamins A, D, E, and possibly others.

The presence of vitamin antagonists in animal and human diets should be considered when adjusting vitamin allowances, as most vitamins have antagonists that reduce their utilization. Mycotoxins are antagonists in the feed that can substantially decrease antioxidant nutrient assimilation and increase their requirements to prevent the damaging effects of free radicals and toxic products. It is now increasingly recognized that at least 25% of the world's grains are contaminated with mycotoxins (Surai, 2003). Mycotoxins cause digestive disturbances such as vomiting and diarrhea, and internal bleeding and interfere with the absorption of dietary vitamins A and vitamins D, E, and K (McDowell, 2006). In broiler chickens, moldy corn (mycotoxins) has been associated with deficiencies of vitamins D (rickets) and E (encephalomalacia) even though these vitamins were supplemented at levels regarded as satisfactory.

Toxic minerals may be antagonists and will likewise increase vitamin requirements. Vitamin E is known to protect against the toxicity of certain heavy metals (e.g., cadmium, mercury, lead), which increases the need for the vitamin (McDowell, 2000a). Lead, for example, has been shown to increase riboflavin requirements (Donaldson, 1986). For chicks, 6.7 mg riboflavin/kg was more effective in suppressing lead toxicity than was 3.0 mg/kg.

Specific vitamins can likewise be antagonistic to other vitamins. Excess vitamin A (40,000–60,000 IU/kg) can affect the metabolism (e.g., absorption) of other fat-soluble vitamins. Large excesses of vitamin E have been shown to result in hemorrhages in some species, apparently by reducing vitamin K absorption. The problem can be eliminated with additional dietary vitamin K (Aburto and Britton, 1998a; Frank *et al.*, 1997).

6. Use of antimicrobial drugs

Some antimicrobial drugs will increase the vitamin needs of animals by altering intestinal microflora and inhibiting the synthesis of certain vitamins. Certain sulfonamides may increase requirements of biotin, folic acid, vitamin K and possibly others when intestinal synthesis is reduced. These gut health issues may be of little significance except when antagonistic drugs toward a particular vitamin are added in excess, i.e., the coccidiostat amprolium versus vitamin B_1 (Scott *et al.*, 1982), sulfaquinoxaline versus vitamin K and sulfonamide potentiators versus folic acid (Perry, 1978).

7. Levels of other nutrients in the diet

The fat level in the diet may affect the absorption of the fat-soluble vitamins A, D, E, and K and the requirements for vitamin E and possibly other vitamins. Fat-soluble vitamins may fail to be absorbed if fat digestion is impaired by liver damage or when the enterohepatic recirculation of bile acids is interrupted. Type (e.g., animal fats, vegetable oils, and blends) and quality (e.g., cis versus trans, saturated versus PUFAs, and oxidized sources) of fats can influence individual vitamin allowances.

For example, a precise vitamin E: PUFA ratio may not apply to all diet and health status types. Therefore, there has been no consensus on the exact vitamin E: PUFA ratio to determine the vitamin requirement. However, the published human data for a diet with an average content of PUFA and containing mainly linoleic acid indicates that the additional vitamin E requirement ranges from 0.4 to 0.6 mg RRR-α-tocopherol/g of PUFA in the diet. A ratio of 0.5 mg RRR-α-tocopherol/g of linoleic acid was used in the diet and the degree of unsaturation of the dietary fatty acids was also considered to evaluate the vitamin E required. Thus, using the proposed equation, humans' estimated requirement for vitamin E varied from 12 to 20 mg/day for a typical range of dietary PUFA intake (Raederstorff *et al.*, 2015). Calculations based on animal diets indicate that high dietary PUFA increases vitamin E requirements by 3 mg/g PUFA (Bieber-Wlaschny, 1988). Many interrelationships of vitamins with other nutrients exist and affect requirements. For example, prominent interrelationships exist for vitamin E with selenium, vitamin D with calcium and phosphorus, choline with methionine, and niacin with tryptophan.

8. Body vitamin reserves

The fat-soluble vitamins A, D, and E, but not vitamin K, are more inclined to remain in the body. This is especially true of vitamin A and carotene, which may be stored by an animal in its liver and fatty tissue in sufficient quantities to meet its requirements for varying periods. Body storage of B group vitamins, except for vitamin B_{12}, is irrelevant. Overall a daily supplementation at the proper levels typical of each species and growth stage is normally recommended in animal husbandry in industrial conditions.

Chapter 4

Vitamin description

FAT-SOLUBLE VITAMINS

Vitamin A

Chemical structure and properties

Vitamin A is used as a generic term for all the non-carotenoid β-ionone derivatives possessing the biological activity of all-trans-retinol (Combs and McClung, 2022). Retinol is the alcohol form of vitamin A. Replacement of the alcohol group (-OH) by an aldehyde group (-CHO) yields retinal, and replacement by an acid group (-COOH) gives retinoic acid (Ross and Harrison, 2013). Vitamin A products for feed use include retinyl acetate, propionate, and palmitate esters (Figure 4.1).

Vitamin A alcohol (retinol) is a nearly colorless, fat-soluble, long-chain, unsaturated compound with 5 bonds. Since it contains double bonds, vitamin A can exist in different isomeric forms. Vitamin A and its precursors, carotenoids, are rapidly destroyed by oxygen, heat, light, and acids. Moisture and trace minerals reduce feed vitamin A activity (Olson, 1984).

Poultry diets are supplemented with synthetic retinol as the contribution of carotenoids from the feed in the formation of vitamin A is minimal (Surai *et al.*, 2003). The combined potency in a feed, represented by its vitamin A and carotene content, is referred to as its vitamin A value. In animal tissues, they exist predominantly as retinal, retinol, retinaldehyde, retinoic, and retinyl esters (Ross and Harrison, 2013).

Vegetables contain a variety of carotenoids. Over 600 forms of carotenoids have been isolated, which differ in molecular structure and biological function (Goodwin, 1984; Ross and Harrison, 2013). In birds, carotenoids function as pigments in feathers and skin, antioxidants, and play various roles in the endocrine and immune systems (Bortolotti *et al.*, 2003; Surai, 2003; Wang *et al.*, 2020).

The carotenes are orange-yellow pigments, mainly in green leaves and to a lesser extent in corn. Four carotenoids, α-carotene, β-carotene, γ-carotene, and cryptoxanthin (one of the main carotenoids of corn), possessing the β-ionone ring (C15=C15), are particularly important because of their provitamin A activity (Surai *et al.*, 2001). Lycopene is an important carotenoid for its antioxidant function but does not possess the β-ionone ring structure, and it is not a precursor of vitamin A.

Vitamin A activity of β-carotene is substantially greater than other carotenoids (Ross and Harrison, 2013). For example, both α-carotene and cryptoxanthin have about one-half the conversion rate of β-carotene (Tanumihardjo and Howe, 2005). Theoretically, 2 molecules of vitamin A could be formed from one molecule of β-carotene. However, biological tests have consistently shown that pure vitamin A has twice the potency of β-carotene on a weight-to-weight basis. The efficacy of β-carotene conversion to vitamin A is greater in birds (2: 1) than in other species, but it falls to 5: 1 with increased ingestion of carotene. Jensen and Edberg (1999)

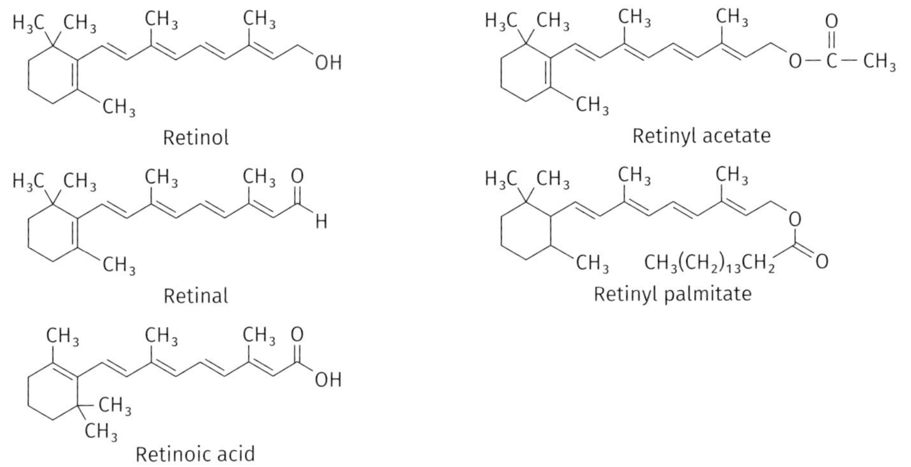

Figure 4.1 Vitamin A chemical structure of some natural and synthetic forms

estimated that, in broilers, 1 mg ß-carotene is equivalent to 393 IU vitamin A, approximately 25% of the normally accepted ratio.

Natural sources

In its active form, vitamin A is scarce in nature, as it is found predominantly as an ester only in fish oil and meat meal. Liver tissue represents the major source along with oilseeds. Green plants contain ß-carotene, the precursor of vitamin A, although the content varies greatly according to the species, state of maturity, and preservation. Maize and its derivatives contain significant quantities of pigmenting carotenoids, with much lower provitamin activity (cryptoxanthin) or not possessing provitamin activity like lutein and zeaxanthin.

The potency of yellow corn is only about one-eighth that of good roughage. There is evidence that yellow corn may lose carotene rapidly during storage. For instance, a hybrid corn high in carotene lost one-half of its carotene in 8 months of storage at 25°C (77°F) and about three-quarters in 3 years. Less carotene was lost during storage at 7°C (45°F) (Quackenbush, 1963). The bioavailability of natural β-carotene was less than chemically synthesized forms (White *et al.*, 1993). Aside from yellow corn and its by-products, practically all concentrates used in feeding animals are devoid of vitamin A value, or nearly so.

Commercial forms

The vitamin A activity contained in ingredients of typical poultry diets is very unpredictable. Therefore, the provision of vitamin A in broilers and turkeys' diets is achieved mainly through synthetic forms. The most convenient and effective means of providing vitamin A to poultry is inclusion in premixes added to feed.

The major sources of supplemental vitamin A used in animal diets are trans-retinyl acetate and trans-retinyl palmitate. The propionate ester is much less common (McGinnis, 1988). These are available in gelatin beadlet product forms for protection against oxidative destruction in premixes, mash, and pelleted and extruded feeds. Carbohydrates, gelatin, and antioxidants are generally included inside the beadlets to stabilize vitamin A to provide physical and chemical protection against factors either normally present in the feed or due to feeding treatment and storage that are destructive to vitamin A.

The vitamin A acetate products most frequently used in poultry feeds contain 500,000 and 1,000,000 IUs or United States Pharmacopeia Units (USP) per gram of product. The values of 1 IU or 1 USP are the same and equal the activity of the 0.3 µg of all-trans-retinol or 0.344 µg of all-trans-retinyl acetate, or 0.6 µg of β-carotene, that is to say, 1 mg of β-carotene is equivalent to 1,667 IU of vitamin A.

Several factors can influence the loss of vitamin A from feedstuffs during storage. The trace minerals in feeds and supplements, particularly copper, are detrimental to vitamin A stability. Dash and Mitchell (1976) reported the vitamin A content of 1,293 commercial feeds over 3 years, and the loss of vitamin A was over 50% in 1 year. Vitamin A loss in commercial feeds was evident even if the commercial feeds contained stabilized vitamin A supplements.

It is therefore important to carefully assess the quality of the commercial product. The gelatin beadlet, in which the vitamin A ester is emulsified into a gelatin-antioxidant viscous liquid formulation and spray dried into discrete dry particles, results in products with good chemical stability, physical stability, and excellent biologic availability (Shields *et al.*, 1982). The reaction between gelatin and sugar makes the beadlet insoluble in water and gives it a more resistant coating that can sustain higher pressure, friction, temperature, and humidity (Frye, 1994).

Vitamin A supplements should not be stored for prolonged periods before feedings. Chen (1990) measured the stability of 3 commercial cross-linked vitamin A beadlets on the market in trace mineral premixes and feeds. After 3 months of storage at high temperature and humidity, vitamin A retention varied from 30 to 80%, depending on the antioxidant present in the beadlet. Vitamin A (and carotene) destruction also occurs from processing feed with steam and pressure. Pelleting effects of vitamin A in the feed are determined by die thickness and hole size, which produce frictional heat and a shearing effect that can break supplemental vitamin A beadlets and expose the vitamin. In addition, steam application exposes feed to heat and moisture. In a 30% concentrate pelleted at 93°C (199°F), after 3 months of storage at high temperature and humidity, retention varied from 57 to 62%. Running fines back through the pellet mill exposes vitamin A to the same factors a second time. Between 14 and 40% of vitamin A present at mixing may be destroyed during pelleting of poultry feed (Kostadinović *et al.*, 2014; Spasevski *et al.*, 2015).

Metabolism

Absorption and transport

Dietary retinyl esters (e.g., acetate) are hydrolyzed to retinol in the intestine by pancreatic retinyl ester hydrolase, absorbed as free alcohol retinol, and then re-esterified in the mucosa, mostly to palmitate. Vitamin A and β-carotene become dispersed in micelles before absorption from the intestine. These micelles are composed of mixtures of bile salts, monoglycerides, and long-chain fatty acids, together with vitamins D, E, and K, all of which influence the transfer of vitamin A and β-carotene to the intestinal cell. Here, most of the β-carotene is converted to vitamin A, which is converted to various esters (Ross and Harrison, 2013).

The retinyl esters are transported mainly in association with lymph chylomicrons to the liver. Hydrolysis of the ester storage form mobilizes vitamin A from the liver as free retinol. Retinol is released from the hepatocyte as a complex with retinol-binding protein (RBP) and transported to peripheral tissues. Retinol, in association with RBP circulates in peripheral tissues complexed to a thyroxine-binding protein, transthyretin (Blomhoff *et al.*, 1991; Ross, 1993). The retinol-transthyretin complex is transported to target tissues, where the complex binds to a cell-surface receptor. The receptor was found in all tissues known to require retinol for their function, particularly the pigment epithelium of the eye (Wolf, 2007). Once the retinoids are transferred into the cell, they are quickly bound by specific binding proteins in the cell cytosol (Figure 4.2).

An enzyme converts β-carotene in feed to retinal in the intestinal mucosa. The retinal is then reduced to retinol (vitamin A). However, extensive evidence exists also for random (excentric) cleavage, resulting in retinoic acid and retinal, with a preponderance of apocarotenals formed as intermediates (Wolf, 1995). The main site of vitamin A and carotenoid absorption is the mucosa of the proximal jejunum. Although carotenoids are normally converted to retinol in the intestinal mucosa, they may also be converted in the liver and other organs, especially in yellow fat species such as poultry (McGinnis, 1988).

Intestinal absorption of vitamin A is calculated to be between 40 and 80%. Many factors may modify it, either positively, such as the inclusion of fats in the diet, the addition of antioxidants, and the use of moderate levels of vitamin E (Abawi *et al.*, 1985; Noel and Brinkhaus, 1998) or negatively, such as high levels of vitamin E, the presence of aflatoxins or enteric infections (West *et al.*, 1992a). Thus, coccidiosis reduces vitamin A (retinol) levels both in plasma and in the hepatic reserves, hence increasing the requirements of vitamin A because of poor absorption and oxidation induced by the cellular immune response (Augustine and Ruff, 1983; Allen, 1988, 1997; Allen *et al.*, 1996). Vitamin A deficiencies reduce resistance to coccidiosis (Chew, 1995; Dalloul *et al.*, 2002; Dalloul and Lillehoj, 2005).

Several factors affect the absorption of carotenoids. Cis-trans-isomerism of the carotenoids is important in determining their absorbability, with the transforms being more efficiently absorbed (Stahl *et al.*, 1995). Dietary fat is important in absorption (Fichter and Mitchell, 1997). Dietary antioxidants (e.g., vitamin E) also affect carotenoids' utilization and perhaps absorption. It is uncertain whether the antioxidants contribute directly to the efficient absorption or whether they protect both carotene and vitamin A from oxidative breakdown. Protein deficiency reduces the absorption of carotene in the intestine.

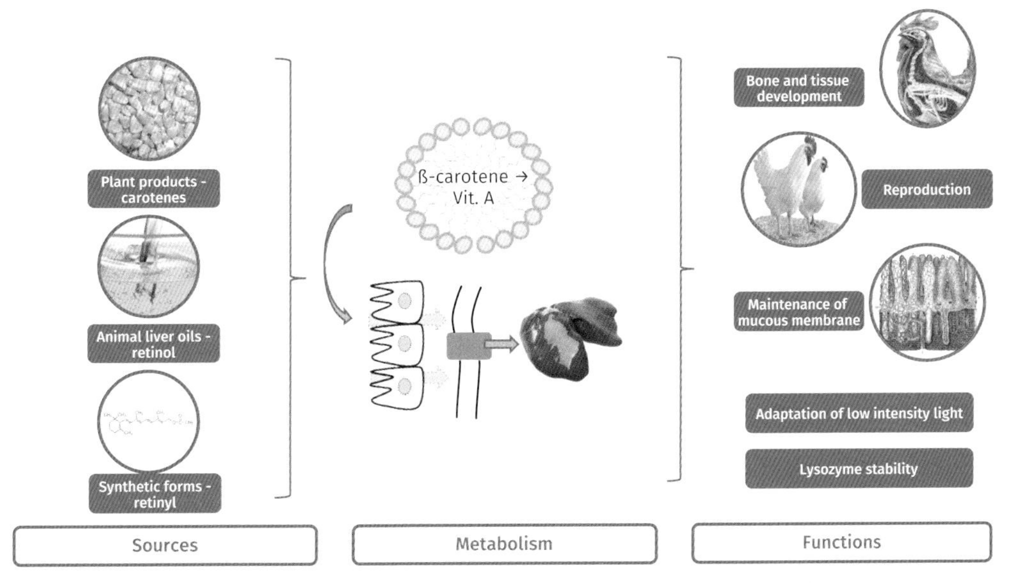

Figure 4.2 Main sources and types of the precursors of vitamin A. Schematic illustration of the absorption, the purpose of the metabolites, and the main functions developed

The intracellular retinoid-binding proteins bind retinol, retinal, and retinoic acid to protect against decomposition, solubilize them in an aqueous medium, render them nontoxic, and transport them within cells to their site of action (Ross and Harrison, 2013). These binding proteins also function by presenting the retinoids to the appropriate enzymes for metabolism (Wolf, 1991, 1993). Some of the principal forms of intracellular (cytoplasmic) retinoid-binding proteins are cellular retinol-binding proteins (CRBP, I and II), cellular retinoic acid-binding proteins (CRABP, I and II), cellular retinaldehyde binding protein (CRALBP), and 6 nuclear retinoic acid receptors (RAR and retinoid X receptor [RXR], with alpha, beta and gamma forms). There are 2 classes of nuclear receptors with all-trans-retinoic acid, the ligand for RAR; 9-cis-retinoic acid is the ligand for RXR (Kasner *et al.*, 1994; Kliewer *et al.*, 1992). Retinol is readily transferred to the egg in birds.

The color of the avian products is a valuable aspect for the consumer. Pigmenting carotenoids are mainly hydroxy carotenoids, e.g., lutein and zeaxanthin, that have no vitamin A activity; they are transferred unchanged to the yolk or the skin resulting in the yellow color of the carcass and eggs. The carotenoid commonly used in laying hen diets, canthaxanthin, is deposited in the yolk at a linearly related level to the diet level (Grashorn and Steinberg, 2002). Other carotenoids that have been considered for inclusion in eggs include lycopene (Kang *et al.*, 2003). In poultry, a single yolk may contain 40–45% of the total carotenoids found in the liver (Surai *et al.*, 1999a; Surai and Speake, 2000), which is the main site of carotenoid accumulation (Surai *et al.*, 2001), and consequently, more than 50% of total carotenoid reserves in the body are in the ovary (Nys, 2000). Carotenoids are also important during the chicken's embryonic development (Klasing, 1998; McDowell, 2004). Finally, vitamin A contributes to maintaining lysozyme stability inside the cells.

Storage and excretion

The liver normally contains about 90% of the total body vitamin A. The remainder is stored in the kidneys, lungs, adrenals, and blood, with small amounts found in other organs and tissues. Several studies have shown that the liver can store enough vitamin A to protect the animal from long periods of dietary scarcity. This large storage capacity must be considered in studies of vitamin A requirements to ensure that intakes that appear adequate for a given function are not being supplemented by reserves stored before the observation period.

Hepatic reserves of vitamin A are usually enough to maintain the production of several eggs with adequate concentrations of this vitamin. In this case, the dietary supply is important during the pre-laying phase to achieve a good reserve level in the hen to deposit during early egg production (Squires and Naber, 1993a). The main excretory pathway for vitamin A eliminates glucuronide conjugates in the bile before fecal excretion.

Biochemical functions

Vitamin A is necessary to support growth, health, and life in all major animal species including poultry (Nabi *et al.*, 2020). Without vitamin A, animals will cease to grow and eventually die. Vitamin A and its derivatives, the retinoids, profoundly influence organ development, cell proliferation, and cell differentiation, and their deficiency originates or predisposes several disabilities (McDowell, 2000a; Esteban-Pretel *et al.*, 2010). During embryogenesis, retinoic acid has been shown to influence processes governing the patterning of neural tissue and craniofacial, eye, and olfactory system development; retinoic acid affects the outcome, regeneration, and well-being of neurons (Asson-Batres *et al.*, 2009; Nabi *et al.*, 2020).

Recent discoveries have revealed that most, if not all, actions of vitamin A in development, differentiation, and metabolism are mediated by nuclear receptor proteins that bind retinoic acid, the active form of vitamin A (Iskakova *et al.*, 2015). A group of retinoic acid-binding proteins (receptors) function in the nucleus by attaching to promoter regions in several specific genes to stimulate their transcription and thus affect growth, development, and differentiation. RAR in cell nuclei are structurally homologous and functionally analogous to the known receptors for steroid hormones, thyroid hormone (triiodothyronine), and vitamin D 1,25 dihydroxy cholecalciferol [1,25$(OH)_2D_3$]. Thus, retinoic acid is now recognized as a hormone regulating many genes' transcription activity (Ross, 1993; Shin and McGrane, 1997; Nabi *et al.*, 2020).

Vision

Retinol is utilized in the aldehyde form (trans-form to 11-cis-retinal) in the retina of the eye as the prosthetic group in rhodopsin for dim light vision (rods) and as the prosthetic group in iodopsin for bright light and color vision (cones). Rhodopsin is important for sight, especially in poultry adapting to low-intensity light in intensive production. Retinoic acid has been found to support growth and tissue differentiation but not vision or reproduction (McDowell, 2000a; Solomons, 2006; Nabi *et al.*, 2020).

Tissue differentiation

Retinoic acid regulates the differentiation of epithelial, connective, and hematopoietic tissues (Safonova *et al.*, 1994). The growth and differentiation response elicited by retinoic acid depends upon cell type. Retinoic acid can be an inhibitor of many cell types, potentially reducing adipose tissues in meat-producing animals (Suryawan and Hu, 1997). Proliferation and cellular aggregation are both critical features for the survival and self-renewal of primordial germ cells (PGCs). With growing chicks, retinoic acid promoted PGCs proliferation and increased intercellular aggregation of PGCs (Yu *et al.*, 2011). Vitamin A-deficient rats fed retinoic acid were healthy in every respect, with normal estrus and conception, but failed to give birth and resorbed their fetuses. When retinol was given even at a late stage in pregnancy, fetuses were saved. Male rats on retinoic acid were healthy but produced no sperm, and without vitamin A both sexes were blind (Anonymous, 1977).

Keratinization of epithelial tissues results in loss of function in the alimentary, genital, reproductive, respiratory, and urinary tracts. Such altered characteristics increase the susceptibility of the affected tissue to infection. Thus, diarrhea and pneumonia are typical secondary effects of vitamin A deficiency.

Immunity

Adequate dietary vitamin A is necessary to help maintain normal resistance to stress and disease. Disease resistance is a function of vitamin A, with the vitamin needed to maintain mucous membranes and the normal function of the adrenal gland (Nabi *et al.*, 2020). Vitamin A deficiency can impair the regeneration of normal mucosal epithelium damaged by infection or inflammation (Ahmed *et al.*, 1990; Stephensen *et al.*, 1996) and thus could increase the severity of an infectious episode and prolong recovery from that episode. An animal's ability to resist infectious disease depends on a responsive immune system; a vitamin A deficiency causes a reduced immune response. In many experiments with laboratory and domestic animals, the effects of both clinical and subclinical deficiencies of vitamin A on the production of antibodies and the resistance of different tissues against microbial infection or parasitic infestation have frequently been demonstrated (Kelley and Easter, 1987; Lessard *et al.*, 1997). Supplemental vitamin A improved the health of animals infected with roundworms and of hens infected with the genus *Capillaria* (Herrick, 1972).

Bone development

Vitamin A plays a role in normal bone development by controlling the activity of osteoclasts of the epithelial cartilage, the cells responsible for bone resorption. In vitamin A deficiency, the activity of osteoclasts is reduced with excessive deposition of periosteal bone due to stimulation of osteoblasts (depositing bone cells) and joint irritation.

Nutritional assessment

Retinol and its fatty acid esters are the compounds relevant for the determination of vitamin A status. Plasma retinol has been used as a general indicator of vitamin A status primarily for determining a vitamin A deficiency defined in humans as a plasma retinol level <0.7 µmol/l or 196 µg/l (Höller *et al.*, 2018). In poultry, a retinol plasma level <1–1.1 µmol/l or 300 µg/l can be considered a deficiency threshold level. However, plasma level is not a good indicator since the plasma concentration is under strict homeostatic control (Tanumihardjo, 2011) and can be influenced by health status, e.g., depression in case of infection or inflammation (Tanumihardjo *et al.*, 2016). As an example, Feng *et al.* (2019) carried out a dose–response experiment with 8 supplemental vitamin A levels (0; 500; 1,000; 1,500; 2,500; 3,500; 7,000, and 14,000 IU/kg) to examine the effects of vitamin A on growth performance and tissue retinol of starter White Pekin ducks. As supplemental vitamin A increased, weight gain and feed intake increased quadratically ($P < 0.05$), and plasma and liver retinol increased linearly or quadratically ($P < 0.05$). In the case of plasma, ducks fed the basal diet with no supplemental vitamin A had 64 µg retinol/l plasma, and the plasma retinol went beyond 300 µg/l when 2,500 IU/kg or above vitamin A was supplemented to basal diets. It reached a plateau when supplemental vitamin A was above 3,500 IU/kg. More precisely at 2,500, 3,500, 7,000, and 14,000 IU/kg plasma retinol was 332, 427, 503, and 572 µg/l.

A more precise assessment of vitamin A status can be achieved by measuring total body stores via biopsies of tissues, like the liver, or using isotope dilution techniques. In blood and tissues, retinol can be determined using reversed-phase high-performance liquid chromatography (HPLC). In the same experiment, Feng *et al.* (2019) showed that liver retinol at the same dosages previously reported were 92, 216, 1,272, and 3,852 µg/g, indicating a linear increase not yet reached a plateau at the highest dosage.

Retinol can be measured using dried blood spots (DBS), providing small blood samples can be collected under field conditions with limited infrastructure. Stability issues have limited the widespread practical application. Still, some improvements have been made, indicating its validity for assessing a low retinol (or a high) status and not a broader evaluation of its nutritional status (Gannon *et al.*, 2020).

The provitamin A carotenoids and especially β-carotene could be used as an indirect measurement of vitamin A status by considering, as discussed in previous paragraphs, that the biological activity of these compounds relative to retinol is estimated to be in the order of 50% for β-carotene and 25% for carotenoids with only one β-ionone end group. Carotenoids are mainly assessed from plasma using HPLC coupled to visible spectrophotometry.

Deficiency signs

Factors causing vitamin A deficiency

Vitamin A deficiency is unlikely in practice (Kidd, 2004), and marginal deficiencies may result when working with minimum levels in feed (Bains, 1997). Under stressful conditions, such as abnormal temperatures or exposure to disease conditions, requirements are higher, as is the probability of deficiency. In poultry, deficiency signs appear quite rapidly, within 2 to 3 weeks.

The efficiency of conversion of ß-carotene to vitamin A is also reduced in situations of stress and illness or due to mycotoxins. Mycotoxins are known to cause digestive disturbances such as vomiting, diarrhea, and internal bleeding. They can also interfere with the absorption of dietary vitamins A, D_3, E, and K (McDowell and Ward, 2008). For example, poultry coccidiosis destroys vitamin A in the gut and injures the microvilli of the intestinal wall.

In chicks, gross signs of vitamin A deficiency are characterized by:

- anorexia
- cessation of growth
- drowsiness
- weakness
- incoordination
- emaciation
- ruffled plumage.

A stratified squamous, keratinizing epithelium replaces the mucous epithelium. The mucous membranes of the nasal passage, mouth, esophagus, and pharynx are affected and develop white pustules (Scott *et al.*, 1982). The kidneys may be distended with uric acid deposits and the epithelium of the eye is affected, producing exudates and eventually xerophthalmia (Figure 4.3).

A severe deficiency will produce ataxia and result in death if not corrected (Hill *et al.*, 1961). Nockels (1988) reported that hypothyroidism is an early indication of vitamin A deficiency in chicks. As vitamin A deficiency progresses in adult poultry, they become emaciated and weak, and their feathers are ruffled. A marked decrease in egg production occurs, and the length of time between clutches increases greatly. Vitamin A deficiency causes at least 5 different and probably physiologically distinct lesions:

- loss of vision due to a failure of rhodopsin formation in the retina
- defects in growth and differentiation of epithelial tissues (frequently resulting in keratinization)
- impairment of immune function
- defects in bone growth

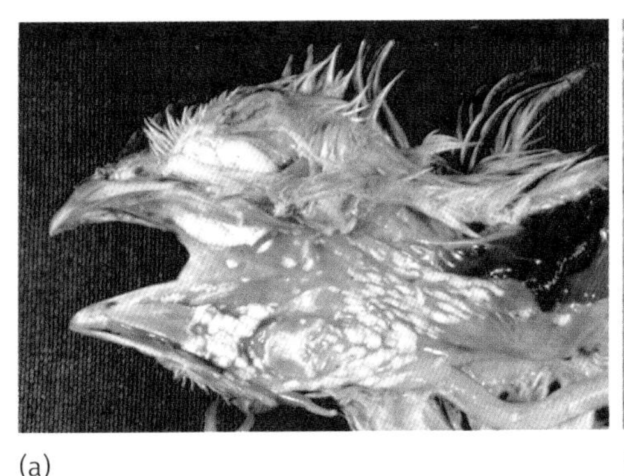

(a)

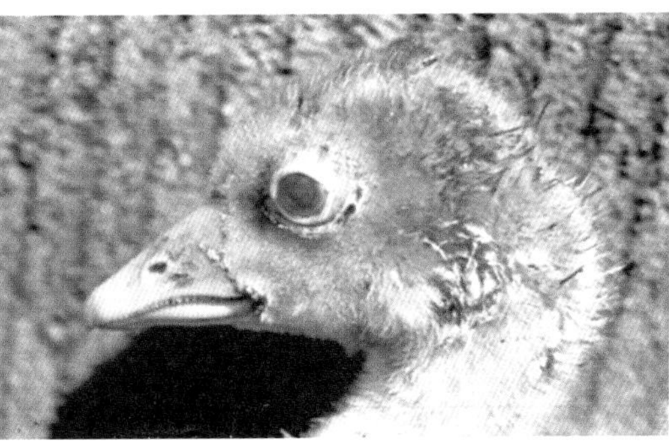

(b)

Figure 4.3 Vitamin A deficiency: (a) hyperkeratosis of the mucous membranes of mouth and esophagus; (b) severe hyperkeratosis of the corneal epithelium in a gosling (source: copyright UK Crown)

- defects in reproduction (i.e., failure of spermatogenesis in the male and resorption of the fetus in the female).

Epithelial tissue disorders

Since the 1930s, vitamin A supplementation has been used to protect the epithelial tissues and mucous membranes, which are natural barriers against pathogens and prevent infections (Latshaw, 1991; Dalloul and Lillehoj, 2005; Eggersdorfer *et al.*, 2012). Severe vitamin A deficiency causes increased intestinal mucosal cell numbers (hyperplasia), reduced intestinal mucosal cell size, the loss of mucosal protein, reduced villus height, and crypt depth, and diminished activities of gut disaccharidases, transpeptidase and alkaline phosphatase (Uni *et al.*, 1998).

There is a breakdown of the epithelium of many systems in the body due to a vitamin A deficiency. Loss of membrane integrity, in turn, alters water retention (López *et al.*, 1973) and impairs the ability to withstand infection (Sijtsma *et al.*, 1989). Bacteria and other pathogenic microorganisms may enter the body and invade tissues, producing infections secondary to original vitamin A deficiency signs.

Impairment of the immune function

Low dietary vitamin A has been shown to cause reduced antibody production, depressed T-cell responses, distributed immunoglobulin metabolism, reduced phagocytosis, and decreased resistance to infection by bacterial and viral pathogens and protozoan enteropathogens (Davis and Sell, 1989; Friedman and Sklan, 1997; Lessard *et al.*, 1997).

Vitamin A deficiency affects the immune function related to the antibody response to T-cell-dependent antigens (Ross, 1992; Nabi *et al.*, 2020). The RAR-alpha mRNA expression and antigen-specific proliferative responses to T-lymphocytes are influenced by vitamin A status *in vivo* and directly modulated by retinoic acid (Halevy *et al.*, 1994). Vitamin A deficiency affects several immune system cells, and repletion with retinoic acid effectively re-establishes the number of circulating lymphocytes (Zhao and Ross, 1995).

A diminished primary antibody response could also increase the severity and duration of an episode of infection. In contrast, a diminished secondary response could increase the risk of developing a second episode of infection. Vitamin A deficiency causes decreased phagocytic activity in macrophages and neutrophils. The secretory immunoglobulin A (IgA) system is an important first line of defense against infections of mucosal surfaces (McGhee *et al.*, 1992). Several studies in animal models have shown that the intestinal IgA response is impaired by vitamin A deficiency (Wiedermann *et al.*, 1993; Stephensen *et al.*, 1996).

Vitamin A is needed for the proper functioning of important lymphoid organs such as the thymus and bursa of Fabricius and modifies leukocyte response, in particular of the CD4+T-cells (Halevy *et al.*, 1994), that is impaired in cases of deficiency (Sklan *et al.*, 1994, 1995; Chew, 1995; Dalloul *et al.*, 2002; Chew and Park, 2004; Klasing, 2007). This has been confirmed by studies with chickens and turkeys using various pathogenic agents (Davis and Sell, 1989; Sijtsma *et al.*, 1990, 1991; Friedman *et al.*, 1991; Chew, 1995; Dalloul *et al.*, 2000; Nabi *et al.*, 2020). Inadequate vitamin A also reduces the immune system's response to challenges and contributes to disease susceptibility (Davis and Sell, 1989). Many experiments have revealed that increased morbidity is observed in chickens experimentally infected with Newcastle disease virus and fed a diet marginally deficient in vitamin A (Sijtsma *et al.*, 1989; Lin *et al.*, 2002). Vitamin A requirements for immunity can be 3 to 10 times greater than that recommended by the NRC (1994) for chickens (Friedman and Sklan, 1989, 1997; Halevy *et al.*, 1994; Lessard *et al.*, 1997).

Viral infections have been found to impair the vitamin A status of chickens (West *et al.*, 1992a). In poultry, carotenoids can directly affect gene expression. This mechanism may enable carotenoids to modulate the interaction between B-cells and T-cells, thus regulating humoral and cell-mediated immunity (Koutsos, 2003; Nabi *et al.*, 2020). A lack of carotenoids was reported to increase parameters of systemic inflammation in growing chicks (Koutsos *et al.*, 2006).

Defects in bone growth

Vitamin A deficiency can cause alterations in bone growth, which creates several areas of compression in the central nervous system with loss of mobility (Howell and Thompson, 1967). Vitamin A deficiency in poultry may act directly on the growth plate in bone development and may also indirectly affect growth by systemic mechanisms. For example, vitamin A appears to be required for growth hormone secretion and thyroid hormone secretion and action (DeLuca *et al.*, 2000).

Defects in reproduction

Vitamin A can be important to the protection of the vascular endothelium of the ovary. Squires and Naber (1993b) report a large incidence of blood spots in eggs from a vitamin A-deficient dietary treatment, which agrees with the results reported by Bearse *et al.* (1960). Gross and histologic examination of the reproductive tract of deficient hens verifies that the ovary is structurally changed by vitamin A deficiency (Bermudez *et al.*, 1993). Hens fed a vitamin A-deficient diet had increased atresic follicles on the ovary, and these follicles had moderate to severe hemorrhage (Bermudez *et al.*, 1993).

In contrast, hens with low egg production rates fed a vitamin A-supplemented diet did not have hemorrhaged ovarian follicles. Conversely, Squires and Naber (1993b) reported that hens fed vitamin A-deficient diets continued to produce eggs through 12 weeks of lay, presumably due to mobilization of liver stores of the vitamin. After this time, the vitamin A content of the yolks of the few eggs produced was similar to the yolk vitamin A content of supplemented hens. Yolk vitamin A content is thus a poor indicator of flock vitamin A status.

Among the first symptoms of vitamin A deficiency to appear is the decrease in sexual activity in males and failure of spermatogenesis, accompanied by a reduction in fertility and the number of hatched eggs. Breeder cocks need to receive sufficient vitamins to support high sexual activity during the breeding period. They usually copulate 20 to 30 times a day, which makes a high rate of sperm synthesis necessary. Supplies of vitamin A above requirements permit an adequate growth rate in breeder males, with an optimum development of the organs and systems involved in reproduction (Damjanov *et al.*, 1980). Reductions in testis size, circulating testosterone, and fertility have been reported during vitamin A deficiency in cockerels (Damjanov *et al.*, 1980). The level of carotenoids to which a developing embryo is exposed affects the subsequent deposition of dietary carotenoids in the tissue of the post-hatch chick. Chicks hatched from carotenoid-depleted eggs will have a compromised immune function. Koutsos *et al.* (2006) reported that chicks from carotenoid-depleted eggs without carotenoid exposure post-hatch increased systemic inflammation parameters.

Hatchability is decreased, and there is an increase in embryonic mortality in eggs from affected birds. A watery discharge from the nostrils and eyes is noted, and eyelids are often stuck together. When day-old chicks are given a vitamin A-free diet, clinical signs may appear at the end of the first week if the chicks are the progeny of hens receiving a diet low in vitamin A. When chicks are the progeny of hens receiving high levels of vitamin A, signs of deficiency may not appear until chicks are 6 or 7 weeks of age, even though they are receiving a diet completely devoid of vitamin A (Scott *et al.*, 1982; West *et al.*, 1992b).

Average survival times of the progeny fed a vitamin A-free diet increased linearly with increasing levels of vitamin A in the maternal turkey diet (Jensen, 1965). The vitamin A level of the hen's diet is positively correlated with the growth of chicks and poults from that hen, and the level of vitamin A in the chick's and poult's diet is positively associated with development.

Safety

In general, the possibility of vitamin A toxicity for poultry is remote. However, vitamins A and D_3 have the greatest chance of being provided in toxic concentrations to poultry. Excess vitamin A has been demonstrated to have harmful effects in most species studied. Presumed safe upper levels are 4 to 10 times the nutritional requirements for poultry and other monogastric (NRC, 1994).

Most of the harmful effects have been obtained by feeding over 100 times the daily requirements for 5 to 6 weeks or more. Thus, small excesses of vitamin A should not be dangerous for short periods. The clinical signs of vitamin A toxicity in poultry include (Scott *et al.*, 1982):

- weight loss
- decreased feed intake
- swelling and crusting of the eyelids to the extent that they become sealed closed
- inflammation of the mouth, adjacent skin, and skin of the feet
- decreased bone strength
- bone abnormalities
- mortality.

Skin lesions at the commissure of the beak, nose, and eyes attributable to mucous membrane hyperplastic activity have been shown to occur in chicks within 72 hours after oral dosing with 60,000 IU of vitamin A (Kriz and Holman, 1969). The release of lysosomal enzymes is believed to be responsible for degradative changes observed in tissues and intact animals suffering from hypervitaminosis A (Fell and Thomas, 1960). In hypervitaminosis A, retinol penetrates the lipid of the membrane and causes it to expand. Because the protein of the membrane is relatively inelastic, the membrane is weakened. Thus, many phenomena in hypervitaminosis can be explained in terms of membrane damage, either in cells or organelles within cells.

Excess vitamin A (10 and 20 g/ml) in a culture medium from broiler chickens showed a down-regulation of alkaline phosphate activity and calcium-binding protein mRNA expression of osteoblasts (Guo *et al.*, 2010). Excess vitamin A affects the metabolism of other fat-soluble vitamins via competition for absorption and transport. Therefore, in diets containing barely adequate levels of vitamins D_3, E, and K, a marked increase in dietary vitamin A in the range of 4, or more, times the recommended dose may cause decreases in growth or egg production due to a deficiency of one or more of the other fat-soluble vitamins rather than a toxic effect of vitamin A.

Dietary vitamin A levels above 20,000 IU/kg impede the utilization of vitamin D_3 in broilers fed with low levels (500 IU/kg) of supplemental vitamin D_3 (Aburto and Britton, 1998a,b). In the presence of low levels of vitamin D_3, the addition of vitamin A reduced body weight and bone ash and resulted in rickets. The supplementation of practical levels of vitamin D_3 (2,000–3,000 IU/kg diet) seems to have prevented much of the body weight depression, produced maximum bone ash and controlled the incidence and severity of rickets.

In another study, Aburto *et al.* (1998) confirmed that high dietary vitamin A (45,000 IU/kg) interferes with the utilization of vitamin D_3 and the vitamin D metabolites 25 hidroxycholecalciferol ($25OHD_3$) and $1,25(OH)_2D_3$, increasing the requirement for each of them.

Moreover, 45,000 IU/kg of dietary vitamin A ameliorated the potentially toxic effects of feeding high levels of vitamin D_3, 25OHD_3, and 1,25$(OH)_2D_3$ to young broiler chickens.

A marked increase in dietary vitamin A has been shown to interfere with the absorption of carotenoids, resulting in decreased poultry pigmentation. Excessive doses of vitamin A to the laying hen result in an adverse effect on vitamin E, carotenoids, and ascorbic acid in the embryonic/neonatal liver and can compromise the antioxidant status of the progeny (Surai *et al.*, 1998a; Grobas *et al.*, 2002).

High dietary vitamin A (40,000 IU/kg) in hen diets significantly lowered egg yolk vitamin E (Grobas *et al.*, 2002). Excess vitamin A (28,000 and 56,000 IU/kg) given to chicks during early postnatal development was associated with inhibiting vitamin E and carotenoid utilization (Surai and Kuklenko, 2000). It was concluded that the effect of vitamin A on the development of the neonatal chick's antioxidant system is dose-dependent and that an excess of vitamin A can compromise the antioxidant defense system. Conversely, high dietary levels of vitamin E or D_3 have been shown to protect the chick from vitamin A toxicosis.

The route of administration of vitamin A influences the toxicity of the vitamin. In chicks and poults, levels of vitamin A that caused adverse changes in body weight, packed cell volume, serum calcium or phosphorus, or bone ash were 100 times the NRC requirement when birds were fed *ad libitum*, but only 10 times the NRC level when birds were fed via force-feeding.

Vitamin D

Chemical structure and properties

The term vitamin D covers a group of closely related compounds possessing antirachitic activity. Provitamin D_2 ergosterol is a sterol found in fungi and yeasts, which undergoes a photochemical reaction caused by ultraviolet (UV) radiation from sunlight to form vitamin D_2 or ergocalciferol. Vitamin D_3 or cholecalciferol is produced only in animals via UV radiation of provitamin D_3 or 7-dehydrocholesterol present in the skin. The provitamin 7-dehydrocholesterol, derived from cholesterol or squalene, is synthesized in the body and present in large amounts in the skin, the intestinal wall, and other tissues. Sterols with vitamin D activity have a common steroid nucleus and differ like the lateral chain attached to carbon 17 (Figure 4.4). Vitamin D precursors have no antirachitic activity.

It is assumed that in birds vitamin D_2 has only 10% of the biological activity of vitamin D_3 (Zheng and Teegarden, 2013; DeLuca, 2014; Combs and McClung, 2022). Four important variables

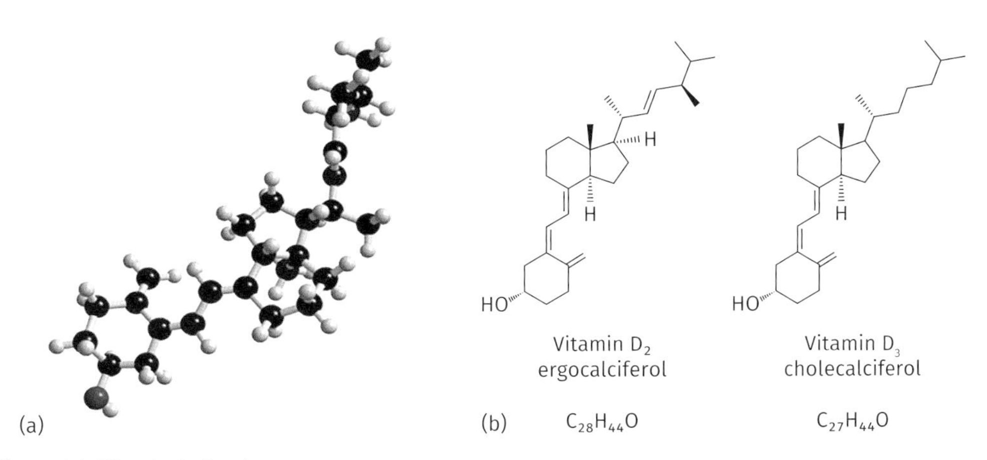

Figure 4.4 Vitamin D structure

selectively determine the amount of vitamin D_3 that will be photochemically produced by skin exposure to sunlight (Norman and Henry, 2007). The 2 principal determinants are the quantity and intensity of UV and the appropriate wavelength of the UV light. The third important variable determining skin vitamin D synthesis is the concentration of 7-dehydrocholesterol present in the skin. The fourth determinant of vitamin D_3 production is the concentration of melanin in the skin (skin color). The darker the skin, the longer time required to convert 7-dehydrocholesterol to vitamin D_3 (Zheng and Teegarden, 2013; Combs and McClung, 2022).

The provitamin 7-dehydrocholesterol is a lipid secreted by the uropygial gland and is present in feathers (Edwards, 2000), the skin's epidermis, and sebaceous secretions. For poultry, Tian *et al.* (1994) reported that the skin of the legs and feet of chickens contains about 30 times as much 7-dehydrocholesterol (provitamin D_3) as the body skin. Birds can obtain vitamin D_3 in quantities equivalent to 20–40 µg/kg through the action of sunlight on 7-dehydrocholesterol. This mechanism is of little significance when animals are kept indoors, so vitamin D_3 must be provided in the feed. Heuser and Norris (1929) showed that 11–45 minutes of sunshine daily were sufficient to prevent rickets in growing chicks. No further improvements in growth were obtained under these conditions by adding cod liver oil (a rich source of vitamin D).

Natural sources

Besides fish oil and meal, vitamin D_3 is scarce in feed ingredients, so supplementation is required. In the great majority of tables comprising the nutritional value of feedstuffs, the vitamin D content is calculated based on the equivalent bioactivity of vitamin D_2 plus D_3. However, vitamin D_2 is a poor source of vitamin D for birds due to its low bioavailability.

Vitamin D occurs as colorless crystals that are insoluble in water but readily soluble in alcohol and other organic solvents in the pure form. Like vitamins A and E, oxidation destroys them unless vitamin D_3 is stabilized. Its oxidative destruction is increased by heat, moisture, over-treatment with UV light, by peroxidation in the presence of rancidifying PUFA and trace minerals. There is less vitamin D_3 in freeze-dried fish meals during drying, possibly because of decreased atmospheric oxygen. There is negligible loss of crystalline cholecalciferol during storage for 1 year or crystalline ergocalciferol for 9 months in amber-evacuated capsules at refrigerator temperatures (Zheng and Teegarden, 2013; Combs and McClung, 2022).

Commercial forms

The majority of vitamin D_3 used to fortify animal feeds is in the form of a spray-dried formulation containing 500,000 IU/g. A combination of vitamin A and D_3, usually in a 5: 1 ratio – i.e., vitamin A 1,000,000 IU/g and vitamin D_3 200,000 IU/g – is also used in feed fortification.

For more than 20 years also, the first metabolite $25OHD_3$ has been largely used as a feed additive (tradename Rovimix® HyD) in spray-dried form (Soares *et al.*, 1995; Ward, 1995). A form of calcitriol as $1,25(OH)_2D_3$ glycoside is also available as feed material. This metabolite is extracted from the plant *Solanum glaucophyllum* (Bachmann *et al.*, 2013). Finally, 1-alpha-hydroxycholecalciferol or 1-alpha-hydroxyvitamin D_3 ($1\alpha OHD_3$), also called alfacalcidol is a is a non-endogenous analogue of vitamin D This molecule can be chemically synthesized by replacing the hydrogen at the 1alpha position with a hydroxy group (Edwards, 1989; Rennie *et al.*, 1993; Combs and McClung, 2022).

Metabolism

Absorption, conversion to active forms, and transport

Vitamin D is absorbed from the intestinal tract in association with fats, as are all the fat-soluble vitamins. Like the others, it requires the presence of bile salts for absorption (Braun, 1986) and is absorbed with other neutral lipids via chylomicron. On average, only 50% of an oral dose of vitamin D is absorbed. However, considering sufficient vitamin D is usually produced by daily exposure to sunlight, it is not surprising that the body has not evolved a more efficient mechanism for dietary vitamin D absorption. Effective treatment of rickets by rubbing cod liver oil on the skin indicates that vitamin D can also be absorbed through the skin (Deluca, 2014).

Vitamin D from the diet is absorbed into the portal circulation from the intestinal tract by passive diffusion and is more likely to be absorbed in the greatest amounts from the ileal portion due to the longer retention time of food in the distal portion of the intestine (Zheng and Teegarden, 2013; DeLuca, 2014; Combs and McClung, 2022; Maurya and Aggarwal, 2017; Swiatkiewicz *et al.*, 2017). Like other steroids, vitamin D and its metabolites circulate in the plasma, bound to the vitamin D-binding protein (VBP or DBP).

By itself, vitamin D is biologically inactive and must be converted to the active form through 2 hydroxylations. The first hydroxylation is catalyzed by the hepatic microsomal enzyme of the cytochrome P450 (CYP) family 25-hydroxylase (CYP2R1 and CYP27A1) with the transformation of cholecalciferol to 25-hydroxycholecalciferol [$25OHD_3$, or calcidiol or calcifediol] which is the circulating and storage form of vitamin D. This conversion step is not metabolically regulated.

$25OHD_3$ is then transported to the kidney, on the VBP, where it can be converted, in the proximal convoluted cells, to a variety of compounds, of which the most important is 1,25-dihydroxycholecalciferol [$1,25(OH)_2D_3$ or calcitriol] by the action of 1α-hydroxylase CYP27B1 (DeLuca, 2008, 2014;). Vitamin C is involved in this stage.

Subsequently, the $1,25(OH)_2D_3$ is transported to the intestine, the bones, or another part of the kidney, which participates in calcium and phosphorus metabolism (Figure 4.5). VBP has the greatest affinity for $25OHD_3$, the main circulating form, then for cholecalciferol, and finally for $1,25(OH)_2D_3$. Another important enzyme is the renal 24-hydroxylase (CYP24A1), catalyzing the first step of its inactivation, from $25OHD_3$ to $24,25\text{-}(OH)_2\text{-}D_3$. The physiological role of this metabolite is less clear: it is considered one of the main metabolites destined for excretion. However, some research (Seo *et al.*, 1998) has identified a potential role in bone mineralization.

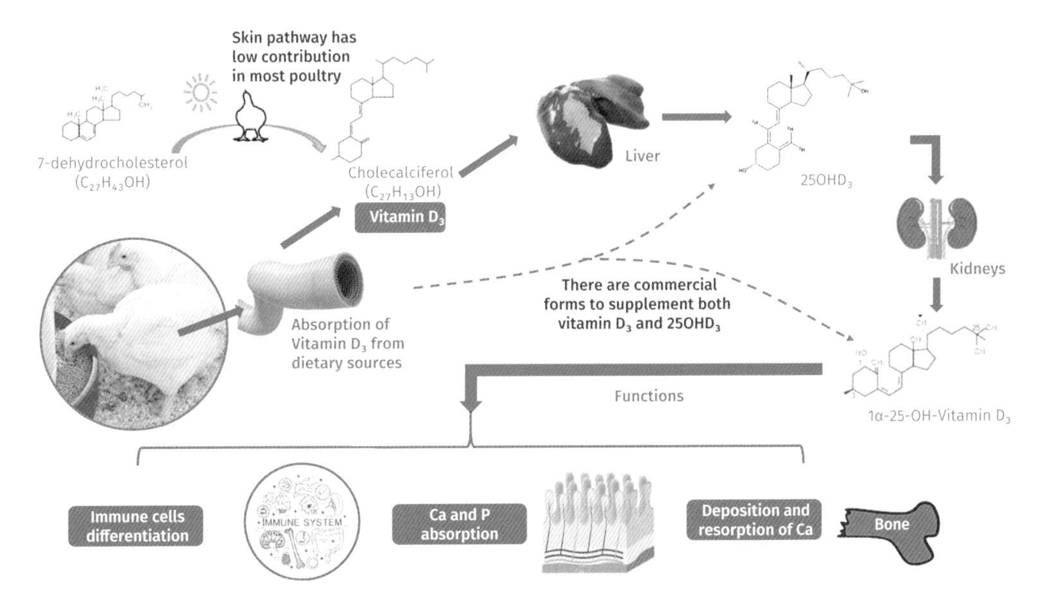

Figure 4.5 Vitamin D metabolism

Although the kidney is the main site of 1-α-hydroxylation, other cells and organs like intestinal cells, immune cells, endothelial cells, brain, mammary glands, pancreatic islets, parathyroid glands, placenta, prostate, and skin express active 1α-hydroxylase (Johnson and Kimlin, 2006; DeLuca, 2008; Shanmugasundaram and Selvaraj, 2012). 1,25$(OH)_2D_3$ acts metabolically as a hormone. Under conditions of calcium stress, parathyroid hormone (PTH) activates renal mitochondrial 1α-hydroxylase, which converts 25OHD_3 to 1,25$(OH)_2D_3$, and inactivates renal and extrarenal 24- and 23-hydroxylases (Goff *et al.*, 1991).

Under conditions with little calcium stress (when little PTH is secreted), the 1-α-hydroxylase can also be directly stimulated by low blood calcium or phosphorus concentration. High plasma 1,25$(OH)_2D_3$ concentration has an inhibitory effect on renal 1-α-hydroxylase and a stimulatory effect on tissue 24-hydroxylase (Engstrom *et al.*, 1987). Thus, the production and catabolism of the hormone 1,25$(OH)_2D_3$ are tightly regulated. It is now known that the most important point of regulation of the vitamin D endocrine system occurs through stringent control of the renal 1-α-hydroxylase activity. In this way, the production of the hormone 1,25$(OH)_2D_3$ can be modulated according to the calcium needs of the organism (Zheng and Teegarden, 2013; DeLuca, 2014).

Storage and excretion

In contrast to aquatic species, which store significant amounts of vitamin D in the liver, land animals do not store appreciable amounts of the vitamin. The body can store vitamin D, although to a much lesser extent than vitamin A, and the principal stores of vitamin D occur in skin, fat, and blood, primarily as 25OHD_3, egg yolk, and liver. It is also found in the lungs, kidneys, and elsewhere in the body.

During times of deprivation, vitamin D is released slowly, especially in skin and adipose, thus meeting the vitamin D needs of the animal over a longer period (Norman and Henry, 2007). The vitamin D_3 level in the hen's diet positively correlates with vitamin D_3 and 25OHD_3 contents within the egg yolk (Mattila *et al.*, 1999). The excretion of absorbed vitamin D and its metabolites occurs primarily in feces with the aid of bile salts (Zheng and Teegarden, 2013; DeLuca, 2014).

Biochemical functions

Classical functions

The classical function of vitamin D is to regulate the absorption, transport, deposition, and mobilization of calcium. The active form is 1,25$(OH)_2D_3$, which acts, together with PTH and calcitonin, similarly to steroid hormones. PTH and calcitonin function in a delicate relationship with 1,25$(OH)_2D_3$ to control blood calcium and phosphorus levels (Engstrom and Littledike, 1986). The production rate of 1,25$(OH)_2D_3$ is under physiological control. When blood calcium is below the normal range, PTH upregulates the production of calcitriol, elevating plasma calcium and phosphorus by stimulating specific ion pump mechanisms in the intestine, bone, and kidney.

These 3 sources of calcium and phosphorus provide reservoirs that enable vitamin D to elevate calcium and phosphorus in blood to levels necessary for normal bone mineralization and other functions ascribed to calcium. Contrary to the other 2, calcitonin regulates high serum calcium levels by depressing gut absorption, halting bone demineralization, and depressing reabsorption in the kidney.

The hormone enters the cell in the target tissue and binds to a cytosolic receptor or a nuclear receptor. 1,25$(OH)_2D_3$ regulates gene expression by binding to tissue-specific receptors and subsequent interaction between the bound receptor and the DNA (Norman, 2006). The receptor-hormone complex moves to the nucleus. It attaches to the chromatin and stimulates the transcription of particular genes to produce specific mRNAs, which code for synthesizing particular proteins. Evidence for transcription regulation of a specific gene typically includes

$1,25(OH)_2D_3$-induced modulation in mRNA levels. Additionally, evidence may consist of measurements of transcription and a vitamin D responsive element within the promoter region of the gene (Hannah and Norman, 1994).

Recent studies have identified a heterodimer of the vitamin D receptor (VDR) and a vitamin A receptor (RXR) within the nucleus of the cell as the active complex for mediating positive transcriptional effects of $1,25(OH)_2D_3$. This classical function is driven by the effects of vitamin D at intestinal, bone, and kidney levels. The 2 receptors (vitamins D and A) selectively interact with specific hormone response elements composed of direct repeats of specific nucleotides located in the promoter of regulated genes. The complex that binds to these elements consists of 3 distinct elements: the $1,25(OH)_2D_3$ hormonal ligand, the VDR, and one of the vitamins A (retinoid) X receptors (RXR) (Kliewer *et al.*, 1992; Whitfield *et al.*, 1995).

Intestinal effects

Vitamin D stimulates the active transport of calcium and phosphorus across the intestinal epithelium. This stimulation does not involve PTH directly but affects the active form of vitamin D (Zheng and Teegarden, 2013). PTH indirectly stimulates intestinal calcium absorption by stimulating the production of $1,25(OH)_2D_3$ under conditions of hypocalcemia.

Vitamin D promotes calcium and phosphorus absorption, however, the mechanism is still not completely understood. Current evidence indicates that $1,25(OH)_2D_3$ is transferred to the nucleus of the intestinal cell, where it interacts with the chromatin material (Wasserman, 1981; Zheng and Teegarden, 2013; Combs and McClung, 2022). In response to the $1,25(OH)_2D_3$, specific RNAs are elaborated by the nucleus. When these are translated into particular proteins by ribosomes, the events leading to calcium and phosphorus absorption enhancement occur (Scott *et al.*, 1982). In the intestine, calcitriol promotes the synthesis of calbindin (calcium-binding protein [CaBP]) and other proteins and stimulates calcium and phosphorus absorption. This calbindin is not present in the intestine of rachitic chicks but appears following vitamin D supplementation.

Originally, it was felt that vitamin D did not regulate phosphorus absorption and transport. In 1963, through an *in vitro* inverted sac technique, it was demonstrated that vitamin D plays such a role (Harrison and Harrison, 1963). A more recently discovered phosphaturic hormone, fibroblast growth factor 23 (FGF23), primarily produced in osteoblast and osteocyte cells, is responsible for P homeostasis through a pathway that involves feedback regulation between FGF23, vitamin D, phosphorus, and calcium (Sitara *et al.*, 2006; David *et al.*, 2013).

Bone effects

Vitamin D_3 plays an essential role in the metabolism and development of the skeleton in chickens and turkeys, maintaining complex balances with calcium and phosphorus. Increasing the dosage of vitamin D_3 increases the plasma concentration of ionized and total calcium and reduces the concentration of phosphorus and sodium (Shafey *et al.*, 1990). It also improves phosphorus absorption and retention, and utilization of phytic phosphorus (Shafey *et al.*, 1990; Mohammed *et al.*, 1991) and intervenes in the differentiation and maturation of chondrocytes (Whitehead *et al.*, 1993a).

It must be noted that other vitamins (B_6, folic acid, C, and K) and mineral trace elements (copper, zinc, magnesium, boron, fluorine, and aluminium) are also involved in the ossification process. Minerals are deposited on the protein matrix (Zheng and Teegarden, 2013; Combs and McClung, 2022). This deposition is accompanied by an invasion of blood vessels that gives rise to trabecular bone. This process causes bones to elongate. This organic matrix fails to mineralize during a vitamin D deficiency, causing rickets in the young and osteomalacia in adults. The active metabolite calcitriol brings about the mineralization of the bone matrix.

Vitamin D has another function in bone: mobilizing calcium from bone to the extracellular fluid compartment. PTH shares this function. It requires metabolic energy and presumably transports calcium and phosphorus across the bone membrane by acting on osteocytes and osteoclasts. Rapid, acute plasma calcium regulation is possible due to the interaction of plasma calcium with calcium-binding sites in bone material as blood comes in contact with bone. Changes in plasma calcium are brought about by a difference in the proportion of high- and low-affinity calcium-binding sites, access to which is regulated by osteoclasts and osteoblasts, respectively (Snow *et al.*, 1986; Bronner and Stein, 1995). Another proposed role of vitamin D is its involvement in bone, namely, in collagen biosynthesis in preparation for mineralization (Gonnerman *et al.*, 1976). $25OHD_3$ is more potent than vitamin D_3 (2.5–4 times more) in improving calcium and phosphorus metabolism.

Kidney effects

There is evidence that vitamin D functions in the distal renal tubules to improve calcium reabsorption and is mediated by the calcium-binding protein calbindin (Bronner and Stein, 1995). It is known that 99% of the renal-filtered calcium is reabsorbed without vitamin D and PTH. Although it is unknown whether they work in concert, the remaining 1% is controlled by these 2 hormonal agents. It has been shown that $1,25(OH)_2D_3$ improves renal calcium reabsorption (Sutton and Dirks, 1978).

Non-classical functions (beyond bone mineralization)

Other functions that we can call non-classical are connected with the discovery of the presence of 1α-hydroxylase and the receptor of the active metabolite in several tissues like the pancreas, bone marrow, cells of the ovary, cells of the brain, breast, and epithelial cells. This function suggests a role in many other aspects like immune system modulation, muscle cell differentiation, and reproduction (Machlin and Sauberlich, 1994; Deluca, 2014). More than 50 genes have been reported to be transcriptionally regulated by $1,25(OH)_2D_3$ (Hannah and Norman, 1994; Zheng and Teegarden, 2013; Combs and McClung, 2022).

Immune system modulation

The actions of $1,25(OH)_2D_3$ are involved in regulating the growth and differentiation of various cell types, including those of the hematopoietic and immune systems (Reinhardt and Hustmeyer, 1987; Lemire, 1992).

Recent studies have suggested $1,25(OH)_2D_3$ as an immunoregulatory hormone, and $25OHD_3$ appears more efficient than vitamin D in modulating immune response (Shanmugasundaram and Selvaraj, 2012; Morris and Selvaraj, 2014; Morris *et al.*, 2015; Shanmugasundaram *et al.*, 2019). Aslam *et al.* (1998) reported that vitamin D deficiency depresses the cellular immune responses in young broiler chicks. Turkey osteomyelitis, a disease that affects commercially produced turkeys, and disease incidence in *E. coli*-challenged birds were also decreased with vitamin D metabolites (Huff *et al.*, 2002). Elevated $1,25(OH)_2D_3$ was also associated with a significant 70% enhancement of lymphocyte proliferation in cells treated with pokeweed mitogen (Hustmyer *et al.*, 1994). Calcitriol has also been credited with functions regulating the cells of the immune system (Mireles, 1997; Aslam *et al.*, 1998).

Muscle cell differentiation

Satellite cells are muscle stem cells giving rise, when activated, to a skeletal muscle cells precursors pool, able to differentiate and fuse to increase the nuclei accretion into existing muscle fibers or to form new fibers. These adult stem cells are involved in normal growth of skeletal muscle as well as regeneration following injury or disease (Berri *et al.*, 2013; Hutton *et al.*, 2014). It has been shown that directly feeding $25OHD_3$ affects broiler chicken vitamin D status (Yarger *et al.*, 1995a) and could stimulate satellite cell-mediated muscle hypertrophy response in the chicken *pectoralis major* muscle.

Reproduction

Vitamin D has also been shown to be required for chick embryonic development. Vitamin D treatment stimulated yolk calcium mobilization, and the vitamin D-dependent Ca^{2+} binding protein, calbindin, is present in the yolk sac (Tuan and Suyama, 1996). These findings strongly suggest that the hormonal action of $1,25(OH)_2D_3$ on yolk sac calcium transport is mediated by the regulated expression and activity of calbindin, analogous to the response of the adult intestine. Calcitriol is also essential for transporting eggshell calcium to the embryo across the chorioallantoic membrane (Elaroussi *et al.*, 1994). $25OHD_3$ is easily deposited into broiler and turkey egg yolk. It is then converted to $1,25(OH)_2D_3$ by the embryonic kidney after day 8 of embryo development to support calcium transfer from the eggshell and assimilation into the embryonic skeleton.

Accordingly, Manley *et al.* (1978) observed a significant improvement in the hatchability of fertile turkey eggs when $25OHD_3$ was added to the diet compared to vitamin D_3. Calcitriol is not transferred into the egg and thus cannot support hatchability in vitamin D deficient hen diets (Sunde *et al.*, 1978).

Nutritional assessment

As previously discussed, in the body, vitamin D undergoes successive metabolic hydroxylation into 25-hydroxy-vitamin D and 1,25-dihydroxy-vitamin D in the liver and kidney, respectively. The first hydroxylation product of vitamin D, 25OHD, is recognized as the best status marker for humans, other mammals, and poultry (Höller *et al.*, 2018). Very briefly, vitamin D cannot be used as it is quickly transformed into $25OHD_3$ through the 25-hydroxylation, and the production of 1,25-dihydroxy-vitamin D is strictly regulated according to calcium and phosphorus plasma levels.

Since the body does not store $25OHD_3$, the concentration in circulation (plasma or serum) can be used for status determination. Both competitive chemiluminescence immunoassays and HPLC coupled with tandem mass spectrometry (HPLC-MS/MS) assays are used in clinical practice. The advantages and disadvantages of both technologies have been reviewed in depth (Van den Ouweland, 2016).

The varying selectivity of the antibodies for $25OHD_3$ (and $25OHD_2$) and the potential for cross-reactivity with related metabolites such as 24,25-dihydroxy-vitamin D impact the repeatability between different immune-based assays. This aspect is extremely critical when using immune assays with animal plasma as most commercial immune kits are based on human antibodies, and few of them are "optimized" for use in poultry or other animal species.

HPLC-MS/MS has been referred to as the gold standard, but, in common with several delicate analyses, the result can also be erroneous as this technique requires the skills of an experienced analyst (Atef, 2018). Vitamin D is stable at room temperature on DBS and was one of the first vitamins analyzed with this sampling method (Eyles *et al.*, 2009). DBS has been successfully tested in broilers allowing a less invasive blood sampling (Falleiros *et al.*, 2019).

Experts still debate what an adequate $25OHD_3$ plasma level is for humans. A 75 nmol/l or 30 ng/ml (conversion factor 2.5) is considered a cut-off between adequate and inadequate vitamin D nutritional status (Holick, 2007). However, some authors and health bodies have placed this threshold at 50 nmol/l (Cashman, 2018), while others consider such values to be the low-end of adequacy (Heaney and Holick, 2011). Levels above 150 nmol/l or 60 ng/ml are considered excessive in humans, although these figures are also a matter of debate. One point of discussion is the fact that vitamin D nutritional status is normally assessed using calcium and phosphorus metabolism and bone status as the endpoint. Research has progressively indicated that besides the endocrine function, vitamin D has broader autocrine and paracrine functions such as immune system modulation and muscle cell development. These functionalities seem to require higher $25OHD_3$ circulating levels to be activated.

A direct transposition of human data to animals is impossible, and the establishment of clinical ranges upon which to adjust dietary supplementation is underway. As a general reference, human cut-off values previously mentioned can be used. Finally, the dietary administration of $25OHD_3$ has been shown in different studies to increase more efficiently than vitamin D_3 the $25OHD_3$ plasma level (see, e.g., Vignale *et al.*, 2015).

Deficiency signs

The primary vitamin D deficiency sign is a bone disorder called rickets in young animals. It is generally characterized by a decreased concentration of calcium and phosphorus in the organic matrices of cartilage and bone. Vitamin D results in clinical signs like those indicating a lack of calcium or phosphorus or both, as all 3 are concerned with proper bone formation.

In the adult, osteomalacia is the counterpart of rickets and, since cartilage growth has ceased, is characterized by a decreased concentration of calcium and phosphorus in the bone matrix (Figures 4.6a and 4.6b). Outward signs of rickets include the following skeletal changes, varying somewhat with species depending on anatomy and severity:

- weak bones causing curving and bending of bones
- enlarged hock and knee joints
- tendency to drag hind legs
- beaded ribs and deformed thorax.

Although there appear to be differences among species in the susceptibility of different bones to such degenerative changes and differences that probably reflect bodily conformation (e.g., dog compared with sheep), there is an apparent common pattern (Abrams, 1978). Spongy parts of individual bones and bones relatively rich in such tissues are generally the first and most severely affected. As in simple calcium deficiency, the vertebrae and the bones of the head suffer the greatest degree of resorption. Next come the scapula, sternum, and ribs.

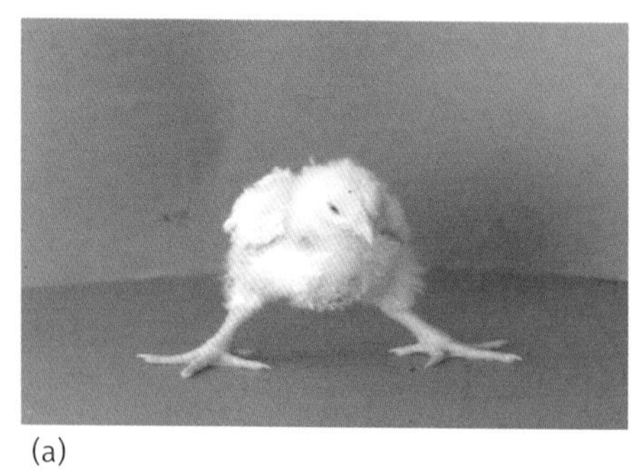
(a)

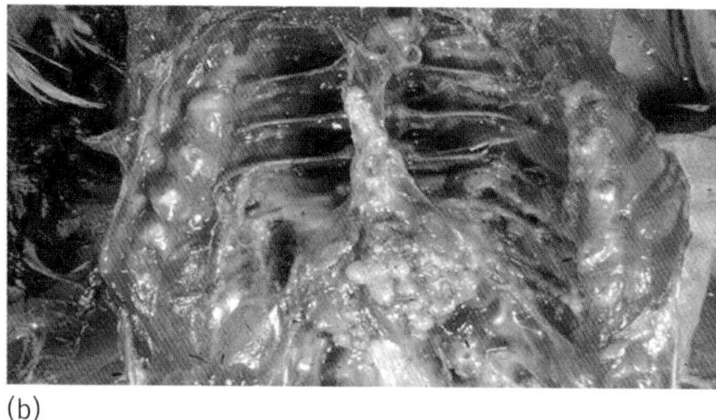
(b)

Figure 4.6 (a) Vitamin D deficiency (source: Dr. H. Weiser, DSM Kaiseraugst); (b) "ricketty rosary," gross enlargement of the costochondral junctions (source: copyright UK Crown)

The most resistant bones are metatarsals and shafts of long bones. Several methods have been used to assess the nutritional status of animals deficient in vitamin D.

Poor growth rates and bone abnormalities in animals and humans are the chief indications when vitamin D deficiency is substantially advanced. The incomplete calcification of the skeleton is easily detectable with X-rays and reduced bone ash but, like other production-related signs, would not be specific for vitamin D deficiency versus other nutrient inadequacies (e.g., calcium and phosphorus). Deviations from normal serum calcium, phosphorus, and alkaline phosphatase are associated with rickets. Serum calcium and inorganic phosphorus concentrations decreased markedly during the acute phase of rickets (Gershoff *et al.*, 1957).

Safety

After vitamin A, vitamin D is the next most likely to be consumed in concentrations toxic to animals (Fraser, 2021). Although vitamin D is toxic at high concentrations, short-term administration of as much as 100 times the required level may be tolerated. For most species, the presumed maximal safe level of vitamin D_3 for long-term feeding conditions (more than 60 days) is 4 to 10 times the dietary requirement. Studies in a number of species indicate that vitamin D_3 is 10 to 20 times more toxic than vitamin D_2 when provided in excessive amounts (NRC, 1987).

Excessive vitamin D intake produces various effects, all associated with abnormal elevation of blood calcium (Fraser, 2021). Elevated blood calcium is caused by greatly stimulated bone resorption and increased intestinal calcium absorption. The main pathological effect of ingestion of massive doses of vitamin D is widespread calcification of soft tissues. Pathological changes in these tissues are observed to be inflammation, cellular degeneration, and calcification. Diffuse calcification affects joints, synovial membranes, kidneys, myocardium, pulmonary alveoli, parathyroids, pancreas, lymph glands, arteries, conjunctivae, and corneas. More advanced cases interfere with cartilage growth. As expected, the skeletal system undergoes a simultaneous demineralization that results in the thinning of bones. Other common observations of vitamin D toxicity are loss of appetite, extensive weight loss, elevated blood calcium, and lowered blood phosphate. Vitamin D toxicity is enhanced by elevated dietary calcium and phosphorus supplies and is reduced when the diet is low in calcium (Fraser, 2021).

In early studies, Lofton and Soares (1986) observed a higher incidence of tibial dyschondroplasia (TD) using 20,000 mg/kg (500 µg/kg) vitamin D_3, and Cruishank and Sim (1987) increased valgus-varus bone deformities with 40,000 mg/kg (100 µg/kg). Subsequently, Yarger *et al.* (1995a) observed no renal calcification until they supplemented the diet with 3,450 µg/kg (138,000 IU/kg), and Qian *et al.* (1997), with 6,600 µg/kg, also indicated no negative consequences. Baker *et al.* (1998), using 1,250 µg/kg (50,000 IU/kg, 250 times the NRC level), found no signs of toxicity or reduced growth; in fact, this dose produced good results in phosphorus-deficient diets. Papesova and Fucikova (2000), with diets supplemented with 2,500–125,000 IU/kg, found toxicity from 25,000 IU/kg. i.e., 10–15 times the normal commercial supplementation, but only after administering it for 3 months.

Signs of toxicity only have been observed at 40 times the commercial level of inclusion. Nain *et al.* (2007a,b) reported that when the researchers used 80,000 IU/kg instead of 5,000 IU/kg in broilers, the higher dosage produced 2.5 times higher mortality from sudden death syndrome. They observed twice the number of birds with moderate arrhythmia and tachycardia after a stress event. Intense and prolonged hypercalcemia caused by the high dose of vitamin D_3 proved harmful since an adequate calcium level is important for the proper functioning of the cardiac muscle.

$25OHD_3$ is absorbed faster and in greater proportion than cholecalciferol, but its safety profile is quite similar to that of cholecalciferol (10 times the recommended dose). Calcitriol is

10 times more efficient than cholecalciferol in preventing and curing rickets (Ameenudin *et al.*, 1985), but its maximum safe concentration is around 2 µg/kg (Rennie *et al.*, 1995). Tsang *et al.* (1990a,b) indicated that 5 µg/kg 1,25$(OH)_2D_3$ is the optimum level to improve eggshell quality and placed the toxic level at 7 µg/kg.

Terry *et al.*'s (1999) study focused on determining the maximum tolerance level for using the 25OHD_3 metabolite in layer diets. They assessed various multiple levels – 41.25, 82.5, 412.5, and 825 µg/kg – and the effect of these levels had on different parameters. The results indicated that 25OHD_3 is safe at a dosage of 82.5 µg/kg, with a margin of safety of approximately 5× between the proposed 1× level of 82.5 µg/kg and the 5× level (412.5 mg/kg feed) that constitutes threshold toxicity in layers. As we have seen, 1,25$(OH)_2D_3$ needs supplements at lower levels than with 25OHD_3, and logically, as indicated by Soares *et al.* (1995), maximum tolerance levels in absolute terms are reached sooner. Hence, the very low dosage and the narrower margin of safety pose a risk in use in the feed of this metabolite.

The potential toxicity of calcitriol and other metabolites like 1αOHD_3, both with a much narrower safety profile, could be increased due to excess calcium in chickens' diet (San Martin, 2018). The synthetic metabolite 1αOHD_3 was evaluated by Edwards *et al.* (2002). It seems to have similar activity to 1,25$(OH)_2D_3$, inducing much faster calcium absorption and mobilization than vitamin D_3. It is 8 times more effective in increasing bone ash content (Świątkiewicz *et al.*, 2017). However, a dietary level of 5 µg 1αOHD_3/kg may be at the upper limit of safety in broiler performance, though higher levels may be needed for overtly toxic effects to be seen. However, the level of 5 µg/kg has been found to be overtly toxic for breeding birds (Rings *et al.*, 2011).

Vitamin E

Chemical structure and properties

The term vitamin E includes all tocopherol and tocotrienol derivatives that qualitatively have α-tocopherol activity. This definition was given by the International Union of Pure and Applied Chemistry-International Union of Biochemistry (IUPAC-IUB) Commission on Biochemical Nomenclature. Both the tocopherols and the tocotrienols consist of a hydroquinone nucleus and an isoprenoid side chain. Tocopherols have a saturated side chain, whereas the tocotrienols have an unsaturated side chain containing 3 double bonds.

There are 4 principal compounds of each of these 2 sources of vitamin E activity (α, β, γ, and δ), differentiated by the presence of methyl (-CH_3) groups at positions 5, 7, or 8 of the chroman ring (Figure 4.7). α-tocopherol, the most biologically active of these compounds, is

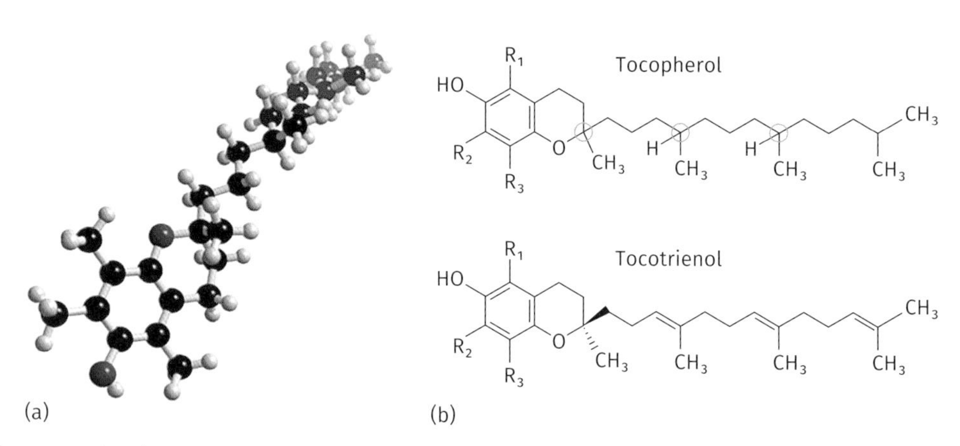

Figure 4.7 Vitamin E structure

the predominant vitamin E active compound in feedstuffs and the form used commercially to supplement animal diets. The biological activity of the other tocopherols is limited, but other functions have been found for non-α-tocopherol forms of vitamin E (Schaffer *et al.*, 2005; Freiser and Jiang, 2009; Traber, 2013).

The tocopherol molecule has 3 asymmetric carbon atoms at 2′, 4′, and 8′ positions. These 3 asymmetric carbon atoms generate 8 forms RRR-, RSR-, RRS-, RSS-, SRR-, SSR-, SRS-, and SSS-α-tocopherol. The d-form of α-tocopherol has all of the methyl groups in these positions facing in one direction and is referred to as the RRR-form, which is the form found in plants. The all-rac (all racemic), or chemically synthesized form of α-tocopherol, has an equal mixture of the R and S configurations at each of the 3 positions (i.e., it contains 8 stereoisomers) (Traber, 2013). Alpha-tocopherol is a yellow oil that is insoluble in water but soluble in organic solvents, resistant to heat but readily oxidized. The relative biological activity of vitamin E is expressed in International Units (IU), 1 IU corresponding to the activity of 1 mg of (all-rac)-α-tocopheryl acetate.

Natural sources

Vitamin E is widespread in nature, with the richest sources being vegetable oils, cereal products containing these oils, eggs, liver, legumes, and, in general, green plants (Chen *et al.*, 2019). In nature, the synthesis of vitamin E is a function of plants; thus, their products are the principal sources. It is abundant in whole cereal grains, particularly in germ, and thus in by-products containing the germ (McDowell, 2000a; Traber, 2006, 2013). Feed Table averages are often of little value in predicting individual content of feedstuffs or bioavailability of vitamins. Vitamin E content of 42 varieties of corn varied from 11.1 to 36.4 IU/kg, a 3.3-fold difference (McDowell and Ward, 2008). There is wide variation in the vitamin content of feeds, with many feeds having a three- to tenfold range in reported α-tocopherol values.

Naturally occurring vitamin E activity of feedstuffs cannot be accurately estimated from earlier published vitamin E or tocopherol values. Alpha-tocopherol is especially high in wheat germ oil and sunflower oil. Corn and soybean oil contain predominantly γ-tocopherol and some tocotrienols (McDowell, 2000a; Traber, 2006, 2013). Cottonseed oil contains both α- and γ-tocopherols in equal proportions. In practice, supplements are added in the more stable form of α-tocopherol acetate.

The stability of all naturally occurring tocopherols is poor, and substantial losses of vitamin E activity occur in feedstuffs when processed and stored and in the manufacturing and storage of finished feeds (Gadient, 1986; Dove and Ewan, 1991; McDowell, 1996). Vitamin E sources in these ingredients are unstable under conditions that promote oxidation of feedstuffs; in the presence of heat, oxygen, moisture, oxidizing fats, and trace minerals. Vegetable oils that normally are excellent sources of vitamin E can be extremely low in the vitamin if oxidation has been promoted. Oxidized oil has little or no vitamin E, and it will destroy the vitamin E in other feed ingredients and deplete animal tissue stores of vitamin E.

Oxidation of vitamin E increases after grinding, mixing with minerals, adding fat, and pelleting for balanced feed. When feeds are pelleted, the destruction of vitamins E and A may occur if the diet does not contain sufficient antioxidants to prevent their accelerated oxidation under moisture and high-temperature conditions. Iron salts (i.e., ferric chloride) can destroy vitamin E.

A study testing vitamin E stability reported that artificial corn drying for 40 minutes at 87°C produced an average 10% loss of α-tocopherol and 12% loss of other tocopherols (Adams, 1973; Adams *et al.*, 1975). When corn was dried for 54 minutes at 93°C, the α-tocopherol loss averaged 41%. Artificial drying of corn results in a much lower vitamin E content. Young *et al.*

(1975) reported a concentration of 9.3 or 20 mg/kg α-tocopherol in artificially dried corn versus undried, respectively. Apparently, the damage is not due to moisture alone but to the combined propionic acid/moisture effect. Further decomposition of α-tocopherol occurs over a more extended time until the grain eventually has α-tocopherol levels of less than 1 mg/kg, commonly found in propionic acid-treated barley.

Commercial forms

Vitamin E is usually incorporated into feeds as all-rac-α-tocopheryl acetate. Other vitamin E esters are produced like propionate or succinate, but the acetate form has been shown to be the one providing the best bioavailability. All-rac-α-tocopheryl acetate, is manufactured by condensing trimethyl hydroquinone and isophytol and conducting ultra-vacuum molecular distillation, producing a highly purified form of α-tocopherol. This material may then be acetylated. As previously stated, all-rac-α-tocopherol is a mixture of α-tocopheryl acetate's 8 stereoisomers (4 enantiomeric pairs). The enantiomeric pairs, racemates, are present in equimolar amounts (Cohen *et al.*, 1981; Scott *et al.*, 1982). This finding indicates that the manufacturing processes lead to all-rac-α-tocopheryl acetate with similar proportions to all 8 stereoisomers (Weiser and Vecchi, 1982).

The vitamin E acetate product form mostly used in animal feeding is an adsorbate that provides good storage stability and responds well to physical treatments applied in feed manufacturing, like pelleting or extrusion with the use of temperature and steam. Vitamin E acetate is also available in the spray-dried form, water-soluble, for application in drinking water or milk replacers. The spray-dried formulation is also indicated when stability may be critical, like aggressive premixes with very high pH or canned pet food.

Commercially there is no truly "natural" tocopherol product available since the d-form or RRR-form of α-tocopherol commercial products are obtained from the original raw material only after several chemical processing steps. Hence, it should be referred to as "naturally derived" and not natural. In addition, the International Unit (IU) is the standard of vitamin E activity; consequently, it is the same regardless of the source.

However, some studies in several species comparing the naturally derived RRR to the synthetic all-rac-α-tocopheryl acetate have shown the former to be more effective in elevating plasma and tissue concentrations when administered on an equal IU basis (Jensen et al., 2006). Research in humans, poultry, sheep, pigs, guinea pigs, fish, and horses, in which the elevation of plasma concentrations was measured, indicated that the biopotency of RRR-α-tocopherol compared to all-rac-α-tocopherol can vary from the "official" Figure of 1.36: 1 up to closer to 2: 1 (Traber, 2013), with differences among species. Considering the 1.36: 1 ratio, 1 mg of all-rac-α-tocopheryl acetate can be replaced by 0.74 mg RRR-α-tocopheryl acetate. In Figure 4.8, the vitamin E activity of different forms are reported relative to dl-α-tocopheryl acetate or all-rac-tocopheryl acetate set at 1.

Metabolism

Absorption and transport

Tocopherol's absorption occurs predominantly in the median portion of the small intestine through the portal vein to the liver. Before absorption, tocopheryl acetate is almost completely hydrolyzed by duodenal pancreatic esterase, the enzyme which releases free fatty acids from dietary triacylglycerides. The ester bond, which increases stability, is hydrolyzed. The resulting alcohol form is absorbed by the enterocytes and transported to the general circulation, thereby permitting the vitamin to function as a biological antioxidant. Any ester form, i.e., tocopheryl acetate, succinate, or propionate, to be absorbed into the body is converted to the

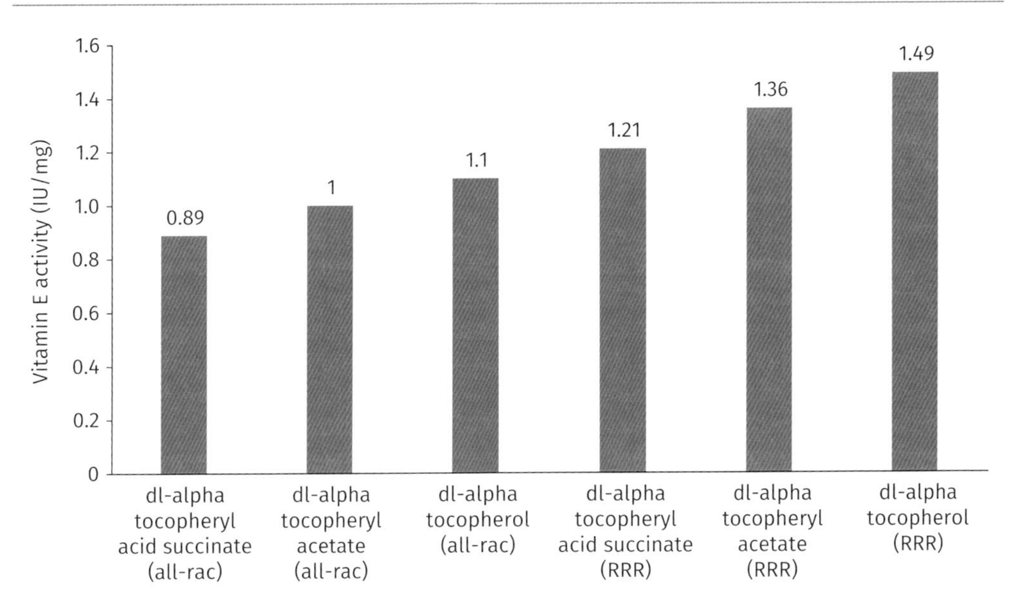

Figure 4.8 Vitamin E Activity of different chemical forms (IU/mg) relative to dl-α-tocopheryl acetate or all-rac-tocopheryl acetate set at 1 (source: United States Pharmacopeia, 1980)

alcohol form, and an α-tocopherol transfer protein has been identified (Traber, 2006, 2013). In young animals, the lower efficiency of the esterase can limit digestion and absorption.

Vitamin E, as all fat-soluble vitamins, carotenoids, and other fat-soluble dietary components, is incorporated into chylomicrons. Vitamin E absorption is related to fat digestion, and is facilitated by bile acids, monoglycerides, free fatty acids, and pancreatic lipase necessary for the solubilization of vitamin E and incorporation into mixed micelles for absorption (Sitrin *et al.*, 1987). This explains why in the case of malabsorption syndrome in birds, the efficiency of vitamin E absorption, as well as that of all fat-soluble vitamins, is impaired.

In healthy conditions, the efficiency of vitamin E absorption is variable from 35 to 50%, lower than that of vitamin A. Medium-chain triglycerides enhance vitamin E absorption, whereas PUFAs reduce it. The animal appears to have a preference for tocopherol versus other tocols. Rates and amounts of absorption of the various tocopherols and tocotrienols are in the same general order of magnitude as their biological potencies. Alpha-tocopherol is absorbed best, with γ-tocopherol absorption slightly less than α-forms but with a more rapid excretion. Generally, most of the vitamin E activity within plasma and other animal tissues is α-tocopherol (Ullrey, 1981).

The mechanisms for uptake of vitamin E absorption into enterocytes are not well understood. According to Reboul and Borel (2011), non-vitamin E specific transporters like cholesterol and lipid transporters should be involved. No plasma-specific vitamin E transport proteins have been described. Vitamin E in plasma is attached mainly to lipoproteins in the globulin fraction within cells and occurs mainly in mitochondria and microsomes. The liver takes the vitamin and is released in combination with low-density and very-low-density lipoproteins (LDL and VLDL) (Traber, 2013).

Plasma vitamin E concentrations depend on α-tocopherol secretion from the liver (Kaempf-Rotzoll *et al.*, 2003). Additionally, the newly absorbed vitamin E, rather than that returning from the periphery, appears to be preferentially secreted into the plasma from the liver (Traber *et al.*, 1998). Thus, the liver, not the intestine, discriminates between tocopherols (Traber, 2013).

In contrast to α-tocopherol, the 7 other vitamers are not recognized by the α-tocopherol transfer protein (α-TTP) in the liver.

After hepatic uptake, the α-tocopherol form of vitamin E is preferentially resecreted into the circulation. The α-tocopherol transfer protein (α-TTP) is a critical regulator of vitamin E status that stimulates the movement of vitamin E between membrane vesicles *in vitro* and facilitates the secretion of tocopherol from hepatocytes. Recent studies have shown that the liver has a critical role in the biodiscrimination of stereoisomers because of the presence of α-TTP, which preferentially transfers α-tocopherol, compared with other dietary vitamin E forms (Panagabko *et al.*, 2002). This protein preferentially selects RRR and 2R α-toc for secretion into plasma (Leonard *et al.*, 2002; Cortinas *et al.*, 2004). Some authors suggested that the metabolism of 2S ST in the liver may be faster than that of 2R ST: thereby, the reduced presence of 2S ST in the liver and other tissues could be caused by faster metabolism rather than the lower affinity of the α-TTC (Kiyose *et al.*, 1995; Kaneko *et al.*, 2000).

It has also been established that there is a negative interaction between vitamin E and vitamin A or β-carotene, as they interfere with each other in their absorption and deposition processes (Haq *et al.*, 1996). This was reported previously by Combs (1976). This author noted that hens fed high vitamin A levels had low plasma levels of vitamin E and, therefore, low concentrations of the latter in egg yolk. Moreover, Surai *et al.* (1998a) concluded that excessive supplementation with vitamin A, above 40,000 IU/kg, in laying hen diets results in an adverse effect on vitamin E in the embryonic/neonatal liver that can compromise the antioxidant status of the progeny.

Storage and excretion

Vitamin E is stored throughout all body tissues, with the highest storage in the liver and the fat (Sunder and Flachowsky, 2001). However, vitamin E is not accumulated in the liver as it contains only a small fraction of total body stores, in contrast to vitamin A, for which about 95% of the body reserves are in the liver.

Subcellular fractions from different tissues vary considerably in their tocopherol content, with the highest levels found in membranous organelles, such as microsomes and mitochondria, that contain highly active oxidation-reduction systems (Taylor *et al.*, 1976; McCay *et al.*, 1981; Traber, 2013; Surai *et al.*, 2019).

Turkeys deposit much less tocopherol than chickens in their tissues. Small amounts of vitamin E will persist tenaciously in the body for a long time. However, stores are exhausted rapidly by PUFA in the tissues. The rate of disappearance is proportional to the intake of PUFA. Major excretion routes of absorbed vitamin E are feces and bile, in which tocopherol appears mostly in the free form (McDowell, 2000a).

Biochemical functions

Vitamin E is essential for the reproductive, circulatory, nervous, immune, and muscular systems (Figure 4.9) (Hoekstra, 1975; Sheffy and Schultz, 1979; Bendich, 1987; McDowell, 2000a). It is one of the vitamins to which the greatest investigative efforts have been dedicated (Surai, 2003; Sirri and Barroeta, 2007; Khan *et al.*, 2012b,c; Surai *et al.*, 2019).

Vitamin E:

- is the main antioxidant in blood and, on a cellular level, it maintains the integrity of the cellular and vascular membranes
- it acts as a detoxifier and takes part in many other biochemical reactions

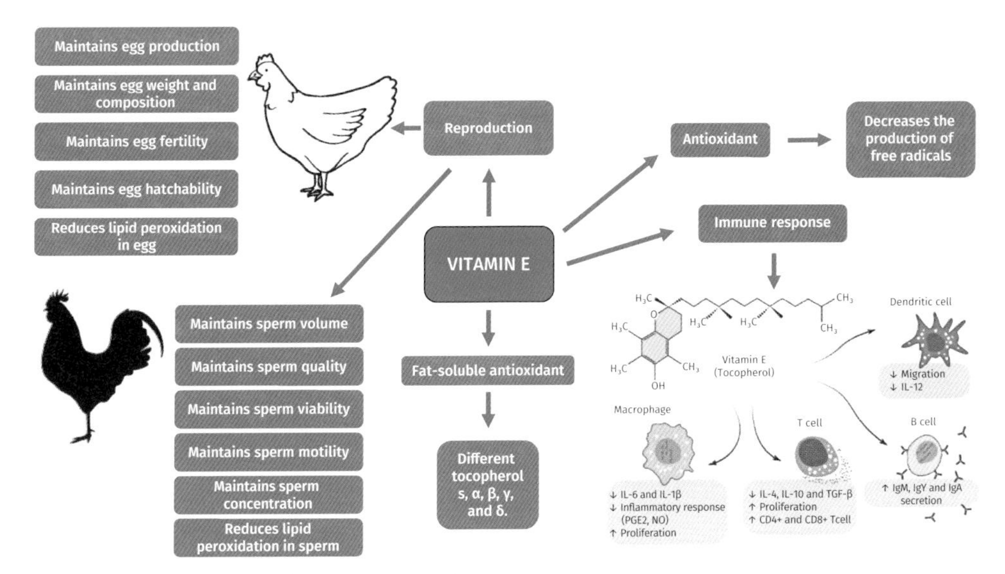

Figure 4.9 Vitamin E functions (source: adapted from Nawab *et al.*, 2019 and Shojadoost *et al.*, 2021)

- is essential for the fertility of adult birds
- it promotes the activity of immune system cells
- can alleviate stress and increase immunocompetence in birds (Cherian and Sim, 1997; Yang *et al.*, 2000; Siegel *et al.*, 2001; Khan *et al.*, 2012c; Surai *et al.*, 2019)
- is also involved in the prevention of cardiovascular and carcinogenic diseases.

Classical α-tocopherol functions of vitamin E

Antioxidant

The relationship between vitamin E consumed and the prevention of oxidation or oxidative distress in biological systems has been studied and extensively reviewed by Surai *et al.* (2019). Under physiological conditions, cells maintain redox homeostasis by producing oxidants, i.e., reactive oxygen species (ROS) and other free radicals, and eliminating them through an antioxidant system. When the balance favors oxidants, we have oxidative distress (Surai *et al.*, 2019).

Free-radical reactions are ubiquitous in biological systems and are associated with energy metabolism, biosynthetic reactions, natural defense mechanisms, detoxification, and intra- and intercellular signaling pathways. Redox homeostasis is an essential mechanism for aerobic organisms (bacteria, plants, animals, and humans). Highly ROS, such as the superoxide anion radical (O_2-), hydroxyl radical (OH), hydrogen peroxide (H_2O_2), and singlet oxygen (O_2-), are continuously produced in the course of normal aerobic cellular metabolism. Additionally, phagocytic granulocytes undergo respiratory bursts to produce oxygen radicals to destroy intracellular pathogens. However, these oxidative products can, in turn, damage healthy cells if they are not eliminated. Antioxidants serve to stabilize these highly reactive free radicals, thereby maintaining the structural and functional integrity of cells (Chew, 1995).

Vitamin E is a quenching agent for free-radical molecules with single, highly reactive electrons in their outer shells. Free radicals attract a hydrogen atom, along with its electron, away from the chain structure, satisfying the electron needs of the original free radical, but leaving the PUFA short one electron. Thus, a fatty acid-free radical is formed that joins with molecular oxygen to form a peroxyl radical that steals a hydrogen-electron unit from yet another PUFA. This reaction can continue in a chain, destroying thousands of PUFA molecules (Gardner, 1989). Free radicals can be extremely damaging to biological systems (Padh, 1991).

Vitamin E has a crucial role within the cellular defense system in the face of oxidation at both intracellular and extracellular levels. α-tocopherol is integrated within the cellular membrane and protects lipids from oxidation, preventing them from being attacked by reactive oxygen and free radicals (Surai *et al.*, 2019). Tocopherols remove the peroxyl radical, donating a hydrogen atom and converting it to peroxide. Support for the antioxidant role of vitamin E *in vivo* also comes from observations that synthetic antioxidants can either prevent or alleviate certain clinical signs of vitamin E deficiency diseases. Therefore, antioxidants are very important to human and animal immune defense and health.

Most vitamin E deficiency symptoms are related to disorders of the cellular membrane due to the oxidative degradation of PUFAs and phospholipids (Chow, 1979) and critical sulfhydryl groups (Brownlee *et al.*, 1977). Orientation of vitamin E within cell membranes appears to be critical to its functionality (Surai *et al.*, 2019). It has been demonstrated how the deposition of α-tocopherol in the animal tissues, as well as in the egg, increases in direct proportion to its supply in the diet and is accompanied by greater oxidative stability (Galobart *et al.*, 2001a,b; Cortinas *et al.*, 2006; Villaverde *et al.*, 2008). Conversely, it is known that susceptibility to oxidation increases as the number of double bonds of fatty acids increases.

As the profile of fatty acids in the ration is reflected in the fatty acid composition of the different tissues of the animal and the eggs, increasing the degree of unsaturation in the feed increases susceptibility to oxidation and reduces the quantity of α-tocopherol deposited in the tissues (Galobart *et al.*, 2001a; Cortinas *et al.*, 2003; Villaverde *et al.*, 2004a,b). Hence, high levels of PUFA in the diet cause an increase in the susceptibility of tissues to lipid oxidation, increasing the requirements for vitamin E (Dutta-Roy *et al.*, 1994; Muggli, 1994).

Vitamin E supplies become depleted when it acts as an antioxidant, which explains the frequent observation that the presence of dietary unsaturated fats (susceptible to peroxidation) increases or precipitates a vitamin E deficiency. Consequently, vitamin E supplementation should increase in parallel to the amount of unsaturated fatty acids and the degree of oxidation of the fat added to the feed. Farm livestock requires 2.5–3.0 mg dl-α-tocopheryl acetate for each gram of PUFA in the diet.

Using blended fats with a 18% PUFA, 5 mg vitamin E should be added for every 1% blended fat. Requirements also depend on the presence or absence of other compounds that intervene in the tissue oxidation defense system, such as selenium. It should be borne in mind that depending on the feed ingredients, and hence the content of tocopherols, carotenoids, and other antioxidants, there will be a variation in the oxidative state of the animal and, therefore, the requirements of antioxidants and specifically of vitamin E (Surai and Sparks, 2001a). Interruption of fat peroxidation by tocopherol explains the well-established observation that dietary tocopherols protect body supplies of oxidizable materials such as vitamin A, vitamin C, and the carotenes.

Relationship with selenium in tissue protection

Vitamin E and selenium share several molecular functions in regulating the encoding of many genes for proteins with potent antioxidant activity. Consequently, both have been included in the study of the selenogenome (Sun *et al.*, 2019). Selenium is part of 25 selenoproteins in avian species. The functions of most remain unknown, although these selenoproteins generally participate in antioxidant and anabolic processes (Hatfield and Gladyshev, 2002; Sun *et al.*, 2019).

Tissue breakdown occurs in most species receiving diets deficient in vitamin E and selenium, mainly through peroxidation. Peroxides and hydroperoxides are highly destructive to tissue integrity and lead to disease development. Selenium has been shown to act in aqueous cell media (cytosol and mitochondrial matrix) by destroying hydrogen peroxide and hydroperoxides via the enzyme glutathione peroxidase (GSH-Px), which is a cofactor (Sun *et al.*, 2019). This capacity prevents the oxidation of unsaturated lipid materials within cells, thus protecting fats within the cell membrane from breaking down. The various GSH-Px enzymes are characterized by different tissue specificities and are expressed from other genes. Different forms of GSH-Px perform their protective functions in concert, each providing antioxidant protection at various body sites.

Therefore, selenium has a sparing effect on vitamin E and delays the onset of deficiency signs. Likewise, vitamin E and sulfur amino acids partially protect against or delay the onset of several forms of selenium deficiency syndromes (Surai *et al.*, 2019). Vitamin E in cellular and subcellular membranes appears to be the first line of defense against the peroxidation of vital phospholipids. Still, even with adequate vitamin E, some peroxides are formed. As part of the enzyme GSH-Px, selenium is a second line of defense that destroys these peroxides before they have an opportunity to cause damage to membranes.

Therefore, through different biochemical mechanisms, selenium, vitamin E, and sulfur-containing amino acids can prevent some of the same nutritional diseases. Vitamin E prevents fatty acid hydroperoxide formation, sulfur amino acids are precursors of GSH-Px, and selenium is a component of GSH-Px (Smith *et al.*, 1974; Surai *et al.*, 2019).

Membrane structure and prostaglandin synthesis

Alpha-tocopherol may be involved in the formation of the structural components of biological membranes, thus exerting a unique influence on the architecture of membrane phospholipids (Ullrey, 1981). It is reported that α-tocopherol stimulated the incorporation of 14C from linoleic acid into arachidonic acid in fibroblast phospholipids (McDowell, 1989c). Also, it was found that α-tocopherol exerted a pronounced stimulatory influence on the formation of prostaglandin E from arachidonic acid, while a chemical antioxidant had no effect (Traber, 2013).

Meat quality and myopathies

To improve oxidative stability and thus increase the shelf life of meat, antioxidants have been successfully added to animal feeds. Several compounds, such as carotenoids, vitamin E, vitamin C, and selenium, are known to have potent antioxidant effects on meat. Of all of them, α-tocopherol has demonstrated the highest biological efficiency in preventing lipid oxidation *in vivo* (Barroeta, 2007).

Myodystrophic tissue is common in cases of vitamin E-selenium deficiency, with leakage of cellular compounds such as creatinine and various transaminases through affected membranes into plasma. The more active the cell (e.g., the cells of skeletal and involuntary muscles), the greater the inflow of lipids for energy supply, and the greater the risk of tissue damage if vitamin E is limited.

Certain consequences of vitamin E deficiency (i.e., muscular dystrophy) can be prevented by diet supplementation with other antioxidant nutrients, which helps validate the antioxidant role of tocopherols. Chemical antioxidants are stored at very low levels and thus are not as effective as tocopherol.

The origin and pathologic traits of current broiler myopathies like wooden breast, white striping (Petracci *et al.*, 2019; Prisco *et al.*, 2021), and spaghetti meat (Baldi *et al.*, 2021) are different from the myodystrophies observed in vitamin E deficiency. However, their severity could be partially alleviated by vitamin E supplementation early in life (Wang *et al.*, 2020a,b).

Immune response

Vitamin E is perhaps the most studied nutrient related to the immune response (Meydani and Han, 2006). Evidence accumulated over the years and from many species indicates that vitamin E is an essential nutrient for the normal function of the immune system. Furthermore, studies suggest that disease-reducing beneficial effects of certain nutrients, such as vitamin E, can affect the immune response (Khan *et al.*, 2012c; Surai *et al.*, 2019).

Considerable attention is presently being directed to vitamin E and selenium's role in protecting leukocytes and macrophages during phagocytosis, the mechanism whereby animals immunologically kill invading bacteria. Vitamin E and selenium may help these cells survive the toxic products produced to effectively kill ingested bacteria (Badwey and Karnovsky, 1980). Macrophages and neutrophils from vitamin E-deficient animals have decreased phagocytic activity (Khan *et al.*, 2012c).

Since vitamin E acts as a tissue antioxidant and aids in quenching free radicals produced in the body, any infection or other stress factor may exacerbate depletion of the limited vitamin E stores from various tissues. The former 2 responses are generally used to determine a nutrient requirement.

During stress and disease, there is an increase in the production of glucocorticoids, epinephrine, eicosanoids, and of phagocytic activity. Eicosanoid and corticoid synthesis and phagocytic respiratory bursts are prominent producers of free radicals, which challenge the animal's antioxidant systems.

Vitamin E also most likely has an immune-enhancing effect by virtue of the alterations it brings to arachidonic acid metabolism and the subsequent synthesis of prostaglandins, thromboxanes, and leukotrienes. Under increased stress conditions, levels of these compounds from endogenous synthesis or exogenous entry may adversely affect immune cell function (Hadden, 1987; Khan *et al.*, 2012c). Vitamin E has been implicated in stimulating serum antibody synthesis, particularly IgG antibodies (Tengerdy, 1980). The protective effects of vitamin E on animal health may reduce glucocorticoids, which are known to be immunosuppressive (Golub and Gershwin, 1985).

Vitamin E and selenium enhance host defenses against infections by improving phagocytic cell function. Both vitamin E and GSH-Px are antioxidants that protect phagocytic cells and surrounding tissues from oxidative attack by free radicals produced by the respiratory burst of neutrophils and macrophages during phagocytosis (Baker and Cohen, 1983; Baboir, 1984; Surai *et al.*, 2019). Hogan *et al.* (1990, 1992, 1996) reported that dietary vitamin E supplementation increased the intracellular kill of *Staphylococcus aureus* and *E. coli* by neutrophils.

Reproduction

Avian semen is rich in PUFAs and consequently susceptible to lipid peroxidation. This peroxidation could be one of the major causes of age-dependent low fertility in male breeders. Vitamin E can provide stability to spermatozoal plasma membranes by inhibiting the generation of free radicals (Khan *et al.*, 2012b). Vitamin E is also important for embryo development and impacts hatchability (Surai *et al.*, 2019).

Blood clotting

Vitamin E is an inhibitor of platelet aggregation (McIntosh *et al.*, 1985). It may do this by inhibiting the peroxidation of arachidonic acid, which is required to form prostaglandins involved in platelet aggregation (Panganamala and Cornwell, 1982; Machlin, 1991; Traber, 2013). The antioxidant property of vitamin E also ensures erythrocyte stability and capillary blood vessel integrity maintenance.

Cellular respiration, electron transport, and deoxyribonucleic acid

Vitamin E is involved in biological oxidation-reduction reactions (Surai *et al.*, 2019). Vitamin E also appears to regulate the biosynthesis of deoxyribonucleic acid (DNA) within cells. Vitamin E seems to be of particular importance in the cellular respiration of the heart and skeletal muscles (Leeson and Summers, 2008).

Relationship to toxic elements or substances

Both vitamin E and selenium protect against the toxicity of various heavy metals (Whanger, 1981). Vitamin E is highly effective in reducing the toxicity of metals such as silver, arsenic, and lead and shows slight effects against cadmium and mercury toxicity. Vitamin E can be effective against other toxic substances (Surai *et al.*, 2019).

Non-α-tocopherol functions of vitamin E

Although α-tocopherol has been the most widely studied form of vitamin E, other tocopherols and tocotrienols have been shown to have biological significance (Qureshi *et al.*, 2001; Eder *et al.*, 2002; McCormick and Parker, 2004; Schaffer *et al.*, 2005; Nakagawa *et al.*, 2007; Sun and Alkon, 2008; Freiser and Jiang, 2009; Traber, 2013; Surai *et al.*, 2019). The greater emphasis on α-tocopherol undoubtedly arises from observations that γ-tocopherol and δ-tocopherol are only 10 and 1% as effective as α-tocopherol, respectively, in experimental animal models of vitamin E deficiency.

Research with tocotrienols and non-alpha tocopherols has been conducted with laboratory animals and *in vitro* studies. Gamma-tocopherol has beneficial properties as an anti-inflammatory and possibly anti-atherogenic and anticancer agent (Wolf, 2006). Tocotrienols have been shown to possess excellent antioxidant activity *in vitro* and have been suggested to suppress reactive oxygen substances more efficiently than tocopherols (Schaffer *et al.*, 2005; Khan *et al.*, 2012b; Surai *et al.*, 2019). Studies have shown that tocotrienols exert more significant neuroprotective, anticancer, and cholesterol-lowering properties than tocopherols (Qureshi *et al.*, 2001; Sun and Alkon, 2008).

Other functions

Additional functions of vitamin E that have been reported (Scott *et al.*, 1982) include a role in (1) normal phosphorylation reactions, especially of high-energy phosphate compounds, such as creatine phosphate and adenosine triphosphate (ATP); (2) synthesis of vitamin C (ascorbic acid); (3) synthesis of ubiquinone; and (4) sulfur amino acid metabolism.

Pappu *et al.* (1978) have reported that vitamin E plays a role in vitamin B_{12} metabolism. A vitamin E deficiency interfered with converting vitamin B_{12} to its coenzyme 5′ deoxyadenosylcobalamin and, concomitantly, metabolism of methylmalonyl-CoA to succinyl-CoA. In humans, Turley and Brewster (1993) suggest that cellular deficiency of adenosylcobalamin may be one mechanism by which vitamin E deficiency leads to neurologic injury.

In rats, vitamin E deficiency has been reported to inhibit vitamin D metabolism in the liver and kidneys by interfering with the formation of active metabolites and decreasing the concentration of the hormone receptor complexes in the target tissue. Liver vitamin D hydroxylase activity decreased by 39%, 1-alpha hydroxylase activity in the kidneys decreased by 22%, and 24-hydroxylase activity by 52% (Sergeev *et al.*, 1990).

Nutritional assessment

Vitamin E encompasses 8 naturally occurring vitamers – 4 tocopherols and 4 tocotrienols but only α-tocopherol is routinely measured and used for status determination since this form is preferably maintained in circulation. α-tocopherol concentrations in plasma allow quantification by HPLC with fluorescence or UV detection. Using normal-phase HPLC, tocopherols and tocotrienols can also be separated. A recently introduced fast and sensitive reversed-phase HPLC method resolves the challenging separation of β- and γ-tocopherol, while the separation and quantification of the 8 stereoisomers of α-tocopherol are much more challenging (Höller *et al.*, 2018).

Further research into the functional markers of vitamin E status (e.g., products of lipid peroxidation) or assay systems would have potential for point-of-care applications. Cell activity assays based on measuring hemolysis of erythrocytes under oxidative stress are another possible functional marker for α-tocopherol (Sauberlich, 1999). There is a relatively high correlation between plasma and liver levels of α-tocopherol and also between the amount of dietary α-tocopherol administered and plasma levels. This has been observed in rats, chicks, pigs, lambs, and calves within rather wide intake ranges. However, plasma tocopherol levels can be affected by blood lipid transport capacity.

Plasma α-tocopherol concentration of 3.5 mg/l (8 µmol/l) is considered deficient in humans, with values of 9 mg/l (20 µmol/l) referred to as acceptable. Similar reference values can be regarded as indicative for assessing vitamin E nutritional status in poultry. For example, Lin *et al.* (2005b) supplemented the breeder's diet with increasing vitamin E doses (0, 40, 80, 120, and 160 mg/kg). The breeder's plasma α-tocopherol concentration significantly increased, returning the following values 0.84, 3.25, 5.68, 8.25, and 10.88 mg/l, respectively, indicating a change from inadequacy to sufficiency when 120 and 160 mg/kg were fed.

Deficiency signs

Specific vitamin E deficiency signs

Vitamin E deficiency in poultry can result in at least 3 specific conditions:

- **exudative diathesis** (Figure 4.10) with signs of subcutaneous edema and, in severe cases, blackening of the affected parts, apathy, and inappetence
- **encephalomalacia** (crazy chick disease) (Figure 4.11), characterized by ataxia, head retraction, and cycling of legs
- **nutritional muscular dystrophy** (Figure 4.12) (Scott *et al.*, 1982; Sun *et al.*, 2019).

Exudative diathesis

Exudative diathesis in chicks is severe edema produced by a marked increase in capillary permeability. The subcutaneous edema soon progresses to a hemorrhagic stage, creating a blue-green skin discoloration (Figure 4.10a). Affected chicks show reduced spontaneous activity and food intake. If not treated with vitamin E or selenium, they usually survive no more than 2 to 6 days. Both vitamin E and selenium are involved in preventing exudative diathesis and nutritional muscular dystrophy. However, vitamin E does not prevent or cure exudative diathesis in diets severely deficient in selenium.

In contrast, adding as little as 0.05 ppm of dietary selenium completely prevents this disease. The combined deficiency of selenium and vitamin E in poults produced a mild type of exudative diathesis (Creech *et al.*, 1957). This condition was characterized by hemorrhaging on the inner margins of the thighs and caudal breast muscles; in contrast to the exudative diathesis of the selenium- and vitamin E-deficient chick, it involved only mild edema.

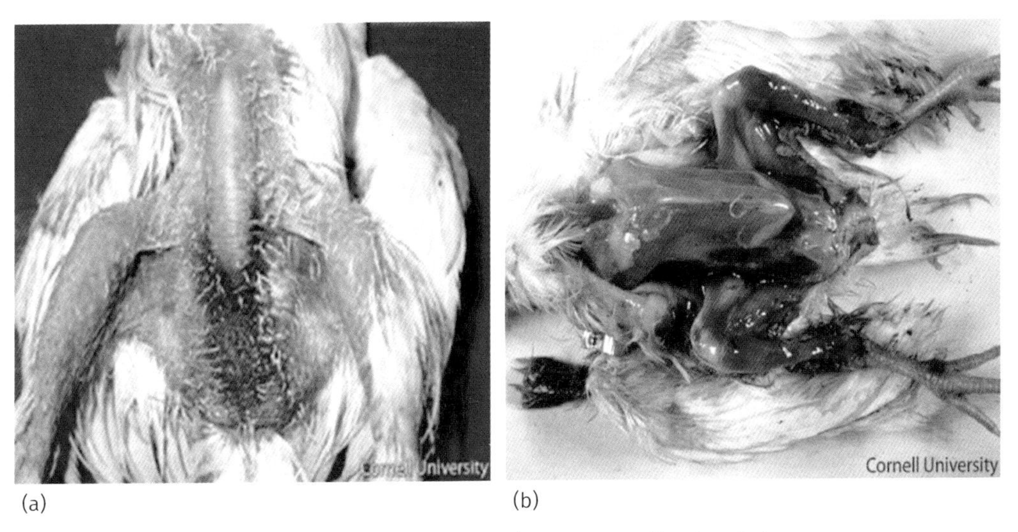

(a) (b)

Figure 4.10 Vitamin E deficiency: exudative diathesis (source: Cornell University)

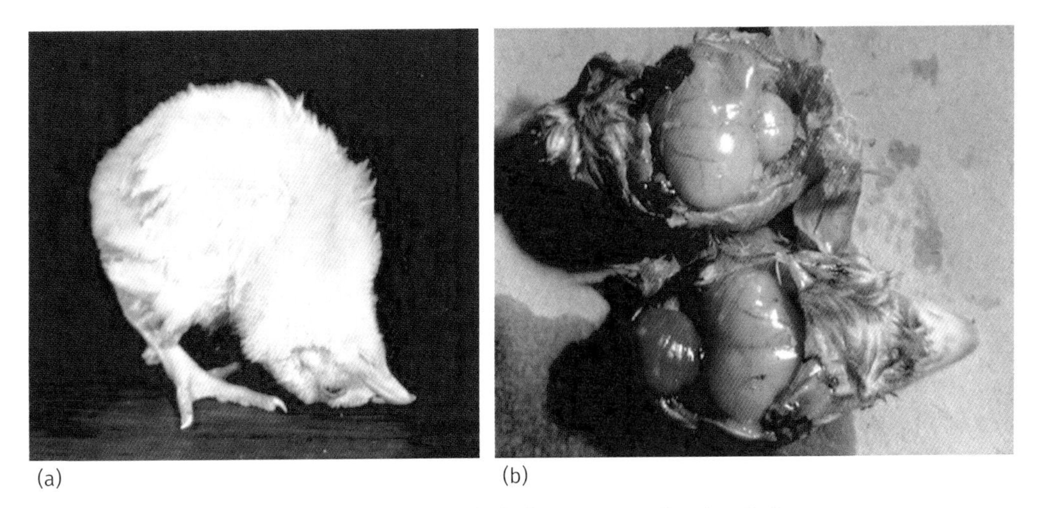

(a) (b)

Figures 4.11 Vitamin E deficiency: encephalomalacia (source: Cornell University)

For ducklings, exudative diathesis would appear to be more similar to that of the chick, i.e., green-colored edema of the subcutaneous tissues can be seen most frequently on the thigh with associated petechial hemorrhages of the thigh musculature (Combs and Combs, 1986). The appearance of exudative diathesis is infrequent and is associated with only the more severe cases of nutritional muscular dystrophy in deficient ducklings (Jager, 1977). For Japanese quail, the combined deficiency of selenium and vitamin E has only produced exudative diathesis in some animals.

Encephalomalacia

Encephalomalacia generally affects chicks from 2 to 6 weeks of age and results from hemorrhages and edema within the cerebellum (Figure 4.11). At least one important function of

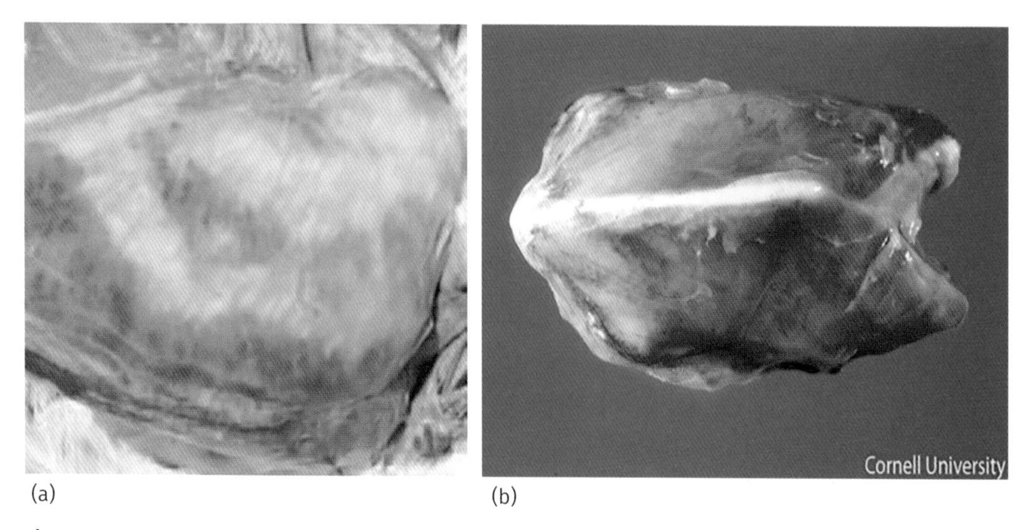

(a) (b)

Figures 4.12 Vitamin E deficiency: nutritional muscular dystrophy (source: Cornell University)

vitamin E is to interrupt the production of free radicals at the initial stage of encephalomalacia. The quantitative need for vitamin E for this function depends on the amount of linoleic acid in the diet. However, Vérice *et al.* (1991) fed diets high in linoleic acid with or without vitamin E supplementation. Chicks receiving diets high in linoleic acid or vitamin E did not develop encephalomalacia pathology.

Furthermore, Fuhrmann and Sallmann (1995) reported little influence of fatty acid type on the development of encephalomalacia. They also stated that the cerebellum is the most susceptible to changes in vitamin E status because of its low vitamin E content. Selenium is ineffective in preventing encephalomalacia, while synthetic antioxidants are partially effective. The fact that low antioxidant levels can prevent encephalomalacia in chicks but fails to avoid exudative diathesis or muscular dystrophy in the same chicks strongly suggests that preventing encephalomalacia vitamin E acts as an antioxidant.

Nutritional muscular distrophy

When a sulfur amino acid deficiency accompanies vitamin E deficiency, chicks show severe nutritional muscular dystrophy, especially in breast muscle, at about 4 weeks (Figure 4.12). Cystine effectively prevents nutritional muscular dystrophy in vitamin E-deficient chicks, and cystine is ineffective in preventing the dystrophic condition in other animals. Although vitamin E and selenium are generally highly effective in preventing exudative diathesis, selenium is only partially effective in protecting against nutritional muscular dystrophy in chicks when added in the presence of a low level of dietary vitamin E. Much larger quantities of selenium are required to reduce the incidence of dystrophy in chicks receiving a vitamin E-deficient diet low in methionine and cystine (Scott *et al.*, 1982).

Degeneration of the smooth muscle of the gizzard is the most characteristic sign of selenium deficiency in the young turkey poult. In marked contrast to the skeletal myopathy of the vitamin E-deficient chick, gizzard myopathy in the selenium- and vitamin E-deficient poult is not prevented by dietary sulfur-containing amino acids but is completely controlled by supplements of selenium (Walter and Jensen, 1963). However, the dietary level of vitamin E affects the amount of selenium required to prevent the disorder. It was necessary to use a basal diet low in methionine, vitamin E, and selenium to experimentally produce gizzard myopathy.

Nutritional muscular distrophy in ducklings is characterized by degeneration of the sarcoplasmic reticulum and mitochondria of the smooth muscle of the duodenum and gizzard. It is prevented with either vitamin E or selenium.

Other deficiency signs

Myopathies

Turkeys suffer from a pale, soft, and exudative (PSE) syndrome-like condition characterized by light-colored breast meat, losing moisture rapidly, and falling apart when sliced. Confirmation of a low vitamin E and selenium status in animals is obtained when specific deficiency diseases are associated with a lack of these nutrients. Likewise, gross lesions and histopathological examinations provide definite evidence of vitamin E and/or selenium deficiency.

Muscular damage resulting from vitamin E and/or selenium deficiencies causes leakage of intercellular contents into the blood. Thus, elevated levels of selected enzymes above normal concentrations for particular species serve as diagnostic aids in detecting tissue degeneration. Serum enzyme concentrations that follow the incidence of nutritional muscular dystrophy include serum aspartate aminotransferase, lactic dehydrogenase, creatine phosphokinase, and malic dehydrogenase. Enzyme tests are very sensitive, and an elevation of enzyme activity in serum is usually discovered before any pathological changes or clinical signs appear (Tollersrud, 1973).

Fertility and reproductive failures

Prolonged vitamin E deficiency can result in reproductive failure and permanent sterility. Rengaraj and Hong (2015) reviewed the effects of vitamin E in poultry species. Vitamin E is essential for normal hatchability (Wilson, 1997). Hatchability of eggs from vitamin E-deficient hens is reduced (NRC, 1994), and embryonic mortality may be high during the first 4 days of incubation and later stages due to circulatory failure. A vitamin E inadequacy caused an increase in embryo mortality during the last week of incubation in White Leghorns and during the second and third weeks of incubation in Rhode Island Reds (Leeson *et al.*, 1979a,b).

Vitamin E showed a protective effect against a decrease in hatchability in diets containing different levels of T-2 toxin, and dietary vitamin E concentration was positively correlated with the hatching percentage ($r = 0.74$) in the first week of an experiment (Tobias *et al.*, 1992). Supplemental vitamin E (80 mg/kg) during the laying period improved the reproductive performance of breeder pullets (Lin *et al.*, 2004). Reproduction of Taiwanese native chicken cockerels was enhanced with supplemental vitamin E (Lin *et al.*, 2005a).

The association between vitamin E deficiency and decreased fertilizing capacity of cockerel spermatozoa was established more than 20 years ago (Surai, 1999b). By acting as a lipid-soluble antioxidant within membranes and preventing reactive chain oxidation (Niki, 1993), vitamin E plays a key role in protecting spermatozoan lipids against peroxidation. For Japanese quail, higher levels of corn oil increased sperm peroxidation, which was controlled by dietary vitamin E (150 mg/kg) (Golzar Adabi *et al.*, 2011). For chickens, vitamin E tended to improve semen quality traits by increasing concentrations of spermatozoa and cell viability (Franchini *et al.*, 2001). Providing high levels of vitamin E (120 to 160 mg/kg) to hens resulted in hatched chicks with enhanced antioxidant capability and a lower oxidative stress level (Lin *et al.*, 2005a).

Vitamin E deficiency also reduces hatchability in turkey eggs (Jensen and McGinnis, 1957a,b). Turkey embryos deficient in vitamin E may have protruding eyes with a bulging cornea. In Japanese quail, embryonic survival (i.e., egg hatchability) was markedly depressed among females reared to maturity with vitamin E- and selenium-deficient diets. Many of the surviving progeny of selenium- and vitamin E-deficient females showed extreme generalized muscle weakness and prostration after hatching (Jensen, 1968). Similarly, sterility in quail was caused by vitamin E deficiency (Price, 1968). Hooda *et al.* (2007) concluded that 75 IU of vitamin E per kilogram of feed was best for male breeder quail, with lower supplementation amounts affecting testicular activity.

Ascites

Mortality in broiler chickens associated with fluid accumulation in the abdominal cavity (ascites) is the ultimate consequence of excessively high blood pressure in the pulmonary circulation, known as pulmonary hypertension syndrome. The ascites are caused by an imbalance between oxygen supply and its requirement to sustain fast growth and high feed efficiency. High levels of vitamin E and C have been shown to protect against ascites. Increased dietary vitamin E (250 mg/kg) plus selenium (Roch *et al.*, 2000a,b) or high levels of vitamins E and C (Broz and Ward, 2007) were able to reduce ascites-related mortality in broiler chickens.

Resistance to stressing conditions

The effect of vitamin E supplementation on egg production in physiologic conditions is often negligible (Hossain *et al.*, 1998). Nevertheless, vitamin E is considered a protective effect against an egg production decline (Scheideler, 1998; Puthpongsiriporn *et al.*, 2001). The depression in egg production in laying hens brought about by heat stress was partially prevented by dietary supplementation with vitamin E (Utomo *et al.*, 1994; Balnave, 2004; Balnave and Brake, 2005). Evidence was also obtained that the mechanism might involve restoring the supply in the circulation of egg yolk precursors, particularly vitellogenin.

A larger-scale experiment was carried out in which hens were housed in 2 climatically controlled houses and exposed to chronic heat stress of 32°C (90°F) from 24 to 28 or 32 to 36 weeks. They were fed diets containing 10, 125, or 500 mg of vitamin E per kilogram of feed from the point of lay and egg production characteristics, and feed intake were measured up to 40 weeks. Egg production was severely depressed by the stress, but the diet containing 500 mg/kg over both periods gave 7% better production than the diet with 10 mg/kg. The diet containing 125 mg/kg gave immediate results (Bollengier-Lee *et al.*, 1998). When flaxseed was fed to laying hens, vitamin E at 50 IU/kg significantly improved egg production compared to 27 IU/kg (Scheideler and Froning, 1996).

Safety

Compared with vitamin A and D, in both acute and chronic toxicity studies with animals, vitamin E is relatively nontoxic but not entirely devoid of undesirable effects. Hypervitaminosis E studies in rats, chicks, and humans indicate maximum tolerable levels in the range of 1,000 to 2,000 IU/kg diet (NRC, 1987). For chickens, the effects of vitamin E toxicity are depressed growth rate, reduced hematocrit, reticulocytosis, increased prothrombin time (corrected by injecting vitamin K), and reduced calcium and phosphorus in dry, fat-free bone ash (NRC, 1987).

Lowered egg production resulted when hens were fed 30,000 IU/kg vitamin E (Mori *et al.*, 2003). Previous studies indicated that extremely high dosages of vitamin E (e.g., 20,000 mg/kg feed) might affect the thyroid hormone concentrations in hatching chicks. Therefore, the chicks might be inhibited in piping the eggshell (Engelmann *et al.*, 2001).

An adverse effect of excessive vitamin E intake is its interference with vitamin D utilization, particularly when the vitamin D level is marginal. In broiler chickens, increasing dietary vitamin E up to 10,000 IU/kg diet adversely affected ($P < 0.01$) bone ash, plasma calcium, and plasma and liver vitamin A concentrations (Aburto and Britton, 1998a,b). Bartov (1997) concluded that vitamin E, at a concentration of 150 mg/kg of diet, did not aggravate a mild vitamin D deficiency. Formulating feed with the proper vitamins A, D_3, and E ratios is important.

Excess supplementation of α-tocopherol could be detrimental to the other vitamin E forms. In humans, extra supplementation of diets with α-tocopherol reduced serum concentrations of gamma and delta tocopherols (Haung and Appel, 2003; Wolf, 2006). The effects of high supplemental α-tocopherol levels on other forms of vitamin E are unknown for livestock.

Vitamin K

Chemical structure and properties

The generic term vitamin K refers to different fat-soluble compounds of the quinone group that exhibits antihemorrhagic effect. The basic molecule is a naphthoquinone (2-methyl-1,4-naphthoquinone), and the various vitamers differ in the nature and length of the side chain (Figure 4.13).

- Vitamin K_1 or phylloquinone derived from plants.
- Vitamin K_2, or menaquinone, is mainly the form produced by bacterial fermentation. Vitamin K_2 can be divided into subtypes indicated with MK-n, where n stands for the number of isoprenoid residues in the aliphatic side chain: for example, short-chain for menaquinone-4 or MK-4 or long-chain for menaquinone-7 or MK-7. MK-4 is synthesized in the liver from ingested menadione or changed to a biologically active menaquinone by intestinal microorganisms (Suttie, 2013).
- Vitamin K_3 or menadione is produced by chemical synthesis. This form, partially water-soluble and highly stable, is the form normally used in compound feeds for animal nutrition.

Vitamin K_1 is a golden yellow, viscous oil. Vitamin K_1 is slowly degraded by atmospheric oxygen but fairly rapidly destroyed by sunlight. The feed industry does not utilize vitamin K_1 due to cost and lack of a stabilized form.

Natural sources

Vitamin K_1 is present in fresh dark-green plants, e.g., alfalfa, and is abundant in pasture and green roughages, thus providing high quantities of vitamin K to grazing livestock. Light is important for its formation, and parts of plants that do not normally form chlorophyll contain little vitamin K. However, the natural loss of chlorophyll as the leaves yellow does not bring about a corresponding change in vitamin K. Cereals and oil cakes contain only small amounts

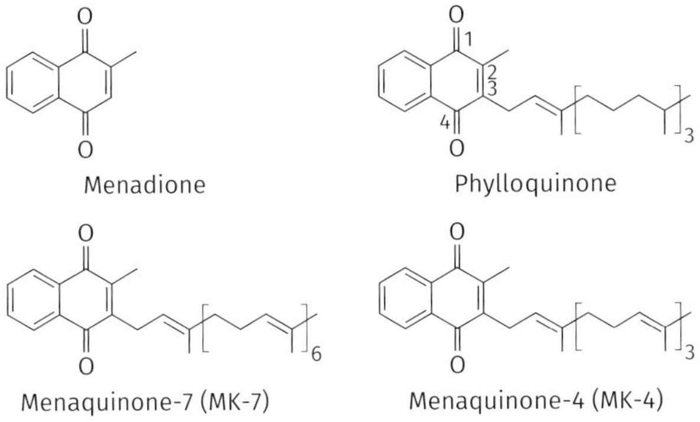

Menadione

Phylloquinone

Menaquinone-7 (MK-7)

Menaquinone-4 (MK-4)

Figure 4.13 Vitamin K structures

of vitamin K: swine poultry and feedlot animals would receive little vitamin K from diets based on grains and oilseed meals.

Vitamin K_2 can be found in all by-product feedstuffs of animal origin, including fish meal and fish liver oils, especially after they have undergone extensive bacterial putrefaction. Vitamin K_2 is also produced by the bacterial flora in birds and is especially important in providing the vitamin K requirements of most mammals. However, chickens do not receive sufficient vitamin K_2 from intestinal microbial synthesis (Scott *et al.*, 1982). In reality, the site of synthesis is the lower gut, an area of poor absorption. Thus, availability to the host is limited unless the animal practices coprophagy, in which case the synthesized vitamin K is highly available. The type of diet, independent of vitamin K concentration, will influence total K_2 synthesis.

Commercial sources

Vitamin K supplementation in animal diets is provided by the synthetic product, namely vitamin K_3, in the form of various bisulfite complexes, which are more stable and potent (Huyghebaert, 1991). The major use of vitamin K in the animal industry is in poultry (Suttie, 2013). The various products used by the feed industry and their respective content in menadione are listed in Table 4.1.

Metabolism

Absorption and transport

Like all fat-soluble vitamins, vitamin K is absorbed in association with dietary fats and requires the presence of bile salts and pancreatic juice for adequate uptake from the alimentary tract. The absorption of vitamin K depends on its incorporation into mixed micelles, and the optimal formation of these micellar structures requires the presence of both bile and pancreatic juice. Thus, any malfunction of the fat absorption mechanism (e.g., biliary obstruction, malabsorption syndrome) reduces the availability of vitamin K (Ferland, 2006). Unlike phylloquinone and the menaquinones, menadione salts, relatively water-soluble, are absorbed satisfactorily from low-fat diets. Male animals are more susceptible to dietary vitamin K deprivation than females, apparently due to a stimulation of phylloquinone absorption by estrogens, and the administration of estrogens increases absorption in both male and female animals (Jolly *et al.*, 1977; Suttie, 2013).

In poultry, portal circulation is the major transport route of absorbed phylloquinone from the intestine. The absorption of various forms differs significantly. An energy-dependent process absorbs ingested phylloquinone from the proximal portion of the small intestine (Hollander, 1973). Shearer *et al.* (1970) demonstrated the association of phylloquinone with serum lipoproteins, but little is known of the existence of specific carrier proteins.

Table 4.1 Menadione salts used for diet supplementation

Vitamin K_3 salt	Menadione (K_3) concentration (%)	Amount of menadione salt to provide 1 g of menadione (K_3) (g)
Menadione sodium bisulfite (MSB)	50	2
Menadione dimethylpyrimidinol bisulfite (MPB)	45.4	2.2
Menadione nicotinamide bisulfite (MNB)	43	2.3
Menadione sodium bisulfite complex (MSBC)	33	3

In contrast to the active transport of phylloquinone, menaquinone is absorbed from the small intestine by a passive noncarrier-mediated process. Menadione can be absorbed from both the small intestine and the colon by a passive process and transformed into a biologically active form. The measured efficiency of vitamin K absorption ranges from 10 to 70%, depending on the form of the vitamin administered. Some reports have indicated that menadione is completely absorbed, whereas phylloquinone is absorbed only at a rate of 50%. The complete absorption of menadione may be due to the aqueous solubility of the menadione salts.

Storage and excretion

Griminger and Brubacher (1966) showed that a major portion of the phylloquinone and menaquinones fed to chicks were retained intact in the liver. In other organs, menaquinones exceed phylloquinone. As such, phylloquinone had equally as good biological activity upon prothrombin synthesis as menaquinone found in the chick's liver following the feeding of menadione. Therefore, MK-4 (menaquinone-4) is most likely produced if menadione is fed or if the intestinal microorganisms degrade the dietary K_1 or K_2 to menadione. However, the formation of MK-4 is not required for the metabolic activity of vitamin K since phylloquinone is equally active in synthesizing the vitamin K-dependent, blood-clotting proteins (Scott *et al.*, 1982).

Menadione is widely distributed in all tissues and is very rapidly excreted. Although phylloquinone is quickly concentrated in the liver, it does not have a long retention time in this organ (Thierry *et al.*, 1970). The inability to rapidly develop a vitamin K deficiency in most species results from the difficulty in preventing the absorption of the vitamin from the diet or intestinal synthesis rather than from significant storage of the vitamin.

Rats were found to excrete about 60% of ingested phylloquinone in the feces within 24 hours of ingestion, but only 11% of ingested menadione (Griminger and Donis, 1960; Griminger, 1984). However, 38% of ingested menadione and only a small amount of phylloquinone were excreted via the kidneys during the same period. The conclusion was that although menadione is well absorbed, it is poorly retained in the liver, while the opposite is true for phylloquinone. Normal human subjects were found to excrete less than 20% of a large (1 mg) dose of phylloquinone in feces. Still, as much as 70 to 80% of the ingested phylloquinone was excreted unaltered in the feces of patients with impaired fat absorption caused by pancreatic insufficiency or adult celiac disease. (Suttie, 2013).

Some breakdown products of vitamin K are excreted in the urine. One of the main excretory products is a chain-shortened and oxidized derivative of vitamin K, which forms γ-lactone and is probably excreted as a glucuronide (Suttie, 2013).

Biochemical functions

The principal function of vitamin K is controlling the blood coagulation period since it activates plasmatic prothrombin. A complex series of reactions are involved in converting circulating fibrinogen into a fibrin clot. Many proteins with different metabolic functions participating in the "cascade" of blood coagulation require vitamin K for their biosynthesis (Figure 4.14).

Vitamin K is required for the synthesis of the active form of prothrombin (Factor II) and other plasma clotting factors, namely Factor VII (proconvertin), Factor IX (Christmas factor), and Factor X (Stuart–Prower factor). These factors are synthesized as inactive precursors (zymogens), and vitamin K is necessary for their conversion into biologically active proteins (Suttie and Jackson, 1977). Thus, in the case of vitamin K deficiency, blood coagulation time increases because of the lack of conversion of these factors. In deficiency, vitamin K administration produces a prompt response in 4 to 6 hours, and in the absence of the liver, this response does not occur (Suttie, 2013).

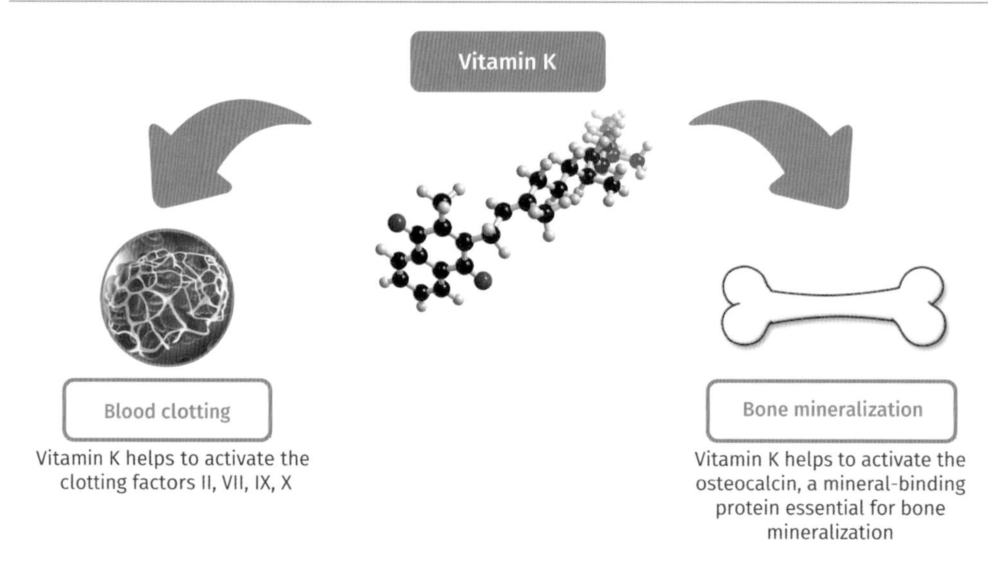
Vitamin K
Blood clotting
Vitamin K helps to activate the clotting factors II, VII, IX, X
Bone mineralization
Vitamin K helps to activate the osteocalcin, a mineral-binding protein essential for bone mineralization

Figure 4.14 Vitamin K functions

Vitamin K-dependent proteins can be identified by γ-carboxyglutamic acid residues (Gla), an amino acid common to all vitamin K proteins. The discovery of this new amino acid clarified the role of vitamin K in blood coagulation and led to the discovery of additional vitamin K-dependent proteins (e.g., bone proteins) (Ferland, 2006; Suttie, 2013).

Bleeding disorders result from an inability of a liver microsomal enzyme, currently called the vitamin K-dependent carboxylase (Esmon *et al.*, 1975), to carry out the normal post-translational conversion of specific glutamyl residues in the vitamin K-dependent plasma proteins to γ-carboxyglutamyl residues (Nelsestuen *et al.*, 1974). Therefore, the result of low vitamin K serves as a cofactor as this enzyme decreases thrombin generation.

Carboxylation allows prothrombin and the other procoagulant proteins to participate in a specific protein-calcium phospholipid interaction necessary for their biological role (Suttie and Jackson, 1977; Suttie, 2013). Four other vitamin K-dependent proteins have also been identified in plasma: proteins C, S, Z, and M. Protein C and protein S play an anticoagulant rather than a procoagulant role in normal hemostasis (Suttie and Olson, 1990). Protein C inhibits coagulation and, stimulated by protein S, promotes fibrinolysis. Also, a protein C-S complex can partially hydrolyze the activated factors V and VIII and thus inactivate them. Protein S can also regulate bone turnover (Binkley and Suttie, 1995). The function of proteins M and Z is unclear, and protein Z has been shown to have an anticoagulant role under some conditions (Suttie, 2013).

The blood-clotting mechanism can be stimulated by either an intrinsic system, in which all the factors are in the plasma, or an extrinsic system. In the extrinsic coagulation system, tissue thromboplastin converts prothrombin in the blood to thrombin in the presence of various elements and calcium. The enzyme thrombin facilitates the conversion of the soluble fibrinogen into insoluble fibrin. Fibrin polymerizes into strands and enmeshes the formed elements of the blood, especially the red blood cells, to create the blood clot (Griminger, 1984). The final active component in both the intrinsic and extrinsic systems appears to activate the Stuart factor, which leads to prothrombin activation.

Vitamin K-dependent reactions are present in most tissues, not just blood, and a reasonably large number of proteins are subjected to this post-translational carboxylation of specific glutamate residues to γ-carboxyglutamate residues (Vermeer, 1986). Atherocalcin is a vitamin

K-dependent protein in atherosclerotic tissue. A vitamin K-dependent carboxylase system in the skin is related to calcium metabolism (de Boer-van den Berg *et al.*, 1986).

Two of the best-characterized vitamin K-dependent proteins not involved in hemostasis are osteocalcin or bone Gla protein and matrix Gla protein, which were initially discovered in bone. Osteocalcin is a protein containing 3 Gla residues that give the protein its mineral-binding properties. Osteocalcin appears in embryonic chick bone and rat bone matrix at the beginning of mineralization of the bone (Gallop *et al.*, 1980). It accounts for 15% to 20% of the non-collagen protein in the bone of most vertebrates and is one of the most abundant proteins in the body.

Osteocalcin is produced by osteoblasts through synthesis controlled by 1,25-dihydroxy vitamin D. About 20% of the newly synthesized protein is released into the circulation and can be used to measure bone formation. As is true for other non-blood vitamin K-dependent proteins, the physiological role of osteocalcin remains largely unknown. However, reduced osteocalcin content of cortical bone (Vanderschueren *et al.*, 1990) and alteration of osteocalcin distribution within osteons (Ingram *et al.*, 1994) are associated with aging. It remains unknown whether any of these findings are related to the age-related increased risk of fracture.

Osteocalcin may play a role in the control of bone remodeling because it has been reported to be a chemoattractant for monocytes, the precursors of osteoclasts. Serum osteocalcin is a good predictor of bone turnover in pigs (Carter *et al.*, 1996). This suggests a possible role for osteocalcin in bone resorption (Binkley and Suttie, 1995; Suttie, 2013). However, in Lavelle *et al.*'s (1994) study, no functional deficiencies were observed in the bone metabolism of breeders or their progeny with vitamin K levels below the minimum requirements. The quantity of vitamin K transferred to the egg depends on the amount of vitamin K ingested by the breeder (Sebrell and Harris, 1971). When supplementation levels in the breeder rations are inadequate; eggs are produced with low vitamin K content, accompanied by high levels of embryonic mortality due to hemorrhagic processes during the final period of incubation (Nelson and Norris, 1960). Hatched chicks show a longer coagulation period than normal, and trauma can provoke fatal hemorrhages (Lavelle *et al.*, 1994).

Several reports have indicated that warfarin, a vitamin K antagonist, alters the functional properties of bone particles prepared from rats. However, vitamin K-deficient chick embryos could mobilize sufficient quantities of calcium for normal skeletal development, although they exhibited a severe reduction in blood clotting and bone osteocalcin concentration (Lavelle *et al.*, 1994).

Several observations in humans indicate that vitamin K could be involved in the pathogenesis of bone mineral loss (Binkley and Suttie, 1995; Cashman and O'Connor, 2008): (1) low blood vitamin K in patients with bone fractures; (2) concentration of circulating under γ-carboxylated osteocalcin associated with age, low bone mineral density, and hip fracture risk; (3) anticoagulant therapy associated with decreased bone density, and (4) decreased bone loss and calcium excretion with vitamin K supplementation.

To date, both *in vitro* and *in vivo* studies suggest a role of vitamin K in regulating multiple enzymes involved in sphingolipid metabolism within the myelin-rich regions in the brain (Denisova and Booth, 2005). The brain is enriched with sphingolipids, which are important membrane constituents and major lipid signaling molecules that have a role in motor and cognitive behavior.

Nutritional assessment

The vitamin K family comprises K_1 (phylloquinone from plants) and K_2 (menaquinone from carnivorous and bacterial sources). Moreover, we must include the other vitamers indicated with MK-n, e.g., MK-4 and MK-7. The various forms have very different pharmacokinetics, with a half-life of 1–2 hours for MK-4 and K_1 and 3 days or more for MK-7 and longer chain MKs (Schurgers and Vermeer, 2002).

Vitamin K status may be assessed by measuring the circulating concentration of each relevant vitamers or by measuring the circulating concentration of uncarboxylated Gla-proteins. Direct measurement of circulating K-vitamers is generally accomplished by reversed-phase HPLC or ultra-performance liquid chromatography with fluorescence or mass spectrometric detection. However, many menaquinones are not available as reference compounds. The concentration in circulation reflects recent dietary exposure rather than true status concentrations (Höller *et al.*, 2018). ELISA-based methods for measuring uncarboxylated Gla-proteins are currently the most reliable for assessing vitamin K status. These tests can determine tissue-specific proteins such as uncarboxylated osteocalcin (ucOC) for bone.

Deficiency signs

The major clinical sign of vitamin K deficiency in all species is impairment of blood coagulation. Other clinical symptoms include low prothrombin levels, increased clotting time, and hemorrhaging. In its most severe form, a lack of vitamin K will cause subcutaneous and internal hemorrhages, which can be fatal. Vitamin K deficiency can result from dietary deficiency, lack of microbial synthesis within the gut, inadequate intestinal absorption, or inability of the liver to use the available vitamin K. In addition, a deficiency can be caused by the ingestion of vitamin K antagonists like dicumarol, or by feeding sulfonamides (in monogastric species) at levels sufficient to inhibit the intestinal synthesis of vitamin K. Supplementation vitamin K will overcome the anticoagulation effect of dicumarol.

Clinical signs of vitamin K deficiency are similar in all poultry species, with most research completed with newly hatched chicks and growing broilers. A deficiency of vitamin K causes a reduction in the prothrombin content of the blood and, in the chick, may reduce the quantity in the plasma to less than 2% of normal. Since the prothrombin content of the blood of normal, newly hatched chicks is only about 40% of that of adult birds, very young chicks are readily affected by a deficiency of vitamin K. A carryover from the parent hen to the chick has been demonstrated (Sebrell and Harris, 1971). Therefore, breeder hen diets should be supplemented with vitamin K to ensure good chick health. Laying hens fed a diet deficient in vitamin K produce eggs low in this vitamin, and when the eggs are incubated, the chicks produced have low reserves and a prolonged clotting time.

The adverse effects on blood clotting are not apparent until after hatching, when hemorrhaging and mortality may occur should trauma be encountered. Consequently, the chicks may bleed to death from an injury as slight as that caused by debeaking or wing banding (Figure 4.15).

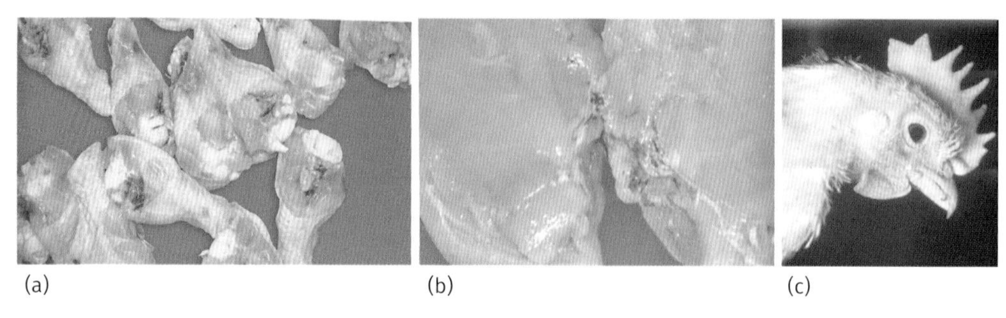

Figure 4.15 Vitamin K deficiency (a and b) hemorrhaging; (c) anemic-looking comb and wattles of deficient fowl (source: Dr. Brubacher, DSM Kaiseraugst)

In very young chicks deficient in vitamin K, blood coagulation time begins to increase after 5–10 days, with clinical signs occurring most frequently in chicks 2–3 weeks after consuming a vitamin K-deficient diet. Hemorrhages often happen in any part of the body, spontaneously or due to an injury or bruise. Postmortem examination usually reveals accumulations of blood in various parts of the body; sometimes, there are petechial hemorrhages in the liver. Almost invariably, there is the erosion of the gizzard lining.

Even though inadequate dietary vitamin K alters bone osteocalcin, signs associated with the skeletal system are not as apparent as blood-clotting problems. Although blood clotting was impaired and there was a reduction in bone γ-carboxyglutamic acid concentrations, vitamin K deficiency did not functionally impair the skeletal metabolism of laying hens or their progeny (Lavelle *et al.*, 1994). Vitamin K-dependent γ-carboxylated proteins have been identified as ligands for a unique family of receptor tyrosine kinases with transforming ability. The involvement of vitamin K metabolism and function in 2 well-characterized birth defects, warfarin embryopathy and vitamin K epoxide reductase deficiency, suggests that developmental signals from vitamin K-dependent pathways may be required for normal embryogenesis (Saxena *et al.*, 1997).

Borderline deficiencies of vitamin K often cause small hemorrhagic blemishes on the breast, legs, and wings, the abdominal cavity, and the intestine's surface. Chicks show anemia that, in part, may be caused by blood loss but also by the development of hypoplastic bone marrow. Even a borderline deficiency of vitamin K is of economic importance in broiler production because the hemorrhagic areas in the legs or throughout the body may result in a high percentage of condemnations during the inspection at the processing plant. A condition manifested by numerous small hemorrhages scattered throughout all muscle tissues has been reported frequently in the commercial broiler industry for many years (Almquist, 1978; Kranen *et al.*, 2000) (Figure 4.15a and b).

Several considerations influence the likelihood of a vitamin K deficiency in poultry, including dietary sources of the vitamin, level of vitamin K in the maternal diet, intestinal synthesis, coprophagy, presence of sulfa drugs, and other non-nutrients in the diet, and disease conditions. Chicks suffering from coccidiosis, which causes severe damage along the intestinal tract, may bleed excessively or fatally.

When sulfaquinoxaline or certain other drugs are present in the feed or in the drinking water or when coccidiosis is being treated, supplementary vitamin K is needed at higher levels, up to 10 times more is required than in the absence of these drugs (Scott *et al.*, 1982). According to Esmail (2002), in the case of coccidiosis, vitamin K requirements rise to 8 mg/kg, which is several times higher than that indicated by the NRC.

Antimicrobial agents suppress intestinal bacteria that synthesize vitamin K (Bains, 1999), and in their presence, the bird may be entirely dependent on dietary vitamin K (NRC, 1994). Arsenilic acid increases the need for dietary vitamin K in both breeder and chick diets.

In poultry, little intestinal synthesis occurs because of the short digestive tract. The young chicken's large intestine or colon, a major area of bacterial activity, comprises less than 6% of the total length of the intestinal tract and just around 7% in adult birds (Griminger, 1984).

Moreover, poultry cannot utilize the vitamin K synthesized by intestinal flora (microbiota) because the synthesis is too close to the distal end of the intestinal tract to permit significant absorption. The rapid rate of food passage through the digestive tract may also influence vitamin K synthesis in poultry. The passage time for chickens would be approximately 3–4 hours compared to 15 hours or more in pigs and other species (Griminger, 1984). Mycotoxins are also antagonists that may cause vitamin K deficiency: for example, its anticoagulant action is impaired by aflatoxins (Daghir, 1996).

Safety

The toxic effects of the vitamin K family are manifested mainly as hematologic and circulatory derangements. Not only is species variation encountered, but profound differences are observed in the ability of the various vitamin K compounds to evoke a toxic response (Barash, 1978).

Vitamin K_1 and Vitamin K_2 are nontoxic at very high dosage levels. The synthetic menadione compounds have shown toxic effects when fed to humans, rabbits, dogs, and mice in excessive amounts. However, the toxic dietary level of menadione is at least 1,000 times the dietary requirement (NRC, 1994).

There is somewhat more information on the interaction of vitamin K with other fat-soluble vitamins. Vitamin K activity is impaired by excessive levels of vitamins A (up to 100,000 IU/kg) and E (4,000 mg/kg), with repercussions on coagulation time (3 times longer) and broiler mortality (Abawi and Sullivan, 1989; Frank *et al.*, 1997).

Menadione compounds can safely be used at low levels to prevent the development of a deficiency but should not be used as a pharmacologic treatment for a hemorrhagic condition. In studies with chicks, the major effect of toxic levels of menadione was hemolytic anemia, with a high mortality rate but at dosage levels are several orders of magnitude greater than the daily requirement of the vitamin (NRC, 1994).

WATER-SOLUBLE VITAMINS

Among the water-soluble vitamins are the B complex vitamins plus choline and vitamin C. Most of them either cannot be synthesized by the birds or can but not in sufficient quantities to cover their requirements in different physiological situations. Some can be supplied through the metabolism of the microbiota of the intestinal tract. Still, since absorption is limited to the posterior sections of the digestive tract, this process is not very efficient and depends on subsequent coprophagy. Generally, they are not stored in significant quantities in the bird (except vitamin B_{12}), which prevents toxicity problems but requires regular supplementation in the ration.

Vitamin B_1 (thiamine)

Chemical structure and properties

Thiamine consists of a molecule of pyrimidine and a molecule of thiazole linked by a methylene bridge and contains both nitrogen and sulfur atoms (Figure 4.16). Thiamine is isolated in pure form as white, crystalline thiamine hydrochloride. The vitamin has a characteristic sulfurous odor and a slightly bitter taste (Bettendorff, 2013).

Thiamine is mainly found in the form of chloride hydrochloride ($C_{12}H_{17}N_4OSCl.HCl$, molecular mass 337.27 g mol^{-1}) that decomposes at 198°C (Bettendorff, 2013). Thiamine hydrochloride is a hydrophilic molecule: it can form a hydrate even under normal atmospheric conditions by absorbing nearly 1 mole of water and has a solubility of ~1 g/ml water at 25°C. Under ordinary conditions, thiamine hydrochloride is more hygroscopic than mononitrate salt. However, both products should be kept in sealed containers.

Thiamine is sparingly soluble in alcohol and insoluble in fat solvents. It is very sensitive to alkali, in which the thiazole ring opens at room temperature when the pH is above 7. In a dry state, thiamine is stable at 100°C for several hours, but moisture greatly accelerates destruction, and thus it is much less stable to heat in fresh than in dry foods. It is destroyed by ultraviolet light.

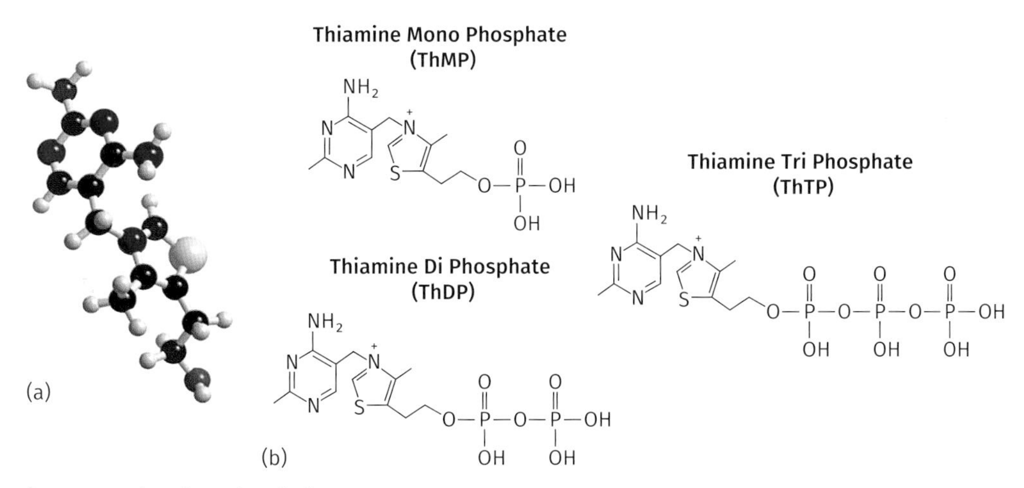

Figure 4.16 Vitamin B_1 chemical structures

Natural sources

Brewer's yeast is the richest known natural source of thiamine. Cereal grains and their by-products, soybean meal, cottonseed meal, and peanut meal, are relatively rich sources of thiamine. Since the vitamin is present primarily in the germ and seed coats, by-products containing the latter are richer than the whole kernel, while highly milled flour is very deficient. In humans, beriberi was prevalent in Orient countries, where polished rice is the dietary staple. Rice may have 5 mg/kg of thiamine, but the content is much lower for polished rice (0.3 mg/kg) and higher for rice bran (23 mg/kg) (Marks, 1975). Wheat germ ranks next to yeast in thiamine concentration. The level of thiamine in grain rises as the protein level rises: depending on species, strain, and use of nitrogenous fertilizers (Bettendorff, 2013).

Nevertheless, the frequent presence of antagonists, such as mycotoxins, and high susceptibility to inactivation by heat must be considered. Reddy and Pushpamma (1986) studied the effects of 1 year of storage and insect infestation on the thiamine content of feeds. Thiamine losses were high in several varieties of sorghum and pigeon pea (40–70%) and lower in rice and chickpea (10–40%). Insect infestation caused the further loss. Since thiamine is water-soluble and unstable in heat, large losses may result during certain feed manufacturing processes (McDowell, 2000a; Bettendorff, 2013).

Commercial sources

Thiamine sources available for addition to feed are the thiamine chloride hydrochloride (337.28 g/mol; 98%) and thiamine mononitrate (327.36 g/mol; 98%) salts (Figure 4.17). Both are fine granular, white to pale-yellow powders. Because of its lower solubility in water, the mononitrate salt has somewhat better stability characteristics in dry products than the hydrochloride (Bettendorff, 2013). Thiamine mononitrate is prepared from thiamine hydrochloride by dissolving the hydrochloride salt in a mildly alkaline solution, followed by precipitation of the nitrate half-salt with a stoichiometric amount of nitric acid.

Metabolism

Absorption and transport

Thiamine appears to be readily digested and released from naturally occurring sources. A precondition for normal thiamine absorption is sufficient stomach hydrochloric acid production.

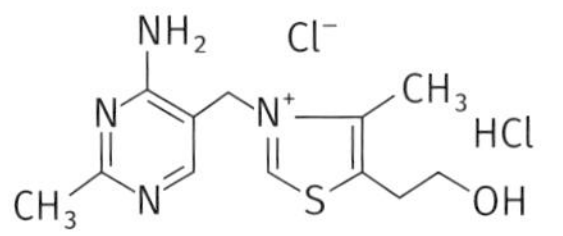

Figure 4.17 Vitamin B_1 forms used in animal nutrition

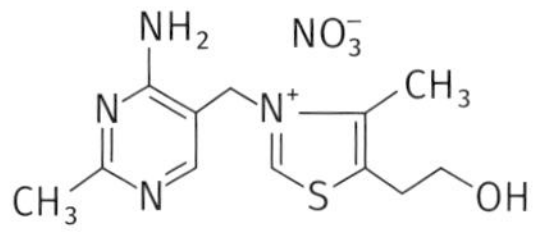

Phosphoric acid esters of thiamine are split in the intestine. The free thiamine formed is soluble in water and easily absorbed, especially in the jejunum. The mechanism of thiamine absorption is not yet fully understood, but active transport and simple diffusion are apparently involved. There is active sodium-dependent transport of thiamine at low concentrations against the electrochemical potential, whereas, at high concentrations, it diffuses passively through the intestinal wall.

Thiamine synthesized by the gut microflora in the cecum, or large intestine, is largely unavailable to animals except by coprophagy. Specific proteins (transporters and carriers) in the cell membrane have binding sites for thiamine, allowing it to be solubilized within the cell membrane. This permits the vitamin to pass through the membrane and ultimately reach the aqueous environment on the other side (Rose, 1990; Bates, 2006). Absorbed thiamine is transported via the portal vein to the liver with the carrier plasma protein. Thiamine is efficiently transferred to the embryo.

Thiamine phosphorylation can occur in most tissues, particularly in the liver. Almost 80% of thiamine in animals is phosphorylated in the liver under the action of ATP to form the metabolically active enzyme form thiamine pyrophosphate (TPP, also named diphosphate or cocarboxylase). Of total body thiamine, about 80% is TPP, about 10% is thiamine triphosphate (TTP), and the remainder is thiamine monophosphate (TMP) and free thiamine.

Storage and excretion

Although thiamine is readily absorbed and transported to cells throughout the body, it is one of the most poorly stored vitamins. Most mammals on a thiamine-deficient diet will exhaust their body stores within 1–2 weeks (Ensminger *et al.*, 1983). The thiamine content in individual organs varies considerably, and the vitamin is preferentially retained in organs with high metabolic activity. Thiamine is contained in the greatest quantities in major organs such as the liver, heart, brain, and kidneys during deficiencies. Although liver and kidney tissues have the highest thiamine concentrations, approximately 50% of the total thiamine body stores are in muscle tissue (Tanphaichair, 1976).

Thiamine intakes above current needs are rapidly excreted. Absorbed thiamine is passed in urine and feces, with small quantities excreted in sweat. Fecal thiamine may originate from feed, synthesis by microorganisms, or endogenous sources (i.e., via bile or excretion through the mucosa of the large intestine). When thiamine is administered in large doses, urinary excretion reaches saturation, and the fecal concentration increases considerably (Bräunlich and Zintzen, 1976).

Biochemical functions

Thiamine is one of the enzymes critical in the metabolism of lysine, branched-chain amino acids, carbohydrates, and lipogenesis (Bettendorff, 2013). The main functions of thiamine are illustrated in Figure 4.18. Primarily, thiamine is important in carbohydrate and energy metabolism, especially in the heart and nervous system. For this reason, thiamine recommendations increase when the main energy source supplied by the feed is carbohydrates.

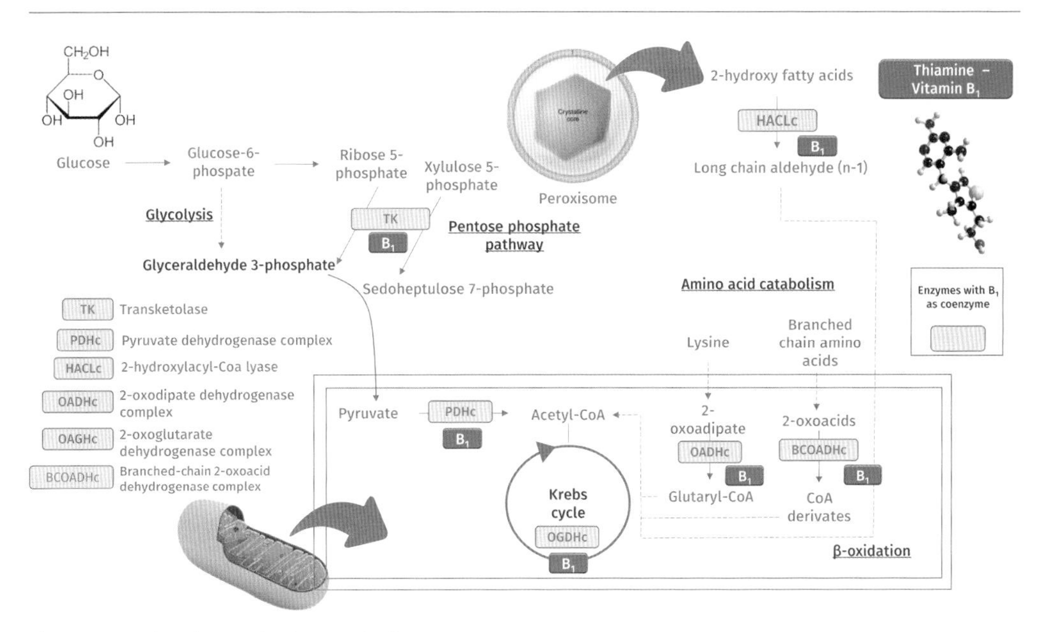

Figure 4.18 Vitamin B_1 roles in metabolism

The TPP is the active thiamine derivative involved in the tricarboxylic acid cycle (TCA, citric acid, or Krebs cycle). Thiamine is the coenzyme for all enzymatic decarboxylations of α-keto acids. Thus, it functions in the oxidative decarboxylation of pyruvate to acetate, which in turn is combined with coenzyme A (CoA) for entrance into the TCA cycle. Thiamine is essential in 2 oxidative decarboxylation reactions in the TCA cycle in cell mitochondria and one in the cytoplasm of the cells.

Decarboxylation in the TCA cycle removes carbon dioxide, and the substrate is converted into the compound having the next lower number of carbon atoms:

1 pyruvate –> acetyl-CoA + CO_2
2 α-ketoglutaric acid –> succinyl-CoA + CO_2.

These reactions are essential for the utilization of carbohydrates to provide energy. Vitamins B_2 (riboflavin), pantothenic acid, and niacin are also involved with thiamine in this biochemical process. Thiamine plays a very important role in glucose metabolism. TPP is a coenzyme in the transketolase reaction that is part of the direct oxidative pathway (pentose phosphate cycle) of glucose metabolism in the liver, brain, adrenal cortex, and kidney cell cytoplasm, but not skeletal muscle. The pentose phosphate cycle is the only mechanism known for ribose synthesis needed for nucleotide formation. This cycle also reduces nicotinamide adenine dinucleotide phosphate (NADPH), essential for lowering intermediates from carbohydrate metabolism during fatty acid synthesis (Bettendorff, 2013).

Thiamine is, together with vitamin B_6 (pyridoxine) and B_{12} (cobalamine), one of the commonly called "neurotropic" B vitamins, playing special and essential roles both in the central nervous system (CNS) and the peripheral nervous system (PNS) (Muralt, 1962; Cooper *et al.*, 1963; Calderón-Ospina and Nava-Mesa, 2020). The maintenance of nerve membrane function and the synthesis of myelin and several types of neurotransmitters (e.g., acetylcholine, serotonin, and amino acids) are essential in transmitting nervous impulses. Another thiamine function in the transmission of nervous impulses is due to its participation in the passive transport of sodium (Na^+) to excitable membranes, which is important for the transmission of impulses at the membrane of ganglionic cells. However, thiamine's role in energy metabolism explains a significant part of its activity in the nervous system by providing energy to nerve cells.

Nutritional assessment

Thiamine nutritional status is typically determined by measuring thiamine-dependent erythrocyte transketolase activity (ETKA) or thiamine (free or phosphorylated) concentrations. The ETKA assay is the most acceptable for a functional assessment of thiamine deficiencies by measuring the relative increase of erythrocyte transketolase activity in response to *in vitro* addition of TDP. However, analytical variability is reported due to standardization and sample stability issues (Sauberlich, 1999; Höller *et al.*, 2018). HPLC-based methods to quantify free thiamine and the phosphorylated form require further improvements.

Deficiency signs

The detailed pathophysiology and biochemistry of thiamine deficiency-induced processes in the brain have been studied in human subjects, animal models, and cultured cells (Gibson and Zhang, 2002; Martin *et al.*, 2003; Ke and Gibson, 2004). Neurodegeneration becomes apparent, initially, as a reversible lesion and later irreversibly in specific areas of the brain, notably the submedial thalamic nucleus and parts of the cerebellum, especially the superior cerebellar vermis (Bates, 2006; Bettendorff, 2013). The classic pathological syndrome or disease caused by thiamine deficiency in humans is called beriberi. It involves both nervous and circulatory systems with symptoms that are also observed in various animal species. This is explained by the fact that the brain satisfies its energy requirement chiefly by the degradation of glucose and is therefore dependent on biochemical reactions in which thiamine plays a key role.

Poultry is more susceptible to neuromuscular effects of thiamine deficiency than most mammals. In chickens and turkeys, there is a loss of appetite, emaciation, impairment of digestion, a general weakness, opisthotonos or stargazing, and frequent convulsions, with polyneuritis as an extreme clinical sign.

Of all nutrients, a thiamine deficiency has the most marked effect on appetite. Animals consuming a low-thiamine diet soon show severe anorexia, lose all interest in food, and will not resume eating unless given thiamine. Thiamine must be force-fed or injected to induce animals to continue eating if the deficiency is severe. Paralysis of the crop, manifested as delayed emptying, accompanies the general neuropathy of experimental thiamine deficiency in chicks (Naidoo, 1956).

Early signs of thiamine deficiency are lethargy and head tremors. Chicks fed very low thiamine (0.4 mg/kg) survived for only 7–10 days. Apparently, only a few days after, the supply of thiamine in the yolk sac was exhausted (Gries and Scott, 1972). Some chicks develop nervous disorders, apathy, and tremor as early as the third or fourth day of life. These signs increased in severity up to ataxia, inability to stand, and high-grade opisthotonos or twisting of the neck. The severity of the spasms increased when the chicks were frightened. Chicks that showed these high-grade nervous disorders died within a few hours.

The classic disease of polyneuritis in birds represents a late stage of thiamine deficiency resulting from peripheral neuritis, perhaps caused by an accumulation of intermediates of carbohydrate metabolism. In mature chickens, polyneuritis (Figure 4.19) is observed approximately 3 weeks after being fed a thiamine-deficient diet (Scott *et al.*, 1982). As the deficiency progresses, paralysis of the muscles occurs, beginning with the flexors of the toes and moving upward, affecting the extensor muscles of the legs, wings, and neck. The chicken sits on its

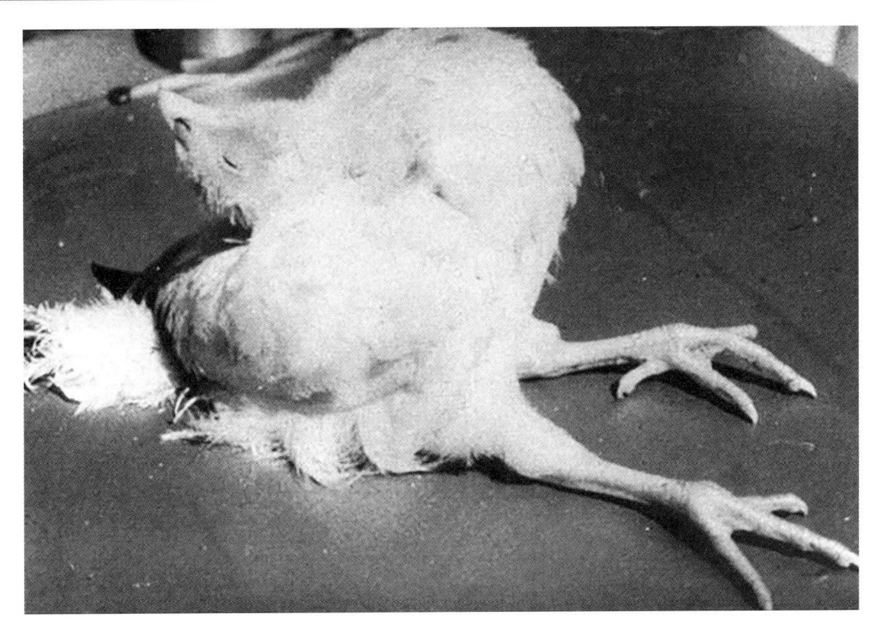

Figure 4.19 Thiamine deficiency: general weakness, polyneuritis paralysis, and opisthotonos (head retraction) (source: Dr. Paul Hibrich, Hanover)

flexed legs and draws back the head in stargazing (opisthotonos) position. Retraction of the head is due to paralysis of the anterior neck muscles. At this stage, the chicken soon loses the ability to stand or sit upright and falls to the floor, where it may lie with the head still retracted.

For chickens with thiamine deficiency, body temperature drops to as low as 36°C (97°F), and respiratory rate progressively decreases (Scott *et al.*, 1982). There is adrenal gland hypertrophy that apparently results in tissue edema, particularly in the skin. Atrophy of genital organs also occurs in chickens with chronic thiamine deficiency, which is more pronounced in the testes than in the ovaries.

According to dietary content, the hen transfers thiamine to the egg (Polin *et al.*, 1963; NRC, 1994; Pérez-Vendrell *et al.*, 2003). Inadequate thiamine to the breeder flock will result in high mortality of embryos before hatching, and chicks that do hatch exhibit polyneuritis (Polin *et al.*, 1962; Charles *et al.*, 1972; Bettendorff, 2013). Deficient birds can rapidly detect and discriminate against feeds that do not provide the vitamin (Hughes and Wood-Gush, 1971) and are high in carbohydrate content (Thornton and Shutze, 1960).

In turkeys, thiamine deficiency also resulted in tissue alteration of amino acids, decreased concentration of epinephrine and ATP, and increased serotonin in the brain of birds (Remus and Firman, 1989, 1990, 1991a,b). In the thiamine-deficient turkey, the onset of anorexia was rapid; by day 4, deficient birds had significantly lower feed consumption (Remus and Firman, 1990). In addition to neurological disease conditions, the other main group of disorders involves cardiovascular damage, and cardiac abnormalities have also been reported in acutely thiamine-deficient chicks (Sturkie *et al.*, 1954). The heart shows a slight degree of atrophy.

Acutely deficient pigeons developed vomiting, emaciation, leg weakness, and opisthotonos, the last of which appeared between days 7 and 12 after beginning the thiamine-free diet (Swank, 1940). Chronic deficiency due to a diet partially inadequate in thiamine resulted in leg weakness but no opisthotonos. Evidence of cardiac failure was also noted. The lesions produced in thiamine-deficient pigeons are reported to be identical to those found in Wernicke's polio encephalitis in humans (Lofland *et al.*, 1963).

Pheasant mycotoxin-induced polyneuritis was eliminated within hours after intraperitoneal injection of thiamine (Cook, 1990). Cereals and soy have a high thiamine content and are thus unlikely to lead to a deficiency: however, on occasion, deficiencies have been confirmed in the field, with symptoms such as anorexia, polyneuritis, and foot problems.

Vitamin B_1 requirements increase if the diet is high in carbohydrates, so the body's reserves are rapidly exhausted if there is a thiamine deficiency. Substances with anti-thiamine activity, hence causing a deficiency, are fairly common and include structurally similar antagonists and structure-altering antagonists. For example, fish meal contains thiaminases. The synthetic compounds pyrithiamin, oxythiamin, and amprolium (an anticoccidial) are structurally similar antagonists. Their mode of action is competitive inhibition, interfering with thiamine at different points in metabolism. Pyrithiamin blocks the esterification of thiamine with phosphoric acid, inhibiting the thiamine coenzyme cocarboxylase. Oxythiamin competitively inhibits thiamine's binding to the carboxylase complex, blocking important metabolic reactions. The coccidiostat amprolium inhibits the intestinal absorption of thiamine and blocks phosphorylation of the vitamin (McDowell, 2000a). Thiaminase activity destroys thiamine by altering the structure of the vitamin (Bettendorff, 2013).

In premixes that include choline and trace minerals, thiamine stability is relatively low, and at ambient temperature, its content may be reduced by up to 50%. This occurs to a greater extent in feed contaminated by mycotoxin-producing fungi such as *Aspergillus* and *Fusarium*, where the B_1 concentration can drop by a factor of up to 10 (Nagaraj *et al.*, 1994). Thiamine content was reduced from 43 to 50% for 2 cultivars of wheat infested with *Aspergillus flavus* compared to the uncontaminated wheat (Kao and Robinson, 1973).

Safety

Thiamine in large amounts orally is not generally toxic; the same is true of parenteral doses (NRC, 1987). In chickens, it takes some 700 times the requirement level of thiamine to induce toxicity. Signs of toxicity are blockage of nerve transmissions and labored breathing, with death usually occurring due to respiratory failure.

Vitamin B_2 (riboflavin)

Chemical structure and properties

Riboflavin exists in 3 forms in nature: free dinucleotide riboflavin and the 2 coenzyme derivatives, flavin mononucleotide (FMN) and flavin adenine dinucleotide (FAD) (Pinto and Rivlin, 2013). Riboflavin is an odorless, bitter, orange-yellow compound that melts at about 280°C. The molecular structure of riboflavin is shown in Figure 4.20.

Riboflavin is only slightly soluble in water but readily soluble in dilute basic or strongly acidic solutions. It is quite stable to heat in neutral and acid but not alkaline solutions, and very little (3–4%) is lost in feed processing (Lewis *et al.*, 2015; Yang *et al.*, 2020). Aqueous solutions are unstable to visible and UV light, and instability is increased by heat and alkalinity. Both light and oxygen have been found to induce riboflavin degradation (Becker *et al.*, 2003). When dry, riboflavin is appreciably less affected by light.

Natural sources

Vitamin B_2 was first isolated from egg albumin in 1933 and subsequently detected in milk and liver. Overall only a few feedstuffs fed to poultry contain enough riboflavin to meet the

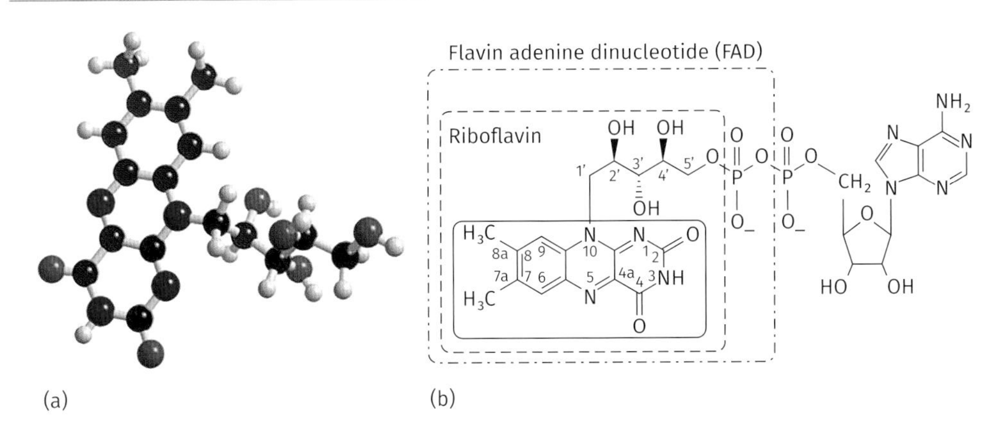

Figure 4.20 Vitamin B_2 chemical structure

requirements of young growing poultry (Cheng *et al.*, 2019; McDowell, 2000a). Riboflavin is found in appreciable quantities in green plants, by-products of animal origin, and dehydrated alfalfa. However, its content is limited to cereals and protein ingredients of plant origin, mostly used in poultry diets. Riboflavin is also synthesized by yeast, fungi, and some bacteria, including intestinal bacteria, e.g., *Fecalibacterium prausnitzii*.

Riboflavin is more bioavailable from animal products than from plant sources as the flavin complexes in plants are more stable to digestion than in animal sources. Corn-soy diets usually contain 2–2.6 mg/kg riboflavin, 60% of which is bioavailable (Chung and Baker, 1990). The increase in pelleting temperatures and the use of expanders to control contamination by *Salmonella* has increased its degradation (Yang *et al.*, 2020). The bioavailability of riboflavin was less for chicks fed corn-soybeans than those fed purified amino acid diets.

Commercial forms

Riboflavin is commercially available to the feed, food, and pharmaceutical industries as a feed-grade crystalline compound produced by chemical synthesis or fermentation, formulated in spray-dried powders containing 80% riboflavin. Riboflavin 5'-phosphate sodium salt (75–79% riboflavin) is available for applications requiring a water-dispersible source of riboflavin. High-potency, USP, or feed-grade crystalline powders are electrostatic, hygroscopic, and dusty and thus do not flow freely and show the poor distribution in feeds. In contrast, 80% of commercial spray-dried powders show reduced electrostaticity and hygroscopicity for better feed flowability and distribution (Adams, 1978).

Metabolism

Absorption and transport

Riboflavin covalently bound to protein is released by proteolytic digestion. Phosphatases hydrolyze phosphorylated forms (FAD, FMN) of riboflavin in the upper gastrointestinal tract to free the vitamin for absorption. Mucosal cells absorb free riboflavin via an active saturable transport system in all parts of the small intestine (Pinto and Rivlin, 2013). Riboflavin is phosphorylated to FMN in mucosal cells by the enzyme flavokinase (Rivlin, 2006). The FMN then enters the portal system, is bound to plasma albumin, transported to the liver, and converted to FAD, the form most present in plasma and tissues.

Transport of flavin by blood plasma involves loose associations with albumin and tight associations with some globulins (McCormick, 1990). A genetically controlled riboflavin-binding protein is present in serum and eggs. There is a hereditary recessive disorder in chickens, renal riboflavinuria, in which the riboflavin-binding protein is absent (White, 1996). Eggs become riboflavin-deficient, and embryos generally do not survive beyond day 14 of incubation (Clagett, 1971; Rivlin, 2006).

Also, if the riboflavin-binding protein is in excess, it can diminish riboflavin availability in the chicken embryo (Lee and White, 1996). Presumably, the lack of the specific vitamin transport protein prevents the adequate transfer of dietary riboflavin to the developing embryo, and riboflavin losses occur via urine. Thyroid hormones, particularly triiodothyronine (T_3), regulate the activities of the flavin biosynthetic enzymes, the synthesis of the apoflavoproteins, and the formation of covalently bound flavins (Pinto and Rivlin, 2013).

Storage and excretion

Hepatic cells from deficient animals have a relatively greater maximal absorption uptake of riboflavin (Rose *et al.*, 1986). Hepatic cell riboflavin absorption occurs via facilitated diffusion. According to Yang and Wang (1996a,b), the maximum deposition of riboflavin in the liver is achieved with 17 ppm in weeks 1 and 6 and 4 ppm in weeks 2 and 3, respectively. Absorption of methionine also increases if the maximum concentration was used.

Pinto and Rivlin (2013) suggested that physiological mechanisms facilitate the transfer of riboflavin from maternal stores to the egg. Animals do not appear to be able to store appreciable amounts of riboflavin, with the liver, kidneys, and heart having the greatest concentrations.

The liver, the major storage site, contains about one-third of the total body riboflavin. Intakes of riboflavin above current needs are rapidly excreted in the urine, primarily as free riboflavin. Minor quantities of absorbed riboflavin are excreted in feces and bile.

Biochemical functions

Riboflavin, in its phosphorylated form (FMN and FAD) or as a constituent of the flavoproteins, is a coenzyme and cofactor of more than 100 enzymes, namely flavoenzymes, involved in the transfer of electrons in redox reactions, in the metabolism of carbohydrates and amino acids and the synthesis and oxidation of fatty acids and transporting proteins (Pinto and Rivlin, 2013). Hence recommendations in poultry rise when the quantity of fat or protein in the feed increases. Interaction of flavin coenzymes with their respective apoflavoprotein involves both noncovalent and covalent associations, but only 25 have been identified to be covalently linked. Figure 4.21 shows the most important functions of riboflavin.

The conversion to FMN and FAD is regulated by nutritional status, particularly protein-calorie malnutrition, metabolic rate, hormones, and drugs. Flavoenzymes function within an eclectic array of cellular processes that involve (Pinto and Rivlin, 2013):

- electron transport
- metabolism of lipids, drugs, and xenobiotic substances
- cell signaling
- protein folding.

If riboflavin levels are low, the respiration process becomes less efficient, and 10 to 15% more feed is required to meet energy needs (Christensen, 1983). The enzymes that function aerobically are called oxidases, and those that function anaerobically are called dehydrogenases. The general function is in the oxidation of substrate and generation of energy (i.e., ATP). Flavoproteins function by accepting and passing on hydrogen by involvement in the hydrogen transport system or cytochrome system. Flavoproteins assist in the generation of ATP.

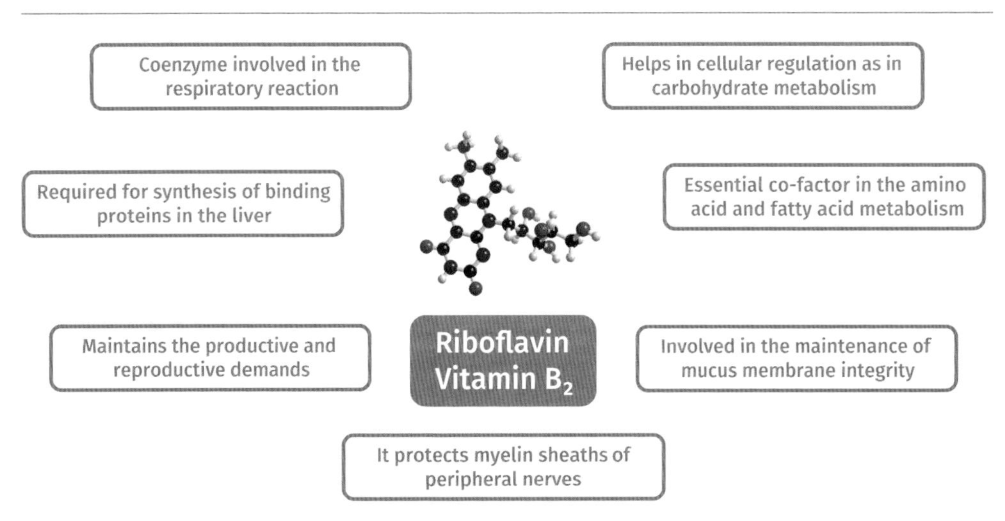

Figure 4.21 Vitamin B_2 functions

Collectively, the flavoproteins show great versatility in accepting and transferring 1 or 2 electrons with various potentials. Many flavoproteins contain a metal (e.g., iron, molybdenum, copper, zinc). The combination of the flavin and metal ion is often involved in adjusting these enzymes in transfers between single- and double-electron donors. Xanthine oxidase contains the metals molybdenum and iron. It converts hypoxanthine to xanthine and the latter to uric acid. It also reacts with aldehydes to form acids, converting retinal (vitamin A aldehyde) to retinoic acid.

Flavoproteins may accept a hydrogen ion (H^+) directly from the substrate, thus catalyzing the oxidation of the substrate, or it may catalyze the oxidation of some other enzyme by accepting a hydrogen ion from it, for example, from the niacin-containing coenzymes, nicotinamide adenine dinucleotide (NADH) and NADPH.

Flavoprotein enzymes may be arbitrarily classified into 3 groups.

1 NADH2 dehydrogenases: reduced pyridine nucleotide is a substrate, and the electron acceptor is either a member of the cytochrome system or some other acceptor besides oxygen.
2 Dehydrogenases: accept electrons directly from the substrate and pass them to one of the cytochromes.
3 Oxidases (true): accept electrons from the substrate and pass them directly to oxygen (O_2 is reduced to H_2O_2); they cannot reduce cytochromes.

Riboflavin functions in flavoprotein-enzyme systems to help regulate cellular metabolism, although they are also specifically involved in the metabolism of carbohydrates. Riboflavin is also an essential factor in amino acid metabolism as part of amino acid oxidases. These enzymes oxidize amino acids, a process which results in the decomposition of the amino acids, yielding ammonia and a keto acid. Distinct oxidized D-amino acids (prosthetic group FAD) and L-amino acids (prosthetic group FMN) are produced.

In the methionine and homocysteine metabolism, riboflavin plays a role as a coenzyme in the same way that cobalamin, folate, and pyridoxine (Pinto and Rivlin, 2013). Riboflavin not only is a key link in the utilization of dietary folates and cobalamins but also controls homocysteine re-methylation and trans-sulfuration in association with methyl donor flavoenzymes within the one-carbon cycle as well as the FAD/FMN diflavin enzyme, MSR, the FAD-dependent 5,10-methylenetetrahydrofolate reductase (MTHFR) necessary for methionine formation. This function affects cardiovascular disease and osteoporosis (Pinto and Rivlin, 2013).

In addition, riboflavin plays a role in fat metabolism (Rivlin, 2006), and a FAD flavoprotein is an important link in fatty acid oxidation. This includes the acyl-coenzyme A dehydrogenases, which are necessary for the stepwise degradation of fatty acids. An FMN flavoprotein is required for the synthesis of fatty acids from acetate. Thus, flavoproteins are needed to degrade and synthesize fatty acids.

Riboflavin and other vitamins play an important role in skin development, tensile strength, and healing rates (Ward, 1993). A riboflavin deficiency can slow the epithelialization of wounds by 4–5 days (Lakshmi *et al.*, 1989), reduce collagen content by 25%, and decrease the tensile strength of injuries by 45%. Riboflavin deficiency can increase skin homocysteine by two- to fourfold, ultimately impairing collagen's cross-link formation (Lakshmi *et al.*, 1990). Marginal field deficiencies of riboflavin could increase skin tears, cause longer healing times, and ultimately increase costly downgrades.

Among the enzymes that require riboflavin is the FMN-dependent oxidase responsible for converting phosphorylated pyridoxine (vitamin B_6) to a functional coenzyme. Riboflavin deficiency also decreases the conversion of the vitamin B_6 coenzyme pyridoxal phosphate to the main vitamin B_6 urinary excretory product of 4-pyridoxic acid.

Riboflavin deficiency affects iron metabolism, with less iron absorbed and an increased rate of iron loss due to an accelerated rate of small intestinal epithelial turnover (Powers *et al.*, 1991, 1993). Riboflavin coenzyme Q10 and niacin are associated with poly (adenosine diphosphate [ADP]-ribose) polymerase (PARP), a family of proteins involved in several cellular processes, which function in post-translational modification of nuclear proteins. The poly ADP-ribosylated proteins function in DNA repair, replication, and cell differentiation (Premkumar *et al.*, 2008; Pinto and Rivlin, 2013). It plays an important role in maintaining the integrity of mucous membranes and the nervous system (Pinto and Rivlin, 2013). It interacts with other vitamins: pyridoxine, niacin, and pantothenic acid. Squires and Naber (1993b) demonstrated that the riboflavin concentration in the egg diminishes as the laying hen gets older.

Nutritional assessment

The assessment of the riboflavin nutritional status is not simple, and it seems that the sensitivity to changes in riboflavin intake is quite low. The typical functional test used the erythrocyte glutathione reductase activity coefficient (EGRac) assay, which allows for determining the degree of tissue saturation with riboflavin (Sauberlich, 1999). The riboflavin vitamers – free riboflavin and the coenzymes FMN and FAD – can be analyzed directly in serum (or homogenized erythrocytes) using liquid chromatography coupled to tandem mass spectrometry (LC-MS/MS), and data can be compared with EGRac. There is a high correlation between plasma riboflavin and EGRac, and all vitamers but not FAD seem suitable to assess riboflavin status (Höller *et al.*, 2018).

Deficiency signs

Riboflavin is more likely than other vitamins to become deficient under practical conditions, especially under stressful conditions (Ruiz and Harms, 1988a, 1989a; Whitehead, 2000b) and when aflatoxins are present (Leeson *et al.*, 1995), for which reason an ample safety margin should be applied in poultry nutrition.

Ruiz and Harms (1988a) observed that riboflavin deficiency is more severe in modern strains of chicks and poults than in those used 40 to 50 years ago, perhaps due to the faster growth rate and improved feed conversion of the modern broiler. A primary deficiency of dietary riboflavin has wide implications for other vitamins, as flavin coenzymes are involved in the metabolism of 5 vitamins: folic acid, vitamin B_6, vitamin K, niacin, and vitamin D (Pinto and Rivlin, 2013).

Chicks fed a diet only marginally deficient in riboflavin often recover spontaneously. The condition is curable in the early stages, but in its acute phase, it is irreversible (NRC, 1994). Deficiency is characterized by dermal and hematological abnormalities, poor plumage, anemia, deterioration in growth rates and feed conversion, neuropathic abnormalities with paralysis and claws curvature, a lowering of resistance to heat stress, enteritis, diarrhea, and an increase in mortality in the first week (Summers *et al.*, 1984; Leeson *et al.*, 1995; Klasing, 1998; Pinto and Rivlin, 2013).

When chicks are fed a diet deficient in riboflavin, their appetite is fairly good, but they grow very slowly and become weak and emaciated. There is no apparent impairment of feather growth. On the contrary, main wing feathers often appear disproportionally long. Increased hematocrit, increased mean corpuscular volume, decreased mean hemoglobin concentration, and a marked heterophil leucocytosis occurred in the chick before neurological manifestations (NRC, 1994). Perhaps due to mitochondrial dysfunction, riboflavin-deficient rats require 15–20% more energy intake than control animals to maintain the same body weight (Rivlin, 2006).

The characteristic sign of riboflavin deficiency in the chick is "curled-toe" paralysis, caused by changes in the sciatic nerves (Figure 4.22). There is marked enlargement of sciatic and brachial nerve sheaths, with sciatic nerves reaching a diameter 4 to 6 times normal. Histologic examinations of affected nerves show definite degenerative changes in myelin sheaths, which, when severe, may pinch the nerve, producing a permanent stimulus that causes the curled-toe paralysis (Scott *et al.*, 1982). When the curled-toe deformity is long-standing, irreparable damage has occurred in the sciatic nerve, and riboflavin administration no longer cures the condition. However, "curled-toe" does not develop in a total riboflavin-free diet or when the deficiency is very marked because the chicks die before it appears. Chicks are first noted

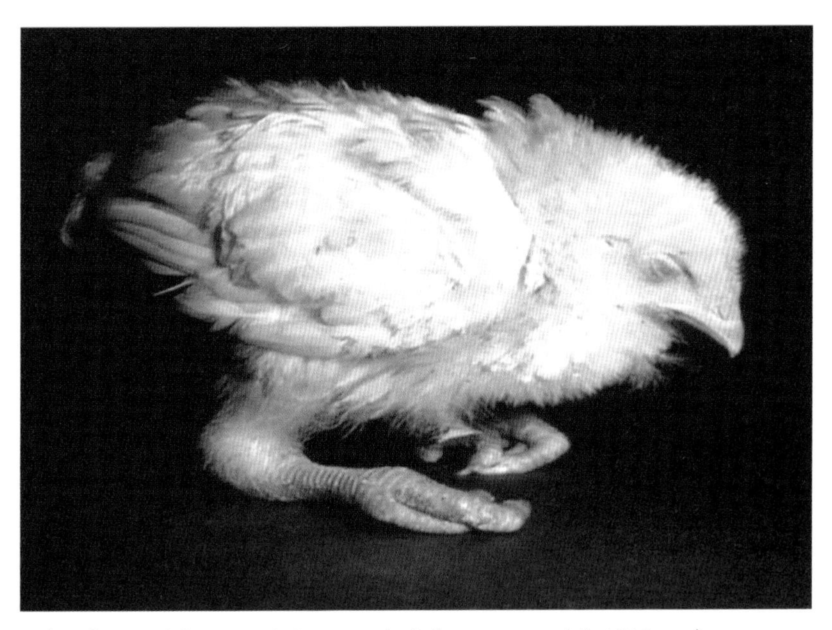

Figure 4.22 Vitamin B_2 deficiency: curled-toe paralysis (source: copyright UK Crown)

walking on their hocks with their toes curled inward. Deficient chicks do not move about except when forced, and their toes are curled inward when walking and resting on their hocks (Scott *et al.*, 1982).

Legs become paralyzed, but the birds may otherwise appear normal. An approximately 10% incidence of curled-toe paralysis was observed among birds fed a diet with no added riboflavin (1.5 mg/kg) (Bootwalla and Harms, 1990). Retarded growth, splay, and hock-resting postures and leg paralysis, rather than curled-toe paralysis, have been reported in some studies as the predominant signs of riboflavin deficiency in chicks (Ruiz and Harms, 1988a; Chung and Baker, 1990).

Hepatic architecture is markedly disrupted in riboflavin deficiency with hepatic lipid peroxidation in experimental animals. Mitochondria in riboflavin-deficient mice progress through a series of morphological changes ranging from elongation of cristae to the development of cristae clusters that result in cup-shaped mitochondria that tend to nest within each other.

Although these structural abnormalities occur, changes in oxidative metabolism appear marginal, as minor losses are observed in the activity of the flavin-dependent components of the electron transport chain, namely, complexes I and II. Other critical organelles markedly impaired during riboflavin deficiency are peroxisomes. These organelles contribute to several crucial metabolic processes such as β-oxidation of fatty acids, biosynthesis of ether phospholipids, and metabolism of ROS. Within erythrocytes, riboflavin deficiency causes a reduction in the activity of glucose-6-phosphate dehydrogenase (Pinto and Rivlin, 2013).

The most critical requirements for riboflavin are those exhibited by the young chick and the breeder hen. There is increasing evidence that the vigor and livability of the baby chicks are directly tied to the amount of riboflavin in the hen's diet. Portsmouth (1996) indicates that riboflavin deficiency can periodically be observed in newly hatched chicks, manifested as clubbed down. However, Whitehead (2004a) points out that according to recent research, the cause of this problem may be not nutrition but infection.

Turkey poults and pheasants exhibit clinical signs similar to those of the chick, whereas ducks and geese are more likely to have bowing of the legs in conjunction with perosis (NRC, 1994). In the poult, dermatitis appears in about 8 days; the vent becomes encrusted, inflamed, and excoriated; growth is retarded or completely stopped by about the seventeenth day, and deaths begin to occur about the twenty-first day. However, when poults were fed a corn-soy diet analyzed to contain 2.7 mg/kg of naturally occurring riboflavin, the only signs exhibited were paralysis of one or both legs, poor feathering, poor growth, and, finally, mortality (Ruiz and Harms, 1989a).

In ducklings, diarrhea and cessation of growth are generally associated with riboflavin deficiency. Other signs of riboflavin deficiency are growth retardation, diarrhea after 8 to 10 days, and high mortality after 3 weeks. In laying poultry, the hatchability of incubated eggs is first reduced, and subsequently, egg production is decreased, roughly in proportion to the degree of deficiency. Embryonic mortality has 2 typical peaks (days 4 and 20 of incubation) and often an intermediate peak on day 14. Embryos that fail to hatch from eggs of hens receiving low-riboflavin diets are dwarfed and exhibit pronounced micromelia; some embryos are edematous. The down fails to emerge properly, thus resulting in a typical abnormality termed "clubbed down," which is most common in neck areas and around the vent. The nervous systems of these embryos show degenerative changes much like those described in thiamine-deficient chicks. When dietary riboflavin provided to breeder hens was decreased from 9.7 to 1.7 mg/kg, embryo mortality increased to 83.3% and hatchability to 3.1%; however, reducing riboflavin from 9.7 to 7.0 or 4.4 mg/kg did not affect these variables (Flores-Garcia and Scholtyssek, 1992).

Naber and Squires (1993b) reported that the riboflavin of egg albumen is a sensitive measurement to determine if riboflavin had been added to the diet of laying hens. Hens fed a riboflavin-deficient diet laid eggs with low concentrations of the vitamin within 4 days. Therefore, the correlation between egg albumen riboflavin content and feed riboflavin content is high. The withdrawal of vitamin B_2 from the diet during the last weeks reduces its content in breast tissue by 37% (Deyhim *et al.*, 1996), which is of interest from the consumer's point of view since normally, 100 g of breast meat contributes 9% of the recommended daily intake of this vitamin.

Safety

A large body of evidence has accumulated that supplementation with riboflavin over nutritional requirements has very little toxicity for animals and humans (Pinto and Rivlin, 2013). There are no reports of riboflavin toxicity studies in poultry. Most data from rats suggest that dietary levels between 10 and 20 times the requirement (possibly 100 times) can be tolerated safely (NRC, 1987). When massive amounts of riboflavin are administered orally, only a small fraction of the dose is absorbed, the remainder being excreted in the feces.

Lack of toxicity is probably because the transport system necessary for riboflavin absorption across the gastrointestinal mucosa becomes saturated, limiting riboflavin absorption (Christensen, 1973). Also, the capacity of tissues to store riboflavin and its coenzyme derivatives appears to be limited when excessive amounts are administered.

Vitamin B_6 (pyridoxine)

Chemical structure and properties

The term vitamin B_6 refers to a group of 3 pyridine derivatives named according to the functional group in the position 4 (Dakshinamurti and Dakshinamurti, 2013):

- pyridoxol or pyridoxine (PN), the alcohol form
- pyridoxal (PL), the aldehyde form
- pyridoxamine, the amine form.

These 3 compounds have a similar vitamin activity in the different species of birds. Pyridoxine is the predominant plant form, whereas pyridoxal and pyridoxamine are vitamin forms generally found in animal products. Three additional vitamin B_6 forms are the phosphorylated forms pyridoxine 5′-phosphate (PNP), pyridoxal-5′-phosphate or codecarboxylase (PLP) and pyridoxamine 5′-phosphate (PMP) The natural, free forms of the vitamers could be converted to the key coenzymatic form, PLP, by the action of 2 enzymes, a kinase, and an oxidase.

Various forms of vitamin B_6 found in animal tissues are interconvertible, with vitamin B_6 metabolically active mainly as PLP and to a lesser degree as PMP (Figure 4.23). Vitamin B_6 is stable in response to heat, acid, and alkali exposure; however, light is highly destructive, especially in neutral or alkaline media. The free base and the commonly available hydrochloride salt are soluble in water and alcohol.

Natural sources

Vitamin B_6 is widely distributed in feedstuffs. Most vitamin B_6 in animal products is pyridoxal and pyridoxamine phosphates, whereas, in plants and seeds, the usual form is pyridoxine (McDowell, 2000a). The vitamin B_6 present in cereal grains is concentrated mainly in bran, with the rest containing only small amounts.

Most of the ingredients are good sources of this vitamin, but its bioavailability is relatively low (40–65%): in soybean meal it is 65% and in corn it varies from 45 to 56% (McDowell and

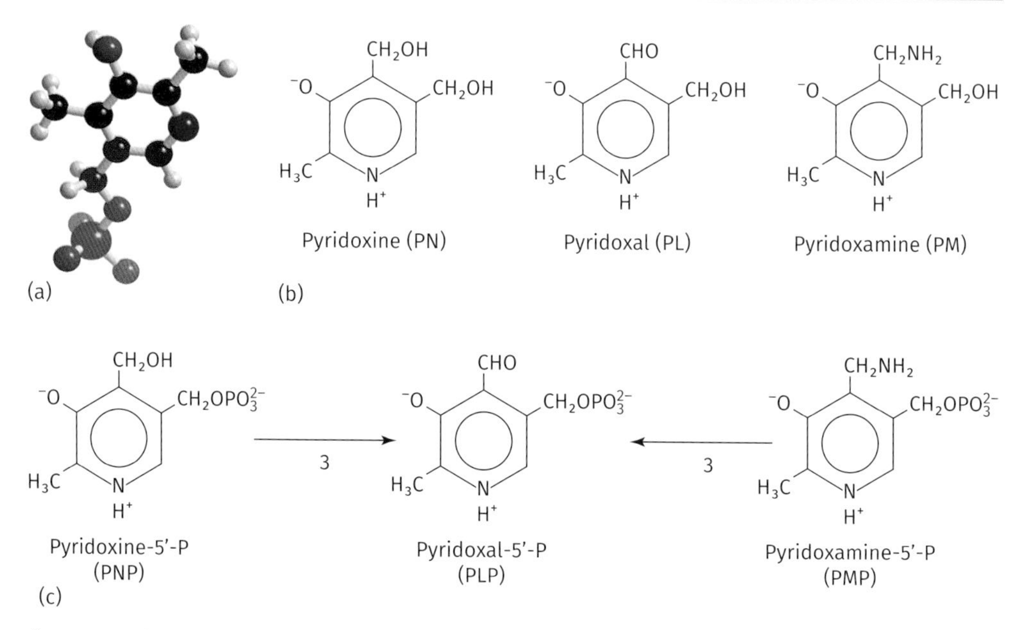

Figure 4.23 Vitamin B_6 chemical structure

Ward, 2008). The levels of vitamin B_6 contained in feedstuffs are also affected by processing, refining, and storage with losses as high as 70% being reported (Shideler, 1983) and with a commonly accepted range of 0 to 40% (Birdsall, 1975). Of the forms, pyridoxine is far more stable than either pyridoxal or pyridoxamine. Therefore, the processing losses of vitamin B_6 tend to be highly variable (9–40%), with plant-derived foods (which mostly contain pyridoxine) losing little if any of the vitamin and animal products (which mostly contain pyridoxal and pyridoxamine) losing large quantities (Lewis *et al.*, 2015; Yang *et al.*, 2020). The bioavailability of feedstuffs can be as low as 40–50% after heating. There was little difference in availability between corn samples not heated and those heated to 120°C (248°F). However, corn heated to 160°C (320°F) contained significantly less available B_6.

Besides heat, losses may be caused by light and various oxidative agents. Blanching of rehydrated lima beans resulted in a loss of 20% of the vitamin B_6, but, more significantly, the availability of the vitamin was reduced by almost 50% (Ekanayake and Nelson, 1990). Irradiation, as a potential method for microbial control of poultry feed, results in a loss of 15% vitamin B_6 potency (Leeson and Marcotte, 1993).

Coprophagy is a source of vitamin B_6 from microbial synthesis. However, it is not demonstrated that vitamin B_6 from posterior digestive tract sections is absorbed and used in significant quantities by monogastric animals.

Pyridoxine-5´-β-D-glucoside (PNG), a conjugated form of vitamin B_6, is abundant in various plant-derived foods (McCormick, 2006). This form of B_6 may account for up to 50% of the total vitamin B_6 content of oilseeds, such as soybeans and sunflower seeds. The utilization of dietary PNG relative to pyridoxine is 30% in rats and 50% in humans (Gregory, 1991a). The glycosylated PNG can quantitatively alter the metabolism of pyridoxine *in vivo*. Hence, it partially impairs the metabolic utilization of co-ingested non-glycosylated forms of vitamin B_6 (Nakano and Gregory, 1995; Nakano *et al.*, 1997).

There are several vitamin B_6 antagonists, which either compete for reactive apoenzyme sites or react with PLP to form inactive compounds. The presence of a vitamin B_6 antagonist in linseed meal is of particular interest to animal nutritionists. This substance was identified in 1967 as linatine, l-((N-γ-L-glutamyl) amino)-D-proline and was found to have antibiotic properties (Parsons and Klostermann, 1967). Pesticides (e.g., carbaryl, propoxur, or thiram) can be antagonistic to vitamin B_6. Feeding a diet enriched with vitamin B_6 prevented disturbances in the active transport of methionine in rats intoxicated with pesticides (Witkowska *et al.*, 1992; Dakshinamurti and Dakshinamurti, 2013).

Commercial forms

Commercially, vitamin B_6 is available as fine crystalline powder of pyridoxine hydrochloride 99% and dilutions. Supplemental vitamin B_6 is reported to have higher bioavailability and stability than the naturally occurring vitamin.

Metabolism

Absorption and transport

Digestion of vitamin B_6 would first involve splitting the vitamin, as it is bound to the protein portion of foods. Vitamin B_6 compounds are absorbed from the diet in dephosphorylated forms. The small intestine is rich in alkaline phosphatases for the dephosphorylation reaction. Sakurai *et al.* (1992) reported that a physiological dose of pyridoxamine was rapidly transformed to pyridoxal in the intestinal tissues and then released in the form of pyridoxal into the portal blood.

Vitamin B_6 is absorbed mainly in the jejunum and the ileum by passive diffusion. Absorption in the colon is insignificant, even though colon microflora synthesize the vitamin. After absorption, B_6 compounds quickly appear in the liver, where they are mostly converted into PLP, considered the most active vitamin form in metabolism. Under normal conditions, most of the vitamin B_6 in the blood is present as PLP that is linked to proteins, largely albumin in the plasma and hemoglobin in the red blood cells (McCormick, 2006). Both niacin (as NADP-dependent enzyme) and riboflavin (as the flavoprotein pyridoxamine phosphate oxidase) are important for the conversion of vitamin B_6 forms and phosphorylation reactions (Kodentsova *et al.*, 1993).

Although other tissues also contribute to vitamin B_6 metabolism, the liver is responsible for forming PLP found in plasma. Pyridoxal and PLP found in circulation are associated primarily with plasma albumin and red blood cell hemoglobin (Mehansho and Henderson, 1980). Pyridoxal phosphate accounts for 60% of plasma vitamin B_6. Researchers do not agree on whether pyridoxal or PLP is the transport form of B_6.

Storage and excretion

Only small quantities of vitamin B_6 are stored in the body, and over half, in the case of birds, is found forming part of enzymes in the muscle and liver. Vitamin B_6 is widely distributed in various tissues, mainly as PLP or pyridoxamine phosphate, mostly stored in muscular tissue.

Pyridoxic acid is the major excretory metabolite of the vitamin, eliminated via urine. Also, small quantities of pyridoxol, pyridoxal, pyridoxamine, and phosphorylated derivatives are excreted in urine (Henderson, 1984). Vitamin B_6 metabolism is altered in renal failure, as observed in rats exhibiting plasma pyridoxal phosphate 43% lower than controls (Wei and Young, 1994).

Biochemical functions

Vitamin B_6, primarily as PLP and, to a lesser extent, as PMP, plays an essential role in the amino acid, carbohydrate, and fatty acid metabolism, and the energy-producing citric acid cycle, with over 60 enzymes known to depend on vitamin B_6 coenzymes.

Pyridoxal phosphate functions in practically all reactions involved in amino acid metabolism, including transamination, decarboxylation, deamination, desulfhydration, and the cleavage or synthesis of amino acids. The largest group of vitamin B_6-dependent enzymes are transaminases. Aminotransferase is involved in the interconversion of a pair of amino acids into their corresponding keto acids, e.g., amino groups transferred from aspartate to α-ketoglutarate forming oxaloacetate and glutamate.

Minimum vitamin B_6 requirements have been proposed for rations with moderate protein levels and a balanced amino acid relationship (Daghir and Shah, 1973). The recommended levels of vitamin B_6 supply increase with feeds with high protein content or with an amino acid profile distant from the ideal protein level since more enzymes are needed to metabolize the excess amino acids, which depend on vitamin B_6. Non-oxidative decarboxylations involve PLP as a coenzyme, e.g., converting amino acids into biogenic amines, such as histamine, serotonin, GABA, and taurine. Vitamin B_6 participates in functions that include (Marks, 1975; McCormick, 2006; Dakshinamurti and Dakshinamurti, 2013):

1. deaminases: for serine, threonine, and cystathionine
2. desulfydrases and transulfurases: interconversion
3. synthesis of niacin from tryptophan: hydroxykynurenine is not converted to hydroxyanthranilic acid but rather to xanthurenic acid due to lack of the B_6-dependent enzyme, kynureninase
4. formation of α-aminolevulinic acid from succinyl-CoA and glycine, the first step in porphyrin synthesis
5. conversion of linoleic to arachidonic acid in the metabolism of essential fatty acids (this function is controversial)
6. glycogen phosphorylase catalyzes glycogen breakdown to glucose-1-phosphate (pyridoxal phosphate does not appear to be a coenzyme for the enzyme but rather affects the enzyme conformation)
7. synthesis of epinephrine and norepinephrine from either phenylalanine or tyrosin – both norepinephrine and epinephrine are involved in carbohydrate metabolism and other body reactions
8. racemases – PLP-dependent racemases enable certain microorganisms to utilize D-amino acids (racemases have not yet been detected in mammalian tissues)
9. transmethylation involving methionine
10. incorporation of iron in hemoglobin synthesis formation of antibodies – B_6 deficiency inhibits the synthesis of globulins that carry antibodies inflammation – higher vitamin B_6 levels were linked to protection against inflammation (Morris et al., 2010).

Neurological functions of pyridoxine

Pyridoxine is a coenzyme of several enzymes involved in the endogenous production of hydrogen sulfide, dopamine, norepinephrine, serotonin (5-HT), and GABA, as well as taurine, sphingolipids, and polyamines, which are molecules involved in cell signaling in the CNS (Dakshinamurti and Dakshinamurti, 2013).

Neurological disorders, including states of agitation and convulsions, result from reduced B_6 enzymes in the brain, including glutamate decarboxylase and γ-aminobutyric acid transaminase. Dopamine release is delayed with a vitamin B_6 deficiency, contributing to motor abnormalities (Tang and Wei, 2004). Maternal restriction of B_6 in rats adversely affected synaptogenesis, neurogenesis, neuron longevity, and progeny differentiation (Groziak and Kirksey, 1987, 1990).

Effects on immunity and as antioxidant

Animal and human studies suggest that a vitamin B_6 deficiency affects both humoral and cell-mediated immune responses. In humans, vitamin B_6 depletion significantly decreased the percentage and the total number of lymphocytes, mitogenic responses of peripheral blood lymphocytes to T- and B-cell mitogens, and interleukin 2 production (Meydani *et al.*, 1991).

The role of PLP in effecting one-carbon metabolism is important in nucleic acid biosynthesis and immune system function. PLP is also needed for gluconeogenesis by way of transaminases acting on glucogenic amino acids and for lipid metabolism that involves several aspects of PLP function: e.g., the production of carnitine needed to act as a vector for long-chain fatty acids for mitochondrial β-oxidation and of certain bases for phospholipid biosynthesis (McCormick, 2006).

Vitamin B_6 exhibits antioxidant properties inhibiting superoxide radicals, preventing lipid peroxidation, protein glycosylation, and Na^+,K^+-ATPase activity in high glucose-treated erythrocytes and hydrogen peroxide-treated monocytes and endothelial cells (Dakshinamurti and Dakshinamurti, 2013).

Metabolism of homocysteine and cardiovascular function

Homocysteine is a sulfur-containing amino acid formed during the metabolism of methionine. Pyridoxine is required as a coenzyme for the 2 key steps of the transsulfuration pathway catalyzed by cystathionine synthetase and cystathionine γ-lyase. In this metabolic pathway, several B vitamins are involved (Figure 4.24).

Pyridoxine deficiency may increase blood pressure by stimulating smooth muscle in the blood vessels and creating endothelial dysfunction, generating ROS, and increasing susceptibility to oxidation. Homocysteine also enhances collagen synthesis, altering the elastin/collagen ratio, which contributes to the changes in the vessel wall that lead to systemic vascular resistance and hypertension (Dakshinamurti and Dakshinamurti, 2013).

Nutritional assessment

The 6 interconvertible forms of vitamin B_6 can be measured in plasma to assess nutritional status. Nonetheless, PLP is the vitamer normally used, and its measurement in erythrocytes seems to provide a more appropriate evaluation (Sauberlich, 1999). However, considering the complex metabolic pathways in which vitamin B_6 is involved, assessing the ratios between metabolites, or the possibility of quantifying numerous amino acids and metabolites related to PLP-dependent pathways, may provide a better insight into nutritional status (Höller *et al.*, 2018).

Deficiency signs

Inadequate vitamin B_6 will lead to inefficiencies in the utilization of protein in the diet, accompanied by a reduction in the capacity for nitrogen retention and an increase in excretion. A reduction of nitrogen retention and consequently growth causes dermatitis, epileptic-like convulsions, anemia, and partial alopecia.

Also, lipid metabolism is affected; that is, desaturation and elongation of fatty acids are impaired in growing chickens (An *et al.*, 1995). Signs of B_6 deficiency in chicks appear very

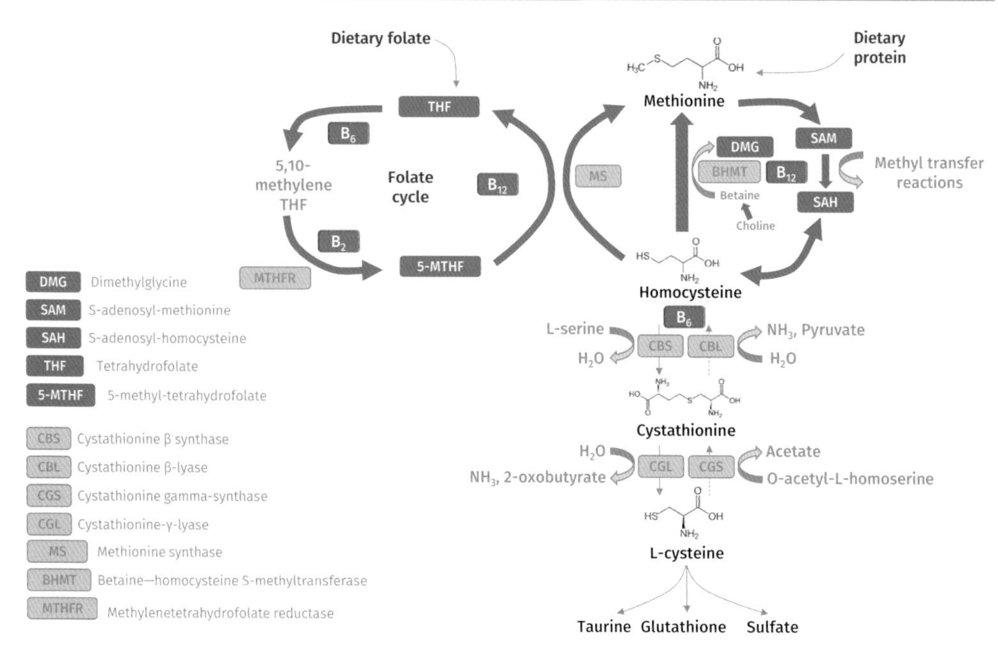

Figure 4.24 Folate, transsulfuration, and choline oxidation pathways are involved in riboflavin, pyridoxine, cyanocobalamin, and choline

rapidly after introducing a B_6-deficient feed. Fuller and Kifer (1959) reported that symptoms of a deficiency appeared on day 8.

Chronic borderline B_6 deficiency produces perosis: usually, one leg is severely crippled, and one or both of the middle toes may be bent inward at the first joint (Gries and Scott, 1972). Vitamin B_6 deficiency in growing chicks caused hyperhomocysteinemia affecting biomechanical properties of tibial bone, with reduced dry weight and cortical thickness (Massé *et al.*, 1994, 1996).

A marked increase in gizzard erosion was found in vitamin B_6-deficient chicks (Daghir and Haddad, 1981). Chicks fed a vitamin B_6-deficient diet have little appetite and grow slowly, with plumage failing to develop fully and exhibiting general weakness after a few days of deprivation (Figure 4.25a).

A more specific sign of B_6 deficiency is the nature of the nervous condition that develops. Deficient chicks are abnormally excitable. As deprivation continues, nervous disorders become increasingly severe (Bräunlich, 1974). There is trembling and vibration of the tip of the tail, with movement stiff and jerky. Chicks run aimlessly about with lowered heads and drooping wings. Finally, convulsions develop, during which chicks fall on their side or back, with the legs scrabbling. Violent convulsions cause complete exhaustion and may lead to death (Leeson and Summers, 2008). These clinical signs may be differentiated from encephalomalacia by the greater activity intensity during a B_6 deficiency seizure, resulting in complete exhaustion and death (Scott *et al.*, 1982). The birds squat in a characteristic posture (Figure 4.25b and c), with wings slightly spread and head resting on the ground (Bräunlich, 1974). Miller (1963) observed high proportions of pendulous crops in vitamin B_6-deficient chicks.

Vitamin B_6 participates in the incorporation of iron into hemoglobin and in the synthesis of immunoglobulins so that deficiency will cause blood alterations. Marginal deficiencies provoke microcytic, normochromic polycythemia (Blalock and Thaxton, 1984), and deficient chicks

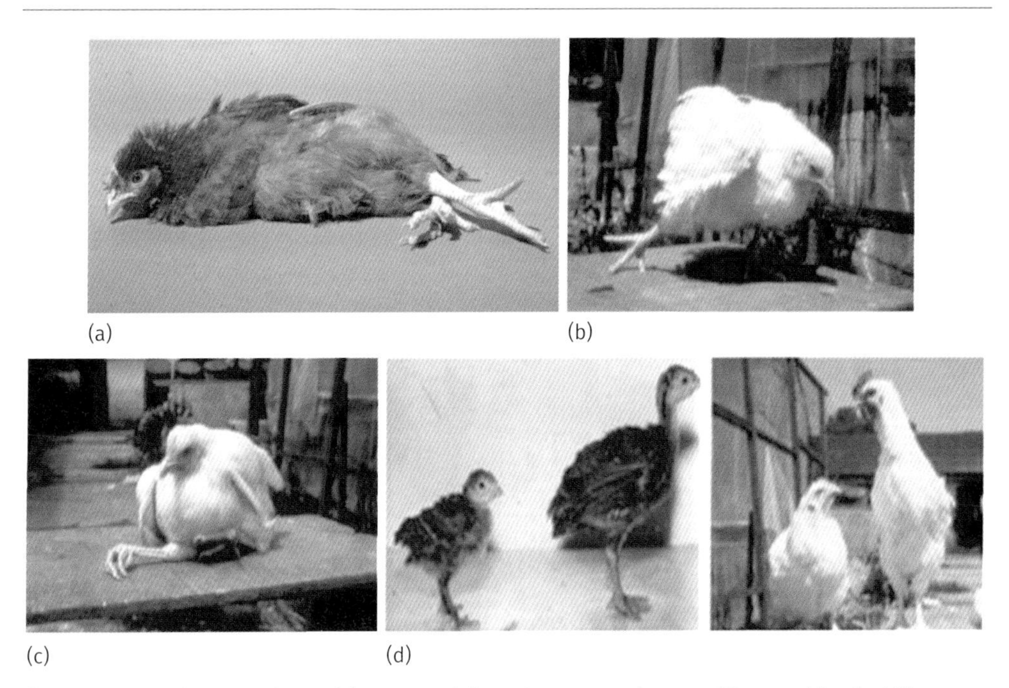

Figure 4.25 Vitamin B_6 deficiency: (a) rough, deficient plumage, weakness, stiff extremities, inability to stand (source: Dr. H. Weiser, Roche Basel); (b and c) neuritis and "squatting position" (courtesy of L.R. McDowell, University of Florida); (d) poor growth in a vitamin B_6-deficient turkey poult (about 4 weeks old) compared with a normal poult at right (courtesy of T.W. Sullivan, University of Nebraska)

show a decreased immunoglobulin M and immunoglobulin G response to antibody challenge (Blalock *et al.*, 1984). An extreme deficiency leads to microcytic, polychromatic, and hypochromic anemia in conjunction with atrophy of the spleen and thymus (Asmar *et al.*, 1968).

Similar signs of a vitamin B_6 deficiency have been observed in turkey poults: loss of appetite, poor growth (Figure 4.25d), oversensitivity, cramps, and eventually death. Vitamin B_6 deficiency reduces egg production and hatchability in broiler breeders and decreases feed consumption, weight loss, and death. A severe deficiency (levels of vitamin B_6 below 0.5 mg/kg) in diet causes rapid involution of the ovary, oviduct, comb, and wattles in mature laying hens. Involution of testes, comb, and wattles occurs in vitamin B_6-deficient adult cockerels (Scott *et al.*, 1982).

Ducklings not receiving enough vitamin B_6 grow slowly, and plumage development is poor. At 5 days of age, ducklings showed retarded growth (Yang and Jeng, 1989). First observed at 7 days, clinical signs were characterized by decreased appetite, extreme weakness, hyperexcitability, convulsions, and death. Hematologic examination at 3 weeks of age indicated that vitamin B_6 deficiency in ducklings resulted in microcytic and hypochromic anemia.

Safety

Insufficient data is available to support estimates of the maximum dietary tolerable levels of vitamin B_6 for poultry. It is suggested, primarily from dog and rat data, that nutritional levels at least 50 times the dietary requirements are safe for most species (NRC, 1987).

Signs of toxicity, which occur most obviously in the peripheral nervous system, include changes in gait and peripheral sensation (Krinke and Fitzgerald, 1988), ataxia, muscle weakness, and incoordination at levels approaching 1,000 times the requirement (Leeson and Summers, 2008; Dakshinamurti and Dakshinamurti, 2013).

Vitamin B_{12} (cyanocobalamin)

Chemical structure and properties

Nutritionists now consider vitamin B_{12} to be the generic name for a group of compounds with vitamin B_{12} activity in which the cobalt atom is in the center of the corrin nucleus (cobalt-containing corrinoids). Cyanocobalamin has a molecular weight of 1,355 and is the most complex structure and heaviest compound of all vitamins (Figure 4.26). The empirical formula of vitamin B_{12} is $C_{63}H_{88}O_{14}N_{14}PCo$.

Vitamin B_{12} is a dark-red crystalline hygroscopic substance, freely soluble in water and alcohol but insoluble in acetone, chloroform, and ether. Oxidizing and reducing agents and exposure to sunlight tend to destroy its activity. Losses of vitamin B_{12} during feed processing are usually not excessive because vitamin B_{12} is stable at temperatures as high as 250°C being the most stable vitamin during feed pelleting and storage processes (Lewis *et al.*, 2015; Yang *et al.*, 2020).

Adenosylcobalamin and methylcobalamin are naturally occurring forms of vitamin B_{12} in feedstuffs and animal tissues. Cyanocobalamin is not a naturally occurring form of the vitamin but is the most widely used form of cobalamin in clinical practice because of its relative availability and stability (Green and Miller, 2013).

Natural sources

Feedstuffs of animal origin – meat, liver, kidney, milk, eggs, and fish – are reasonably good sources of vitamin B_{12}. The kidney and liver are excellent sources; ruminants' organs are richer in vitamin B_{12} than those of monogastrics. Vitamin B_{12} presence in the tissues of animals follows from ingestion of vitamin B_{12} in animal feeds or from intestinal synthesis. The richest sources are fermentation residues, activated sewage sludge, and manure.

Plant products are practically devoid of B_{12}. The vitamin B_{12} reported in higher plants in small amounts may result from synthesis by soil microorganisms, excretion of the vitamin onto the soil, with subsequent absorption by the plant. The root nodules of certain legumes contain small quantities of vitamin B_{12}. Certain seaweed species (algae) have been reported to contain appreciable amounts of vitamin B_{12} (up to 1 µg/gram solids). Seaweed itself does not synthesize vitamin B_{12}; it is synthesized by the bacteria associated with seaweed and then

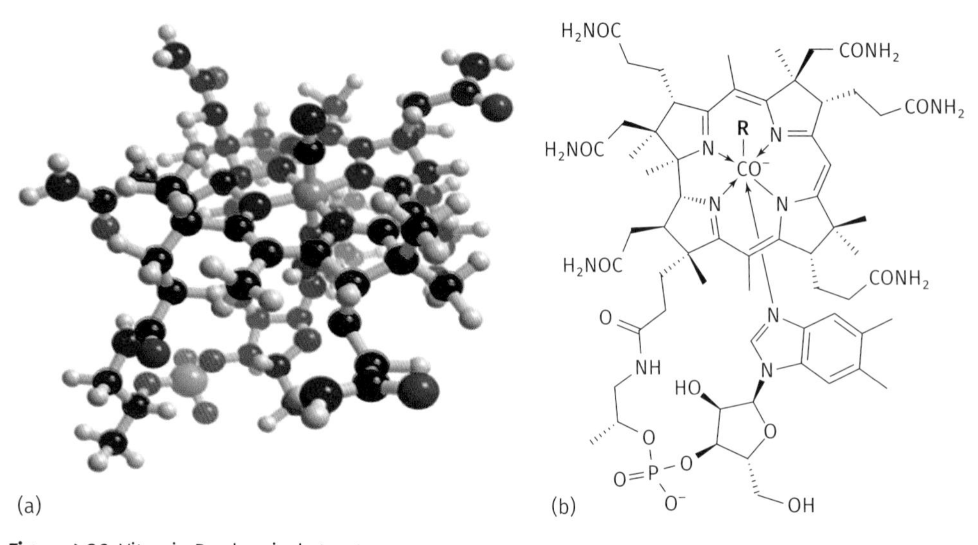

Figure 4.26 Vitamin B_{12} chemical structure

concentrated by the seaweed (Scott *et al.*, 1982). Dagnelie *et al.* (1991) reported that vitamin B_{12} from algae is largely unavailable.

Bedding can be a source of vitamin B_{12} for birds housed on solid floors, although there are no data relating to its absorption level. Microorganisms synthesize vitamin B_{12} in the intestinal tract. However, cobalamin produced in the colon is not bioavailable because the receptors necessary for absorbing the vitamin are found in the small intestine, upstream of the site of corrinoid production (Seetharam and Alpers, 1982). This cobalamin can be made available to the host via coprophagy.

Commercial forms

Commercial sources of vitamin B_{12} are produced from fermentation products, and it is available as cyanocobalamin, the most stable form of this vitamin. Little is known about the bioavailability of orally ingested B_{12} in feeds.

Metabolism

Absorption and transport

The absorptive site for vitamin B_{12} is the lower portion of the small intestine. Substantial amounts of B_{12} are secreted into the duodenum and then reabsorbed in the ileum. Passing vitamin B_{12} through the intestinal wall is a complex procedure and requires the intervention of certain carrier compounds able to bind the vitamin molecule (McDowell, 2000a). In most species, for the absorption of vitamin B_{12}, the following is required (Green and Miller, 2013):

- production of the intrinsic factor for absorption of vitamin B_{12} through the ileum
- functional pancreas (trypsin secretion) required for release of bound vitamin B_{12} before combining the vitamin with the intrinsic factor
- functional ileum with receptor and absorption sites.

Gastric juice defects are responsible for most cases of food-vitamin B_{12} malabsorption in monogastrics (Carmel, 1994). Factors that diminish vitamin B_{12} absorption include protein, iron, and vitamin B_6 deficiencies, thyroid removal, and dietary tannic acid (Hoffmann-La Roche, 1984).

The absorption of vitamin B_{12} is limited by the number of intrinsic factor-vitamin B_{12} binding sites in the ileal mucosa so that not more than about 1 to 1.5 μg of a single oral dose of the vitamin in humans can be absorbed (Bender, 1992). The absorption is also slow: peak blood concentrations of the vitamin are not achieved for some 6 to 8 hours after an oral dose.

There are structural differences in vitamin B_{12} intrinsic factors among species. Intrinsic factors have been demonstrated in humans, monkeys, pigs, rats, cows, ferrets, rabbits, hamsters, foxes, lions, tigers, and leopards. They have not yet been detected in guinea pig, horses, sheep, chickens, and other species. Therefore, intrinsic factor concentrates prepared from the stomach of one animal species do not always increase B_{12} absorption in different animal species or humans. Similarly, there are species differences in vitamin B_{12} transport proteins (Polak *et al.*, 1979; Green and Miller, 2013). Vitamin B_{12} is bound to transcobalamin (TC) and haptocorrin (HC) for transport in the blood, with about 20% being attached to TC and the rest to HC. The TC-bound cobalamin is the form most actively transported into tissues.

Storage and excretion

The storage of vitamin B_{12} is found principally in the liver. Other storage sites include the kidney, heart, spleen, and brain (Green and Miller, 2013). Even though vitamin B_{12} is water-soluble, Kominato (1971) reported a tissue half-life of 32 days, indicating considerable tissue storage.

Biochemical functions

Although the most important tasks of vitamin B_{12} concern the metabolism of nucleic acids and proteins, it also functions in the metabolism of fats and carbohydrates. Overall, protein synthesis is impaired in vitamin B_{12}-deficient animals (Friesecke, 1980). Moreover, the promotion of red blood cell synthesis and the maintenance of nervous system integrity are functions attributed to vitamin B_{12} (McDowell, 2000a). Vitamin B_{12} is metabolically related to other essential nutrients, such as choline, methionine, and folic acid. (Savage and Lindenbaum, 1995; Stabler, 2006).

A summary of vitamin B_{12} functions includes (Figure 4.27):

- purine and pyrimidine synthesis
- transfer of methyl groups
- formation of proteins from amino acids
- carbohydrate and fat metabolism.

Vitamin B_{12} is an important cofactor in the following functions:

- the maintenance of normal DNA synthesis: failure of this metabolic pathway can lead to megaloblastic anemia
- the regeneration of methionine for the dual purposes of maintaining protein synthesis and methylation capacity
- the avoidance of homocysteine accumulation, an amino acid metabolite implicated in vascular damage, thrombosis, and several associated degenerative diseases, including coronary artery disease, stroke, and osteoporosis (Green and Miller, 2013).

Gluconeogenesis and hemopoiesis are critically affected by cobalt deficiency, and carbohydrate, lipid, and nucleic acid metabolism are all dependent on adequate B_{12} and folic acid metabolism. Cyanocobalamin is involved in the metabolism of fatty acids, the synthesis of proteins, and reactions involving the transfer of methyl and hydrogenated/hydrogen groups (Green and Miller, 2013).

Vitamin B_{12} is a cofactor of 2 important metabolic reactions in cells, one involving mitochondrial adenosylcobalamin and the other cytoplasmic, mostly related to methylcobalamine.

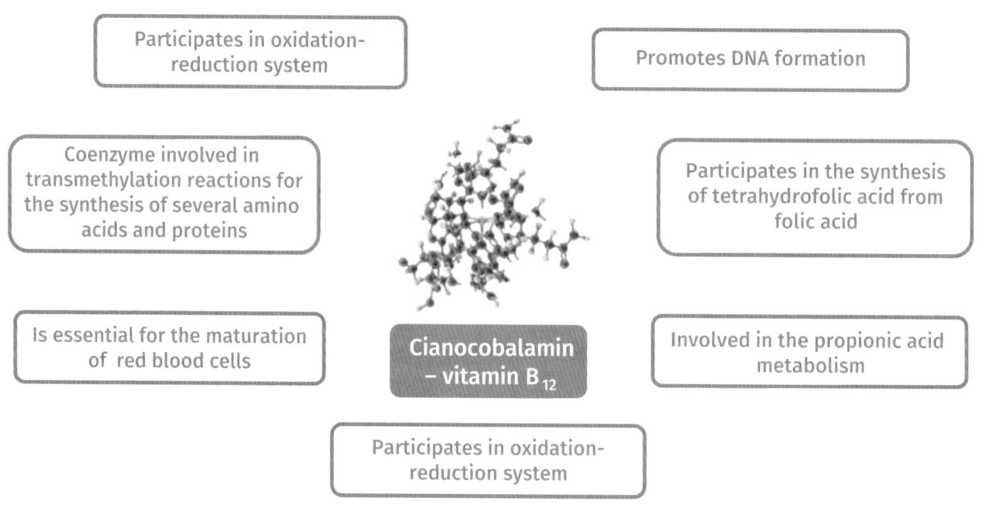

Figure 4.27 Vitamin B_{12} functions

In the mitochondrial reaction, B_{12} in the form of 5′-deoxyadenosylcobalamin is required for the enzyme methylmalonyl-CoA mutase, a vitamin B_{12}-requiring enzyme (5′-deoxyadenosylcobalamin) that catalyzes the conversion of methylmalonyl-CoA to succinyl-CoA (Green and Miller, 2013). This is an intermediate step in transforming propionate to succinate during the oxidation of odd-chain fatty acids and the catabolism of ketogenic amino acids. In animal metabolism, propionate of dietary or metabolic origin is converted into succinate, entering the tricarboxylic acid (Krebs) cycle.

In the cytoplasmic reaction, B_{12} in the form of methylcobalamin is required in the folate-dependent methylation of the sulfur amino acid homocysteine to form methionine catalyzed by the enzyme methionine synthase. Apart from being necessary for adequate protein synthesis, methionine is also a key precursor for the maintenance of methylation capacity through the synthesis of the universal methyl donor S-adenosylmethionine. Additionally, the methionine synthase reaction is finally necessary for normal DNA synthesis.

The methyl group transferred to homocysteine during methionine synthesis is donated by the folate derivative methyltetrahydrofolate (methyl-THF), forming THF. THF is later transformed to 5,20-methylenetetrahydrofolate (methylene-THF) by a one-carbon transfer during serine conversion to glycine. Methylene-THF can be reduced again to form methyl-THF. Still, it also serves as the critical one-carbon source for the *de novo* synthesis of thymidylate from deoxyuridylate, required for DNA replication. Finally, an additional function of vitamin B_{12} relates to immune function. In mice, vitamin B_{12} deficiency affected immunoglobulin production and cytokine levels (Funada *et al.*, 2001).

Nutritional assessment

Historically, vitamin B_{12} was measured using microbiological assays such as the *Lactobacillus delbrueckii* method, which was later adapted for high-throughput use (Sauberlich, 1999). Measuring the total vitamin B_{12} concentration in serum is the first-line clinical test for determining vitamin B_{12} deficiency. The current assays are mostly based on the competitive binding of the serum vitamin to intrinsic factor, followed by radiometric or fluorescence-based detection (Höller *et al.*, 2018).

TC-bound cobalamin, the form most actively transported into tissues, can be measured and is considered a relevant marker of vitamin B_{12} status. A newer method estimates holotranscobalamin (holoTC) as a fraction of vitamin B_{12} carried by TC in serum and, therefore, available for tissue uptake (Höller *et al.*, 2018).

Deficiency signs

The most common cause of clinically evident B_{12} deficiency is malabsorption either due to gastric issues affecting intrinsic factors – including pernicious anemia, an autoimmune loss of intrinsic factor responsible for uptake of cobalamin that is fatal if untreated – or ileal mucosa issues, although inadequate dietary intake cause or contribute to B_{12} deficiency.

Vitamin B_{12} deficiency has profound pathophysiological effects on the blood, nervous system, and possibly organs. The most noticeable effect of vitamin B_{12} deficiency is megaloblastic anemia, caused by the disruption of DNA synthesis. Vitamin B_{12} deficiency reduces bodyweight gain, feed intake, and feed conversion in growing chicks, turkey poults, and quail. Poor feathering and mortality are the most obvious signs of a vitamin B_{12} deficiency, and gizzard erosions may also appear (NRC, 1994).

Vitamin B_{12} deficiency in growing chicks and turkeys may result in a nervous disorder and defective feathering. It has also been related to leg weakness and perosis, this appears to be a secondary effect when the diet lacks choline, methionine, or betaine as a source of methyl groups. The addition of B_{12} may prevent perosis under these conditions because of its effect on the synthesis of methyl groups (Figure 4.28). Additional clinical signs of B_{12} deficiency include anemia, gizzard erosion, and fatty deposits in the heart, liver, and kidneys.

The reduction of methylene-THF to methyl-THF is an irreversible reaction under physiological conditions. Consequently, when B_{12} is deficient and THF synthesis is impaired through interdiction of the methionine synthase reaction, methyl-THF has no metabolic outlet, forward to THF or backward to methylene-THF, and it becomes trapped (Green and Miller, 2013).

Deficiency of vitamin B_{12} will induce folic acid deficiency by blocking the utilization of folic acid derivatives: folic acid remains trapped as methylfolate and thus becomes metabolically useless. This explains why the hematological damage of vitamin B_{12} deficiency is indistinguishable from that of folacin deficiency, resulting in an inadequate quantity of methylene-THF to participate adequately in DNA synthesis. Vitamin B_{12} deficiency can be generated with the addition of high dietary levels of propionic acid.

In hens, body weight and egg production are maintained despite a deficiency, but B_{12} influences egg size (Scott *et al.*, 1982). However, Squires and Naber (1992) reported that both egg production and hen weight increased with vitamin B_{12} supplementation, as did hatchability and egg weight. The hatchability of incubated eggs may be severely reduced if the breeder diet contains inadequate vitamin B_{12} (Squires and Naber, 1992; Zhang *et al.*, 1994). Changes that manifest themselves in vitamin B_{12}-deficient chick embryos (Olcese *et al.*, 1950) may be summarized as:

- general hemorrhagic condition
- fatty liver in varying degrees
- the heart is often enlarged and irregular in shape
- kidneys pale or yellow, sometimes hemorrhagic
- incidence of perosis
- myoatrophy of the leg

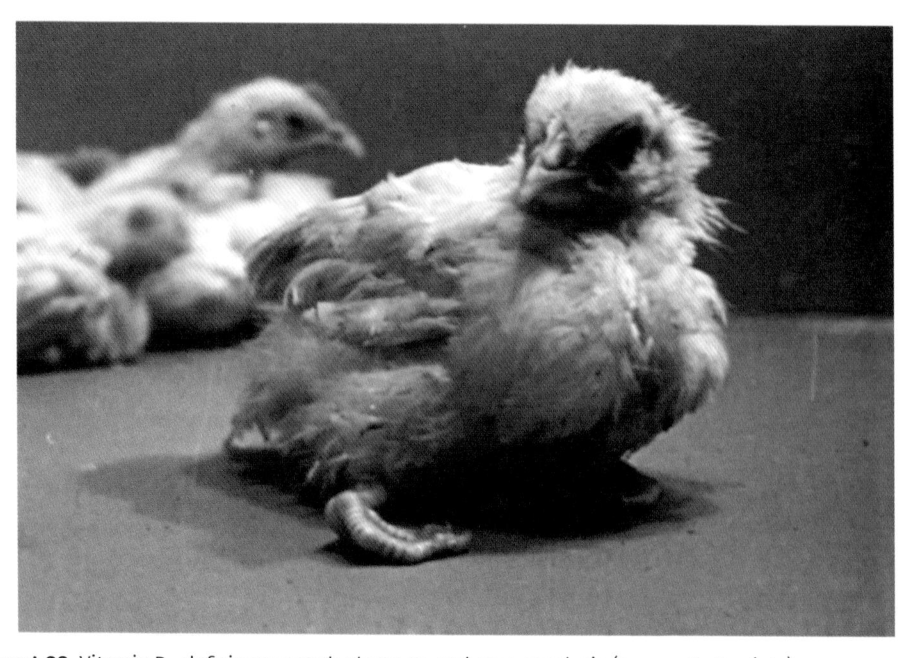

Figure 4.28 Vitamin B_{12} deficiency: rough plumage, curly toe paralysis (source: E. Gerriets)

- fewer myelinated fibers in the spinal cord
- high incidence of embryonic malpositions.

Hypertrophy of the thyroid gland has also been repeatedly observed (Ferguson and Couch, 1954). The most obvious change in B_{12}-deficient embryos is myoatrophy of the leg, characterized by atrophy of thigh muscles (Olcese *et al.*, 1950).

A period of 2–5 months may be needed to deplete hens of vitamin B_{12} stores to such an extent that progeny will hatch with low vitamin B_{12} reserves. The depletion rate is most rapid when hens are fed high-protein diets (Scott *et al.*, 1982). Chicks that hatch without good carry-over of vitamin B_{12} from the dam have a high mortality rate. Vitamin B_{12}-deficient embryos die at about day 17.

Safety

Adding vitamin B_{12} to feeds in amounts far above requirement or absorbability appears to be without hazard. Dietary levels of at least several hundred times the requirement are considered safe for most species (NRC, 1987). Vitamin B_{12} is reported to be toxic with around 5 mg/kg diet. Signs of toxicity are unclear, especially with many older reports, since results are likely confounded with toxic effects of fermentation residues, inadvertently included with B_{12} during manufacture (Leeson and Summers, 2008).

Niacin (vitamin B_3)

Chemical structure and properties

The 2 forms of niacin or vitamin B_3, nicotinic acid (pyridine-3-carboxylic acid) and nicotinamide (or niacinamide; pyridine-3-carboxylic acid amide) are functional parts of the coenzymes nicotinamide adenine dinucleotide (NAD) and NADP, involved in the cellular respiration processes (Kirkland, 2013).

The empirical formula is $C_6H_3O_2N$ (Figure 4.29). Nicotinic acid and nicotinamide correspond to 3-pyridine carboxylic acid and its amide. Both are white, odorless, crystalline solids soluble in water and alcohol. They are resistant to heat, air, light, and alkali and thus are stable in feeds. Niacin is also stable in the presence of the usual oxidizing agents: however, it will undergo decarboxylation at a high temperature in an alkaline medium.

An additional source of supplemental niacin would be the vitamin K supplement menadione nicotinamide bisulfite (MNB), with a content ≥31% nicotinamide. Results with chicks suggest MNB is fully effective as a source of vitamin K and niacin activity (Oduho *et al.*, 1993).

Natural sources

Niacin is widely distributed in feedstuffs of both plant and animal origin. Good sources are animal and fish by-products, distiller grains and yeast, various distillation and fermentation

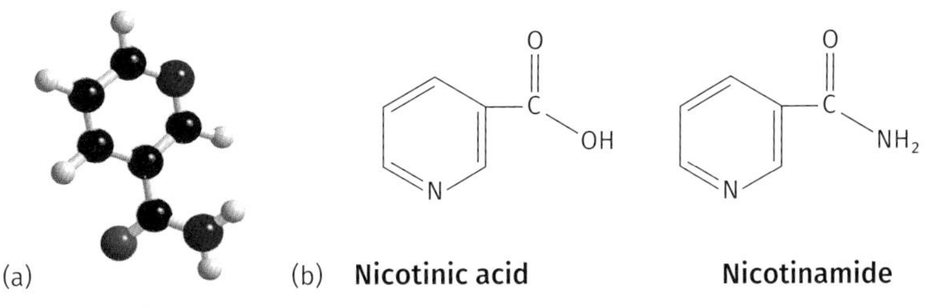

Figure 4.29 Niacin chemical structure

solubles, cereals, and certain oilseed meals. Niacin is fairly stable under normal conditions, but its bioavailability is low, at least in monogastric animals, especially in wheat and sorghum (10–15%) and in corn (0% to 30%), as it is found in combination with a peptide or a carbohydrate (Luce *et al.*, 1966; 1967). In oilseeds, bioavailability is 40%. Oilseeds contain about 40% of their total niacin in bound form, while only a small proportion of the niacin in pulses, yeast, crustacean, fish, animal tissue, or milk is bound.

Two types of bound niacin were initially described: (1) a peptide with a molecular weight of 12,000 to 13,000, the so-called niacinogens; and (2) a carbohydrate complex with a molecular weight of approximately 2,370 (Darby *et al.*, 1975). The name niacytin has been used to designate this latter material from wheat bran. Using a microbiological assay, Ghosh *et al.* (1963) reported that 85 to 90% of the total nicotinic acid in cereals is in a bound form. Using a rat assay procedure, for 8 samples of mature cooked cereals (corn, wheat, rice, and milo), only about 35% of the total niacin was available (Carter and Carpenter, 1982).

Therefore, in calculating the niacin content of formulated diets, probably all the niacin from cereal grain sources should be ignored or at least given a value no greater than one-third of the total niacin. In immature seeds, niacin is part of biologically available coenzymes necessary for seed metabolism. Niacin binding to carbohydrates by ester linkages may cause it to be retained in the mature seed until it is utilized. Hence, the vitamin availability for man and animals is thus impaired. In rat growth assays for available niacin, corn harvested immaturely ("milk stage") gave values from 74 to 88 µg/gm. In contrast, corn harvested at maturity gave assay values of 16 to 18 µg/gm (Carpenter *et al.*, 1988).

Most species can use the essential amino acid tryptophan from which niacin can be synthesized. Because tryptophan can give rise to body niacin, both the niacin and tryptophan content should be considered together in expressing niacin values of feeds. However, tryptophan is preferably used for protein synthesis (Kodicek *et al.*, 1974; Kirkland, 2013). Consequently, it is unlikely that tryptophan conversion greatly contributes to the niacin supply since feedstuffs used in most diets tend to be low in tryptophan. Furthermore, the efficiency of the biochemical conversion is low (Scott *et al.*, 1982). Chicken meat is an excellent source of niacin, providing some 14 mg/100 g (78% of recommended daily intake).

Commercial forms

Nicotinic acid and niacinamide are both available commercially as fine granular-powder formulations containing 99% activity.

Metabolism

Absorption and transport

Nicotinic acid and nicotinamide are rapidly absorbed from the stomach and the intestine at either physiological or pharmacologic doses (Nabokina *et al.*, 2005; Jacob, 2006). In the gut mucosa nicotinic acid is converted to nicotinamide (Stein *et al.*, 1994). Niacin in foods occurs mostly in its coenzyme forms. Pyrophosphatase activity in the upper small intestine metabolizes NAD and NADP to yield nicotinamide, which is then hydrolyzed to form nicotinamide riboside and eventually free nicotinamide, and which seems to be absorbed as such without further hydrolysis in the gastrointestinal tract (Kirkland, 2013).

Intestinal absorption of both nicotinic acid and nicotinamide at low concentrations appears via sodium-dependent high-affinity transporters. Once absorbed from the lumen into the enterocyte, nicotinamide may be converted via the Preiss–Handler pathway to NAD or released into the portal circulation. Although some nicotinic acid moves into the blood in its native form, the enterocyte's bulk of nicotinic acid is converted to NAD. The intestinal mucosa contains niacin conversion enzymes such as NAD glycohydrolase (Henderson and Gross, 1979). As required, NAD glycohydrolases in the enterocytes release nicotinamide from NAD into the plasma, as the principal circulating form of niacin, for transport to tissues that synthesize NAD as needed.

Blood transport of niacin is associated mainly with red blood cells. Erythrocytes effectively take up nicotinic acid and nicotinamide by facilitating diffusion, converting them to nucleotides to maintain a concentration gradient. However, niacin rapidly leaves the bloodstream and enters the kidney, liver, and adipose tissues.

The amino acid tryptophan is a precursor for niacin synthesis in the body. There is considerable evidence that synthesis can occur in the intestine, and there is also evidence that synthesis can take place elsewhere within the body. The extent to which the metabolic requirement for niacin can be met from tryptophan will depend first on the amount of tryptophan in the diet and second on the efficiency of conversion of tryptophan to niacin (Linh *et al.*, 2021). The kynurenine pathway of tryptophan conversion to nicotinic acid and finally NAD in the body is shown in Figure 4.30.

The conversion of tryptophan to nicotinic acid-NAD is irreversible (Kirkland, 2013). Protein, energy, vitamin B_6, and vitamin B_2 nutritional status and hormones affect one or more steps in the conversion sequence and hence can influence the yield of niacin from tryptophan. Two enzymes require iron to convert tryptophan to niacin with a deficiency reducing tryptophan utilization. At low levels of tryptophan intake, the conversion efficiency is high, and it decreases when niacin and tryptophan levels in the diet are increased (Linh *et al.*, 2021).

Tryptophan is converted into niacin at a ratio of 45–50 : 1 in chickens (Whitehead and Portsmouth, 1989) or 102–119 : 1 in turkeys (Ruiz and Harms, 1988b). Conversion of tryptophan to niacin among species is probably due to inherent differences in liver levels of picolinic acid carboxylase, the enzyme that diverts one of the intermediates (2-amino, 3-acroleylfumaric acid) to the picolinic acid pathway instead of allowing this compound to condense to quinolinic acid, the immediate precursor of nicotinic acid (Kirkland, 2013).

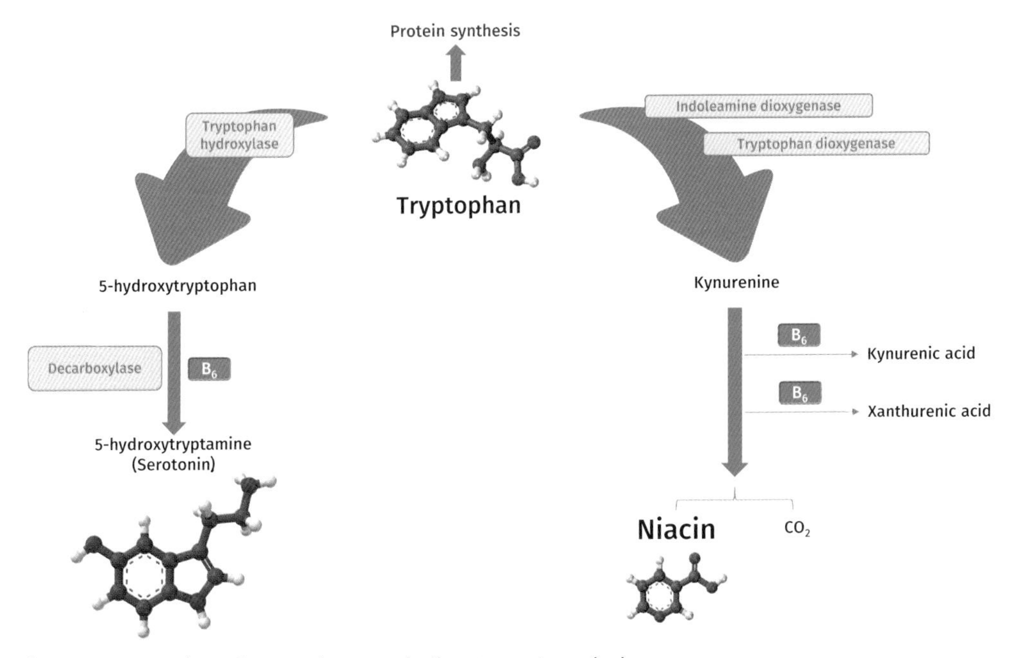

Figure 4.30 Overview of tryptophan metabolism to produce niacin

Picolinic acid carboxylase activity in livers of various species has a positive correlation to experimentally determined niacin requirements. The rat diverts very little of its dietary tryptophan to carbon dioxide and water and thus is relatively efficient in converting tryptophan to niacin. The duck has a very high niacin requirement, approximately twice as high as chickens, with considerably higher levels of picolinic acid carboxylase activity (Scott *et al.*, 1982).

In practice, the production of niacin from tryptophan is minimal since this amino acid is not normally found in excess in diets. Moreover, high levels of fat in feed, especially saturated fat, will inhibit this reaction (Whitehead, 2001; Kirkland, 2013).

Finally, tryptophan is preferably used for protein synthesis (Kodicek *et al.*, 1974; Kirkland, 2013). Consequently, it is unlikely that tryptophan conversion greatly contributes to the niacin supply since feedstuffs used in most diets tend to be low in tryptophan.

Storage and excretion

Although niacin coenzymes are widely distributed in the body, no true storage occurs. The liver is the site of the greatest niacin concentration in the body, but the amount stored is minimal. The tissue content of niacin and its analogs, NAD and NADP, is a variable factor dependent on the diet and several other factors, such as strain, sex, age, and treatment of animals (Hankes, 1984). The liver is a central processing organ for niacin. Aside from its role in converting tryptophan to NAD, it receives nicotinamide and some nicotinic acid via the portal circulation and nicotinamide released from other extrahepatic tissues. In the liver, nicotinic acid and nicotinamide are metabolized to NAD or to yield compounds for urinary excretion, depending on the niacin status of the organism.

Urine is the primary pathway of excretion of absorbed niacin and its metabolites. In the chicken, nicotinic acid is conjugated with ornithine as either αα- or ∂-nicotinyl ornithine or dinicotinyl ornithine. The excretion of these metabolites is measured in studies of niacin requirements and niacin metabolism.

Biochemical functions

There are 14 known metabolic reactions in which niacin participates, forming part of the NAD and NADP coenzymes. Therefore, it is essential in the metabolism of carbohydrates, amino acids, and fatty acids and for obtaining energy through the Krebs cycle. NAD and NADP coenzymes are especially important in the metabolic reactions that furnish energy to the animal.

Like the riboflavin coenzymes, the NAD and NADP containing enzyme systems play an important role in biological oxidation-reduction, including more than 200 reactions in the metabolism of carbohydrates, fatty acids, and amino acids, due to their capacity to serve as hydrogen transfer agents. Hydrogen is effectively transferred from the oxidizable substrate to oxygen through a series of graded enzymatic hydrogen transfers. Nicotinamide-containing enzyme systems constitute one such group of hydrogen transfer agents.

Important metabolic reactions catalyzed by NAD and NADP are summarized as follows (McDowell, 2000a; Kirkland, 2013):

1 carbohydrate metabolism:
   - glycolysis: anaerobic and aerobic oxidation of glucose
   - TCA or Krebs cycle

2 lipid metabolism:
   - glycerol synthesis and breakdown
   - fatty acid oxidation and synthesis
   - steroid synthesis

3 protein metabolism:
   - degradation and synthesis of amino acids
   - oxidation of carbon chains via the TCA cycle
4 photosynthesis
5 rhodopsin synthesis

Niacin, riboflavin, and coenzyme Q_{10} are associated with poly ADP-ribose synthesized in response to DNA strand breaks and involved in the post-translational modification of nuclear proteins (Kirkland, 2013). The poly ADP-ribosylated proteins function in DNA repair, DNA replication, and cell differentiation (Carson *et al.*, 1987; Premkumar *et al.*, 2008). These functions may be important in tissues with high turnover rates like the skin, intestines, and CNS (Kirkland, 2013; Gasperi *et al.*, 2019). Rat data have shown that even a mild niacin deficiency decreases liver poly ADP-ribose concentrations, and those levels are also altered by feed restriction (Rawling *et al.*, 1994). Zhang *et al.* (1993) suggested that a severe niacin deficiency may increase the susceptibility of DNA to oxidative damage, likely due to the lower availability of NAD.

Protein turnover rates in Japanese quail have been related to niacin deficiency; a high turnover rate due to the deficiency was primarily attributed to enhanced degradation rate of proteins rather than enhanced synthesis rate of proteins (Park *et al.*, 1991).

Nutritional assessment

Niacin and its metabolites can be measured in plasma via gas chromatography (GC), HPLC, or simultaneously via LC-MS/MS. However, the main gap is the lack of reliable ranges, even in humans, making the assessment extremely complicated (Höller *et al.*, 2018).

Deficiency signs

There is good evidence that poultry, even chick, and turkey embryos can synthesize niacin, but the synthesis rate may be too slow for optimal growth. The deficiency could be found in animal populations depending on feed ingredients, particularly corn, which is low in available niacin and its precursor tryptophan (Kirkland, 2013). It has been claimed that tryptophan must first be deficient before there can be a marked deficiency of niacin in the chicken. Chicks at hatch have considerable tryptophan contained in the protein of the yolk. Thus, a niacin deficiency will not readily occur unless the feed is low in amino acids and vitamins (NRC, 1994).

Niacin deficiency is characterized by severe metabolic disorders in the skin, digestive organs, and neurological system. The first signs of loss of appetite, retarded growth, weakness, dermatitis, digestive disorders, and diarrhea (Figure 4.31).

The deficiency results in "black tongue," a condition characterized by tongue and mouth cavity inflammation. At about 2 weeks of age, the entire mouth cavity and the esophagus become distinctly inflamed, growth is retarded, and feed consumption is reduced. Experiments using diets containing a limited amount of tryptophan have shown that the chick does require niacin and that a deficiency produces an enlargement of the tibiotarsal joint, bowing of the legs, poor feathering, and dermatitis (Scott *et al.*, 1982). Oloyo (1997) noted that supplementing a niacin-deficient broiler diet with 15.0 mg/kg niacin prevented dermatitis, but 22.5 mg/kg niacin was required to prevent leg deformities.

The main clinical sign of niacin deficiency in young chicks is an enlargement of the hock joint and bowing of the legs, similar to perosis. The main difference between this condition and the perosis of manganese or choline deficiency is that the Achilles' tendon rarely slips from its condyles in niacin deficiency. In niacin-deficient laying hens, there is weight loss, and egg production and hatchability are reduced.

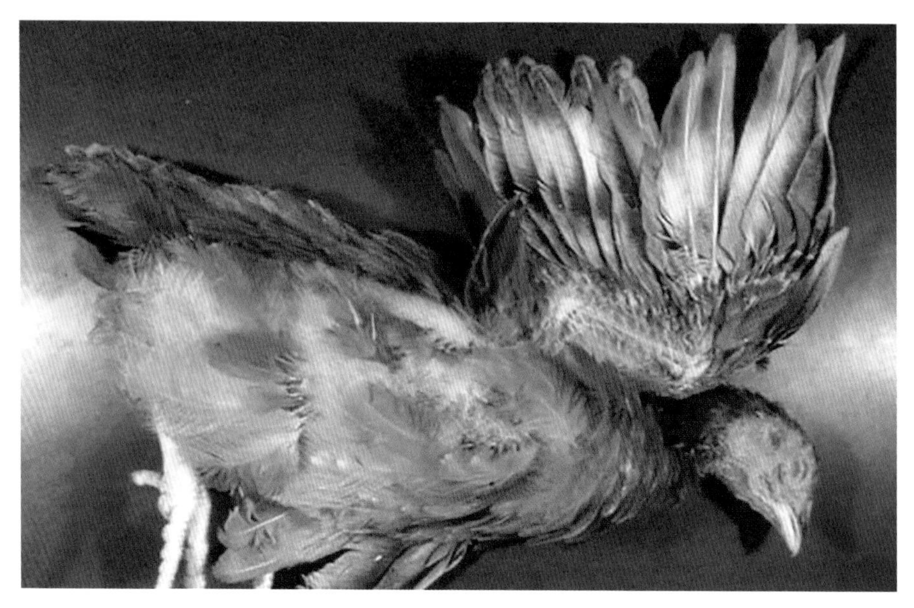

Figure 4.31 Niacin deficiency: dermatitis (source: copyright UK Crown)

Turkey poults, pheasant chicks, ducklings, and goslings expressed perosis as the primary niacin deficiency sign (NRC, 1994). Compared to the chick, the turkey poult, duckling, pheasant chick, and gosling have higher requirements for niacin. This higher requirement is related to these species' less efficient conversion of tryptophan to niacin. Symptoms of niacin deficiency in turkeys and ducks are much more severe, similar to those in chickens. Ducks receiving low-niacin diets show severely bowed legs and ultimately become so crippled and weak that they cannot walk. Niacin deficiency in the turkey is also characterized by a severe bowing of the legs and enlargement of the hock joint. Goslings on purified diets developed perosis and hock deformities that were prevented with nicotinic acid administration (Briggs *et al.*, 1953). There are antivitamins or antagonists for niacin. These compounds have the basic pyridine structure, and 2 of the important antagonists of nicotinic acid are 3-acetyl pyridine and pyridine sulfonic acid.

Safety

Research indicates that nicotinic acid and nicotinamide have a high safety margin, being toxic at dietary intakes greater than about 350 mg/kg bodyweight per day (NRC, 1987).

Clinical signs for niacin toxicosis in chicks include reduced egg production, growth retardation, short legs, and coarse, dense feathering. High dietary levels of niacin (0.75 to 2.0%) fed to broilers were detrimental to bone dimensions and mechanical properties (Johnson *et al.*, 1992, 1995; Leeson and Summers, 2008). There was no change in the mineral content of the tibia, but bone strength decreased with increased susceptibility to fracture.

Pantothenic acid (vitamin B_5)

Chemical structure and properties

In popular literature, pantothenic acid is often referred to as vitamin B_5, though the origin of this designation is obscure (Rucker and Bauerly, 2013). Pantothenic acid is an amide consisting of pantoic acid joined to β-alanine found forming part of the coenzymes, especially coenzyme

A (CoA), containing the vitamin as an essential component, and the acyl groups carrier protein (ACP). The structural formula and crystalline structure are shown in Figure 4.32.

The free acid of the vitamin is a viscous, pale-yellow oil readily soluble in water and ethyl acetate. It crystallizes as white needles from ethanol and is reasonably stable to light and air. The oil is extremely hygroscopic and easily destroyed by acids, bases, and heat. Maximum heat stability occurs at pH 5.5 to 7.0.

Pantothenic acid is optically active (characteristic of rotating a polarized light). It may be prepared either as the pure dextrorotatory (d) form or the racemic mixture (dl) form. The racemic form has approximately one-half the biological activity of d-calcium pantothenate, the commercial form used in poultry nutrition. Only the dextrorotatory form, d-pantothenic acid, is effective as a vitamin.

Natural sources

Pantothenic acid is widely distributed in feedstuffs of animal and plant origin. Corn and soybean meal diets are likely to be low in pantothenic acid. Alfalfa hay, peanut meal, cane molasses, yeast, rice bran, green leafy plants, wheat bran, brewer's yeast, fish solubles, and rice polishings are good sources of the vitamin for animals. Milling by-products, such as rice bran and wheat bran, are good sources, 2 to 3 times higher than the respective grains. Many poultry diets are borderline in supplying pantothenic acid requirements, and many are deficient in this vitamin.

The biological availability of pantothenic acid is high in corn and soybean meal but low in barley, wheat, and sorghum, approximately 60%. (Southern and Baker, 1981). Changing processing methods can greatly alter vitamin feed levels. For example, with changes in sugar technology, literature values for pantothenic acid content of beet molasses have decreased from 50 to 100 mg/kg in the 1950s to 1–4 mg/kg (Palagina *et al.*, 1990).

Pantothenic acid is fairly stable in feedstuffs during long storage periods (Scott *et al.*, 1982). Heating during processing may cause considerable losses, especially if temperatures attain 100–150°C for long periods and pH values above 7 or below 5. Gadient (1986) considers pantothenic acid slightly sensitive to heat, oxygen, or light but very sensitive to moisture. As a general guideline, pantothenic acid activity in normal pelleted feed over 3 months at room temperature should be 80–100%. Although this vitamin is found in practically all feedstuffs, complementary supplementation is advisable in rations for birds to ensure a high production level.

Commercial forms

Pantothenic acid is available as a commercially synthesized product for feed, known as d- or dl-calcium pantothenate. Because livestock and poultry can biologically utilize only the

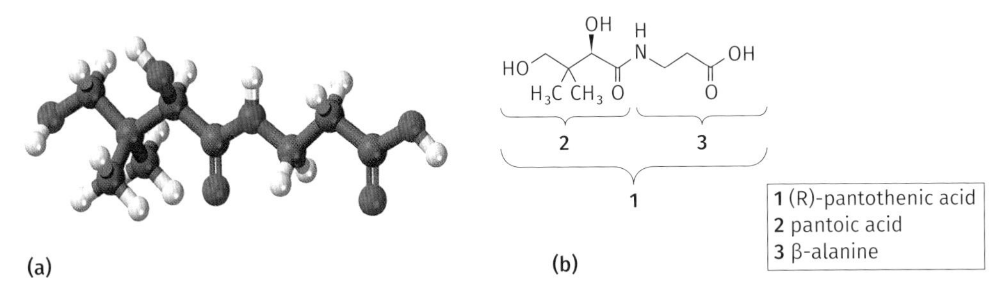

Figure 4.32 The structure of pantothenic acid

d-isomer of pantothenic acid, nutrient requirements for the vitamin are routinely expressed in the d-form. One gram of d-calcium pantothenate is equivalent to 0.92 gm of d-pantothenic acid activity. Therefore 1.087 g of d-calcium pantothenate is required to get the activity of 1 g of d-pantothenic acid.

Sometimes a racemic mixture (i.e., equal parts d- and dl-calcium pantothenate) is offered to the feed industry. The racemic mixture of 1 g of the dl-form has 0.46 g of d-pantothenic acid activity. Hence with this product, 2.174 g is needed to get the activity of 1 g of d-pantothenic acid. Products sold based on racemic mixture content can be misleading and confusing to a buyer not fully aware of the biological activity supplied by d-calcium pantothenate. To avoid confusion, the label should clearly state the grams of d-calcium pantothenate or its equivalent per unit weight and the grams of d-pantothenic acid. Moreover, because of its hygroscopic and electrostatic properties, the racemic mixture can create handling problems.

Losses of calcium pantothenate may occur in premixes that are extremely acidic. Verbeeck (1975) reported calcium pantothenate to be stable in premixes with or without trace minerals, regardless of the mineral form. Recently Lewis *et al.* (2015) and Yang *et al.* (2020) reported that pelleting causes only small losses of pantothenic acid.

Metabolism

Absorption and transport

Pantothenic acid is found in feeds in both bound (largely as CoA) and free forms. It is necessary to liberate the pantothenic acid from the bound forms in the digestive process before absorption. Work with chicks and rats indicated that pantothenic acid, its salt, and the alcohol are absorbed primarily in the jejunum by a specific transport system that is saturable and sodium ion-dependent (Fenstermacher and Rose, 1986; Miller *et al.*, 2006). The alcohol form, panthenol, oxidized to pantothenic acid *in vivo*, appears to be absorbed somewhat faster than the acid form.

After absorption, pantothenic acid is transported to various tissues in the plasma. Most cells take it up via another active-transport process involving cotransport of pantothenate and sodium in a 1 : 1 ratio (Olson, 1990). Pantothenic acid is converted to CoA and other compounds within tissues where a vitamin is a functional group (Sauberlich, 1985).

Storage and excretion

Livestock does not appear to have the ability to store appreciable amounts of pantothenic acid: organs such as the liver and kidneys have the highest concentrations. Most pantothenic acid in blood exists in red blood cells as CoA, but free pantothenic acid is also present. The serum does not contain CoA but does contain free pantothenic acid.

Urinary excretion is the major route of body loss of absorbed pantothenic acid, and excretion is prompt when the vitamin is consumed in excess. Most pantothenic acid is excreted as a free vitamin, but some species (e.g., dogs) pass it as β-glucuronide (Taylor *et al.*, 1972). Pearson *et al.* (1953) found that pantothenic acid's urinary and fecal excretion was 4 to 6 times the intake when semi-synthetic diets were fed. Pantothenic acid excretion increased with increased crude protein intakes. An appreciable quantity of pantothenic acid (~15% of daily intake) is completely oxidized and excreted across the lungs as CO_2.

Biochemical functions

Pantothenic acid is involved in several metabolic pathways important in endogenous metabolism energy exchange in all tissues. Its main functions include (Rucker and Bauerly, 2013):

- utilization of nutrients
- synthesis of fatty acids, cholesterol, and steroid hormones
- synthesis of neurotransmitters, steroid hormones, porphyrins, and hemoglobin
- participation in the citric acid cycle or Krebs cycle, as a constituent of acetyl-coenzyme A and other enzymes and coenzymes
- energy-yielding oxidation of fats, carbohydrates, and amino acids
- involved in the production of antibodies, the adrenal glands' activity, and the acetylation of choline for nerve impulse transmission
- relationship with vitamin B_{12}; if the latter is deficient, it accentuates the lack of pantothenic acid
- interactions with folic acid, biotin, and copper.

CoA's most important function is acting as a carrier mechanism for carboxylic acids (Lehninger, 1982; Miller *et al.*, 2006; Rucker and Bauerly, 2013). When bound to CoA, such acids have a high potential for transfer to other groups, and such carboxylic acids are normally referred to as "active." The most important of these reactions is the combination of CoA with acetate to form "active acetate" with a high-energy bond that renders acetate capable of further chemical interactions. Combining CoA with two-carbon fragments from fats, carbohydrates, and certain amino acids to form acetyl-CoA is essential in their complete metabolism because the coenzyme enables these fragments to enter the TCA cycle. For example, acetyl-CoA is utilized directly by combining with oxaloacetic acid to form citric acid, entering the TCA cycle. Coenzyme A, along with ACP, functions as a carrier of acyl groups in enzymatic reactions involved in synthesizing fatty acids, cholesterol, and other sterols; oxidation of fatty acids, pyruvate, and α-ketoglutarate; and biological acetylations. Decarboxylation of α-ketoglutaric acid in the TCA cycle yields succinic acid, which is then converted to the "active" form by linkage with CoA. Active succinate and glycine are involved in the first step of heme biosynthesis.

In the form of acetyl-CoA, acetic acid can also combine with choline to form acetylcholine, a chemical transmitter at the nerve synapse, and can be used to detoxify various drugs such as sulfonamides. Pantothenic acid also stimulates the synthesis of antibodies, increasing animal resistance to pathogens. It appears that when pantothenic acid is deficient, the incorporation of amino acids into the blood albumin fraction is inhibited, which would explain why there is a reduction in the titer of antibodies (Axelrod, 1971).

Nutritional assessment

Early assays use pantothenic acid-dependent microorganisms such as *Lactobacillus plantarum* for quantification (Sauberlich, 1999). This assay is prone to various interferences, and therefore more specific radioimmunoassays (RIA) or enzyme-linked immunosorbent assay (ELISA) tests have been developed (Sauberlich, 1999) and used to measure it in blood plasma to determine body status (Höller *et al.*, 2018).

Deficiency signs

The primary lesions of pantothenic acid deficiency for poultry appear to involve the nervous system, adrenal cortex, and skin (Scott *et al.*, 1982). In chickens, a growth decline is followed by a decrease in feed conversion and retardation of feather growth. Plumage becomes rough and ruffled, and feathers become brittle and may fall; next, dermatitis rapidly develops in chicks. Corners of the beak and the area below the beak are most affected, but the disorder is also observed in the feet. Outer layers of skin between toes and on the bottoms of feet peel off, and small cracks and fissures appear.

In some cases, skin layers of feet thicken and cornify, and wart-like protuberances develop on the balls of the feet. The foot problem is usually exacerbated by bacterial invasion of the lesions. Within 12 to 14 days after chickens begin a deficient diet, the margins of the eyelids are sealed closed by a thick discharge. Figure 4.33 illustrates the chick's typical deficiency syndrome.

Pantothenic acid concentrations in the liver are reduced during deficiency, and the liver becomes hypertrophied and varies in color from faint yellow to dirty yellow. Nerves and fibers of the spinal cord show myelin degeneration, and these degenerating fibers occur in all cord segments down to the lumbar region (Scott *et al.*, 1982).

In young chicks, pantothenic acid deficiency signs are difficult to differentiate from biotin deficiency since both cause severe dermatitis, broken feathers, perosis, poor growth, and mortality. In pantothenic acid deficiency, dermatitis of the feet is evident over the toes, in contrast to biotin deficiency, which primarily affects the footpads and is often more severe than a deficiency of pantothenic acid (McDowell, 2000a).

Young ducks do not show the signs usually seen in chickens and turkeys except for retarded growth; however, their mortality rate is very high. Like those in young chickens, signs of pantothenic acid deficiency in young turkeys include general weakness, dermatitis and sticking together of eyelids (Figure 4.33b). Poor feathering is the most prevalent deficiency sign in pheasants and quail (Scott *et al.*, 1964).

Pantothenic acid deficiency does not normally affect egg production but severely depletes hatchability, and hatch chicks may be too weak to survive. Embryos from pantothenic acid-deficient hens have been observed to have subcutaneous hemorrhages and severe edema, with most of the mortality showing up during the latter part of the incubation period (Leeson and Summers, 2008). Embryonic mortality in pantothenic acid deficiency usually occurs during the last few days of incubation. A direct linear relationship exists between dietary pantothenic acid and hatchability. Beer *et al.* (1963) fed White leghorn hens a purified diet that contained pantothenic acid at 0.9 mg/kg of diet. They found that the hens required the addition of 1 mg/kg of diet for optimum egg production, at least 4 mg/kg of diet for maximum hatchability, and 8 mg/kg of diet for optimum hatchability and viability of offspring. Dawson *et al.* (1962) reported that turkey breeder hens fed a diet deficient in pantothenic acid demonstrated high embryonic mortality during the first week of development. After 17 days, the surviving embryos were small and poorly feathered, showing signs of edema, hemorrhaging, fatty livers, and pale, dilated hearts.

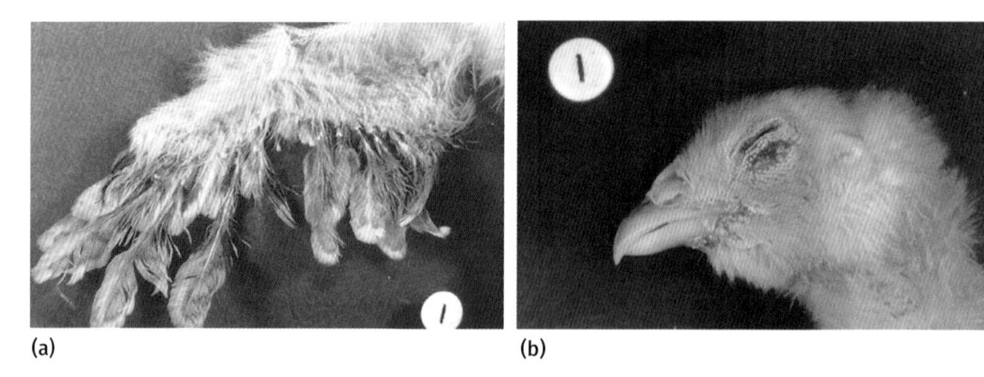

(a) (b)

Figure 4.33 Pantothenic acid deficiency: (a) faded and rough plumage (source: Copyright UK Crown); (b) (b) inflammation at the corner of the beak and the eyelids (source: copyright UK Crown)

The most common antagonist of pantothenic acid is Ω-methyl-pantothenic acid which has been used to produce a vitamin deficiency in humans (Hodges *et al.*, 1958). Other antivitamins include pantoyltaurine, phenylpantothenate hydroxocobalamin (c-lactam), an analog of vitamin B_{12}, and anti-metabolites of the vitamin containing alkyl or aryl ureido and carbamate components in the amide part of the molecule (Fox, 1991; Brass, 1993; Rucker and Bauerly, 2013).

Safety

Pantothenic acid is generally regarded as nontoxic. Excesses are mostly excreted in the urine. Pantothenic acid can become toxic at around 2,000 mg/kg. First, diarrhea and gastrointestinal disturbances can be observed followed by a reduced growth rate associated with liver damage (Leeson and Summers, 2008; Rucker and Bauerly, 2013). These levels are around 100 times the recommended supplementation for all species. Calcium pantothenate, sodium pantothenate, and panthenol are not mutagenic in bacterial tests.

Biotin (vitamin B_7)

Chemical structure and properties

The chemical structure of biotin includes a sulfur atom in its ring (like thiamine) and a transverse bond across the ring (Figure 4.34). Biotin is a bicyclic compound, a monocarboxylic acid with sulfur as a thioether linkage. One of the rings contains a ureido group (-N-CO-N-), and the other is a tetrahydrothiophene ring. The tetrahydrothiophene ring has a valeric acid side chain. With its rather unique structure, biotin contains 3 asymmetric carbon atoms; therefore, 8 different isomers are possible. Of these isomers, only d-biotin has vitamin activity (Mock, 2013).

Biotin crystallizes from water as long, white needles. Its melting point is 232–233°C. Free biotin is soluble in dilute alkaline solutions and hot water and practically insoluble in fats and organic solvents. Biotin is quite stable under ordinary conditions. It is destroyed by nitric acid, other strong acids, strong bases, and formaldehyde and is inactivated by oxidative rancidity reactions (Scott *et al.*, 1982). It is gradually destroyed by UV radiation.

Structurally related biotin analogs can vary from no activity to partial replacement of biotin activity to anti-biotin action. Mild oxidation converts biotin to the sulfoxide, and strong oxidation converts it to sulfone. Strong agents result in sulfur replacement by oxygen, resulting in oxybiotin and desthiobiotin. Oxybiotin has some biotin activity for chicks (one-third) but less for rats (one-tenth).

Natural sources

Biotin is present in common poultry feedstuffs: however, corn, wheat, other cereals, meat, and fish are relatively poor sources of biotin (Table 4.2). Of all the vitamins present in feed

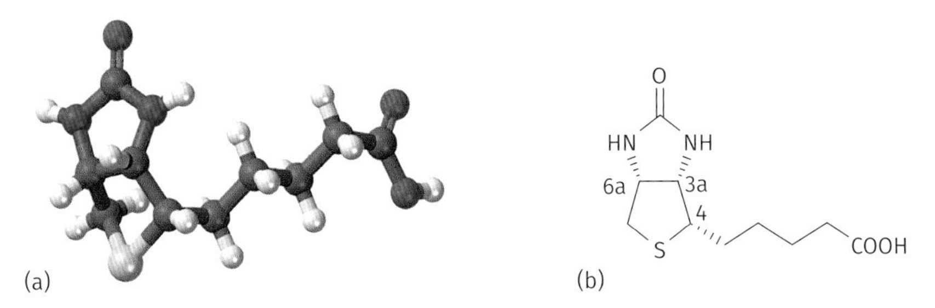

Figure 4.34 d-biotin chemical structures

Table 4.2 Biotin content in feedstuffs (source: adapted from Frigg, 1987)

Feedstuffs	Mean bioavailable biotin content (ug/kg)	Feedstuffs	Mean bioavailable biotin content (ug/kg)
Barley	14	Safflower seed meal	305
Corn	79	Sunflower seed meal	346
Corn gluten meal	189	Fish meal	135
Oats	86	Meat meal > 50% CP	88
Rye	0	Meat and bone meal < 50% CP	76
Rice polishings	74	Skim milk powder	165
Sorghum	58	Whey powder	316
Wheat	0	Cassava meal	3
Wheat bran	72	Grass meal	238
Wheat middlings	17	Alfalfa	407
Wheat germ	150	Molasses, beet	331
Rapeseed meal	68	Molasses, cane	1080
Soybean meal	270	Brewer's yeast	634

ingredients of plant origin, biotin is the one that presents the most variable content, being affected by numerous environmental factors (Frigg, 1976, 1984, 1987; Whitehead *et al.*, 1982; Misir and Blair, 1984; Mock, 2013; Cheng *et al.*, 2019). For example, 59 samples of corn analyzed for biotin varied between 56 and 115 µg/kg, and 62 samples of meat meal ranged from 17 to 323 µg (Frigg, 1987). Compared to cereal grains, oilseed meals are better sources of total biotin. Soybean meal, for instance, contains a mean biotin content of 270 µg/kg with a range of 200 to 387 µg/kg (Frigg and Völker, 1994). Milling wheat or corn reduced biotin concentrations (Bonjour, 1991).

Biotin is present in feedstuffs and yeast in both bound and free forms: therefore, it is important to know the form of biotin, i.e., bound or unbound, and its overall content in the feed. Much of the bound biotin to protein or lysine is unavailable to animal species as covalent bonds hinder its digestion and availability for the animal. For poultry, and presumably other species, often less than one-half of the microbiologically determined biotin in a feedstuff is biologically available (Scott, 1981; Whitehead *et al.*, 1982; Frigg, 1984, 1987). For alfalfa meal, corn, cottonseed meal, and soybean meal, the bioavailability of biotin is estimated at 100%. However, biotin availability is variable for other feedstuffs, for example, 11–50% in barley, 62% in corn gluten meal, 30% in fish meal, 10–60% in sorghum, 32% in oats, and 0–62% in wheat (Whitehead *et al.*, 1982; Buenrostro and Kratzer, 1984; McDowell, 2004). Diets based on these cereals without biotin supplementation lead to higher mortality and slower growth rates.

Other factors influencing biotin availability (and requirement) are some nutrients, such as fiber, which interfere with its intestinal absorption (Misir and Blair, 1984; Oloyo, 1991), protein level, with greater requirements at 18 than at 22% (Whitehead and Blair, 1974), the level of choline and the other water-soluble vitamins, which at high levels reduce the bioavailability of biotin (Whitehead *et al.*, 1976a,b; Whitehead and Randall, 1982); the proportion of added fat (Whitehead *et al.*, 1976a,b) and even the composition of the fat.

The cecal microbiota of the bird can synthesize biotin, but the quantity is variable, and the importance of its utilization by the host is unknown (Scott, 1981). As with the majority of the vitamins of the B group, there is a certain amount of recycling through coprophagy, but at 3 weeks, this is not very important, and at 7 weeks, it only amounts to 0.01 mg/kg (Whitehead and Bannister, 1980).

Biotin is unstable in oxidizing conditions and, therefore, is destroyed by heat, especially under conditions that support simultaneous lipid peroxidation, by solvent extraction and improper storage conditions. Steam pelleting does not affect the stability of biotin (Whitehead and Bannister, 1980; McGinnis, 1986) and there has even been an increase of 10% measured in its bioavailability (Buenrostro and Kratzer, 1984).

Commercial forms

Biotin is commercially available as a 100% crystalline product or as various dilutions, premixed, and low potency spray-dried preparations. The d-form of biotin is the biologically active form. It is the form that occurs in nature and is also the commercially available form. A 2% spray-dried biotin product is also commercially available in feed or drinking water.

Metabolism

Absorption and transport

In most species that have been investigated, physiological concentrations of biotin are absorbed from the intestinal tract by a sodium-dependent active-transport process, which is inhibited by dethiobiotin and biocytin (Said and Derweesh, 1991). Biotinidase, present in pancreatic juice and intestinal mucosa, catalyzes the hydrolysis of biocytin (a bound form of biotin) to biotin and free lysine during the luminal phase of proteolysis. Absorption of biotin by a Na^+-dependent process was noted to be higher in the duodenum than in the jejunum, which was, in turn, more elevated than that in the ileum. It was concluded that the proximal part of the human small intestine was the site of maximum biotin transport (Said *et al.*, 1988; Said, 2011).

Biotin is absorbed intact in the first third to half of the small intestine (Bonjour, 1991). Also, biotin is absorbed from the hindgut of the pig, with 50–61% of infused biotin disappearing between the cecum and feces. This is accompanied by a more than fourfold increase in plasma biotin concentration and a sixfold increase in urinary biotin excretion (Barth *et al.*, 1986). Biotin exits the enterocyte across the basolateral membrane. This transport is also carrier-mediated. However, this carrier is Na^+ independent, is electrogenic, and cannot accumulate biotin against a concentration gradient (Said, 2011). Biotin transport is regulated by multiple factors, including biotin nutritional status, enterocyte maturity, anatomic location, and ontogeny (Said, 2011). Biotin transport is more active in the villus cells than in the crypt cells. Transport is most active in the upper small intestine and progressively less active aborally into the colon.

Biotin appears to circulate in the bloodstream free and bound to a serum glycoprotein, which also has biotinidase activity and catalyzes biocytin's hydrolysis. In humans, 81% of biotin in plasma was free and the remainder bound (Mock and Malik, 1992; Mock, 2013). In the plasma of chickens, 2 biotin-binding proteins have been detected, which appear to be functionally different. Information on biotin transport, tissue deposition, and storage in animals and humans is very limited. Mock (1990) reported that biotin is transported as a free water-soluble component of plasma, is taken up by cells via active transport, and is attached to its apoenzymes. Said *et al.* (1992) reported that biotin is transported via a specialized, carrier-mediated transport system into the human liver. This system is Na^+ gradient-dependent and transports biotin via an electroneutral process (Mock, 2013).

Storage and excretion

All cells contain some biotin, with larger quantities in the liver and kidney. Intracellular distribution of biotin corresponds to known locations of biotin-dependent carboxylase enzymes, especially the mitochondria (Mock, 2013).

Investigations of biotin metabolism in animals are difficult to interpret, as biotin-producing microorganisms are present in the intestinal tract distal to the cecum. The amount of biotin excreted in urine and feces often exceeds the total dietary intake, whereas urinary biotin excretion is usually less than intake. Efficient conservation of biotin and the recycling of biocytin released from the catabolism of biotin-containing enzymes may be as important as the intestinal bacterial synthesis of the vitamin in meeting biotin requirements (Bender, 1992). 14C-labeled biotin showed the major portion of intraperitoneally injected radioactivity to be excreted in the urine and none in the feces or as expired carbon dioxide (Lee *et al.*, 1973). Biliary excretion of biotin and metabolites in rats and pigs is negligible (Zempleni *et al.*, 1997).

Biochemical functions

Biotin is a coenzyme essential for gluconeogenesis, lipogenesis, and the elongation of essential fatty acids. It converts carbohydrates to protein and vice versa, transforming protein and carbohydrate into fat. Biotin is important for the normal functioning of the reproductive and nervous systems and the thyroid and adrenal glands.

Biotin also plays an important role in maintaining normal blood glucose levels from the metabolism of protein and fat when the dietary intake of carbohydrates is low. As a component of 5 carboxylating enzymes, it can transport carboxyl units and fix carbon dioxide (bicarbonate) in tissue (Camporeale and Zempleni, 2006; Mock, 2013).

The 5 biotin-dependent carboxylases are:

1. propionyl-CoA carboxylase (PCC)
2. methylcrotonyl-CoA carboxylase (MCC)
3. pyruvate carboxylase (PC)
4. acetyl-CoA carboxylase 1 (ACC1)
5. acetyl-CoA carboxylase 2 (ACC2).

All except ACC2 are mitochondrial enzymes. In carbohydrate metabolism, biotin functions in both carbon dioxide fixation and decarboxylation, with the energy-producing citric acid cycle dependent upon the presence of this vitamin. The hydrolysis of ATP drives the reaction to ADP and inorganic phosphate. Specific biotin-dependent reactions in carbohydrate metabolism are:

- carboxylation of pyruvic acid to oxaloacetic acid (PC, E.C. 6.4.1.1)
- conversion of malic acid to pyruvic acid
- interconversion of succinic acid and propionic acid
- conversion of oxalosuccinic acid to α-ketoglutaric acid. In protein metabolism, biotin enzymes are important in protein synthesis, amino acid deamination, purine synthesis, and nucleic acid metabolism.

Biotin is required for transcarboxylation in the degradation of various amino acids. The vitamin deficiency in mammals hinders the normal conversion of the deaminated chain of leucine to acetyl-CoA (MCC, E.C. 6.4.1.4). Depleting hepatic biotin reduces the hepatic activity of methylcrotonyl-CoA carboxylase, which is needed for leucine degradation (Mock and Mock, 1992; Mock, 2013). Likewise, the ability to synthesize citrulline from ornithine is reduced in liver homogenates from biotin-deficient rats. The urea cycle enzyme ornithine transcarbamylase was significantly lower in the livers of biotin-deficient rats (Maeda *et al.*, 1996).

Acetyl coenzyme A (CoA)-carboxylase catalyzes the addition of carbon dioxide to acetyl-CoA to form malonyl CoA, the first reaction in the synthesis of fatty acids. Biotin is required for normal long-chain unsaturated fatty acid synthesis and is important for essential fatty acid metabolism. Deficiency in rats and chicks inhibited arachidonic acid (20:4) synthesis from linoleic acid (18:2) while increasing linolenic acid (18:3) and its metabolite (22:6) (Watkins and Kratzer, 1987a). The reduced synthesis of arachidonic acid (20:4) in chicks reduces plasma prostaglandin E_2 (PGE_2) since arachidonic acid is a precursor of prostaglandin (20:4) (Watkins and Kratzer, 1987b,c; Watkins, 1989a,b).

Evidence has emerged that biotin plays unique roles in cell signaling, epigenetic control of gene expression, and chromatin structure (Rodríguez-Meléndez and Zempleni, 2003). In rats, biotin regulates the genetic expression of holocarboxylase synthetase and mitochondrial carboxylases (Rodríquez-Meléndez *et al.*, 2001). Manthey *et al.* (2002) report that biotin affects the expression of biotin transporters, biotinylations of carboxylases, and metabolism of interleukin-2 in Jurat cells.

Nutritional assessment

Biotin status analysis can be measured in plasma using different methods, including microbiological, GC, avidin binding, colorimetric, polarographic, and isotope dilution assays (Sauberlich, 1999). Research is ongoing in humans on several markers of biotin status, but more clinical validation is needed (Höller *et al.*, 2018).

Deficiency signs

Biotin deficiency in chicks and poults results in a wide range of clinical signs with considerable variation in the appearance of individual signs (NRC, 1994). Principal effects in both species are reduced growth rate and feed efficiency (Figure 4.35a), disturbed and broken feathering, dermatitis, and leg and beak deformities (Bain *et al.*, 1988).

Its effect on the cutaneous system is most dramatic since severe dermatitis is the major obvious clinical sign of biotin deficiency in livestock and poultry. The first signs of a deficiency are usually growth depression and loose feathering. Signs of dermatitis appear next (Figure 4.35b), and finally, disorders of the leg (perosis) and beak become apparent (Figure 4.35c and 4.35d). However, Li and Huang (1994) noted that the first signs of biotin deficiency in broiler chicks were lesions on the footpads in the second week, while growth reduction did not occur until the third week.

With dermal lesions, the bottoms of feet become rough and callused and contain deep fissures that show some hemorrhaging. Foot problems are usually exacerbated by bacterial invasion of lesions. Also, toes may become necrotic and slough off. Tops of feet and legs generally show only a dry scaliness (Figure 4.35e).

Lesions appear in the corner of the mouth and slowly spread to the whole area around the beak. Eyelids eventually swell and stick together (Figure 4.35d). Dermal lesions have a characteristic order of appearance, although the speed of onset depends on the severity of deficiency. For chicks fed severely biotin-deficient diets, dryness and flakiness of the feet first become noticeable at about 14 days of age, and slight encrustations and superficial fissures develop on the undersurfaces of the feet at about 18 days (Whitehead, 1978). When the fissures are hemorrhagic, these lesions increase in severity by about 25 days. Between 3 and 4 weeks, dermatitis may also appear on the eyelids, and as this develops, the bird becomes unable to keep the lids apart, eventually sticking together.

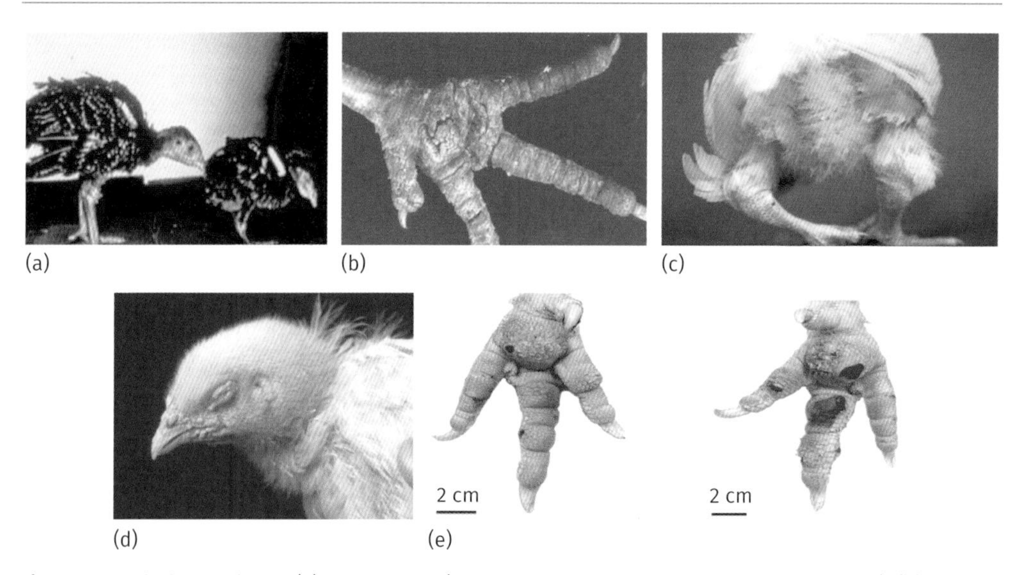

Figure 4.35 Biotin deficiency: (a) poor growth (courtesy of D.C. Dobson, Utah State University); (b) dermatitis with encrustation and cracking on the toes and balls of the feet (source: copyright UK Crown); (c) severe perosis with lateral distortion and shortening of the tibia; hyperkeratosis of the skin of the legs (source: Dr. A. Bollinger, Roche Basel); (d) encrustations at the corner of the beak and around the eyes (source: Prof. C. Whitehead); (e) turkeys foot problems

Dermal lesions are similar to those of pantothenic acid deficiency. However, with biotin deficiency, lesions occur first on the feet and later around the beak and eyes. In contrast, in pantothenic acid deficiency, signs arise first in the corners of the mouth and eyes and only in prolonged cases appear on the feet. Because of the difficulty of making a differential diagnosis between the 2 vitamins, it is often necessary to examine the diet composition and decide which is more likely to be deficient. Both vitamins should be supplemented in a corn-soybean meal ration in commercial poultry production.

Biotin deficiency is a cause of hock disorders in both poults and chicks. The major deficiency sign affecting market turkeys is severe leg weakness. Lesions caused by biotin deficiency are brought about by chondrodystrophy, a condition in which bone mineralization is normal, but linear growth of long bones is impaired. Chondrodystrophy caused by biotin deficiency can shorten metatarsal bones and perosis. Perosis occurs when irregular bone development results in enlargement and deformity of the hock joint (Figure 4.35c). Crippling in turkeys can occur as early as 3 to 4 weeks of age. Often it seems to disappear at 6 to 7 weeks. Then it reappears with great severity between 13 and 16 weeks (Scott, 1981). The birds cannot walk and thus be trampled or cannibalized by other turkeys at this stage. Perosis can occur at any stage. In general, young chickens are less susceptible to leg disorders than poults, although biotin deficiency does cause problems of the same type in chicks as in poults (Whitehead, 1978). Once the deformities of perosis occur, biotin administration is not effective.

Bain *et al.* (1988) reported that "twisted leg" is one of the most common limb disorders in broiler chicken and that biotin deficiency adversely affected tibiotarsal bone growth. Then biotin deficiency could be one of the causes. Tibiotarsal bones are frequently longitudinally distorted in biotin-deficient poultry. Presumably, reduced biotin prevents the ready formation of prostaglandins from essential fatty acids, and bone growth fails to respond to stresses during development (Watkins, 1989b).

Low dietary fat and the necessity for fatty acid synthesis led to an abnormal array of fatty acids and predisposes poultry to a fatty liver and kidney syndrome (FLKS) (Whitehead *et al.*, 1976a,b). FLKS commonly affects 2–5-week-old chicks and is characterized by a lethargic appearance followed by death within a few hours. It manifests as a disrupted metabolic process resulting in fat accumulation in the liver and kidneys. This condition, which has caused heavy economic losses in commercial broiler flocks, was found to be due to suboptimal dietary biotin causing an imbalance between 2 enzymes biotin-dependent and coupled with certain nutritional and environmental stress factors. Situations increasing the metabolic rate of biotin-dependent enzymes, such as low fat or protein levels, aggravate the condition. The signs of FLKS – sudden signs of paralysis, rapid death, pale, swollen liver and kidneys, and abnormal amounts of fat in the liver, kidney, heart, and skeletal muscle – are not those of classic biotin deficiency. They can be virtually eliminated by supplementing chick starter or breeder diets with biotin.

Biotin acts as a cofactor for many enzymes that participate in the metabolism of carbohydrates, lipids, and proteins, which are important for synthesizing long-chain fatty acids. In cases of biotin deficiency, specific alterations have been described in the lipid profile of bird tissues, consisting of a proportional reduction in the concentrations of fatty acids with a greater number of carbon atoms (Watkins and Kratzer, 1987a,b,c; Watkins, 1989a,b; Chee and Chang, 1995). Hypoglycemia is also typical since biotin helps maintain glucose levels when low carbohydrate intake (Balnave *et al.*, 1977).

Biotin requirements in the turkey are higher than that of the chick, so more field problems with biotin deficiency have arisen in turkeys. For turkeys, dry and brittle feathers usually accompany the other signs of clinical biotin deficiency. Bronze poults can exhibit white barring of the feathers, generally affecting just tom turkeys. Likewise, deficient chicks have rough and broken feathering, with head and breast feathers often having a spiky, matted appearance.

Poor egg production and hatchability result from clinical biotin deficiency (Robel, 1991; NRC, 1994). For breeder chickens, biotin deficiency reduces hatchability but is less likely to affect egg production. The biotin content in hatchable eggs increases with the hen's age (Whitehead *et al.*, 1985).

Clinical signs and conditions associated with biotin deficiency in chick embryos and/or newly hatched chicks include bone deformities (perosis), impaired muscular coordination (ataxia), skeletal deformities (e.g., crooked legs), extensive foot webbing, abnormal cartilage development (chondrodystrophy), embryonic mortality, malformed beak ("parrot beak") and reduced size.

Ferguson *et al.* (1961) reported that biotin deficiency in turkeys resulted in a marked decrease in hatchability and a high rate of embryonic mortality during the first week of incubation. At the end of the second week, hatchability decreased from 83 to 14%. At the end of week 3, hatchability was zero. Embryonic mortality because of inadequate biotin occurs largely during the last 3 days of incubation. Feeding the biotin-deficient diet resulted in an abrupt decrease in egg production after 13 weeks (Mock, 2009, 2013).

Several factors can contribute to biotin deficiencies in modern poultry production.

- Increased confinement decreases the opportunity for coprophagy (feces containing biotin synthesized in the intestines).
- Increased use of grain-soybean meal diets, with less biotin-rich feeds including whey, fermentation by-products, yeast, dehydrated alfalfa, and pasture.
- Biotin antagonists in feeds include streptavidin, certain antimicrobial drugs, and dieldrin (a pesticide). Streptomyces are molded, affecting biotin availability found in soil, moldy feeds, manure, and litter.

- Rancidity in feeds causes biotin to be readily destroyed. Biotin in feedstuffs may be destroyed by heat curing, solvent extraction, pelleting, and improper storage conditions. Length of storage, temperature, and humidity result in biotin loss.
- Reduced intestinal synthesis and (or) absorption of biotin from diseases and other conditions affecting the gastrointestinal tract.
- Improved genetic characteristics (breed and type) and intensified production for faster weight gains and better feed conversion.
- Decreased level of biotin or its availability in feeds because of new plant varieties, new feed production practices, and processing methods.
- Reduced feed consumption and consequently reduced biotin intake.
- Interrelationships between biotin and other nutrients affect requirements. Dietary fats, pantothenic acid, vitamin B_6, vitamin B_{12}, folic acid, thiamine, riboflavin, myo-inositol, and ascorbic acid are related to biotin requirements and metabolism.
- Lower levels and availability of biotin in feeds. Different batches of the same feed may vary considerably in biotin. Biotin in feeds exists in both free and bound forms. Certain feeds have a low availability (e.g., wheat, barley, sorghum). A shift from corn, soybean and cottonseed meals often results in diets with less available biotin.

Safety

Studies with poultry indicate that these species can safely tolerate dietary biotin levels 4 to 10 times their nutritional requirements (NRC, 1994). In some studies with poultry, detrimental effects of toxic levels of biotin resulted in lowered egg production and fertility. Birds are very tolerant of high levels of biotin, and because the vitamin is excreted intact, toxicity is very rare (Leeson and Summers, 2008; Mock, 2013).

Folic acid (vitamin B_9)

Chemical structure and properties

Folacin is the generic descriptor for the original vitamin folic acid and related compounds that qualitatively show folic acid activity. The terms folacin, folate, and folic acid can be used interchangeably and refer to many compounds that possess folic acid's biological activity.

Folic acid is structurally one of the most complex vitamins. The pure substance is designated pterylomonoglutamic acid. The basic folate molecule is 5,6,7,8-tetrahydropteroylglutamate, also referred to as tetrahydrofolate (THF) monoglutamate, which consists of a 2-amino-4-hydroxy-pteridine (pterin) moiety linked via a methylene group at the C-6 position to a p-aminobenzoyl-glutamic acid.

Its chemical structure contains 3 distinct parts: glutamic acid, a para-aminobenzoic acid (PABA) residue, and a pteridine nucleus (Figure 4.36).

In most naturally occurring folates, the number of glutamate units in the side chain varies from 5 to 8. The PABA portion of the vitamin structure was once considered a vitamin. Research has shown that if the folic acid requirement of the organism is met, there is no need to add PABA to the diet. Folic acid is a synthetic, fully oxidized monoglutamate form of the vitamin used commercially in supplements and fortified/enriched foods and feeds (Bailey *et al.*, 2013).

Folic acid is a yellowish-orange crystalline powder that is tasteless, odorless, and insoluble in alcohol, ether, and other organic solvents. It is slightly soluble in hot water in the acid form but quite soluble in the salt form. It is fairly stable to air and heat in neutral and alkaline solution but unstable in acid solution. From 70 to 100% of the folic acid activity is destroyed on autoclaving at pH 1 (O'Dell and Hogan, 1943).

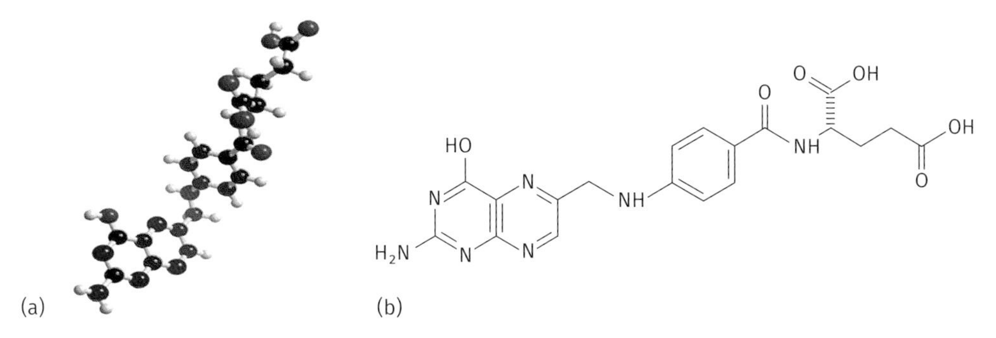

Figure 4.36 Folic acid chemical structure

It is readily degraded by light and UV radiation, and heating can considerably reduce the folic acid activity, particularly under oxidative conditions (Gregory, 1989). Sulfonamides are the folic acid biosynthetic intermediate PABA analogs widely used as antibacterial agents (Brown, 1962). By competing with PABA, sulfonamides prevent folic acid synthesis so that microorganisms cannot multiply, reducing or eliminating an important source of folic acid to the animal.

Natural sources

Much of the naturally occurring folic acid in feedstuffs is conjugated with varying numbers of different glutamic acid molecules, reducing its absorption efficiency. Folic acid is present in most of the ingredients of poultry diets, almost exclusively THF acid derivatives, especially in animal origin, but in insufficient quantity (Bains, 1999). Good sources are also soybeans, other beans, nuts, and cereal grains. The stable THF acid derivatives have a methyl or formyl group in the 5-position and generally possess 3 or more glutamic acid residues in glutamyl linkages. Only limited amounts of free folic acid occur in natural products, and most feed sources contain predominantly polyglutamyl folic acid.

The mean availability of folic acid in 7 separate food items was found to be close to 50%, ranging from 37 to 72% in the monoglutamate form (Babu and Skiikantia, 1976). The bioavailability of orally administered 5-methyl folic and 5-formyl folic acid was equal to folic acid for rats (Bhandari and Gregory, 1992). Folic acid bioavailability in various foods generally exceeded 70% (Clifford *et al.*, 1990). The bioavailability of monoglutamate folic acid is substantially greater than polyglutamyl forms (Clifford *et al.*, 1990; Gregory *et al.*, 1991b).

A considerable loss of folic acid (50–90%) occurs during feed manufacturing. Folic acid is sensitive to light and heating, particularly in acid solutions. Under aerobic conditions, the destruction of most folic acid forms is significant with heating. Chicken meat contains some 12 mg/100 g, providing 6% of the recommended daily intake in humans.

Commercial forms

Spray-dried folic acid and dilutions of crystalline folic acid are the most widely used product forms in animal feeds. Several lines of evidence indicate higher bioavailability of added folic acid than naturally occurring folates in many foods, with approximately 50% lower availability (Gregory, 2001). Synthesized folic acid is the monoglutamate form.

Supplementation with folic acid and 5-methyltetrahydrofolate had equivalent effects in enhancing egg folic acid concentrations and improving folic acid status in laying hens (Tactacan *et al.*, 2010a). Although folacin is only sparingly soluble in water, sodium salt is quite soluble and is used in injections and feed supplements (McGinnis, 1986).

Metabolism

Absorption and transport

Polyglutamate forms of folic acid are digested via hydrolysis to pteroylmonoglutamate before transport across the intestinal mucosa. The enzyme responsible for the hydrolysis of pteroyl-polyglutamate is a carboxy-peptidase known as folate conjugase (Baugh and Krumdieck, 1971). Most likely, several conjugase enzymes are responsible for the hydrolysis of the long-chain folate polyglutamates to the monoglutamates, which then enter the mucosal cell (Rosenberg and Neumann, 1974).

Pteroylmonoglutamate is absorbed predominantly in the duodenum and jejunum, apparently by an active process involving sodium. Using an everted intestinal sac model, Tactacan *et al.* (2010b) reported the presence of a folic acid transport system in the entire intestine of the laying hen. Uptake of folic acid in the cecum raises the likelihood of absorption of bacterial-derived folic acid. Kesavan and Noronha (1983) suggested from rat results that luminal conjugase is a secretion of pancreatic origin and that the hydrolysis of polyglutamate forms of folic acid occurs in the lumen rather than at the mucosal surface or within the mucosal cell.

After hydrolysis and absorption from the intestine, dietary folates are transported in plasma as monoglutamate derivatives, predominantly as 5-methyltetrahydrofolate. The monoglutamate derivatives then enter cells by specific transport systems. The pteroylpolyglutamates, the major folic acid form in cells, are built up stepwise by an enzyme, folate polyglutamate synthetase. Polyglutamates keep folic acid within the cells since only the monoglutamate forms are transported across membranes, and only monoglutamates are found in plasma and urine (Wagner, 2001).

Storage and excretion

Studies showed that 79–88% of labeled folic acid is absorbed, and absorption is rapid since serum concentrations usually peak about 2 hours after ingestion. Folic acid is widely distributed in tissues, largely in the conjugated polyglutamate forms of folic acid, generally containing 3 to 7 glutamyl residues linked by peptide bonds. The natural coenzymes are abundant in every tissue examined (Wagner *et al.*, 1984). Specific folate-binding proteins (FBPs) that bind folic acid mono- and polyglutamate exist in many tissues and body fluids, including liver, kidney, small intestinal brush border membranes, leukemic granulocytes, blood serum, and milk (Tani and Iwai, 1984). The physiological roles of these FBPs are unknown. However, they have been suggested to play a role in folic acid transport analogous to the intrinsic factor in the absorption of vitamin B_{12}.

Urinary excretion of folic acid represents a small fraction of total excretion. Fecal folic acid concentrations are quite high, often higher than intake, meaning not only undigested folic acid but, more importantly, the many bacterial syntheses of the vitamin in the intestine. Bile contains high levels of folic acid due to enterohepatic circulation, with most biliary folic acid reabsorbed in the intestine (Bailey *et al.*, 2013).

Biochemical functions

The principal functions of folic acid are related to:

- the synthesis of protein and purines, and pyrimidines, which make up the nucleic acids needed for cell division (Bailey *et al.*, 2013)
- the interconversions of various amino acids
- the maturation process of red corpuscles and the functioning of the immune system.

This means that there are multiple coenzyme forms in transferring one-carbon activity (Bailey *et al.*, 2013). In forms 5, 6, 7, 8-tetrahydrofolic acid (THF), folic acid is indispensable in transferring single-carbon units in various reactions, a role analogous to that of pantothenic acid in the transfer of two-carbon units (Bailey and Gregory, 2006; Bailey *et al.*, 2013). The one-carbon teams can be formyl, methylene, or methyl groups. Some biosynthetic relationships of one-carbon units are shown in Figure 4.37.

The major *in vivo* pathway providing methyl groups involves the transfer of a one-carbon unit from serine to tetrahydrofolate to form 5,10-methylenetetrahydrofolate, which is subsequently reduced to 5-methyltetrahydrofolate. Methyltetrahydrofolate then supplies methyl groups to remethylate homocysteine in the activated methyl cycle, providing methionine for synthesizing the important methyl donor agent S-adenosylmethionine (Krumdieck, 1990; Jacob *et al.*, 1994; Bailey *et al.*, 2013).

The important physiological function of THF consists of binding the single-carbon (C_1) units to the vitamin molecule, thus transforming them to "active formic acid" or "active formaldehyde." These are interconvertible by reduction or oxidation and transferable to appropriate acceptors. Folic acid polyglutamates work at least as well as or better than the corresponding monoglutamate forms in every enzyme system examined (Wagner, 1995). It is now accepted that the pteroylpolyglutamates are the acceptors and donors of one-carbon units in amino acid and nucleotide metabolism, while the monoglutamate is merely a transport form.

Specific reactions involving single-carbon transfer by folic acid compounds are:

- purine and pyrimidine synthesis
- interconversion of serine and glycine
- glycine–carbon as a source of C_1 units for many syntheses
- histidine degradation
- synthesis of methyl groups for such compounds as methionine, choline, and thymine (a pyrimidine base).

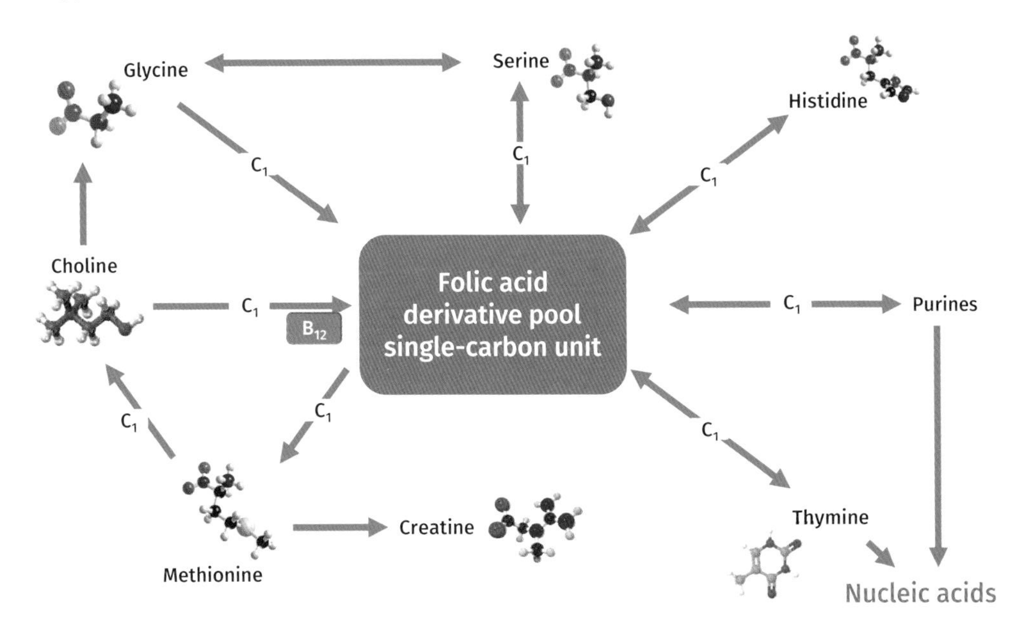

Figure 4.37 Folic acid metabolism requires single-carbon units

As folacin is involved in the interconversion of serine and glycine, in the degradation of histidine, and in the addition of methyl groups to compounds such as methionine, choline, and thiamine, inadequate levels of other methyl group donors – such as vitamin B_{12}, serine, methionine, betaine, and choline – increase folic acid requirements (Bailey *et al.*, 2013). This interaction with other nutrients is especially important in birds, as nitrogen is excreted as uric acid, which entails a high expenditure of methionine and cysteine. Furthermore, methionine tends to be the first limiting amino acid in bird feeding, which entails increasing the requirements of other sources of methyl group donors. Logically, high protein levels in the diet raise the dietary recommendations for folate.

Folic acid is also essentially involved in all the reactions of labile methyl groups. The metabolism of labile methyl groups plays an important role in methionine biosynthesis from homocysteine and choline from ethanolamine. Folic acid has a sparing effect on the requirements of choline. The critical role of both folic acid and vitamin B_{12} in synthesizing choline is discussed in the choline section. Folic acid is needed to maintain the immune system. The blastogenic response of T-lymphocytes to certain mitogens is decreased in folic acid-deficient humans and animals, and the thymus is preferentially altered (Dhur *et al.*, 1991).

Nutritional assessment

Serum/plasma folate is a good indicator of current folate status and is used as a first-line clinical indicator of folate deficiency (Sauberlich, 1999). Folates can be measured using HPLC-MS/MS, electrochemical or fluorescence-based techniques, radio- and immuno-based assays, and the traditional *Lactobacillus casei* growth assay. This microbiological approach measures all biologically active folate species, including di- and tri-glutamates of the species, but cannot differentiate between the species (Höller *et al.*, 2018).

As folate and cobalamin (vitamin B_{12}) jointly participate in one-carbon metabolism and thus have close biological links, both are usually measured concurrently since the deficiency will interact with the blood status markers of the other (Höller *et al.*, 2018).

Deficiency signs

With a folic acid deficiency, there is a reduction in the biosynthesis of nucleic acids essential for cell formation and function. Hence, vitamin deficiency leads to impaired cell division and alterations in protein synthesis. These effects are most noticeable in rapidly growing tissues such as red blood cells, leukocytes, intestinal mucosa, embryos, and fetuses. In the absence of adequate nucleoproteins, normal maturation of primordial red blood cells does not occur, and hematopoiesis is inhibited at the megaloblast stage. As a result of this megaloblastic arrest for normal red blood cell maturation in bone marrow, the first sign of folic acid deficiency is represented by characteristic macrocytic anemia. White blood cell formation is also affected, resulting in thrombopenia, leukopenia, and multi-lobed neutrophils. Vitamin B_{12} is necessary to reduce one-carbon compounds in the oxidation stage of formate and formaldehyde. In this way, it participates with folic acid in the biosynthesis of labile methyl groups (Savage and Lindenbaum, 1995).

Poultry is more susceptible to a lack of folic acid than other farm livestock, as a deficiency can readily be produced by feeding a folic acid-deficient diet. As indicated by retarded growth and feed efficiency, the folic acid deficiency could be made in 15-day-old chicks fed corn-soybean meal diets (Pesti *et al.*, 1991), and it is characterized by poor growth, very poor feathering, anemic appearance, and perosis (Figure 4.38a). The chicks become lethargic, and feed intake declines. As anemia develops, the comb becomes waxy white, and the mucous membrane of the mouth becomes pale (Siddons, 1978).

Turkey poults fed a folic acid-deficient diet have reduced growth rates and increased mortality (Figure 4.38b). The birds develop a spastic type of cervical paralysis in which the neck is stiff and extended but with only a moderate degree of anemia. Poults with cervical paralysis die within 2 days after the onset of these signs unless folic acid is administered immediately (Scott *et al.*, 1982). Erythrocytes of deficient birds tend to be large in diameter, and their nuclei are less dense than those of birds receiving supplementary folic acid (Schweigert *et al.*, 1948).

Folic acid deficiency also results in poor feather development for chicks and turkeys, with weak and brittle shafts. Folic acid, lysine, and iron are required for feather pigmentation: hence depigmentation occurs in colored feathers during a vitamin deficiency. It appears that egg production is less affected by folic acid deficiency than the development of the chick or poult. Egg and poult weights were significantly increased when turkey hens received higher dietary folic acid and when eggs were injected with folic acid (Robel, 1993a). Inadequate folic acid provided to the hen impairs the oviduct's response to estrogen and ability to form albumen (NRC, 1994). An inadequate intake of folic acid by breeding hens results in poor hatchability and a marked increase in embryonic mortality (Figure 4.38c), which occurs during the last days of incubation. A deformed beak and bending of the tibiotarsus are signs of embryonic deficiency. Chicks that successfully emerge are stunted, have poorly developed feathers, and are abnormally pigmented (NRC, 1994).

Folic acid deficiency has sometimes been associated with perosis or slipped tendon. Pollard and Creek (1964) demonstrated histologically that folic acid-deficient bones and cartilage lesions are different from those produced by choline or manganese deficiencies. The abnormal

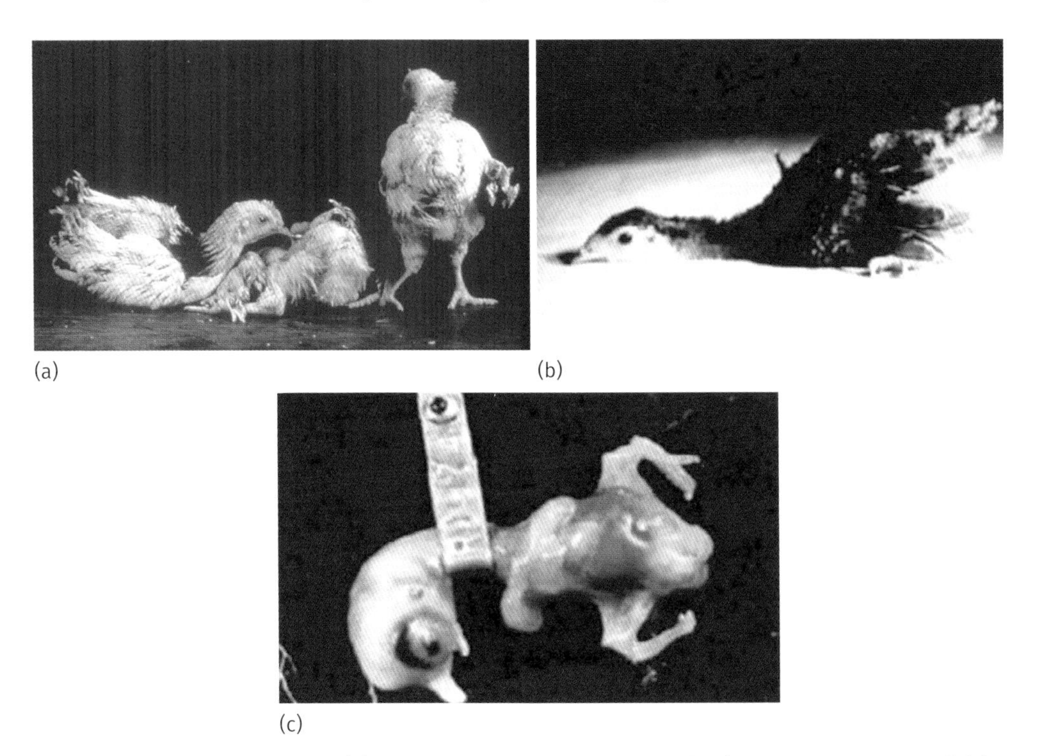

(a) (b) (c)

Figure 4.38 Folic acid deficiency: (a) retarded growth and poor feathering (source: UK Crown copyright); (b) deficiency in poults (source: courtesy of M.L. Sunde, University of Wisconsin); (c) abnormal embryo from an egg laid by a hen fed a diet low in folic acid (source: courtesy of M.L. Sunde, University of Wisconsin)

structure of the hyaline cartilage is found in folic acid-deficient chicks, and ossification is retarded. These disorders are not found in chicks deficient in choline or manganese, although bone deformities and slipped tendons are found in both disorders. However, Bechtel (1964) claimed that choline effectively prevents perosis only when sufficient folic acid is present in the diet. Dietary choline content has been shown to affect the chicks' requirement for folic acid. When the diet contained adequate choline, the folic acid requirement was 0.47 mg/kg diet, but this increased to 0.96 mg/kg diet when the diet was choline-deficient (Young *et al.*, 1955).

Increasing the protein content of the diet has also been shown to increase the incidence and severity of perosis in chicks receiving low levels of dietary folic acid. It is suggested that this increased requirement for folic acid in high-protein diets for poultry results from greater demand for folic acid in uric acid formation (Creek and Vasaitis, 1963).

Folic acid appears to be necessary for cell mitosis. In the absence of folic acid, oviduct growth is not increased in estrogen-treated chicks. The production of water-soluble proteins (particularly the albumen fraction) in the hormone-stimulated oviduct is also greatly reduced, and there is an alteration in the amino acid composition of these proteins. The percentages of arginine, leucine, serine, and tryptophan are decreased, and those of glycine and methionine increased (Siddons, 1978).

The effects of folic acid deficiency on humoral immunity have been more thoroughly investigated in animals than humans. The antibody responses to several antigens have been shown to decrease. As *de novo* synthesis of methyl groups requires the participation of folic acid coenzymes, the effect of folic acid deficiency on pancreatic exocrine function was examined in rats (Balaghi and Wagner, 1992; Balaghi *et al.*, 1993). Pancreatic secretion was significantly reduced in the deficient group compared with the pair-fed control groups after 5 weeks.

Safety

Folic acid is generally considered a nontoxic vitamin (NRC, 1987). Birds are very tolerant of high levels of folic acid, with up to 5,000 times the normal intake needed to induce toxicity. Renal hypertrophy has been described under such conditions (Leeson and Summers, 2008).

Vitamin C

Chemical structure and properties

Vitamin C is named ascorbic acid, and there are 4 stereoisomers: D- and L-ascorbic acid, and D- and L-isoascorbic acid (with the D-form also named erythorbic acid). However, the term vitamin C refers only to the compounds with L-ascorbic acid activity, which are biologically active, and it includes 2 forms (Figure 4.39):

- L-ascorbic acid: reduced form
- dehydro-L-ascorbic acid: oxidized form

Although in nature, the vitamin is primarily present as ascorbic acid, and both forms are, as said, biologically active (but not the D-isomers). In nature, the reduced form of ascorbic acid may reversibly oxidize to the dehydroxidized form, i.e., dehydroascorbic acid (Johnston *et al.*, 2013), and dehydroascorbic acid is irreversibly oxidized to the inactive diketogulonic acid. The latter can be further oxidized to oxalic acid and L-threonic acid. Since this change takes place readily, vitamin C is susceptible to destruction through oxidation, accelerated by heat and light.

Reversible oxidation-reduction of ascorbic acid with dehydroascorbic acid is vitamin C's most important chemical property and the basis for its known physiological activities and

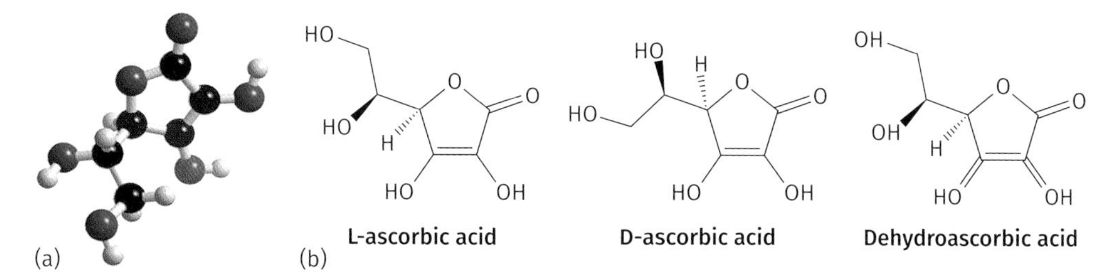

Figure 4.39 Vitamin C chemical structure

stabilities (Moser and Bendich, 1991). Vitamin C is a white to yellow-tinged crystalline powder. It crystallizes, out of the water, like square or oblong crystals. It is slightly soluble in acetone and has lower alcohols. A 0.5% solution of ascorbic acid in water is strongly acid with a pH of 3. The vitamin is more stable in acid than in an alkaline medium.

Crystalline ascorbic acid is relatively stable in the air without moisture. However, vitamin C is the least stable and, therefore, most easily destroyed of all the vitamins. Several chemical substances, such as air pollutants, industrial toxins, heavy metals, and some pharmacologically active compounds, are antagonistic to vitamin C and can lead to increased vitamin requirements (Johnston *et al.*, 2013).

Natural sources

The main sources of vitamin C are fruits and green plants, but some foods of animal origin contain more than traces of the vitamin. Vitamin C occurs in significant quantities in animal organs, such as the liver and kidney, but in only small amounts in meat. However, vitamin C is very low in cereals and oil seeds used in poultry nutrition. Post-harvest storage values vary with time, temperature, damage, and enzyme content (Zee *et al.*, 1991; Johnston *et al.*, 2013).

Commercial forms

Ascorbic acid is commercially available as:

- 100% crystalline L-ascorbic acid
- Sodium ascorbate
- 97.5% L-ascorbic acid – ethyl cellulose-coated (EC)
- 35% phosphorylated Na/Ca salt of L-ascorbic acid ($C_6H_9O_9P$ molecular mass 256.11 g/mol)
- 50% phosphorylated Na salt of L-ascorbic acid ($C_6H_6O_9Na_3P{\cdot}H_2O$ molecular mass 358.08 g/mol).

When providing supplemental ascorbic acid in heat-treated feeds, it is strongly advisable to use a stabilized form like EC-coated or phosphorylated forms. In storage experiments, ascorbic acid protected in this manner was 4 times more stable than untreated ascorbic acid crystals (Kolb, 1984). Adams (1978) reported that EC-coated ascorbic acid showed higher retention after processing than the crystalline form, 84% versus 48%. Retention of ascorbic acid in mash feed was fairly good, but stability was poor in crumbled meals with elevated storage time and temperature.

Crystalline L-ascorbic acid and L-ascorbyl-2-polyphosphate forms had similar bioavailability for broiler chicks (Pardue *et al.*, 1993). However, a wide variation has been observed in the level of these responses and, therefore, in the zootechnical results obtained, which may be due to diverse factors:

- low stability of vitamin C in feed, which improves significantly in phosphorylated forms (Whitehead and Keller, 2003) and also in drinking water, especially if alkaline and/or unchlorinated (Pardue, 1989; Krautmann, 1989)
- level and duration of dosage
- the age of the birds (van Niekerk *et al.*, 1989)
- the intensity and combination of stress factors (McKee and Harrison, 1995; Teeter and Belay, 1996; Balnave, 2004).

Metabolism

Absorption and transport

Vitamin C is absorbed like carbohydrates (monosaccharides). Intestinal absorption in vitamin C-dependent animals (e.g., primates and most species of fish) appears to require sodium-dependent vitamin C transporters (SVCT1 and 2) (Johnston, 2006; Johnston *et al.*, 2013). It is assumed that those not scurvy-prone species like poultry have an absorption mechanism by diffusion mostly in the duodenum and jejunum (Spencer *et al.*, 1963). However, the presence of SCTV1 in the chick renal proximal tubule has been identified. Vitamin C transport and conservation by the kidney is likely to be especially critical in birds due to high plasma glucose levels and resulting high levels of ROS (Johnston and Laverty, 2007).

Ascorbic acid is readily absorbed when quantities ingested are small, but limited intestinal absorption occurs when excess ascorbic acid is ingested. The bioavailability of vitamin C in feeds is limited, but 80 to 90% apparently appears to be absorbed (Kallner *et al.*, 1977). The absorption site in the guinea pig is in the duodenal and proximal small intestine, whereas the rat showed the highest absorption in the ileum (Hornig *et al.*, 1984).

In its metabolism, ascorbic acid is first converted to dehydroascorbate by several enzymes or non-enzymatic processes and can then be reduced back to ascorbic acid in cells (Johnston *et al.*, 2013). Absorbed vitamin C readily equilibrates with the body pool of the vitamin. No specific binding proteins for ascorbic acid have been reported, and it is suggested that the vitamin is retained by binding to subcellular structures.

Storage and excretion

Ascorbic acid is widely distributed throughout the tissues in animals capable of synthesizing vitamin C and in those dependent on an adequate dietary amount of the vitamin. In experimental animals, the highest concentrations of vitamin C are found in the pituitary and adrenal glands, and high levels are also found in the liver, spleen, brain, and pancreas. Vitamin C also tends to localize around healing wounds. Tissue levels are decreased by virtually all forms of stress, which also stimulates the biosynthesis of the vitamin in those animals capable of synthesis.

Ascorbic acid is excreted mainly in the urine, with small amounts in sweat and feces. In guinea pigs, rats, and rabbits, oxidation to carbon dioxide is the major excretory mechanism for vitamin C. Primates do not normally utilize the carbon dioxide catabolic pathway, with the major loss occurring in the urine. Urinary excretion of vitamin C depends on body stores, intake, and renal function.

Biochemical functions

Ascorbic acid is involved in fundamental biological and metabolic processes, and its function is related to its reversible oxidation and reduction characteristics. Thus, its action is important in:

- calcification processes
- immune response
- adaptation to stress
- maintenance of electrolytic balance.

Vitamin C's biochemical and physiological functions have been copiously reviewed (Pardue and Thaxton, 1986; Moser and Bendich, 1991; Padh, 1991; Gershoff, 1993; Whitehead and Keller, 2003; Johnston, 2006; Johnston *et al.*, 2013). However, the exact role of this vitamin in the living system is not completely understood since a coenzyme form has not yet been reported.

In more detail, the main biochemical functions of vitamin C are (Figure 4.40):

- antioxidant and immune role (stimulation of phagocytic activity)
- biosynthesis of collagen
- control of glucocorticoid synthesis
- conversion of vitamin D_3 to its active form
- absorption of minerals (iron).

Antioxidant and immune role (stimulation of phagocytic activity)

One of the most interesting properties of vitamin C is its ability to act as a reducing agent or electron donor. It reacts rapidly with free radicals and works synergistically with vitamin E, facilitating the regeneration of the reduced form of αα-tocopherol in biological systems (Rocha *et al.*, 2010), hence accounting for the observed sparing effect on this vitamin (Jacob, 1995). In the process of sparing fatty acid oxidation, tocopherol is oxidized to the tocopheryl free radical. Ascorbic acid can donate an electron to the tocopheryl free radical, regenerating the reduced antioxidant form of tocopherol.

Tissue defense mechanisms against free-radical damage generally include vitamin C, vitamin E, and β-carotene as the major vitamin antioxidant sources. In addition, several metalloenzymes that include glutathione peroxidase (selenium), catalase (iron), and superoxide

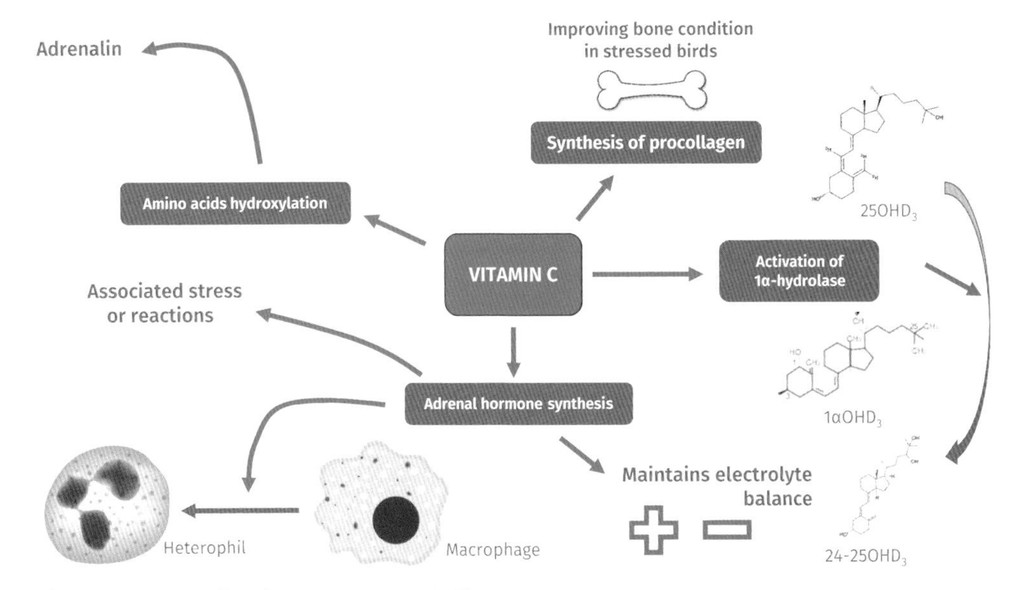

Figure 4.40 Some vitamin C roles on metabolism

dismutase (copper, zinc, and manganese) are also critical in protecting the internal cellular constituents from oxidative damage.

The dietary and tissue balance of all these nutrients is important in protecting tissue against free-radical damage. Both *in vitro* and *in vivo* studies showed that the antioxidant vitamins generally enhance cellular and noncellular immunity aspects. The antioxidant function of these vitamins could, at least in part, enhance immunity by maintaining the functional and structural integrity of important immune cells. A compromised immune system will reduce animal production efficiency through increased susceptibility to diseases, thereby leading to increased animal morbidity and mortality.

Ascorbic acid is reported to have a stimulating effect on the phagocytic activity of leukocytes, the function of the reticuloendothelial system, and the formation of antibodies. Ascorbic acid levels are very high in phagocytic cells, with these cells using free radicals and other highly reactive oxygen-containing molecules to help kill pathogens that invade the body. As an effective scavenger of ROS, ascorbic acid minimizes the oxidative stress associated with activated phagocytic leukocytes' respiratory burst, thereby controlling the inflammation and tissue damage associated with immune responses (Chien *et al.*, 2004).

Biosynthesis of collagen

The beneficial effects of ascorbic acid in the collagen biosynthesis are extensively documented and represent the most clearly established role for vitamin C. Collagens are the tough, fibrous, intercellular materials (proteins) that are the principal components of skin and connective tissue, the organic matrix of bones and teeth and the ground substance between cells.

In the case of vitamin C deficiency, the impairment of collagen synthesis appears to be due to lowered ability to hydroxylate lysine and proline. In addition to the relationship of ascorbic acid to hydroxylase enzymes, Franceschi (1992) suggests that vitamin C is required for the differentiation of connective tissue such as muscle, cartilage, and bone derived from mesenchyme (embryonic cells capable of developing into connective tissue). It is proposed that the collagen matrix produced by ascorbic acid-treated cells provides a permissive environment for tissue-specific gene expression. A common finding in all studies is that vitamin C can alter the expression of multiple genes as cells progress through specific differentiation programs (Ikeda *et al.*, 1997).

Beneficial effects result from ascorbic acid synthesizing "repair" collagen. Alteration of basement membrane collagen synthesis and its integrity in the mucosal epithelium during vitamin C restriction might explain the mechanism by which the capillary fragility is induced in scurvy and the increased incidences of periodontal disease under vitamin C deprivation. Failure of wounds to heal and gum and bone changes resulting from vitamin C undernutrition are direct consequences of reducing insoluble collagen fibers. Ascorbic acid is a cofactor in extracellular matrix metabolism because it affects collagen, laminin, various cell surface integrins, and elastin. Vitamin C is a cofactor for enzymes key to the post-translational modification of matrix proteins (Johnston *et al.*, 2013).

Control of glucocorticoid synthesis

Vitamin C controls the synthesis of glucocorticoids and norepinephrine in the adrenal gland. The protective effects of vitamin C (also vitamin E) on health may partially result from reducing glucocorticoid circulating levels (Nockels, 1990). During stress conditions (e.g., heat stress), glucocorticoids, which suppress the immune response, are elevated. Vitamin C reduces adrenal glucocorticoid synthesis, helping to maintain immunocompetence.

Conversion of vitamin D_3 to its active form

Vitamin C, because of its relationship to hydroxylation enzymes, has a direct effect on C-1 hydroxylation of 25OHD$_3$ to the active form 1,25(OH)$_2$D$_3$ (Suter, 1990; Cantatore *et al.*, 1991). Weiser *et al.* (1990) reported that 100 mg/kg ascorbic acid in chick diets increased plasma concentrations of 1,25(OH)$_2$D$_3$, which led to elevated activities of duodenal calcium-binding protein and greater weights and breaking strength of bones. It is possible that the many cases of "field rickets" in poults may be due to stress-induced deficiency of vitamin C. Vitamin C has been shown to influence the developmental process in the growth plate for bone growth (Farqhuarson *et al.*, 1998).

Absorption of minerals (iron)

Ascorbic acid has a role in metal ion metabolism due to its reducing and chelating properties. This results in enhanced absorption of minerals from the diet and their mobilization and distribution throughout the body. Ascorbic acid promotes non-heme iron absorption from food (Olivares *et al.*, 1997). It reduces the ferric iron at the acid pH in the stomach and forms complexes with iron ions that stay in solution at alkaline conditions in the duodenum. Some other functions of ascorbic acid are the following.

1. Owing to the ease with which ascorbic acid can be oxidized and reversibly reduced, it probably plays an important role in reactions involving electron transfer in the cell. Almost all terminal oxidases in plant and animal tissues can directly or indirectly catalyze the oxidation of L-ascorbic acid. Such enzymes include ascorbic acid oxidase, cytochrome oxidase, phenolase, and peroxidase. In addition, its oxidation is readily induced under aerobic conditions by many metal ions and quinones.
2. Ascorbic acid has a role in the metabolic oxidation of certain amino acids, including tyrosine.
3. Carnitine is synthesized from lysine and methionine and is dependent on 2 hydroxylases containing ferrous iron and L-ascorbic acid. Vitamin C deficiency can reduce the formation of carnitine, resulting in the accumulation of triglycerides in the blood and the physical fatigue and lassitude associated with scurvy (Ha *et al.*, 1994). About 98% of total body carnitine is in muscle; skeletal and heart muscle carnitine concentrations are reduced by 50% in vitamin C-deficient guinea pigs compared with controls (Johnston, 2013).
4. Interrelationships between vitamin C to B vitamins are known: tissue levels and urinary excretion of vitamin C are affected in animals in case of deficiencies of thiamine, riboflavin, pantothenic acid, folic acid, and biotin.
5. Vitamin C has been demonstrated to inhibit nitrosamines, which are potent carcinogens (Aseltine, 1990).
6. Ascorbic acid is found in up to a tenfold concentration in seminal fluid compared to serum levels, and decreasing levels have caused nonspecific sperm agglutination. In a review of ascorbic acid and fertility, Luck *et al.* (1995) suggested 3 of ascorbic acid's principal functions: its promotion of collagen synthesis, its role in hormone production, and its ability to protect cells from free radicals, which may explain its reproductive actions.
7. Vitamin C has a biological role in keratinocytes. Because skin must provide the first line of defense against environmental free-radical attack (e.g., sunburn, skin aging, and skin cancer), it has developed a complex antioxidant network that includes enzymatic and non-enzymatic components. The epidermis is composed of several layers of keratinocytes supplied with enzymes (superoxide dismutase, catalase, thioredoxin reductase, and glutathione reductase) and low-molecular-weight antioxidant molecules (tocopherol,

glutathione, and ascorbic acid) (Podda and Grundmann-Kollmann, 2001). Furthermore, since ascorbic acid is especially important in collagen formation, its presence increases the capacity to heal wounds (Rajkhowa *et al.*, 1996). In keratinocytes, vitamin C counteracts oxidative stress via transcriptional and post-translational mechanisms. Vitamin C can: (a) act directly by scavenging ROS generated by stressors; (b) prevent ROS-mediated cell damage by modulating gene expression; (c) regulate keratinocyte differentiation by maintaining a balanced redox state; and (d) promote cell cycle arrest and apoptosis in response to DNA damage (Catani *et al.*, 2005).

8 Vitamin C is also involved in many hormone activation processes. Hormones like melanotropins, calcitonin, growth hormone-releasing factors, corticotrophin and thyrotropin, vasopressin, oxytocin, cholecystokinin, and gastrin undergo amidations where ascorbic acid serves as a reductant to maintain copper in a reduced state at the active site of the enzyme (Johnston *et al.*, 2013).

Nutritional assessment

Several biological compartments such as whole blood, erythrocytes, leucocytes, and plasma or serum can be used to assess vitamin C status. However, serum or plasma concentration of ascorbate is the most reliable marker. Analysis of ascorbic acid in biological samples is complicated by the high susceptibility of this compound to oxidation which requires the use, for example, of EDTA (Höller *et al.*, 2018). Several approaches have been developed to measure vitamin C in biological materials: HPLC provides an efficient means to quantify vitamin C with good selectivity and sensitivity (Höller *et al.*, 2018).

Deficiency signs

Under normal conditions, poultry can synthesize vitamin C in the kidney from carbohydrate precursors, including glucose and galactose; thus, it is assumed they do not require dietary sources of the vitamin. However, it should be borne in mind that the ability to do this is reduced in the first week of life, especially in males, as manifested by the decline in its concentration in plasma; after that, it progressively increases (Bains *et al.*, 1998). Pardue and Thaxton (1982) estimated that day-old chicks could only synthesize 16 and 33% of what they later could at 20 and 30 days, respectively.

Vitamin C synthesis also falls during stress (Pardue and Thaxton, 1986; Hooper *et al.*, 1989; Pardue, 1989; Seemann, 1991; Jones, 1996), increasing the probability of vitamin C deficiency. The chick is subject to considerable stress, including rapid growth, exposure to hot or cold temperatures, starvation, vaccination, and disease conditions such as coccidiosis. Pardue and Williams (1990) reported that plasma ascorbic acid levels in poults were depressed significantly by cold stress, beak trimming, and injection at 1 and 14 days old.

Disease conditions have been found to affect vitamin C metabolism in poultry. When chicks were infected with fowl typhoid, their plasma vitamin C concentrations were reduced (Hill and Garren, 1958). The vitamin C concentrations in plasma and tissue were also reduced in chicks infected with intestinal coccidiosis (Kechik and Sykes, 1979). Dietary ascorbate was shown to prevent this and contributed to intestinal repair. Ascites, a costly metabolic disease in chickens resulting from pulmonary hypertension, can be modified by vitamin C. Adding vitamin C to broiler diets significantly reduces the ascites mortality (Xiang *et al.*, 2002; Broz and Ward, 2007).

Therefore, in newly hatched chicks and birds exposed to various stressors, vitamin C status can be insufficient either because of a reduced synthetic ability or an increased requirement. In poultry, this can lead to growth, egg production, and eggshell quality deterioration.

Moreover, inflammation and decreased immune competence can be observed in stress or disease situations. This is why, even in poultry, a dietary supplementation with vitamin C is recommended in the first week of age and when stressing factors (e.g. heat or vaccination) can impact endogenous synthesis.

Safety

In general, high intakes of vitamin C are considered low toxicity. Several studies with chickens and turkeys had shown no effect when birds were fed with ascorbic acid at up to 3.3 g/kg feed for 32 weeks or 1.3 g/kg feed for one year (NRC, 1987). Dietary supplementation of ascorbic acid, even at levels as high as 3%, had no appreciable effects on body weight gain, feed intake, and feed efficiency of growing chicks (Nakaya *et al.*, 1986). Leeson and Summers (2008) note that toxic levels of vitamin C interfere with oxidase systems in the liver, and one sign is the excess accumulation of iron in the liver.

Choline

Chemical structure and properties

Choline is considered a vitamin, although it does not fulfill some of the prerequisites of this definition. For example, birds require high quantities of choline (less than 1%), similar to amino and essential fatty acids. It can be synthesized in the liver of birds from serine and methyl groups, requiring 3 moles of methionine for each mole of choline synthesized. However, for most metabolic processes, the quantity and rate of synthesis are insufficient to cover requirements, especially when the supply of precursors such as methionine, vitamin B_{12}, or folacin is limited.

Choline is a β-hydroxyethyl-trimethyl-ammonium hydroxide (Figure 4.41). Pure choline is a colorless, viscous, strongly alkaline liquid that is notably hygroscopic. Choline is soluble in water, formaldehyde, and alcohol and has no definite melting or boiling point. The chloride salt of this compound, choline chloride, is produced by chemical synthesis for use in the feed industry, although there are other forms. Choline chloride consists of deliquescent white crystals, which are very soluble in water and alcohol. Aqueous solutions are almost pH neutral (Jiang *et al.*, 2013).

Natural sources

All naturally occurring fats contain some choline, and thus, it is supplied by all feeds that contain fat. Egg yolk, glandular meats, and the brain are the richest animal sources, whereas the germ of cereals, legumes, and oilseed meals are the best plant sources (DuCoa, 1994). Corn is low in choline, with wheat, barley, and oats containing approximately twice as much choline as corn.

Since betaine can spare the choline requirements, it would be useful to know the concentrations of betaine in feeds. Unfortunately, most feedstuffs contain only small amounts of betaine. However, wheat and wheat by-products contain over twice as much betaine as

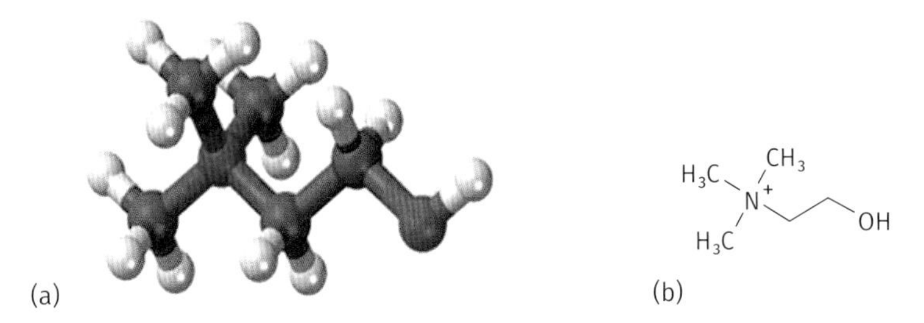

Figure 4.41 Choline structure

choline. Thus, the choline needs of swine or poultry fed with wheat-based diets would be much lower than those provided based on other grains. Sugar beets are also high in betaine.

Little is known of the biological availability of choline in natural feedstuffs. Using a chick assay method, soybean, canola, and peanut meals obtained a substantial proportion of unavailable choline (Emmert and Baker, 1997). Bioavailability of choline is 100% in corn, while in dehulled regular soybean meal and whole soybeans, availability ranged from 75 to 100% (Molitoris and Baker, 1976; Menten *et al.*, 1997; Simon, 1999; McDowell and Ward, 2008). However, soybean lecithin products are equivalent to choline chloride in bioavailability (Emmert *et al.*, 1997). Although 3 times as rich in total choline as soybean meal, canola meal has less bioavailable choline (Emmert and Baker, 1997). In their work with chicks, the production of trimethylamine (resulting from bacterial degradation of choline) in the intestine was greater in chicks fed canola meal than in those fed soybean meals.

Commercial forms

Commercially, choline is produced by chemical synthesis, and choline salts are used in dietary supplementation. The available forms are:

- choline chloride 75% solution in water
- choline chloride on a carrier (50–70 wt. %)
- choline chloride crystals (>95%)

The 75% liquid is very corrosive and requires special storage and handling equipment. It is not suitable for inclusion in concentrated vitamin premixes but is most economical to add directly to concentrate feed mixtures.

Metabolism

Absorption and transport

Choline is present in the unsupplemented diet mainly in phosphatidylcholine or lecithin, with less than 10% present either as the free base or as sphingomyelin. Choline is released from lecithin and sphingomyelin by hydrolysis by digestive enzymes of the gastrointestinal tract, although 50% of ingested lecithin enters the thoracic duct intact (Chan, 1991). Both pancreatic secretions and intestinal mucosal cells contain enzymes capable of hydrolyzing lecithin in the diet. Phospholipase A_2 cleaves the αα-fatty acid within the gut mucosal cell, and phospholipase B cleaves both fatty acids. Quantitatively, digestion by pancreatic lipase is the most important process (Zeizel, 1990). The net result is that most ingested lecithin is absorbed as lysophosphatidylcholine.

These lipid components are incorporated into mixed micelles and enter the enterocytes, mainly within the duodenum and jejunum, by passive diffusion. Choline is also absorbed in the jejunum and ileum primarily by the energy and sodium-dependent carrier mechanism. Only one-third of ingested choline in monogastric diets appears to be absorbed intact.

The extent to which choline is absorbed from raw materials is doubtful (Workel *et al.*, 1999). Absorbed choline is transported into the lymphatic circulation primarily in lecithin bound to chylomicra and is transported to the tissues predominantly as phospholipids associated with the plasma lipoproteins (De La Huerga and Popper, 1952). Phospholipase C cleaves lecithin yielding a diglyceride and phosphorylcholine. Free choline can be oxidized in the mitochondria to yield betaine aldehyde further converted into betaine, which is the actual source of methyl groups. The small fraction of choline acetylated provides the important neurotransmitter acetylcholine.

Storage and excretion

Most of the choline deposited in tissues exists in esterified forms, particularly phosphatidylcholine and phospholipids, accounting for 90% of all choline in the liver. Glycerophosphocholine and betaine are overrepresented in the kidney, whereas acetylcholine is found in relatively high amounts in the brain (Jiang *et al.*, 2013). Free choline accounts for only 0.5–1% of the total choline deposited.

Dietary choline is the main factor governing excretion. Two-thirds of ingested choline is metabolized by microbiota to trimethylamine and excreted in the urine within 6 to 12 hours after ingestion (De La Huerga and Popper, 1952). When an equivalent amount of choline is ingested as lecithin, trimethylamine excretion is lesser and appears within 12 to 24 hours after intake.

Biochemical functions

Choline is ubiquitously distributed in all plant and animal cells, mostly in the form of the phospholipids phosphatidylcholine (lecithin), lysophosphatidylcholine, choline plasmalogens, and, to a lesser extent, in free form or as sphingomyelin–essential components of all membranes (Zeisel, 1990).

Lecithin is most mammalian membranes' predominant phospholipid (>50%). In the lung, desaturated lecithin is the major active component of surfactant (Brown, 1964), lack of which results in a respiratory distress syndrome in premature infants. The main functions of choline can be grouped into 6 categories (Zeisel, 2006; Garrow, 2007; Jiang *et al.*, 2013):

It is a metabolic essential for building and maintaining cell structure

As a phospholipid component, choline is a structural part of lecithin, certain plasmalogens, and sphingomyelins. Lecithin is a part of animal cell membranes and lipid transport moieties in cell plasma membranes. Both phosphatidylcholine and sphingomyelin are preferentially localized to the outer leaflet of the lipid bilayer, thereby contributing to the lipid asymmetry of cellular membranes. These choline-containing phospholipids undergo dynamic trans- and intermembrane movements, facilitating membrane trafficking (Jiang *et al.*, 2013). Choline is required as a constituent of the phospholipids needed for the normal maturation of the cartilage matrix of the bone. Various metabolic functions and synthesis of choline are depicted in Figure 4.42.

Choline plays an essential role in fat metabolism in the liver

It prevents abnormal accumulation of fat (fatty livers) by promoting its transport as lecithin or increasing the utilization of fatty acids in the liver itself (Xu *et al.*, 2010). Phosphatidylcholine is the major phospholipid on the surface of VLDLs: it is packaged with triglyceride droplets in the Golgi cisternae, producing VLDLs that are exported out of the liver. Choline is thus referred to as a "lipotropic" factor due to its acting on fat metabolism by hastening removal or decreasing fat deposition in the liver. Phosphatidylcholine is also the major phospholipid (>95%) in bile and is derived primarily from HDL-phosphatidylcholine (Jiang *et al.*, 2013). In broiler liver, fat content was reduced by adding choline at 760 mg/kg diet for birds fed different energy sources (Rao *et al.*, 2001).

Forming acetylcholine

Choline is essential for forming acetylcholine, a substance that allows the transmission of nerve impulses. Acetylcholine is the agent released at the termination of the parasympathetic nerves. With acetylcholine, nerve impulses are transmitted from presynaptic to postsynaptic fibers of the sympathetic and parasympathetic nervous systems.

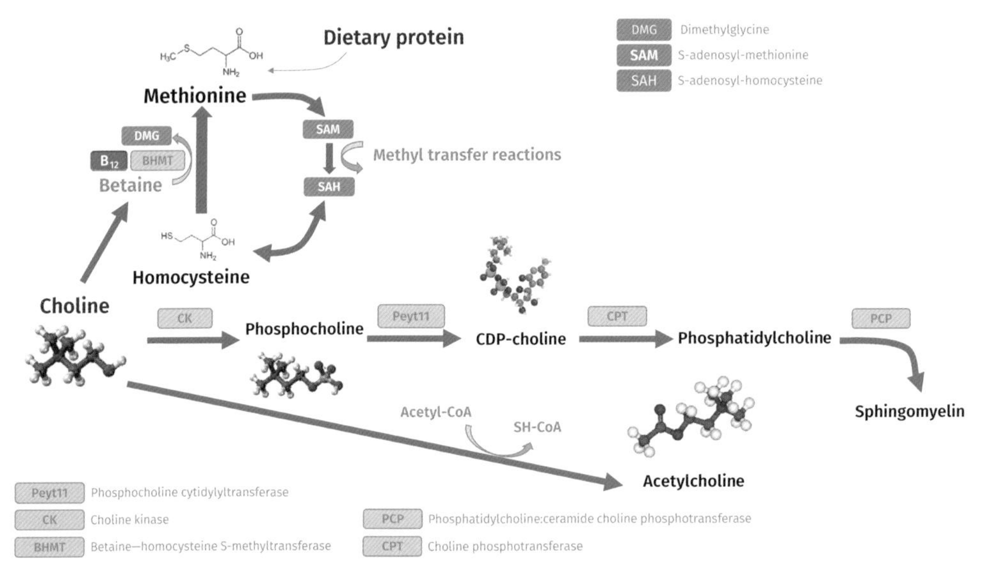

Figure 4.42 The metabolic pathway for the synthesis of choline and related compounds

Metabolites as second messengers

Phosphatidylcholine and sphingomyelin contained in cellular membranes are sources of choline-derived second messengers, including lysophosphatidylcholine, lysosphingomyelin, arachidonic acid, DAG, phosphatidic acid, ceramide, and sphingosine. These second messengers influence signaling pathways involved in inflammation, growth, differentiation, eicosanoid generation, cell cycle arrest, and apoptosis.

Platelet-activating factor

The platelet-activating factor (PAF) is produced from phosphatidylcholine. PAF is involved in processes like platelet activation, blood pressure regulation, and inflammation. PAF releases arachidonic acid to form eicosanoids (Jiang *et al.*, 2013).

Methyl groups

Choline is a source of labile methyl groups or methyl group donors for transmethylation reactions important in forming many substances. Choline furnishes labile methyl groups to form methionine from homocysteine and creatine from guanidino acetic acid. This is a role it shares with methionine and betaine, which means that all these substances can partially substitute for each other. However, their interrelations, reviewed by Simon (1999), are complex (Pillai *et al.*, 2006a,b).

Folic acid and vitamin B_{12} also take part in these reactions. Thus, their requirements increase with insufficient choline supply (Ryu *et al.*, 1995). Methyl groups function in synthesizing purine and pyrimidine, which are used to produce DNA. Methionine is converted to S-adenosylmethionine in a reaction catalyzed by methionine adenosyl transferase. S-adenosylmethionine is the active methylating agent for many enzymatic methylations. A disturbance in folic acid or methionine metabolism changes choline metabolism and vice versa (Zeisel, 1990). The involvement of folic acid, vitamin B_{12}, and methionine in methyl group metabolism and *de novo* choline synthesis may allow these substances to substitute in part for choline. A severe folic acid deficiency has been shown to cause secondary liver choline deficiency in rats (Kim *et al.*, 1994).

The demand for choline as a methyl donor is probably the major factor determining how rapidly a diet deficient in choline will induce pathology. The pathways of choline and one-carbon metabolism intersect at the formation of methionine from homocysteine. Methionine is regenerated from homocysteine in a reaction catalyzed by betaine: homocysteine methyltransferase, in which betaine, a metabolite of choline, serves as the methyl donor (Finkelstein *et al.*, 1982). Large increases in chick hepatic betaine-homocysteine methyltransferase can be produced under methionine-deficient conditions, especially in the presence of excess choline or betaine (Emmert *et al.*, 1996). To be a source of methyl groups, choline must be converted to betaine, which has been shown to perform methylation functions in some cases. However, betaine fails to prevent fatty livers and hemorrhagic kidneys. Since choline contains biologically active methyl groups, methionine can partly be spared by choline and homocysteine (Jiang *et al.*, 2013).

Choline is involved in forming the cartilaginous matrix, which facilitates the growth of the bones. In some trials, choline and the folic acid increase have decreased foot problems (Ryu *et al.*, 1995). Choline has been shown to influence brain structure and function. For rodents, choline was critical during fetal development, affecting stem cell proliferation and apoptosis, thereby altering brain structure and function. Memory is permanently enhanced in rodents exposed to choline during the latter part of gestation (Zeisel and Niculescu, 2006; Jiang *et al.*, 2013). Finally, choline does not affect immunity (Wang *et al.*, 1987).

Nutritional assessment

Plasma choline (and betaine) concentrations are strongly correlated with choline intake amounts, but in severe deficiency, choline concentrations do not fall according to the low nutritional intake.

Deficiency signs

Birds can synthesize choline; this capacity increases with age as it is generally impossible to produce a deficiency over 8 weeks. However, the amounts and the speed at which they are synthesized may sometimes be inadequate. It was observed that methylation of aminoethanol to methylamino ethanol seems to be the rate-limiting step in choline biosynthesis for young birds. Therefore, high levels of dietary methionine or other methyl donors cannot completely spare the chick's dietary choline requirement, which contrasts with the situation with growing mammals such as the pig or the rat.

Growth retardation and perosis result from choline deficiency in young poultry. Perosis is the primary clinical sign of a choline deficiency in chicks and turkey poults. Although perosis commonly refers to many hock abnormalities, true perosis is described as the classic choline deficiency sign. Perosis is first characterized by pinpoint hemorrhages about the hock joint, followed by an apparent flattening of the tibiometatarsal joint (Scott *et al.*, 1982). Progressively, the Achilles' tendon slips from its condyles, thus rendering the bird relatively immobile. Some studies indicated that in the prevention of perosis, choline is required for the phospholipids needed for normal maturation of the cartilage matrix of bone.

Miles *et al.* (1983) demonstrated that adding 0.11% choline plus 0.1% sulfate could essentially spare all supplemental methionine in broiler diets. However, in turkey poult diets (Miles and Harms, 1984), sulfate and choline addition responses were not equivalent to supplemental methionine. Pesti *et al.* (1980), using young chicks, found that supplementation with methyl donors from either 0.23% choline or 0.23% betaine was equivalent to supplementation with 0.23% methionine in 21-day chick experiments using basal diets containing 0.31% methionine and 0.43% cystine. Spires *et al.* (1982) found that supplemental choline could replace up to two-thirds of the supplemental methionine required in broiler diets from 0 to 47 days in diets containing 0.30% methionine and 0.43% cystine in the starter phase and 0.25% and 0.42% methionine and cystine, respectively, in the finisher phase.

Choline requirement of laying hens can be influenced by choline level in the diet of the growing pullet (Scott *et al.*, 1982). Hens that received choline-free diets after 8 weeks of age could synthesize all the choline required for good egg production. Those who received choline supplements in the needed growing diet supplemental choline in the laying diet for maximum egg production. The deficiency signs noted in these hens were a reduction in egg production and an increase in liver fat content. Even with choline deficiency, however, the choline content of the egg was not affected by low dietary choline. Despite the lack of evidence that laying chickens require a dietary source of choline for maximum egg production, adding choline to practical diets markedly reduces the amount of fat in the liver (NRC, 1994). However, several reports with chicks and turkey poults did not find fatty livers with deficiency (Ruiz *et al.*, 1983). A choline response in laying chickens is likely to occur only if inadequate daily sulfur amino acids are provided. The addition of 0.1% of supplemental methionine resulted in no response in laying hens to supplemental choline (Crawford *et al.*, 1969). It appears that benefits from supplemental choline in layer diets occur mainly when supplemental methionine is adequate to meet methionine requirements.

Minimal dietary choline does not affect hatchability with either chickens or turkeys, but Japanese quail and their developing embryos readily express general signs of deficiency (Latshaw and Jensen, 1972; NRC, 1994). Supplementary choline may be necessary to maintain egg size in quail (NRC, 1994). Ducks fed choline-free diets had reduced growth rates and developed severe perosis (Hsu *et al.*, 1988), whereas Bobwhite quail developed enlarged hocks and bowed legs (NRC, 1994). Contrary to some reports, 500 mg/kg of supplemental choline to leghorn hens increased egg weight while reducing specific gravity (Tapia Romero *et al.*, 1985). Also, the choline growth requirement for quail is higher than for chicks or poults.

Safety

Studies with chickens suggest that dietary choline at twice the requirement is safe (NRC, 1994). Some of the chicken data indicate a growth reduction and interference with the utilization of vitamin B_6 when the dietary level of choline exceeds twice the required level. Other research suggests that birds tolerate high choline levels because content of 20,000–30,000 mg/kg diet was needed to induce toxicity (Leeson and Summers, 2008). Clinical signs included a reduced red blood cell number.

Derilo and Balnave (1980) reported a reduced gain and efficiency in young broiler chicks fed a level of choline of 1,771 mg/kg feed, only slightly over the requirement, but with low total sulfur amino acids (6.4 g/kg). When amino acids were supplied at a normal level of 8.4 g/kg, the same choline dosage did not negatively affect performance.

Chapter 5

Optimum vitamin nutrition in poultry breeders

INTRODUCTION

Reproduction is a crucial physiological process for poultry companies' productivity, food quality, and economic performance, and for the welfare and health of their animals. The animals selected for breeding require specialized attention, precise management practices, good health status, and diets of high nutritional quality, which should be strictly controlled (Safari Asl *et al.*, 2018; van Emous *et al.*, 2021). The broiler breeder roosters and hens face an age-related drop in reproductive performance. Therefore, it seems necessary to find approaches to protect them from the oxidative process that cause these damages (Abbaspour *et al.*, 2020). A decreased fertility in roosters older than 45 weeks is one of the main problems observed in breeder farms. In such roosters, sperm quality is reduced to a level that could not be economically valuable for breeder operations (Safari Asl *et al.*, 2018; van Emous *et al.*, 2021).

An adequate and continuous supply of nutrients is necessary for good breeding performance. In particular, vitamins are essential nutrients for developing the reproductive organs, maintaining their functional capacity, and developing zygotes and embryos. Developing and maintaining an adequate muscular and skeletal frame fitted for reproduction is also important, together with a satisfactory feather cover. Breeders also transfer immunity and microflora to their progeny. The critical roles of vitamins on the normal function of the immune system have been extensively studied and are now better understood.

This chapter will focus on data on the beneficial effects of OVN™ levels to maximize breeders' productivity while supporting the welfare, health, and sustainability of breeder farming. The information about vitamin active forms, units of quantification, conversion factors, functions, metabolism, signs of vitamin deficiencies, and general factors that influence vitamin requirements and vitamin utilization were discussed in Chapter 4.

Additional information on the importance of vitamins in the feeding of breeder birds is available in the reviews by Whitehead (1988a), Larbier and Leclercq (1994), Klasing (1998), Fisher and Willemsen (1999); McDowell (2000a, 2004), Kidd (2003), Surai (2003), Calini and Sirri (2007), Leeson and Summers (2008), Rocha *et al.* (2010), Marriott *et al.* (2020), and Shojadoost *et al.* (2021).

GENERAL ASPECTS OF VITAMIN SUPPLEMENTATION

Under practical commercial conditions, an optimum supply of vitamins or at least the minimum requirement is recommended to obtain advantages at different levels. Optimum vitamin supplementation allows for better nutrient utilization, an adequate growth rate leading to a fitting physical condition, good health status, and effective immune response. Furthermore, in broiler breeders, it also has a positive effect on the development and functionality of the reproductive system and the quality and viability of the embryo, with an influence on the weight, livability, nutritional reserves, immunological status, and subsequent development of the chicken.

To achieve these objectives, breeders must receive the vitamin supply to express their genetic potential. The appropriate intake and availability of vitamins may be affected by numerous factors, such as variability and bioavailability in feed ingredients, the presence of antagonists, and the interactions between nutrients and feed processing and storage. These factors indicate that it is not recommended to rely solely on vitamin supply through feed materials under practical commercial conditions, and that adequate vitamin supplementation is needed.

In broiler breeders, only a few studies have been conducted to evaluate the requirements of all nutrients and even fewer on the requirements for vitamins. Thus, most recommendations are based on estimates or extrapolations from other types of birds, and the data proposed are quite old in some cases. It is evident that these values are not completely adequate for current conditions in the poultry sector and that those recommendations should be increased.

The NRC (1994) provided vitamin requirements for broiler breeders based on leghorn hens and only indicated the requirements of biotin proposed by Whitehead *et al.* (1985). No studies were undertaken on broiler breeder males; consequently, no minimum vitamin requirement levels were suggested at that time. Genetic selection is continually advancing, and breeder strains are changing. Growth rate and reproduction indicators are improving progressively, which results in parallel increases in these animals' nutritional and vitamin requirements. However, metabolism has also changed in broiler breeders due to genetic selection (Buzała *et al.*, 2015; Hartcher and Lum, 2020; van Emous *et al.*, 2021).

Furthermore, the greatest rates of production and reproduction in current strains tend to compromise the metabolic capacity of birds. Consequently, we have animals more susceptible to stress caused by different physiological, immunological, and environmental factors. Despite low growth rates and feed intake, pullet breeders under feed restriction can suffer disturbance of plasma metabolites and oxidative stress under acute heat stress. In contrast, chronic heat stress causes tissue damage reflected by increased plasma lactate dehydrogenase, glutamic-oxaloacetic transaminase, and creatine kinase (Xie *et al.*, 2015). Hens and roosters during the breeding phase are even more susceptible to these stresses (Khan *et al.*, 2012a; Jena *et al.*, 2013). For this reason, the availability and activity of vitamins related to metabolism and antioxidant defense are of great importance.

The supply of micronutrients, especially vitamins, is fundamental for breeder males and females. Vitamins have clear repercussions on the growth and size of the male reproductive organs and, in consequence, the quantity of semen produced and the motility and viability of the spermatozoa. Broiler breeder hens usually are discarded around 65–70 weeks of age. After the peak of egg production, which occurs about 30–35 weeks of age, egg production gradually declines and falls to less than 50% after 60 weeks (Liu *et al.*, 2018; van Emous *et al.*, 2021), since the fecundity of females and males is negatively correlated with chronological age (Mol and Zoll, 2015; Liu *et al.*, 2018; Qazi *et al.*, 2021).

The reduced reproductive performance in old broiler breeder hens is predominantly characterized, among others, by a decline in the functionality of the ovary and liver accompanied by hormonal or endocrine changes, reduction in antioxidant capacity, decrease in vitellogenesis, lipogenesis, the transport and accumulation of yolk precursors in the oocyte and reduction in ovarian follicular reserve with decreased oocyte quality (Ishii *et al.*, 2012; Yang *et al.*, 2019; Qazi *et al.*, 2021; van Emous *et al.*, 2021). Therefore, Amevor *et al.* (2021) concluded that enhancing the antioxidant defense system of these organs and promoting the endocrine and transcription factors of the aging breeder hens to promote yolk precursor synthesis and follicle formation should be a major focus for chicken breeders. Vitamins are involved in all these processes and participate in metabolic aspects such as the synthesis and activity of hormones that influence the reproductive system, with vital importance for libido and fertility.

The studies and reviews by Rebel *et al.* (2004), Rocha *et al.* (2010), Khan *et al.* (2012b, 2014), Jena *et al.* (2013), Kazemi-Fard *et al.* (2013), Chang *et al.* (2016), and Yaripour *et al.* (2018) demonstrate that supplementing breeder feed with vitamin doses above the minimum requirements benefited the immune system, reduced stress consequences, or delayed and overcome some deleterious effects of aging of parent stock and its implications in the progeny.

It is known that the vitamin requirements for the production of hatching eggs are higher than for table eggs. Adequate vitamin intake has positive effects on the laying of eggs and their fertility and hatchability, and the subsequent embryonic and post-hatch development of the chick (Fisher and Kemp, 2000; Rocha *et al.*, 2010; Khan *et al.*, 2012b, 2014; Jena *et al.*, 2013; Chang *et al.*, 2016; Yaripour *et al.*, 2018).

It has been indicated that vitamin levels supplied in the feed has an inverse correlation with the incidence of embryo mortality during the intermediary phase of incubation (between 7 and 14 days). Remember that a fertile egg should contain all the nutrients necessary for the development and viability of the chick. During the incubation process, there is no continuous external supply of nutrients. It solely depends on the composition of the egg. It is evident that the hen's nutrition has very important repercussions on the health and development of its progeny, and out of the various nutrients, vitamins play a fundamental role.

It has been demonstrated that there is a direct relationship between the vitamin content of an egg and the hen's intake of these essential nutrients. One especially important and topical issue is that by providing nutrients, especially vitamins, to breeders some aspects related to the well-being of the chickens and the quality of the final product can be modified. Further investigation is needed.

Vitamins as micronutrients represent around 0.05% of the diet and 2–3% of the total cost of breeder feed. However, the absence or inadequate intake of a single vitamin damages health, growth, and reproduction. Vitamin supplementation should be adjusted when feed intake is lower to ensure that the quantity of vitamins ingested permits maximum production potential. The specific situation of restricted feeding of breeder hens entails the risk of marginal ingestion of vitamins which can be avoided by fortifying the vitamin content of the feed. Furthermore, stress situations such as higher temperatures in the summer months represent a challenge to the birds' immunological system, which provokes a fall in feed consumption, compromising the intake of vitamins.

CURRENT VITAMIN RECOMMENDATIONS FOR BREEDERS

Given all the aspects mentioned in the previous section, it would be advisable to adopt a balanced vitamin supplementation program, over and above the minimum requirements, which would allow maintaining the best cost–benefit ratio. This process involves applying safety margins that compensate for the variation in feed ingredients, strains, and production systems found in the market. In practice, the feed industry includes vitamin levels in feeds for broiler breeders that are twice as high as commercial egg-laying hens.

Likewise, commercial feed for breeders has been formulated for decades with vitamin levels above the minimum requirements set by the NRC (1994) and by using high safety margins, above all, for vitamins A, E, D, K, and niacin. Ward conducted in 2014 and 2022 the most recent surveys of vitamin supplementation in broiler breeders in the US market (Table 5.1). These data

Table 5.1 US Survey – vitamin supplementation for commercial breeder feed (Ward, 2014, 2022)

	Commercial broiler breeders (unit per kg feed)		
	Unit/kg	2014	2022
Vitamin A	IU	11,000	10,703
Vitamin D_3	IU	4,050	4,321
Vitamin E	mg	62.0	68.0
Vitamin K	mg	2.7	3.3
Vitamin B_1	mg	2.9	3.1
Vitamin B_2	mg	10.9	11.1
Vitamin B_6	mg	4.4	4.8
Vitamin B_{12}	mg	0.023	0.027
Niacin	mg	45.0	54.0
D-pantothenic acid	mg	17.0	17.5
Folic acid	mg	1.8	2.1
Biotin	mg	0.254	0.267

indicate one of the highest supplementation levels among all poultry feeds. Comparing 2014 and 2022 all vitamin levels have been increased with the only exception of a small reduction of vitamin A. However, Ward observed a great deal of variation with a coefficient of variance in the range of 30%.

We will now describe the most relevant aspects of each vitamin, with specific reference to the reproduction process, showing the results of optimum supplementation of the different vitamins in feed for breeders and their repercussions on aspects of fertility, hatchability, quality, and viability of the chicks, but also of the well-being and health of the animals.

However, let us first review the vitamin levels recommended by the various official bodies and genetic and feed additive companies for female and male broiler breeder strains. The current recommendations for pullet and cockerel broiler breeder supplementation during the starter and growing phase are presented in Table 5.2. It is evident that genetic companies recommend higher supplementation levels than scientific groups, like Rostagno *et al.* (2017) and FEDNA (2018). Considerable differences are observed in vitamin E and choline levels, the latter depending on recommending the quantity added or referring to the total choline.

A similar situation is observed in Table 5.3 for vitamin supplementation recommendations during the laying/breeding phase for broiler breeder hens. Compared to levels recommended by DSM Nutritional Products (2022) OVN™, these levels have been increased in small amounts, except for choline, which doubled. More importance is given to vitamin E during the starter and growing period because the recommendation also doubles.

The current recommendations for male breeders during the mating phase are presented in Table 5.4. Vitamins supplementation for roosters has been considered important for many decades, and levels have changed much in the past 10 years. But some small increments in recommendations are observed in B complex vitamins, and choline recommendation is also doubled by most of the sources revised.

The information for turkey breeders is presented in Table 5.5. There is a close agreement on the recommended dietary levels among the limited sources that recommend vitamin

Table 5.2 Current recommended vitamin levels (IU or mg/kg air-dry feed) for broiler breeders by various sources during starter and grower phases

	Broiler breeders (added per kg feed)									
	Starter-grower phases									
	Unit/kg	NRC, 1994	FEFANA, 2015	Rostagno *et al.*, 2017	FEDNA, 2018	Hubbard Breeders Nutrition Guide, 2019	Cobb-Vantress 2020	Aviagen, 2021	OVN™ (DSM Nutritional Products, 2022)	Poultry breeder references
Vitamin A	IU	3,000	10,000–14,000	9,637	10,000	12,000	11,000	13,100	10,500–13,100	Squires and Naber (1993a) 16,000 IU egg hatchability; Yuan *et al.* (2014) 15,000 IU egg fertility
Vitamin D_3	IU	300	3,000–5,000	2,409	2,800	3,200	3,500	4,000	3,150 –5,200	Atencio *et al.* (2005a) 4,000 IU heavier progeny, higher bone ash and lower TD incidence
$25OHD_3$ (HyD)	mg	–	0.07	–	–	–	–	–	0.069	Lin *et al.* (2019) 0.069 mg, improve survival breeder rate with restricted and ad-libitum intake; Araújo *et al.* (2019b) 0.069 mg
Vitamin E	mg	10	30–50	36.1	30	60–100	100	100	105–160	Siegel *et al.* (2001) 300 mg more eggs; Yang *et al.* (2020a,b) 400 mg maternal dietary vitamin E increased 42d body weight of offspring
Vitamin K	mg	1	3–5	1.93	2.1	5	3	6	3.2–6	Fares *et al.* (2018) 11 mg decreased embryonic mortality
Vitamin B_1	mg	0.7	3–3.5	2.59	1.1	3.5	2.75	5	2.5–5	Olkoswki and Classen (1999) 8 mg increased thiamine metabolism of the offspring
Vitamin B_2	mg	3.6	12–16	6.44	7	12	8	15	9–15	Leeson (2005) 7 mg Influence on hatchability, vigor and survival of the chick
Vitamin B_6	mg	4.5	4–6	3.61	2.7	6	3	5	4.2–6.2	Robel (1992, 2002) 6.2 mg higher hatchability (turkey breeders)

Table 5.2 (continued)

	Broiler breeders (added per kg feed)									
	Starter-grower phases									
	Unit/ kg	NRC, 1994	FEFANA, 2015	Rostagno *et al.*, 2017	FEDNA, 2018	Hubbard Breeders Nutrition Guide, 2019	Cobb-Vantress 2020	Aviagen, 2021	OVN™ (DSM Nutritional Products, 2022)	Poultry breeder references
Vitamin B_{12}	mg	0.008	0.02–0.04	0.016	0.017	0.035	0.025	0.050	0.025–0.05	Panic *et al.* (1970) 0.02 mg better hatchability
Niacin	mg	10.00	50–60	39.2	25	60	40	50	32–62	Leeson (1991) 132 mg improved shell quality
D-panthothenic acid	mg	7	10–15	12.95	12	16	15	20	15–20	Goeger and Ascott (1984) 24 mg, increased semen quantity and quality
Folic acid	mg	0.35	1.5–2	0.9	1	2.5	2	3	1.6–3	Robel (2002) 7.4 mg improved hatchability, higher body weight and offspring vitality (turkey breeders)
Biotin	mg	0.10–0.16	0.2–0.4	0.09	0.11	0.3	0.3	0.3	0.26–0.42	Robel (1989) 0.44 mg better hatchability in broiler breeders; Robel (2002) 0.8 mg better hatchability in turkey breeders; Daryabari *et al.* (2014) 0.45 mg improved fertility
Vitamin C	mg		100–150	–	–	–	–	–	105–160	Monsi and Onitchi (1991) 500 mg increased semen volume, motile sperm per ejaculate and sperm number per ejaculate; Asensio *et al.* (2020) 200 mg improved tail and wing feather score (stress and welfare indicator)
Choline	mg	1,000	350–700	392	250	750	500	1,400	370–740	Rama-Rao *et al.* (2001) 760 mg

Table 5.3 Recommended vitamin levels (IU or mg/kg air-dry feed) for broiler breeders by various sources during the laying/breeding phase

	Broiler breeders (added per kg feed)									
		Laying/Breeding phase								
	Unit/kg	NRC, 1994	FEFANA, 2015	Rostagno *et al.*, 2017	FEDNA, 2018	Hubbard Breeders Nutrition Guide, 2019	Cobb-Vantress 2020	Aviagen, 2021	OVN™ (DSM Nutritional Products, 2022)	Poultry breeder references
Vitamin A	IU	3,000	10,000–14,000	11,000	10,000	12,000	13,000	15,000	12,600–15,700	Squires and Naber (1993a) 16,000 IU egg hatchability; Yuan *et al.* (2014) 15,000 IU egg fertility
Vitamin D_3	IU	300	3,000–5,000	3,000	2,800	3,200	3,500	5,000	3,150–5,200	Atencio *et al.* (2005a) 4,000 IU heavier progeny, higher bone ash and lower TD incidence
$25OHD_3$ (HyD)	mg	–	0.069	–	–	–	–	–	0.069	Lin *et al.* (2019) 0.069 mg, improve survival breeder rate with restricted and ad-libitum intake; Araújo *et al.* (2019b) 0.069 mg
Vitamin E	mg	10	30–50	50	30	60–100	100	130	105–160	Siegel *et al.* (2001) 300 mg more eggs; Yang *et al.* (2020a,b) 400 mg maternal dietary vitamin E increased 42d body weight of offspring
Vitamin K	mg	1	3–5	3	2.1	5	6	9	6–9	Fares *et al.* (2018) 11 mg decreased embryonic mortality
Vitamin B_1	mg	0.7	3–3.5	2.8	1.1	3.5	3	6	3.5–6	Olkoswki and Classen (1999) 8 mg increased thiamine metabolism of the offspring
Vitamin B_2	mg	3.6	12–16	8	7	12	13	20	13–20	Leeson (2005) 7 mg Influence on hatchability, vigor and survival of the chick
Vitamin B_6	mg	4.5	4–6	3	2.7	6	6	8	5–8	Robel (1992, 2002) 6.2 mg higher hatchability (turkey breeders)

Table 5.3 (continued)

	Broiler breeders (added per kg feed)									
		Laying/Breeding phase								
	Unit/kg	NRC, 1994	FEFANA, 2015	Rostagno *et al.*, 2017	FEDNA, 2018	Hubbard Breeders Nutrition Guide, 2019	Cobb-Vantress 2020	Aviagen, 2021	OVN™ (DSM Nutritional Products, 2022)	Poultry breeder references
Vitamin B_{12}	mg	0.008	0.02–0.04	0.025	0.017	0.035	0.035	0.07	0.035–0.07	Panic *et al.* (1970) 0.02 mg better hatchability
Niacin	mg	10	50–60	35	25	60	50	70	55–70	Leeson (1991) 132 mg improved shell quality
D-panthothenic acid	mg	7	10–15	15	12	16	20	25	16–25	Goeger and Ascott (1984) 24 mg, increased semen quantity and quality
Folic acid	mg	0.35	1.5–2	1.1	1	2.5	3	5	2.5–5	Robel (2002) 7.4 mg improved hatchability, higher body weight and offspring vitality (turkey breeders)
Biotin	mg	0.10–0.16	0.2–0.4	0.11	0.11	0.3	0.375	0.6	0.3–0.6	Robel (1989) 0.44 mg better hatchability in broiler breeders; Robel (2002) 0.8 mg better hatchability in turkey breeders; Daryabari *et al.* (2014) 0.45 mg improved fertility
Vitamin C	mg	–	100–150	–	–	–	–	–	105–160	Monsi and Onitchi (1991) 500 mg increased semen volume, motile sperm per ejaculate and sperm number per ejaculate; Asensio *et al.* (2020) 200 mg improved tail and wing feather score (stress and welfare indicator)
Choline	mg	1,000	350–700	450	250	750	500	1,600	370–740	Rama-Rao *et al.* (2001) 760 mg

Table 5.4 Recommended vitamin levels (IU or mg/kg air-dry feed) by various sources for male broiler breeders (mating period)

	Male broiler breeders mating period (added per kg feed)							
	Unit/kg	FEFANA, 2015	Rostagno, 2017	FEDNA, 2018	Hubbard Breeders Nutrition Guide, 2019	Cobb-Vantress 2020	Aviagen, 2021	OVN™ (DSM Nutritional Products, 2022)
Vitamin A	IU	10,000–14,000	9,637	10,000	12,000	11,000	13,000	12,600–15,700
Vitamin D_3	IU	2,300–5,000	2,409	2,800	3,200	3,500	4,000	3,150–5,200
$25OHD_3$ (HyD)	mg	0.069	–	–	–	–	–	0.069
Vitamin E	mg	30–50	36.1	30	60–100	100	100	105–160
Vitamin K	mg	3–5	1.93	2.1	5	3	6	6–9
Vitamin B_1	mg	3–3.5	2.59	1.1	3.5	2.75	5	3.5–6
Vitamin B_2	mg	12–16	6.44	7	12	8	15	13–20
Vitamin B_6	mg	4–6	3.61	2.7	6	3	5	5–8
Vitamin B_{12}	mg	0.02–0.04	0.016	0.017	0.035	0.025	0.05	0.035–0.07
Niacin	mg	50–60	39.2	25	60	40	50	55–70
D-panthothenic acid	mg	10–15	12.95	12	16	15	20	16–25
Folic acid	mg	1.5–2	0.903	1	2.5	2	3	2.5–5
Biotin	mg	0.2–0.4	0.09	0.11	0.3	0.3	0.3	0.3–0.6
Vitamin C	mg	100–150	–	–	–	–	–	105–160
Choline	mg	350–700	392	250	750	500	1,400	370–740

Table 5.5 Recommended vitamin levels (IU or mg/kg air-dry feed) by various sources for turkey breeders

	Turkey breeders (added per kg feed)						
		Starter				Grower	
	Unit/kg	FEFANA, 2015	Hendrix-Genetics, 2016	Aviagen, 2020	OVN™ (DSM Nutritional Products, 2022)	FEFANA, 2015	Hendrix-Genetics 2016
Vitamin A	IU	11,000–15,000	12,000	12,000	12,600–14,700	11,000–15,000	9,600
Vitamin D_3	IU	4,000–5,000	5,000	5,000	4,200–5,200	4,000–5,000	4,800
25OHD_3 (HyD)	mg	0.092	–	–	0.092	0.092	–
Vitamin E	mg	40–60	100	100	105–160	40–60	60
Vitamin K	mg	4–5	4	4	4.2–5.2	4–5	3
Vitamin B_1	mg	4–5	4.5	4	4.7–5.2	4–5	2
Vitamin B_2	mg	15–20	15	15	16–21	15–20	12
Vitamin B_6	mg	6–7	5	7	6.5–7.5	6–7	3.5
Vitamin B_{12}	mg	0.04–0.05	0.04	0.04	0.042–0.052	0.04–0.05	0.02
Niacin	mg	100–150	110	110	105–160	100–150	85
D-panthothenic acid	mg	25–35	28	30	32–37	25–35	23
Folic acid	mg	4–6	3.5	4	4.2–6.2	2–3	2.5

		Laying/breeding phase				
Aviagen, 2020	OVN™ (DSM Nutritional Products, 2022)	FEFANA, 20151	Hendrix-Genetics, 2016	Aviagen, 2020	OVN™ (DSM Nutritional Products, 2022)	Poultry breeder references
8,000	8,400–10,500	11,000–15,000	12,000	12,000	12,600–14,700	Squires and Naber (1993a) 16,000 IU egg hatchability; Yuan *et al.* (2014) 15,000 IU egg fertility
4,000	4,200–5,200	4,000–5,000	5,000	5,000	4,200–5,200	Atencio *et al.* (2005a) 4,000 IU heavier progeny, higher bone ash and lower TD incidence
–	0.092	0.092	–	–	0.092	Lin *et al.* (2019) 0.069 mg, improve survival breeder rate with restricted and ad-libitum intake; Araújo *et al.* (2019b) 0.069 mg
50	65–85	40–60	100	120	105–160	Siegel *et al.* (2001) 300 mg more eggs; Yang *et al.* (2020a,b) 400 mg maternal dietary vitamin E increased 42d body weight of offspring
2	2.2–4.2	4– 5	5	5	4.2–5.2	Fares *et al.* (2018) 11 mg decreased embryonic mortality
1	2.2–3.2	4–5	4.5	4	4.2–5.2	Olkoswki and Classen (1999) 8 mg increased thiamine metabolism of the offspring
5	11–16	15–20	18	20	16–21	Leeson (2005) 7 mg Influence on hatchability, vigor and survival of the chick
5	6.5–7.5	6–7	5	7	6.5–7.5	Robel (1992, 2002) 6.2 mg higher hatchability (turkey breeders)
0.02	0.032–0.042	0.04–0.05	0.04	0.04	0.042–0.052	Panic *et al.* (1970) 0.02 mg better hatchability
55	65–85	100–150	110	90	85–125	Leeson (1991) 132 mg improved shell quality
16	26–31	25–35	30	30	32–37	Goeger and Ascott (1984) 24 mg, increased semen quantity and quality
2	2.2–3.2	2–3	4.5	6	4.2–6.2	Robel (2002) 7.4 mg improved hatchability, higher body weight and offspring vitality (turkey breeders)

Table 5.5 (continued)

	Turkey breeders (added per kg feed)						
		Starter				Grower	
	Unit/kg	FEFANA, 2015	Hendrix-Genetics, 2016	Aviagen, 2020	OVN™ (DSM Nutritional Products, 2022)	FEFANA, 2015	Hendrix Genetics 2016
Biotin	mg	0.4–0.6	0.3	0.4	0.42–0.62	0.4–0.6	0.17
Vitamin C	mg	100–200	–	–	105–210	100–200	–
Choline	mg	1,000–1,200	1,200	1,200	1,050–1,250	1,000–1,200	600

supplementation levels for turkeys. The levels during the past 10 years have changed very little despite the advances in growth and yield due to genetics, the higher stocking densities used nowadays, more disease challenges, and the climatic change with more extreme weather conditions.

Finally, Table 5.6 provides the recommended vitamin supplementation in layer breeders. There's a good alignment among the major genetic companies, and all of them have recently updated their vitamin recommendations with a major focus on vitamin E, vitamin B_1, B_2, and pantothenic acid.

OPTIMUM VITAMIN NUTRITION FOR BREEDERS

Fat-soluble vitamins

All vitamins are important for parent development, growth, immunity, reproduction, and embryo development. In the following paragraphs, we will discuss some of these functions.

However, it is important to highlight the great amount of information generated in the previous years in research using *in ovo* feeding technology. Injection of nutrients *in ovo* is still not used commercially in the hatchery industry despite decades of research and some commercial application in the US and worldwide for more than 30 years (Ricks *et al.*, 1999; Williams and Zedek, 2010; Peebles, 2018; Tufarelli *et al.*, 2021). The main limitations for implementation of *in ovo* feeding on a commercial scale include: (1) the embryonic age proven to be effective for injection of nutrients, probiotics, or other compounds; (2) the discrepancy between the optimum time for nutrient injection with the optimum time for egg transfer from setters to hatchers and *in ovo* vaccination, which is between embryonic day 18.5 and 19.5

		Laying/breeding phase				
viagen, 2020	OVN™ (DSM Nutritional Products, 2022)	FEFANA, 20151	Hendrix-Genetics, 2016	Aviagen, 2020	OVN™ (DSM Nutritional Products, 2022)	Poultry breeder references
0.3	0.42–0.62	0.4–0.6	0.5	0.45	0.42–0.62	Robel (1989) 0.44 mg better hatchability in broiler breeders; Robel (2002) 0.8 mg better hatchability in turkey breeders; Daryabari *et al.* (2014) 0.45 mg improved fertility
–	105–210	100–200	–	–	105–210	Monsi and Onitchi (1991) 500 mg increased semen volume, motile sperm per ejaculate and sperm number per ejaculate; Asensio *et al.* (2020) 200 mg improved tail and wing feather score (stress and welfare indicator)
800	1,050–1,250	1,000–1,200	1,200	1,000	525–1,050	Rama-Rao *et al.* (2001) 760 mg

(Fernandes *et al.*, 2016); and (3) the incompatibility between osmolarity and pH stability of nutrient solutions and vaccine optimum conditions.

In Table 5.7 lists a summary of the latest research results of *in ovo* feeding with several liposoluble vitamins. The day of injection (DOI) was several days before the egg transfer to hatchers in all projects. This timing will complicate egg management in hatcheries, especially in those with single-stage production, which should maintain a profile of temperatures, humidity, and carbon dioxide according to embryo age.

However, the positive results observed on several aspects of embryo development, progeny viability, performance post-hatch, immunity, and health give us strong evidence that embryos may benefit from a higher content of vitamins in the egg than the hen can provide even if their diets have increased levels of these vitamins and fertile eggs enriched with specific vitamins. The design of optimum supplements for breeders is still unclear, but the following research can provide ideas for its development under particular conditions.

Vitamin A

> Details about current vitamin A recommendations for breeders, provided by institutional sources and genetic companies, can be found in Tables 5.2 to 5.6.

Vitamin A has important effects on bone growth and thus the development of young animals, the quantity and quality of semen produced, and the growth and differentiation of epithelial tissues of the reproductive system and the embryo, among other factors. In this regard, it has

Table 5.6 Recommended vitamin levels (IU or mg/kg air-dry feed) by various sources for layer breeders (including male breeders)

	Layers breeders (added per kg feed)					
		Starter and growing phase				
	Unit/kg	Novogen, 2020	Hendrix Genetics, 2020	Hy-Line, 2022	OVN™ (DSM Nutritional Products, 2022)	Novogen, 2020
Vitamin A	IU	12,000	15,000	10,000	12,600–15,700	12,000
Vitamin D_3	IU	3,200	3,500	3,300	3,200–4,800	3,200
$25OHD_3$ (HyD)	mg	–	–	(part of vitamin D_3 as $25OHD_3$)	0.069	–
Vitamin E	mg	50–100	100–105	30 (200 in heat stress)	55–105	50–100
Vitamin K	mg	5	5	4	2.1–5.2	5
Vitamin B_1	mg	3	5	3	2.6–5	3
Vitamin B_2	mg	10	12	10	10.5–15	10
Vitamin B_6	mg	5.5	6	6	5.2–7	5.5
Vitamin B_{12}	mg	0.03	0.04	0.03	0.022–0.05	0.03
Niacin	mg	45	66	50	47–66	45
D-panthothenic acid	mg	16	17	15	15.8–21	16
Folic acid	mg	2.5	3.4	1.2	2.1–3.4	2.5
Biotin	mg	0.3	0.3	0.12	0.26–0.42	0.3
Vitamin C	mg	–	150	(150–200 in heat stress)	160–210	–
Choline	mg	500	750	–	315–525	500

Laying/breeding phase			
Hendrix Genetics, 2020	Hy-Line, 2022	OVN™ (DSM Nutritional Products, 2022)	Poultry breeder references
13,600	12,000	12,600–15,700	Squires and Naber (1993a) 16,000 IU egg hatchability; Yuan *et al.* (2014) 15,000 IU egg fertility
3,750	4,400	3,200–4,800	Atencio *et al.* (2005a) 4,000 IU heavier progeny, higher bone ash and lower TD incidence
–	(part of vitamin D_3 as 25OHD$_3$)	0.069	Lin *et al.* (2019) 0.069 mg, improve survival breeder rate with restricted and ad-libitum intake; Araújo *et al.* (2019b) 0.069 mg
100–105	85 (200 in heat stress)	55–105	Siegel *et al.* (2001) 300 mg more eggs; Yang *et al.* (2020a,b) 400 mg maternal dietary vitamin E increased 42d body weight of offspring
5	5	2.1–5.2	Fares *et al.* (2018) 11 mg decreased embryonic mortality
5	4	2.6–5	Olkoswki and Classen (1999) 8 mg increased thiamine metabolism of the offspring
12	15	10.5–15	Leeson (2005) 7 mg Influence on hatchability, vigor and survival of the chick
7	7	5.2–7	Robel (1992, 2002) 6.2 mg higher hatchability (turkey breeders)
0.05	0.035	0.022–0.05	Panic *et al.* (1970) 0.02 mg better hatchability
55	65	47–66	Leeson (1991) 132 mg improved shell quality
17	21	15.8–21	Goeger and Ascott (1984) 24 mg, increased semen quantity and quality
3.4	3	2.1–3.4	Robel (2002) 7.4 mg improved hatchability, higher body weight and offspring vitality (turkey breeders)
0.4	0.35	0.26–0.42	Robel (1989) 0.44 mg better hatchability in broiler breeders; Robel (2002) 0.8 mg better hatchability in turkey breeders; Daryabari *et al.* (2014) 0.45 mg improved fertility
150	(150–200 in heat stress)	160–210	Monsi and Onitchi (1991) 500 mg increased semen volume, motile sperm per ejaculate and sperm number per ejaculate; Asensio *et al.* (2020) 200 mg improved tail and wing feather score (stress and welfare indicator)
1,000	–	315–525	Rama-Rao *et al.* (2001) 760 mg

Table 5.7 Effects of liposoluble vitamins injection *in ovo* on offspring

In ovo injection characteristics	Species/Study characteristics/Injection day	Result	References
Uninjected/corn oil/corn oil + 10 mg vitamin E/ saline solution/saline solution + vitamin C	Muscovy ducks. Hatchability and performance. DOI 12 d	Vitamin E and C injections increased hatch and final body weight and feed intake. The feed conversion ratio was improved by them only at the starter phase.	Selim *et al.* (2012)
No injection/physiology serum/vitamin E (15 or 30 mg)	Broilers. Serum post-hatch immunological parameters and broiler chicken performance. DOI 14 d	Both vitamin E levels improved hatchability and IgG 42 d while antibodies (avian influenza, infectious bronchitis) and IgM and IgA were improved only by 30 mg injection at 21 and 42 d.	Salary *et al.* (2014)
Diluent or 0.6 µg 25OHD$_3$	Broilers. Determination of sex, yolk weight, BW, serum CA and phosphorous concentrations, and yolk CA, phosphorous, moisture, dry matter, and lipid concentrations. DOI 18 d.	25OHD$_3$ reduced yolk CA differences associated with embryo sex.	Bello *et al.* (2015)
Vitamin E (0, 27.5, 38.5, 49.5 and 60.4 UI)	Broilers. Incubation results, quality, and oxidative state of newborn chicks. DOI 17.5 d	Better body weight, length, newborn chick quality score, higher chick weight/egg weight ratios, and intestine development were obtained with vitamin E injection.	Araujo *et al.* (2019a)
No injection/oil-injected sham/vitamin E (0.037 or 0.074 IU)	Broilers. Immunity and growth performance of broilers reared at heat stress. DOI 17.5 d	Cellular immunity was increased by 0.037 IU and decreased by 0.074 IU, decreasing day 10 bodyweight.	Heidari *et al.* (2021)
No injection/diluent/ 2.4 µg D$_3$ or 2.4 µg 25OHD$_3$ or 2.4 µg D$_3$ + 2.4 µg 25OHD$_3$	Broilers. Performance, breast meat yield, and inflammatory responses.	25OHD$_3$ alone reduced inflammatory response, had greater body weight, and increased breast meat yield.	Fatemi *et al.* (2021a)
No injection/diluent/2.4 µg D$_3$ or 2.4 µg 25OHD$_3$ or 2.4 µg D$_3$ + 2.4 µg 25OHD$_3$	Broilers. Performance, carcass characteristics, and woody breast myopathy incidence. Fed with commercial diet or diet restricted in calcium and phosphorus.	25OHD$_3$ injection alone increased breast meat yield without interaction with calcium and phosphorus restriction.	Fatemi *et al.* (2021b)
No injection/diluent/ 2.4 µg D$_3$ or 2.4 µg 25OHD$_3$ or 2.4 µg D$_3$ + 2.4 µg 25OHD$_3$	Broilers. Performance, breast meat yield, intestinal lesion score after coccidiosis challenge.	*Pectoralis major* muscle tended to increase belonging to the 25OHD$_3$ group, showing that this vitamin may increase body weight and breast meat yield regardless of the challenge.	Fatemi *et al.* (2021c)

PBS (C), PBS with 40 ng 1,25OH$_2$D$_3$ (1,25D-L), 200 ng 1,25OH$_2$D$_3$ (1,25D-H), 40 ng 25OHD$_3$ (25D-L), or 200 ng 25OHD$_3$ (25D-H)	Broilers. Expression of key genes related to osteogenesis, adipogenesis, myogenesis, and vitamin D$_3$. DOI 3 d.	Both 1,25OH$_2$D$_3$ and 25OHD$_3$ induced chicken embryo osteogenesis and adipogenesis but inhibited myogenesis during early chicken embryo development.	Chen C. *et al.* (2021)
No injection or injection of 0, 1.2, 2.4 or 3.6 μg of 25OHD$_3$	Broilers. Incubation parameters of bone mineral composition, mineral density, and bone-breaking strength in post-hatch broilers. DOI 8 d	Tibial and femur bone mineral density was quadratically affected when injections of 0.47 and 0.68 μg of 25OHD$_3$ increased tibia and femur bone mineral density.	Quadros *et al.* (2021)
No injection/deionized water/1 mg of Vitamin A or D$_3$ or E or folic acid	Fayoumi breeders. Hatchability, embryonic growth, and hatchling status.	Hatchability, residual yolk, embryo length and weight, hatchling weight, and the assessed health status indices were increased.	Gouda *et al.* (2021)
No injection/distilled water/vitamin E and nano-selenium (15 or 30 or 45 mg each)	Hatchling status, growth performance, and tissue glycogen level. DOI 17.5 d	The hatch and 48 hour weight were increased with all vitamin levels, increasing the muscle glycogen content.	Kadhim *et al.* (2021)

been observed that vitamin A has a morphogenetic activity, with responsibility for the differentiation of cells during the embryonic development of the chicken (Klasing, 1998, McDowell 2004) and positively influences egg production (i.e., number, weight, or egg quality) and hatchability (Yaripour *et al.*, 2018).

Among the first apparent symptoms of vitamin A deficiency is a decrease in sexual activity in males and failure of spermatogenesis, accompanied by a reduction in fertility and the number of hatched eggs. Roosters need to receive sufficient vitamins to maintain high sexual activity during breeding. They usually copulate 20 to 30 times a day, which makes a high rate of sperm synthesis necessary. Supplies of vitamin A above requirements permit an adequate growth rate in breeder males, with an optimum development of the organs and systems involved in reproduction (Damjanov *et al.*, 1980).

Gao *et al.* (2021) formulated experimental diets for layer breeder roosters, with levels of several vitamins, including vitamin A (20,000 IU), in order to investigate astaxanthin enhanced antioxidant capacity and improved semen quality.

Hepatic reserves of vitamin A are usually enough to maintain the production of several eggs with adequate concentrations of this vitamin. In this case, the dietary supply is important during the pre-laying phase to achieve a good reserve level to carry it through the subsequent breeding phase (Surai *et al.*, 1998a).

Chen *et al.* (2016), when evaluating the reproductive performance of offspring hepatic vitamin A content and hatchling weight, indicated that the optimal dietary vitamin A level for Chinese yellow-feathered broiler breeders from 46 to 54 weeks of age was 10,800 IU/kg. It was demonstrated that dietary vitamin A supplementation elevated follicle-stimulating hormone receptor, luteinizing hormone receptor (LHR), growth hormone receptor (GHR), insulin-like growth factor 1 receptor (IGF-IR), retinoic acid receptor α (RAR), retinoid X receptor (RXR) transcripts and decreases the apoptosis-related genes caspase-3 and Fas in the ovaries of breeders. These results indicated the potential of retinoic acid to regulate ovarian expression of hormone receptors and inhibit apoptosis utilizing the active metabolite.

During laying it is recommended to supply doses of vitamin A above the minimum requirements to avoid deficiency symptoms, prevent problems due to reduced absorption or insufficient reserves, and ensure an adequate content in the fertile egg. Retinol is the initial form of vitamin A transferred to the egg as it binds with protein. Vitamin A is mainly in the aqueous part of the yolk and is gradually transferred to the embryo during incubation (Vieira *et al.*, 1995).

It has been observed that when breeders consume marginal quantities of vitamin A, their progeny have lower vitamin reserves, and disorders manifest after hatching (Hill *et al.*, 1961). Bermudez *et al.* (1993) indicated that insufficient levels of vitamin A are often accompanied by increased atresia. Clagett-Dame and Knutson (2011) added that this deficiency also causes ovulation of degenerated eggs and abnormal embryo development. On the other hand, excessive vitamin A intake (45,000–135,000 IU/kg feed) may decrease egg production and increase congenital abnormalities in embryos (Yuan *et al.*, 2014).

Yaripour *et al.* (2018) showed that a combination of dietary supranutritional levels of vitamins A and E allowed extension of the laying period and reduced fertility decline in older breeder hens at the end of the laying phase, with acceptable productive and fertility parameters. In particular, among the tested treatments, feeding a supranutritional level of 100% (3 mg/kg) vitamin A and 200% (74 mg/kg) vitamin E of Ross recommendations led to the best results.

In the study by Yuan *et al.* (2014), increasing vitamin levels from 5,000 IU/kg to 35,000 IU/kg did not affect the hatchability of eggs. However, supplementing vitamin A at 45,000 IU/kg significantly decreased hatchability at week 24 (Figure 5.1).

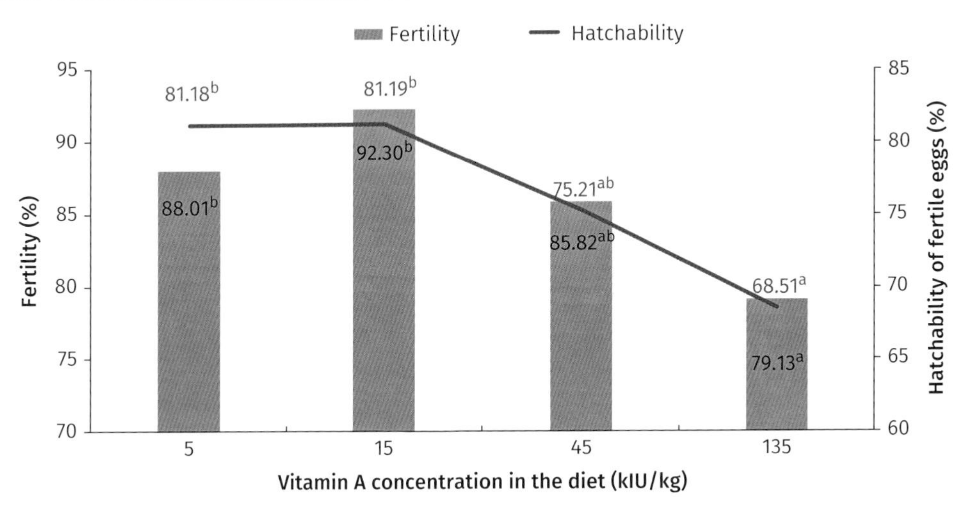

Figure 5.1 Effect Vitamin A supplementation in the diet on fertility and hatchability in broiler breeders at week 24, values with no common superscripts differ significantly, $P < 0.05$ (adapted from Yuan *et al.*, 2014)

Surai *et al.* (1998a) study demonstrated a direct relationship between the quantity of vitamin A in the breeder's diet deposited in the eggs and in the hen liver. Adequate vitamin A content in the hatching egg results in a better growth rate, greater capacity for immune response, and prevents pigmentation problems in the chicken.

Bhanja *et al.* (2012) also concluded that 100 IU vitamin A injected *in ovo* might influence embryonic development. The embryo uses a relatively small and constant quantity of vitamin A during its development. The remaining store would be accessible to nourish the chick in the first days after hatching. The work by Squires and Naber (1993a) demonstrated that after 25–27 weeks of administering feed with different doses of vitamin A, the eggs of the breeders supplemented with 16,000 IU/kg contained 10 times more vitamin A (24 IU vitamin A/gram of yolk) than the fertile eggs of the hens without supplementation. Similarly, more eggs were laid and hatched.

Vitamin A is required for embryonic development. It is necessary to prevent growth abnormalities (Chen *et al.*, 2016), and it is involved in the antioxidant defense of the developing embryo (Gaal *et al.*, 1995). When evaluating vitamin A supplementation in day-old chicks, Fan *et al.* (2015) found an increase in the concentration of immunoglobulin A as hen dietary levels increased.

Vitamin A inclusion in the diet can minimize heat stress in laying hens and strengthen the immune system against parasites, viruses, and bacteria. It exerts a protective effect on mucous membranes and adrenal glands. Vitamin A improves both the innate immune system and the adaptive immune system against infections (Haq *et al.*, 1996; Wiseman *et al.*, 2017). In addition, retinoic acid increased the response of T-lymphocytes (Abd El-Hack *et al.*, 2017).

The properties of vitamin A, including the mechanisms by which vitamin A affects the immune system, are well defined and are mediated through interactions of retinoic acid with nuclear-hormone receptors in immune system cells. The general effects of vitamin A on the immune system have been illustrated in Figure 5.2. Passive diffusion is the main mechanism by which immune system cells acquire vitamin A. Post entry it binds to its nuclear receptor, RXR, which modulates specific immune system cells subset. Vitamin A activates (upregulation of MHC-II, CD-80, CD86, IL-12) innate immune cells (macrophages and dendritic cells). Treatment increases mucin and secretory IgA antibody production in mucosal sites such as the lungs

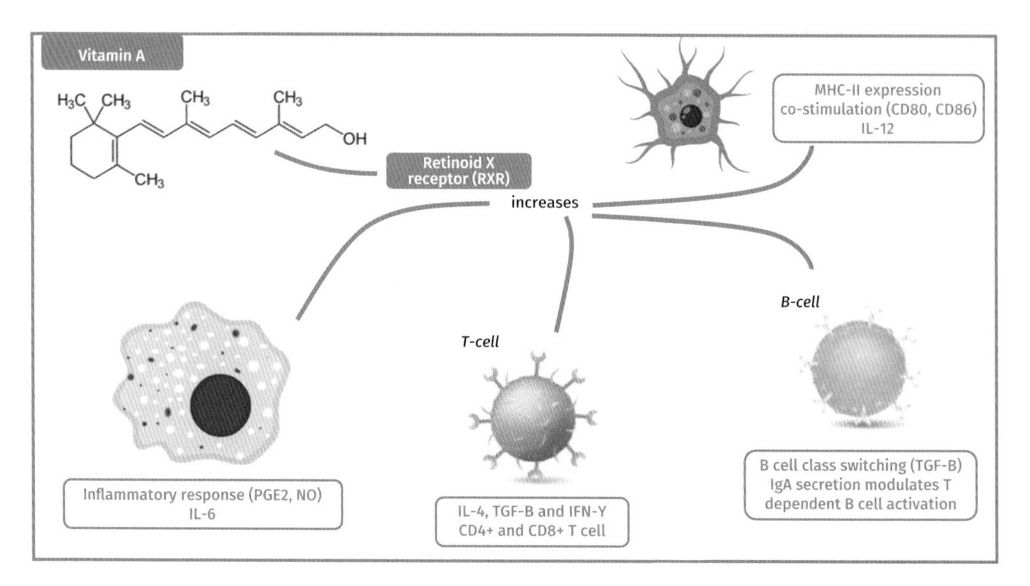

Figure 5.2 Effect of vitamin A on the immune system (adapted from Shojadoost *et al.*, 2021)

and gut. The activity of this vitamin is highly dose-dependent, as low and high doses induce inflammatory and anti-inflammatory responses, respectively (Shojadoost *et al.*, 2021).

Khoramabadi *et al.* (2014) reported that vitamin A supplementation in broilers reduced intestinal epithelial erosions and increased weight gain, it also positively affected the digestibility of proteins and lipids. Prabakar *et al.* (2018) found that combined supplementation of the carotenoids canthaxanthin and apo-carotenoid, each at 6 mg/kg, to the basal diet enhanced the hematological parameters and thereby increased the health and welfare of broiler breeders during heat stress.

An excess of vitamin A can provoke pigmentation problems and deficiencies in other fat-soluble vitamins. For this reason the maximum tolerance level is set at 40,000 IU/kg (NRC, 1987). More recently, Yuan *et al.* (2014) observed that the maximum tolerable dose of vitamin A on Ross 308 broiler breeders was 35,000 IU/kg.

The deposition level of carotenoids in tissues (plasma and yolk) is indicative of variation in dietary availability and physiological demands, such as reproduction. It can be used as an indicator of an animal's health status. Bortolotti *et al.* (2003) demonstrated that plasma carotenoids at the end of the laying period were strongly correlated with the number of eggs laid. Souza *et al.* (2008) added 6 mg canthaxanthin/kg feed to the broiler breeder diet observing a reduction in infertile eggs and embryonic mortality and improved hatchability.

Some authors have concluded that carotenoids can modulate the antioxidant system of the embryo and hatched chick and help maintain the system's efficiency. High concentrations of PUFAs characterize embryonic tissues; thus, adding vitamins and minerals with antioxidant activity to broiler breeder diets improves the oxidative protection of the newly hatched chick (Rocha *et al.*, 2010). The high concentration of PUFAs in embryonic tissues (Surai *et al.*, 1997a) is associated with increased oxygen consumption and respiration toward the end of the incubation period (Wilson *et al.*, 1997), which are accompanied by changes in the concentration of antioxidant enzymes in the embryonic tissues (Surai, 1999b).

The antioxidant enzymes superoxide dismutase, glutathione peroxidase, and catalase protect embryonic tissues against lipid peroxidation during incubation and are the principal antioxidant defense system at hatch (Surai *et al.*, 1999a,b). Surai and Sparks (2001a) confirmed that maternal diet has an important role in the formation of antioxidant systems during embryonic development and confirmed that the antioxidant potential of the egg yolk and embryonic tissues were increased with a diet based on corn (11.8 mg carotenoids/kg diet) compared to a diet based on wheat (5.6 mg carotenoids/kg diet). It has been demonstrated that the enrichment of broiler breeder diets with carotenoids is the main factor influencing the carotenoid concentration in chicken tissues during the first weeks of life (Koutsos *et al.*, 2003; Karadas *et al.*, 2005).

Rosa *et al.* (2012) evaluated the supplementation of 6 mg/kg of canthaxanthin in breeders from 46 to 66 weeks of age. Their results indicated that canthaxanthin improved the hatchability rate of fertile eggs from 91.3 to 93.69%, fertility from 90.98 to 92.11%, reducing mortality from 5.46 to 3.72%, especially early mortality, and reduced the presence of thiobarbituric reactive substances (TBARS) in eggs and chick blood sera when stored for 4 days.

In a subsequent experiment, the same research group (Bonilla *et al.*, 2017) evaluated the same level of canthaxanthin supplementation (6 mg/kg) in breeder diets based on corn or sorghum from 42 to 65 weeks of age. These authors reported a significant improvement in egg production from 54.35 to 57.21% during 54 to 65 weeks of age, independently of grain type. Yolk egg color and numbers of first-quality chicks were also improved.

Rosa *et al.* (2017) reported that canthaxanthin was well absorbed from the diet and effectively transferred to the egg yolk, increasing its concentration. This conferred resistance to oxidative stress to the yolk and later to the developing embryo, reducing the mortality of offspring from 64-week-old breeders (Table 5.8).

In a comprehensive review, Nabi *et al.* (2020) concluded that carotenoids are powerful antioxidants that can alleviate the adverse effect of oxidative stress via several mechanisms, including scavenging free radicals and activating phase II cytoprotective response and down-regulating signaling pathways. Feeding trials in poultry have shown benefits in productive and reproductive performance and improved the oxidative stability of poultry products such as eggs and meat.

Canthaxanthin supplementation has shown a positive effect on vitamin E concentration in 3 ways (Surai *et al.*, 2003).

Table 5.8 Effects of canthaxanthin in broilers breeders (adapted from Rosa *et al.*, 2012, 2017; Bonilla *et al.*, 2017)

Exp	Feed ingredient	Age	Corn		Sorghum	
	Canthaxanthin (mg/kg)	(wk)	0	6	0	6
1	Hatchability of fertile eggs (%)	44–66	91.30	93.69	–	–
	Mortality (%)		5.46	3.72	–	–
	Thiobarbituric reactive substances (TBARS) after 4 days		20.87	15.54	–	–
2	Egg production (%)	42–65	54.35	57.21	54.35	57.21
	Yolk color		9.00	14.00	3.00	14.00
	First quality chick/hen		21.00	24.00	21.00	24.00
3	Yolk canthaxanthin (mg/kg)	54–65	3.36	25.4	0.49	30.4

- Increased assimilation of γ-tocopherol in the diet and its transfer to the egg yolk, increasing concentrations of this substance in the liver of the embryo and hatching chick.
- Increased α-tocopherol concentrations in tissues and plasma of hatched chicks because canthaxanthin acts as an antioxidant during embryonic development, leaving fewer free radicals available to react with vitamin E. Thus, vitamin E is conserved, and its concentration is increased.
- It possibly contributed to the regeneration of vitamin E through electron transfer from the carotenoids to the α-tocopherol radical.

Based on the important role of carotenoids as antioxidants and immune-stimulating agents immediately after hatching, the authors concluded that the consumption of carotenoids by broiler breeders, in addition to influencing the incorporation of these substances by progeny tissues, may increase chicken viability.

Breeders supplemented with canthaxanthin (6 g) + 25OHD$_3$ (69 μg) showed higher egg production, hatchability, hatchability of fertile eggs, and lower early embryo mortality than those fed the control diet. Broilers from breeders fed canthaxanthin + 25OHD$_3$ and supplemented with this additive up to 21 days of age presented a better FCR and higher carcass and breast yields than those derived from non-supplemented breeders (Araujo *et al.*, 2019b).

Vitamin D

> Details about current vitamin D recommendations for breeders, provided by institutional sources and genetic companies, can be found in Tables 5.2 to 5.6.

Broiler breeders are kept indoors during rearing and laying phases without sunlight. As a result, vitamin D$_3$ synthesis is insufficient to cover requirements, and they must receive an external supply in their feed. Vitamin D is an essential component in the bird's endocrine system, regulating calcium and phosphorus homeostasis with bone mineralization and eggshell formation. The active form of vitamin D, 1,25(OH)$_2$D$_3$, acts as a steroid hormone. In Figure 5.3 the main functions of calcitriol in poultry are illustrated.

It should be remembered that the formation of an egg entails the deposition of around 2 g of calcium. The calcium deposited in the eggshell can be from 2 sources: the diet or the mobilization of the calcium reserves stored in the medullary bone, which is affected by the union of the parathyroid hormone and the 1,25(OH)$_2$D$_3$ to the bone cells.

Laying hens have a unique vitamin D$_3$ binding protein with an affinity mainly for vitamin D$_3$ (cholecalciferol) and 25OHD$_3$, which binds phosvitin – one of the egg yolk phosphoproteins – and liberates vitamin D$_3$ to the ovarian follicles, constituting future egg yolk (Fraser and Emtage, 1976; Norman and Hurwitz, 1993). The embryo uses yolk vitamin D$_3$ during its development. There is a positive correlation between the vitamin D$_3$ content in hen feed and the content of vitamin D$_3$ and 25OHD$_3$ in the egg (Mattila *et al.*, 1999).

The embryo's enzymes start to be competent from 1 to 2 weeks of incubation when they become capable of converting cholecalciferol to 25OHD$_3$ in the liver and 25OHD$_3$ to 1,25(OH)$_2$D$_3$ in the kidney (Moriuchi and Deluca, 1974; Kubota *et al.*, 1981). Having reached this stage 1,25(OH)$_2$D$_3$ regulates the homeostasis of calcium, activating the absorption of calcium from the yolk membrane, where the vitamin D-dependent calcium-binding protein calbindin is present (Tuan and Suyama, 1996). As the embryo's calcium requirements increase, the 1,25(OH)$_2$D$_3$ also facilitates calcium absorption from the shell via the chorioallantoic membrane (Hart and Deluca, 1985; Narbaitz, 1987; Clark *et al.*, 1990; Elaroussi *et al.*, 1994).

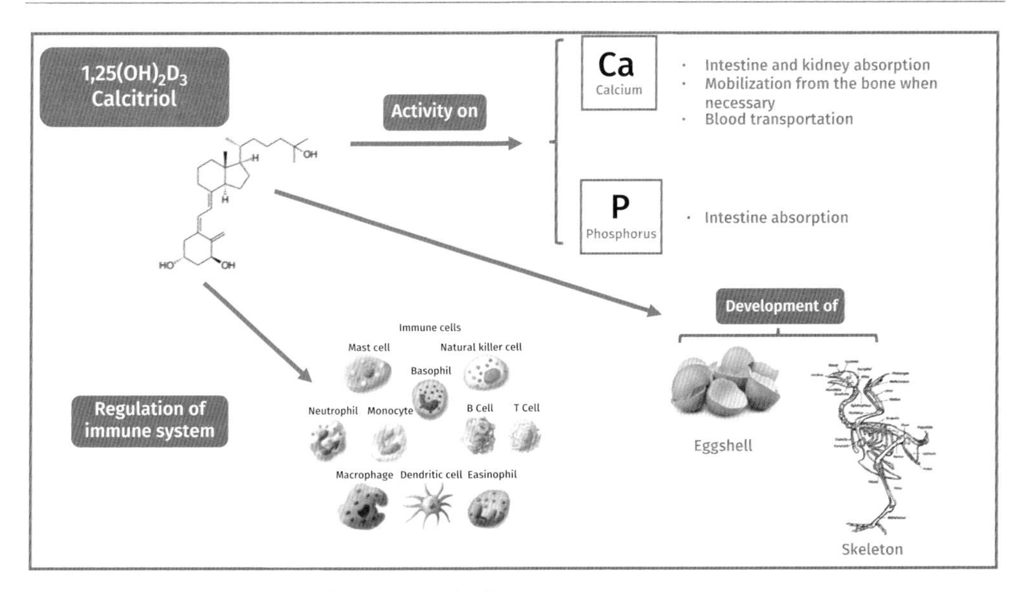

Figure 5.3 Main functions of calcitriol ($1,25(OH)_2D_3$) in poultry

However, recent publications (Chen *et al.*, 2021) indicated that the conversion of $25OHD_3$ to $1,25(OH)_2D_3$ could affect embryo development even during the first 3 days. *In ovo* administration of both sources (40 ng $1,25(OH)_2D_3$ (1,25D-L), 200 ng $1,25(OH)_2D_3$ (1,25D-H), 40 ng $25OHD_3$ (25D-L), or 200 ng $25OHD_3$) induced chicken embryo osteogenesis and adipogenesis but inhibited myogenesis during early chicken embryo development. The latter finding contrasts with other studies in which vitamin D_3 and $25OHD_3$ were given to breeders through the feed (Hutton *et al.*, 2014).

In some species of birds, when the yolk has low vitamin D content, the incubation process is disrupted from day 5 (Millar *et al.*, 1977, Scott *et al.*, 1982). In this case, there is a disturbance in the transportation of calcium from the eggshell via the chorioallantoic membrane; consequently, the embryo's bones are poorly calcified. When the lack of vitamin D is widespread, many of the chicks die at the end of incubation as they are incapable of completing the hatching process. The hatched chicks tend to be weak and present ossification problems (Shen *et al.*, 1981; Narbaitz, 1987). The greater the reserve of vitamin D in the yolk sac, the better prepared the future chick will be for developing the bone tissue, which requires high levels of calcium mobilization.

The studies of Edwards (1995a) and Driver *et al.* (2004, 2006) demonstrated that chickens from breeders with more than 50 weeks' old and fed diets containing 2,000 IU/kg of vitamin D_3 had higher growth rates and better bone formation than those from breeders fed diets with marginal supplies of this vitamin (250–500 IU/kg). Other authors have indicated increases in the production and hatchability of eggs and a reduction in embryo mortality by increasing vitamin D levels in the feed of breeders (Sunde *et al.*, 1978; Abdulrahim *et al.*, 1979). Better bone development and density have been observed in the progeny and a lower incidence of TD (Griminger, 1966; Ameenudin *et al.*, 1985).

Atencio *et al.* (2005a,b,c, 2006) conducted several experiments to elucidate the requirements of broiler breeders. They determined that the requirements increased with age and depended on the parameter used. Between 27 and 36 weeks of age, maximum egg production and hatchability were obtained with vitamin D_3 between 1,390 and 1,424 IU/kg. Between weeks

37 and 66, the vitamin D_3 requirements rose to approximately 2,800 IU/kg. These authors also demonstrated that chicks from breeders that consumed high levels of vitamin D_3 (2,000–4,000 IU/kg) and were fed with different calcium levels presented the highest live weights, a higher ash level in the tibia, and fewer leg problems.

More recent studies, such as those carried out by Saunders-Blades and Korver (2014), investigated the effects of maternal dietary $25OHD_3$ on broiler breeder egg quality and hatchability and progeny bone mineral density and performance. In a field study, all hens were fed vitamin D_3 at 3,000 IU/kg feed, and half of the hens also received, in addition, 34.5 µg of $25OHD_3$ per liter in the drinking water. They concluded the following.

1 Supplementing breeder hens with $25OHD_3$ and sufficient levels of dietary vitamin D_3 had a protective effect on the developing embryo from 0 to 7 days of incubation. The measured 30% reduction in early embryonic mortality could increase the overall productivity of broiler breeder flocks.
2 Based on the increase in hatchability – which approached significance – the rise in shell weight and the protective effect against early embryonic mortality, either $25OHD_3$ has effects beyond that of a sufficient dietary vitamin D_3 level, the requirement of the hen to maximize these functions is higher than 3,000 IU/kg of feed, or both.
3 Although maternal $25OHD_3$ supplementation positively influenced some early chick characteristics, no consistent, long-lasting effects on broiler performance were observed.

Results presented by Araujo *et al.* (2019b) showed that the supplementation of broiler breeder diets with a combination of canthaxanthin (4.55 mg/kg of feed) and $25OHD_3$ (71 µg/kg of feed) improved egg production, broiler breeders' reproductive performance, (Figures 5.4, 5.5 and 5.6) and the performance of their progenies with a lower FCR and higher carcass and breast yields.

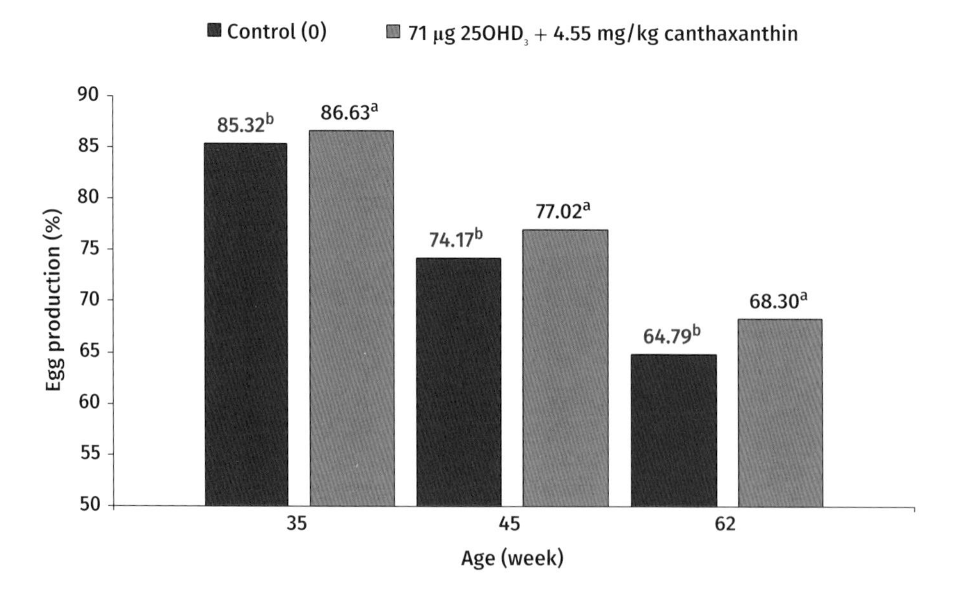

Figure 5.4 Performance of broiler breeders fed diets supplemented or not (control) with canthaxanthin and $25OHD_3$ – egg production, values with no common superscripts differ significantly, $P < 0.05$ (adapted from Araujo *et al.*, 2019b)

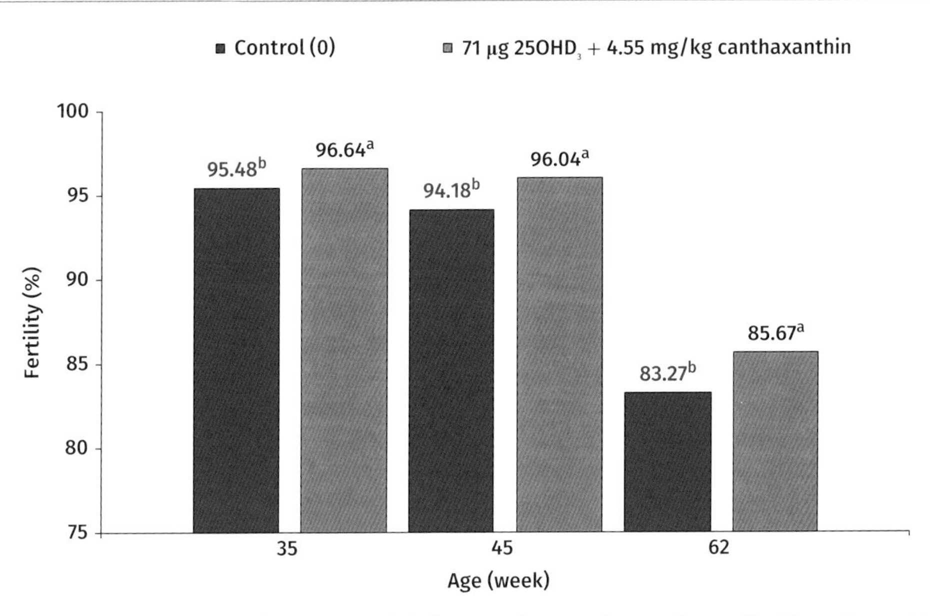

Figure 5.5 Performance of broiler breeders fed diets supplemented or not (control) with canthaxanthin and $25OHD_3$ – fertility, values with no common superscripts differ significantly, $P < 0.05$ (adapted from Araujo *et al.*, 2019b).

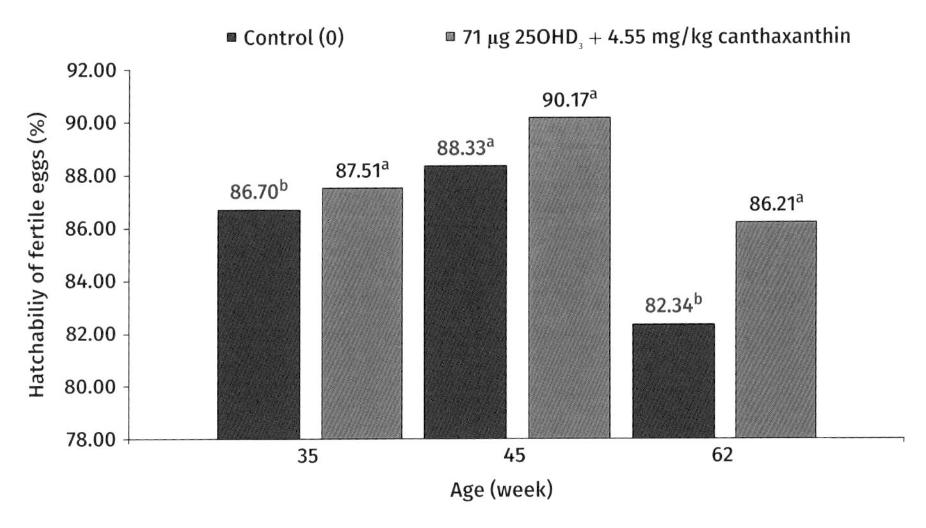

Figure 5.6 Performance of broiler breeders fed diets supplemented or not (control) with canthaxanthin and $25OHD_3$ – hatchability of fertility eggs, values with no common superscripts differ significantly, $P < 0.05$ (adapted from Araujo *et al.*, 2019b).

In a study comparing the supply of 2,760 UI of vitamin D_3 and 60 µg $25OHD_3$/kg feed, Saunders-Blades and Korver (2015) observed a reduction in embryo mortality during the entire incubation period. According to those authors, $25OHD_3$ is transported to the fertile egg, potentially increasing vitamin D status and the efficiency of vitamin D-dependent functions, such as calcium metabolism and homeostasis, and bone growth regulation, thereby improving incubation efficiency.

Vitamin D supplementation is especially important in the final phases of the laying period when there is a decrease in hatchability associated with the lower quality of the shell deposited on the egg. Torres *et al.* (2009) found that the dietary supplementation of $25OHD_3$ at 35 or 69 µg/kg feed of $25OHD_3$ resulted in better quality eggshells and lower embryo mortality in week 2 of development from hens more than 60 weeks of age, regardless of the dosage.

Lin *et al.* (2019) addressed the hen mortality issues related to sudden death caused by compromised cardiac function in one study. The authors observed that additional supplementation of 69 µg/kg feed of $25OHD_3$ to the basal diet effectively ameliorated cardiac pathogenesis and prevented sudden death in broiler breeder hens. A follow-up of this project (Yeh *et al.*, 2020) indicated that the supplementation of 69 µg $25OHD_3$/kg feed modulates vasodilation at the level of the renin-angiotensin system and nitric oxide availability and vascular remodeling relieve arterial pressure to reduce cardiac issues. In the same way, Chou *et al.* (2020) concluded that dietary supplementation of 69 µg $25OHD_3$/kg feed improved livability in broiler breeder hens. The $25OHD_3$ caused sustained activation of autophagy during endoplasmic reticulum stress functions as an antiapoptotic process to prevent cell death by removing damaged proteins/organelles (Sozen *et al.*, 2015).

Supplementation with adequate levels of vitamin D_3 or metabolites with a greater vitamin activity such as $25OHD_3$ (Saunders-Blades and Korver, 2006), is necessary to prevent problems in the development and maintenance of the bone structure. It is not common to supplement breeder diets with $1{,}25(OH)_2D_3$, as this metabolite is neither transferred to the yolk nor participates in embryo development and has possible toxicity problems. Vitamin D requirements are raised when the calcium supply is low, and the calcium-phosphorus ratio is unbalanced.

Vitamin E

Details about current Vitamin E recommendations for breeders, provided by institutional sources and genetic companies, can be found in Tables 5.2 to 5.6.

Vitamin E is one of the compounds that has received the most attention in breeder nutrition because of its role in improving poultry's stress resistance. As the knowledge of the metabolic actions of vitamin E continues to advance, recommendations for incorporating it in feed continue to strengthen. Different institutions have increased the recommendations of vitamin E for the breeding stages to combat the free radicals generated by physiological and environmental stress situations, making it possible to obtain good reproductive and productive performance in the progeny.

The tables published in the year 2000 recommended levels of vitamin E in breeder feed between 30 and 75 mg/kg, reaching 100 mg/kg in the case of turkey breeders. Doses between 100 and 200 mg/kg are necessary for a good immune response.

Among diverse functions, vitamin E is necessary for the integrity and normal physiology of the reproductive system (Figure 5.7). Several authors reported that dietary vitamin E could increase sex hormones (Franchini *et al.*, 1991), hatchability, and fertility (Ipek and Dikmen, 2014). Broiler breeder roosters encounter an age-related reduction in reproductive performance, which becomes more prominent after 45 weeks of age (Abbaspour *et al.*, 2020). A portion of the roosters has reduced sperm quality and libido. Consequently, fertility is reduced to a level that could impact the costs of the flock (Safari Asl *et al.*, 2018).

On the other hand, aging broiler breeder hens have a natural decline in the functionality of the ovary and liver accompanied by hormonal or endocrine changes. There is also a reduction in antioxidant capacity and a decrease in folliculogenesis. Therefore, improving

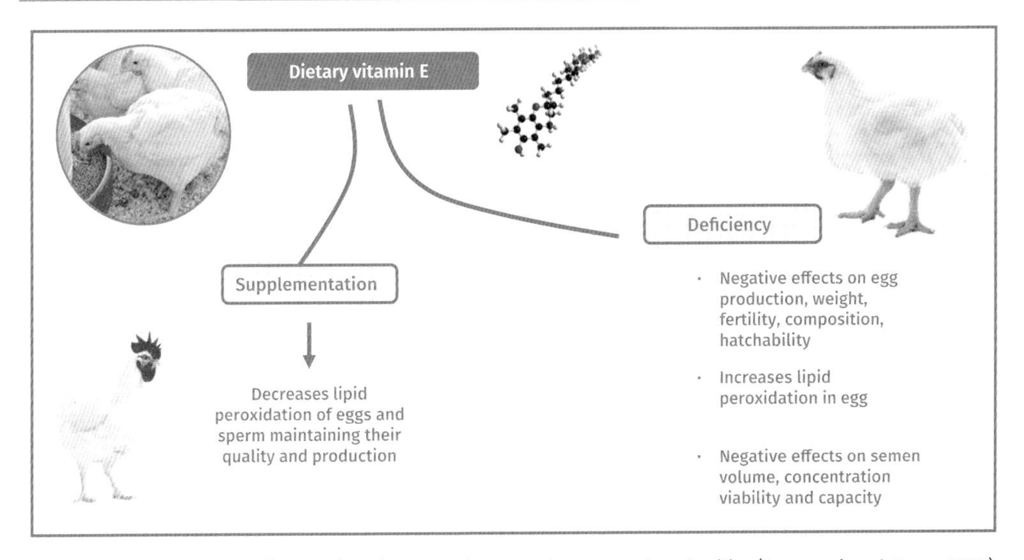

Figure 5.7 Main effects of dietary vitamin E supplementation on poultry fertility (Rengaraj and Hong, 2015)

the reproductive function in aging breeder hens using dietary strategies is of great concern (Amevor *et al.*, 2021).

Vitamin E effect on fertility, hatchability, and day-old chick quality

Supplementing vitamin E above the minimum requirement improves ovulation during the last phase of the laying period, improving the bird's defense system and averting negative consequences on egg production in environmental stress situations (Siegel *et al.*, 2001). Similarly, it has been observed that an inadequate level of vitamin E in the diets of breeders is detrimental to fertility and hatchability. Vitamin E protects against sperm, egg yolk, and embryonic tract oxidation. In breeders, the dietary vitamin E supplementation, once absorbed, is transported to the liver and, from there, to the developing oocyte by VLDL.

It has been demonstrated that there is high efficiency in incorporating α-tocopherol from the maternal feed into the yolk of the chicken egg (Surai, 2003). The quantity of vitamin E in the egg increases linearly with the consumption of vitamin E by the hen. It has been confirmed that the degree of transfer from the feed to the egg and from the egg to the embryo differs for each vitamin E stereoisomer. Among the various isomers of vitamin E deposited in the egg yolk and embryonic tissues, α-tocopherol is the most abundant form. Moreover, although α-tocotrienol is present in lower concentration, it also has an important role in the antioxidant defense of the developing embryo, and synergistic antioxidant action with α-tocopherol has been described. However, there are still many gaps in the knowledge of the transfer and metabolic activity of the different stereoisomers of vitamin E (Cortinas *et al.*, 2004).

Adding vitamin E to the diet of broiler breeder hens can reduce fractional yolk weight. Therefore, it is a good tool for manipulating egg quality in aged broiler breeder hens (Zaghari *et al.*, 2013). These authors showed that feeding vitamin E at 400 *vs.* 100 mg/kg diet, which is 4 times above the value recommended by the genetic strain management guide, can decrease blood triacylglycerol concentration and change the metabolic direction of cholesterol in heavy broiler breeder hens. Recently, Yang *et al.* (2020) concluded that based on optimizing the antioxidant status of egg yolks and newly hatched chicks, the suitable vitamin E concentration in the molted broiler breeder hen (beyond week 70) diet is at least 200 mg/kg.

Changing broiler breeders' production and reproduction characteristics are possible by manipulating dietary antioxidant compounds. The dietary supplementation of zinc-L-selenomethionine, as an organic selenium source, and high vitamin E levels could improve egg characteristics of older breeders and hatchability and hatchling weight, particularly of eggs laid by young broiler breeders (Urso *et al.*, 2015).

The quantity of vitamin E in the egg is double that in the hen's liver. Hence, the supply of vitamin E in the feed should be continuous, as the hepatic reserve is insufficient to maintain an adequate vitamin concentration in the egg. These hepatic reserves diminish rapidly if there is no external supply (Surai *et al.*, 1998b,c, 1999a,b). The vitamin E in the egg yolk is absorbed through the yolk sac membrane and subsequently, during the last week of incubation, transferred to the liver, the embryo's principal reserve organ (Surai *et al.*, 1996).

Increasing the quantity of vitamin E consumed by the breeder has been shown to increase α-tocopherol, as does the oxidative stability of the hatching egg and the developing embryo (Meydani *et al.*, 1988; Surai *et al.*, 1999b). High oxidation levels in the yolk sac membrane of fertile eggs stored for 2 weeks correlate with a decrease in their hatchability (Donaldson *et al.*, 1996). A good antioxidant defense system in the fertile egg is important in counteracting stress situations during embryo development. Vitamin E plays an essential role in this process. Inadequate vitamin E in the diet of breeders gives rise to eggs with low hatchability and high mortality in the last phase of incubation due to failures related to the circulatory system. The existence of a positive correlation between vitamin E in breeder feed and the hatchability and viability of the chicks produced has been demonstrated by Stoianov and Zhekov (1982) and An *et al.* (2010). Other authors have observed similar results in breeders of laying strains (Leeson *et al.*, 1979a,b), breeders of broiler strains (Kristiansen, 1973; Tengerdy and Nockels, 1973; Siegel *et al.*, 2001), and turkey breeders (Atkinson *et al.*, 1955; Jensen and McGinnis, 1957a,b; Jensen, 1968). Hossain *et al.* (1998), in their research with different levels of vitamin E in breeder feed, observed improvements in the immune development of the chicks with doses of 100 mg/kg of vitamin E.

Vitamin E supplementation has also been effective in counteracting the negative effects on hatchability caused by stress conditions, such as heat, presence of toxins (Tobias *et al.*, 1992), antinutritional factors, such as vicine (Muduuli *et al.*, 1982), or aging (Siegel *et al.*, 2001; Amiri *et al.*, 2006). Thus, an adequate supply of vitamin E in the breeder diets has a clear effect on their progeny. The physical reserves of newly hatched chicks are very important as their immune, digestive, and endocrine systems, among others, are not completely developed until they are 7–10 days old. In particular, vitamin E is important for preventing lipid oxidation and stimulating immune defenses during and after hatching.

Hatching and the neonatal period are critical times during which pulmonary respiration starts and changes occur in the metabolism, triggering a rapid tissue growth rate, which involves the chick being highly susceptible to oxidation. The presence of antioxidants, in particular α-tocopherol, in the yolk and integrated into the different embryonic tissues has the benefit of protecting against oxidative destruction (Gaal *et al.*, 1995; Speake *et al.*, 1996; Cherian *et al.*, 1996a,b; Surai *et al.*, 1999b; Surai and Sparks, 2001a). A direct relationship has been demonstrated between the level of vitamin E in the liver of a day-old chick and its viability (Yaroshenko *et al.*, 1995; Surai, 2000). In the initial phases of a chicken's life, the digestion of lipids, including fat-soluble vitamins, is limited, so the chick's vitamin E reserves depend on their egg concentration and hen's consumption. Hassan *et al.* (1990) observed that when the hen's diet contained sufficient vitamin E, the chick's embryonic development was adequate, and its reserves were maintained up to 2 weeks of age. However, chicks from breeders who consumed diets deficient in vitamin E presented exudative diathesis at hatching. In other words, the deficiency had arisen during incubation.

Increased vitamin E concentration in the egg yolk due to dietary supplementation was associated with an increased α-tocopherol concentration in the tissues of the developing embryos and newly hatched chicks resulting in increased antioxidant defenses and decreased lipid peroxidation. Furthermore, increased vitamin E transfer from the feed to egg yolk and further to the developing embryo was associated with the upregulation of antioxidant enzymes reflecting antioxidant system regulation and adaptation. Using 3 model systems, including poultry breeders/males, semen, and chicken embryo/postnatal chickens, the possibility of modulation of the antioxidant defense mechanisms has been demonstrated. For the last 3 decades, vitamin E recycling in the cells as an effective mechanism of the antioxidant defenses has received substantial attention.

Vitamin E effect on egg storage

Prolonged egg storage time (14 *vs.* 0 days) increased embryonic mortality, decreased the hatchability traits, and impaired the antioxidant status of egg yolks and newly hatched chicks. Yang *et al.* (2020a,b) conducted a study to investigate the effects of broiler breeder dietary vitamin E and egg storage time on the egg characteristics, hatchability, and antioxidant status of the egg yolks and newly hatched chicks where the breeder hens were fed the same basic diets containing 6 or 100 mg/kg vitamin E for 12 weeks. Those authors concluded that prolonged egg storage time (14 *vs.* 0 days) increased embryonic mortality, decreased hatchability, and impaired the antioxidant status of egg yolks and newly hatched chicks. At the same time, adding broiler breeder dietary vitamin E (100 *vs.* 6 mg/kg) could partly relieve these adverse impacts induced by long-term egg storage (Figure 5.8).

Vitamin E in ovo feeding

Research has been carried out on incorporating different nutrients in the fertile egg during its incubation through *in ovo* injection. The inclusion of vitamin E in the fertile egg had a

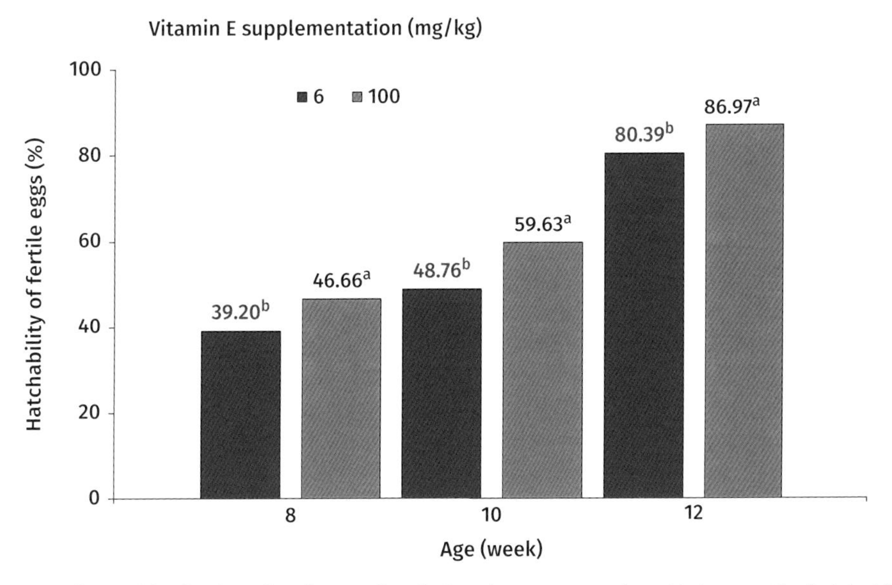

Figure 5.8 Effects of broiler breeder dietary vitamin E and egg storage time, 14 days, on the hatchability of fertile eggs, values with no common superscripts differ significantly, $P < 0.05$ (adapted from Yang *et al.*, 2020b)

positive effect on the physical and immune development of the progeny. However, the effects on hatchability remain to be elucidated. In weight gain and feed conversion at 28 and 42 days, improvements have been observed in meat chickens hatched from eggs inoculated with vitamin E (Hossain *et al.*, 1998; Bhanja *et al.*, 2006).

Parolini *et al.* (2017) reported that the *in ovo* injection of vitamin E increased hatchlings' plasma total antioxidant capacity (T-AOC). Surai *et al.* (1999a,b) and Surai (2000) indicated that increasing the broiler breeder's dietary vitamin E levels improved the vitamin E concentration and reduced the malondialdehyde (MDA) content in chick tissues.

Recently, Araujo *et al.* (2019a) concluded that up to 60.4 IU *in ovo* vitamin E injection improved newly hatched chicks' oxidative state, thus enabling better physical quality. Improvement of neonatal chick characteristics enabled better initial broiler chicken performance. Studies are needed to evaluate *in ovo* feeding of vitamin E on live performance during the grower and finisher phases of broilers.

Vitamin E and male fertility

The relationship between levels of vitamin E and the fertilizing capacity of spermatozoa from breeder males is well established. Vitamin E exerts its antioxidant action on 2 levels: first, on the testicles, where it protects the biological membranes from lipid peroxidation during spermatogenesis. Second, in the seminal plasma, vitamin E protects against the free radicals that attack the lipids (Surai *et al.*, 1998d; Danikowski *et al.*, 2002; Eid *et al.*, 2006). Dietary manipulation can modify the polyunsaturated fatty acid composition of the sperm of broiler and turkey breeder males, improving fertility. The lipid part of the membrane of spermatozoa has a high proportion of PUFAs, which gives them fluidity and flexibility, facilitating their mobility and the fertilization of the ovum. But these positive effects are only achieved in the presence of antioxidants, in the specific case of vitamin E at a dosage between 120 and 300 mg/kg feed (Surai *et al.*, 1997a, 2000; Zanini *et al.*, 2003a,b; Cerolini *et al.*, 2003, 2005; Biswas *et al.*, 2007, 2009). Thus, it is important to incorporate antioxidants such as vitamin E to prevent the oxidation of the semen of breeders.

The study carried out by Khan *et al.* (2013) found increased cellular morphometry of lactotrophs in the vitamin E supplemented group (100 mg/kg). From this study, the authors inferred that the best semen quality in the vitamin E supplemented group is associated with the larger size and area of lactotrophs, and based on those findings, they can conclude that vitamin E has beneficial effects on the morphometry of reproductive hormones, especially for FSH and LH gonadotropes which may result in an optimal release of these hormones necessary to improve semen production.

At 45 weeks of age, when roosters experience reduced reproductive function, Lotfi *et al.* (2021) fed roosters with diets especially enriched in omega-3 to improve reproductive performance. The supplementation of vitamin E at 200 mg/kg improved semen quality parameters and reproductive performance in that study. It could be concluded that vitamin E is an antioxidant that could remarkably improve the effects of omega-3 on sperm characteristics and sexual hormone levels in aged breeder roosters.

Shabani *et al.* (2022) investigated the effect of dietary supplementation of different levels of soybean lecithin and vitamin E on semen quality parameters and some reproductive hormones in Hubbard grandparent roosters. Roosters were fed 3 amounts of soybean lecithin (0, 1, and 2%) and 2 amounts of vitamin E (0 and 300 mg/kg). Adding 1% soybean lecithin and vitamin E into the diet increased semen volume and sperm concentration, membrane integrity, and viability ($P < 0.05$). Vitamin E significantly increased the amplitude of lateral head displacement (ALH) of sperm ($P < 0.05$). MDA concentration was significantly lower in all 3 treatments containing vitamin E ($P < 0.05$). The authors concluded that supplementing rooster diets with vitamin E and 1% lecithin can improve fertility-related parameters in Hubbard grandparent roosters.

The quantity of α-tocopherol in male sperm is dependent on the availability of vitamin E in the diet (Cerolini *et al.*, 2003, 2005, 2006). Incorporating vitamin E in the diet of breeders has effectively avoided loss of fertility (Arscott and Parker, 1967; Yoshida and Hoshii, 1976; Friedrichsen *et al.*, 1980). Thus, when breeders are deficient in vitamin E, the males are less fertile due to the lower quantity and quality of sperm produced (Jensen, 1968; Arscott and Kuhns, 1969). Friedrichsen *et al.* (1980) indicated that a prolonged vitamin E deficiency in the feed of breeders could give rise to permanent sterility. In a study with turkey breeders, Surai (1992) observed that the best quality of semen was obtained when the feed of males was supplemented with 80 mg/kg of vitamin E and the quantity of vitamin E in the semen was between 3.2 and 6.9 µg/ml compared to 1.6 µg/ml in unsupplemented birds (Blesbois *et al.*, 1993). Some studies have included 200–300 mg/kg of vitamin E in the feed, attaining 174 and 188 ng of α-tocopherol/10^9 sperm cells (Surai *et al.*, 1997b; Cerolini *et al.*, 2006; Zaniboni and Cerolini, 2006). Khan *et al.* (2012a,b) demonstrated that vitamin E (100 mg/kg feed) and vitamin C (500 mg/kg feed) or their combination was the most potent nutrients to improve semen traits and seminal biochemical characteristics in roosters after Zn-induced molting.

In a recent review, Surai *et al.* (2019) concluded that vitamin E supplementation of roosters was associated with significant increases in the α-tocopherol level in semen and increased resistance to oxidative stress imposed by various external stressors, especially heat stress. Ebeid (2012) reported that the combination of vitamin E (200 mg α-tocopherol acetate/kg diet) and organic selenium (0.3 mg/kg diet) enhances the antioxidative status and quality of chicken semen under high ambient temperature.

The quantity of vitamin E integrated into the membrane of the spermatozoa may be related to their capacity for fertilization. Supplementation with vitamin E in the final phase of breeding improves the quality and quantity of the semen produced and the antioxidant defenses during their storage *in vivo* (Surai *et al.*, 2000; Bréque *et al.*, 2003). However, this dose-response relationship in young males is not linear (Lin *et al.*, 2005a).

It has also been demonstrated that vitamin E provides additional protection under conditions in which semen is manipulated *in vitro,* including dilution, storage, and freezing (Surai, 2003; Zaniboni and Cerolini, 2009). Some authors point out that breeders need vitamin E at a dosage of more than 160 mg/kg to ensure hatchability maintenance (Lin *et al.*, 2005b). All of the above manifests the important role of vitamin E in the structure and functioning of spermatozoa.

In general, system enhancement due to dietary vitamin E supplementation was mainly manifested via increased concentration of α-tocopherol in different tissues. This direct antioxidant effect of vitamin E (Figure 5.9) is well researched and explained (Surai *et al.*, 2019). However, vitamin E also has an indirect impact on the efficiency of antioxidant defense networks in different tissues, and this includes modulation of:

1. superoxide dismutase (SOD) – the main adaptive enzyme of the first level of antioxidant defense, responsible for detoxification of the main biological radical, namely superoxide radical
2. glutathione peroxidase (GSH-Px) and catalase (CAT) – 2 other important enzymes of the first level of antioxidant defense essential for the completion of superoxide radical detoxification with a conversion of toxic H_2O_2 into the water
3. glutathione (GSH) – one of the most important cellular antioxidants participating in maintaining redox balance in the cell being co-substrate of GSH-Px

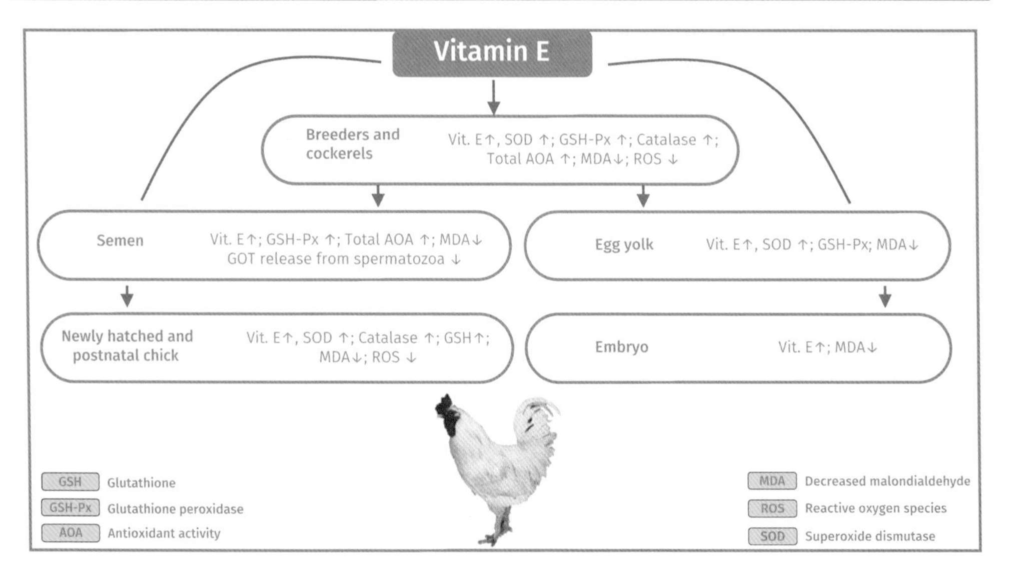

Figure 5.9 Modulation of the antioxidant system by dietary vitamin E in avian reproduction

4 total antioxidant activity (T-AOC) – an important index of the antioxidant defense system that reflects a cell's redox (antioxidant–pro-oxidant) balance.

Vitamin E and immunity

The relationship between vitamin E and the immune system has also been an object of great interest. It has been pointed out that supplementation with vitamin E at levels above the minimum requirements indicated by the NRC (1994), either administered in the hen's feed or utilizing injection *in ovo,* increases the immune response of the progeny (Jackson *et al.*, 1978; Haq *et al.*, 1996; Erf *et al.*, 1998; Hossain *et al.*, 1998; Boa-Amponsem *et al.*, 2001; Amiri *et al.*, 2006). Jackson *et al.* (1978) demonstrated that the production of antibodies was greater in chicks produced by breeders fed 150 mg vitamin E/kg feed. These results were later confirmed by Surai *et al.* (1999a,b) and Surai (2000).

The mechanisms responsible for the immunomodulatory effects of vitamin E have been explored in cell-based, animal, and human studies. Vitamin E has direct and indirect effects on immune cells, with most evidence obtained from studies focused on the impact on T-cell function. It is generally recognized that, similar to the effects on other cells, the scavenging of ROS and reducing oxidative stress play a key role in vitamin E's effects on the immune system. Membrane integrity, inflammation, signal transduction, and cell cycle division are all sensitive processes to oxidative stress (Min *et al.*, 2018; Lewis *et al.*, 2019).

Following a trial, Ajafar *et al.* (2018) concluded that α-tocopherol acetate (α-TOH) dietary supplementation of 300 or 400 mg/kg, 3–4 times more than the required amount of broiler breeder males, showed beneficial effects on immune response parameters. However, the interaction effects of body weight and α-TOH levels did not significantly affect the immune responses of broiler breeder males. Body weight only affected cutaneous basophil hypersensitivity and cell-mediated immunity.

Vitamin K

Details about current vitamin K recommendations for breeders, provided by institutional sources and genetic companies, can be found in Tables 5.2 to 5.6.

The principal function of vitamin K is controlling the blood coagulation period since it activates plasmatic prothrombin. It has also been observed that many proteins with different metabolic functions require vitamin K for their biosynthesis. Thus, most tissues have relationships depending on vitamin K.

Especially remarkable in the case of breeders is the dependence on vitamin K of osteocalcin, a mineral-binding protein present in the bones of chicken embryos and the bone matrix. Osteocalcin is essential for the bone mineralization process. However, in Lavelle *et al.*'s (1994) study, no functional deficiencies were observed in the bone metabolism of breeders or their progeny with vitamin K levels below the minimum requirements.

The quantity of vitamin K transferred to the egg depends on the amount of vitamin K ingested by the breeder (Sebrell and Harris, 1971). When the supplementation levels in the breeder feed are inadequate, eggs are produced with low vitamin K content, accompanied by high levels of embryonic mortality due to hemorrhagic processes during the final period of incubation (Nelson and Norris, 1960; Griminger and Brubacher, 1966). Hatched chicks show a longer coagulation period than normal, and any trauma can provoke fatal hemorrhages (Lavelle *et al.*, 1994).

In the study conducted by Fernandes *et al.* (2009), the objective was to evaluate the effect of 4 levels – 0, 2, 8, and 32 mg/kg feed – of dietary vitamin K on production, egg quality, and bone structure of laying hens near the end of the production cycle. Results indicated that dietary vitamin K supplementation for leghorn hens at the end of the laying phase influenced egg production and bone mineralization without any influence on the eggshell quality.

The lack of consistency in the efficiency of supplementary vitamin K on eggshell quality can be due to the age of the hens. Thus, it could be theorized that if vitamin K supplementation was performed during the pre-laying period when the medullar bone is formed, more consistent results could have been obtained at the final phase of the laying cycle.

Fares *et al.* (2018) studied the direct influence of supplementing vitamin K_3 in breeder layer diets in the last egg production phase on productive performance, eggshell parameters, tibia bone composition, histological observation, hatching traits, and some blood parameters. They used 155 chicken females with 30 males individually housed in cages from 55 to 67 weeks of age. In conclusion, supplementing the layer diet with 11 or 15 mg vitamin K_3/kg could improve egg production, eggshell, bone quality, fertility, hatchability, and embryo mortality (Figure 5.10).

Water-soluble vitamins

Most B group vitamins act as coenzymes on different metabolic pathways, and their presence is fundamental for the organism's normal functioning. An insufficient supply of B group vitamins is usually related to the epithelium and immune system problems. Different authors have demonstrated that the content of most water-soluble vitamins depends on the level consumed by the breeder (Souci *et al.*, 1989; Squires and Naber, 1993a,b). Some B group vitamins require between 7 and 10 days to reach the maximum level of deposition in the egg. It is known that the reduced production of hatching eggs by breeders at the start and the end of the laying period is related to the composition of the egg, and vitamin composition has been pointed out as a key factor. Nutrition is, therefore, important not only during the reproduction phase but also during the growth of the breeders, as is covering vitamin requirements with safety margins, especially in the pre-laying phase and at the end of laying (Leeson and Summers, 2008).

In this respect, supplementation with B group vitamins in drinking water has turned out to be beneficial in chicken flocks coming from young breeders who otherwise have higher mortality early and poor productive performance (Bains, 2001).

In the study by Leeson and Summers (2008), the incubation rate responded to the absence or reintroduction of different vitamins in the feed (Figure 5.11). The lack over 3 weeks of the

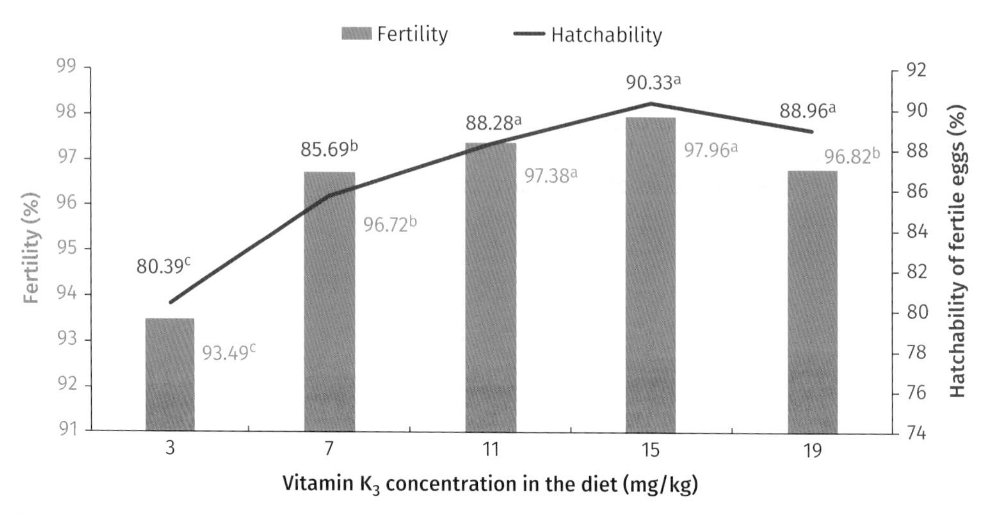

Figure 5.10 Effect of the addition of vitamin K in the diet on fertility and hatchability in breeders from 55 up to 67 weeks of age, values with no common superscripts differ significantly, $P < 0.05$ (Fares *et al.*, 2018)

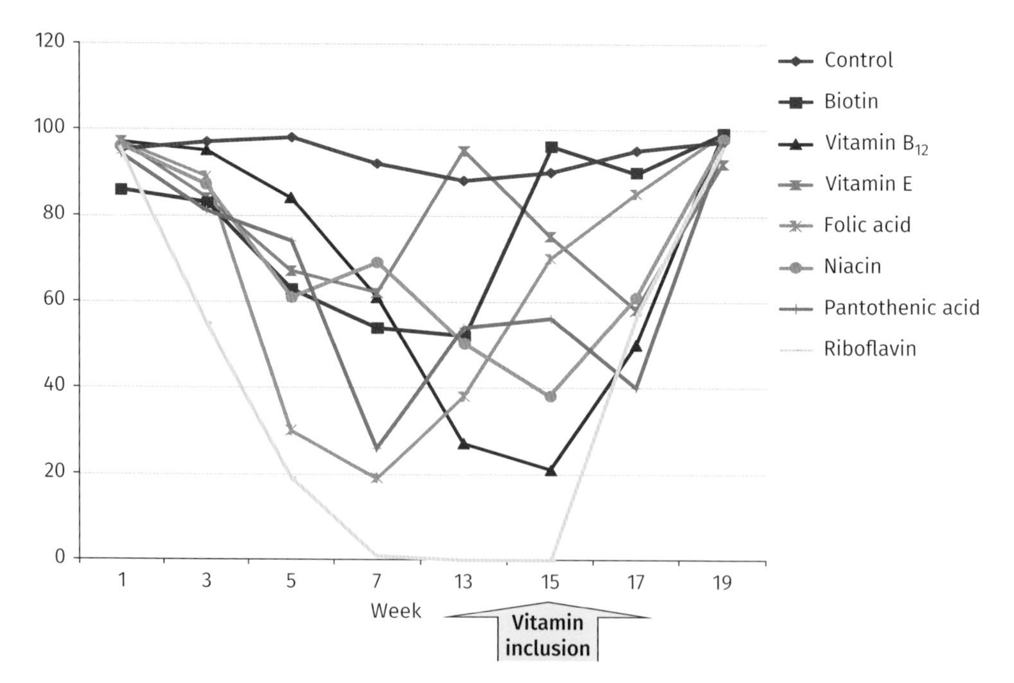

Figure 5.11 Percentage of fertile eggs from breeders fed individual B group vitamins deficient diets. The arrow at 15 weeks of production indicates the introduction in the diet of the vitamin being studied, which was absent at the start of the experiment (source: adapted from Leeson and Summers, 2008)

majority of the B group vitamins, individually, caused more than a 10% reduction in hatchability. After 15 weeks of feeding with deficient diets, the missing vitamin was reintroduced. After 4 weeks of receiving the proper level of all vitamins, the breeders regained the standard levels of production and hatchability.

The NRC (1994) highlighted that the vitamin levels needed to produce table eggs might be lower than those required for hatching eggs. It indicates that water-soluble vitamins, especially riboflavin, pantothenic acid, and vitamin B_{12}, are critical for good hatchability. It is important to remember that the data supplied by NRC (1994) refer to laying breeder strains that produce hens for white table eggs. In the case of biotin, are minimum requirements specified for breeders of broiler strains producing meat chickens.

The *in ovo* injection of several water-soluble vitamins at different periods of embryonic development has been demonstrated to have several positive effects. Table 5.9 describes some of the most updated research in this area. *In ovo* feeding is continuously non-feasible for commercial poultry conditions due to the logistic and technical conflicts with *in ovo* vaccination. However, the positive results of specific vitamins on embryo development indicate that strategic supplementation of broiler breeders could have several benefits for the hens, roosters, egg and eggshell quality, egg storage, embryo development, and offspring live performance and health in the life after hatch.

Vitamin B_1 (thiamine)

> Details about current vitamin B_1 recommendations for breeders, provided by institutional sources and genetic companies, can be found in Tables 5.2 to 5.6.

Thiamine consumed by the hen is transported to the egg yolk associated with thiamine binding proteins. The research conducted by Polin *et al.* (1962) and Charles *et al.* (1972) demonstrated that an inadequate supply of thiamine to breeder hens resulted in high embryonic mortality and chicks with polyneuritis. Olkowski and Classen (1999) studied the response of broiler chickens to a wide range of thiamine supplementation in the breeder diet – 0, 2, 8, 32 mg/kg supplemented to the basal diet – and they observed that 8 ppm B_1 of supplementation increase the thiamine status indices and thiamine metabolism in the offspring.

Although embryos can synthesize thiamine from 5 to 7 days of incubation (Backermann *et al.*, 2008), the quantity of thiamine deposited in the egg is important. It allows the newly hatched chick to have a reserve during the first days. This reserve is important for the initial development of the chick and has repercussions on its subsequent growth. Thus, Bhanja *et al.* (2007) observed that chickens from eggs with an extra quantity of vitamin B_1 that had been incorporated *in ovo* injection were heavier at 28 days of age.

Thiamine is important to the embryo and for egg production and its quality. Unfortunately, research has not been conducted on broiler breeders or turkey breeders. Still, in laying ducks (22–42 weeks of age), Chen W. *et al.* (2018) observed that supplementation with 0.93 mg thiamine/kg maximized laying performance and egg quality without affecting the antioxidant defense system.

Broiler breeders are less efficient in incorporating thiamine in the egg, so their requirements will be higher than those referenced in light breeder hens, such as those indicated by the NRC (1994) set at 0.7 mg/kg. However, although little work has been done concerning thiamine requirements in this type of bird, most tables published by recognized bodies recommend levels between 3 and 6 mg/kg for breeder feeds.

Table 5.9 Effects of *in ovo* injection of water-soluble vitamins to embryos

In ovo injection characteristics	Species/Study characteristics/Injection day	Result	References
50 mg vitamin C or 100 μg vitamin B_1 or 100 μg vitamin B_6 or water or no injection	Broiler. Hatchability, embryo development, and broiler performance. DOI 14 d	Vitamin C injection increased chicken weight to egg weight ratio. Vitamin B_1 improved 28d body weight.	Bhanja *et al.* (2012)
Uninjected/corn oil/corn oil + 10 mg vitamin E/ saline solution/saline solution + vitamin C	Muscovy ducks. Hatchability and performance. DOI 12 d	Vitamin E and C injections increased hatch and final body weight and feed intake. The feed conversion ratio was improved by them only at the starter phase.	Selim *et al.* (2012)
Broilers – vitamin C 3 and 6 mg; ducks – vitamin C 4 and 8 mg	Broilers and Pekin ducks. Hatchability evaluation. DOI 13, 15, and 17 (broilers); DOI 12 and 20 (Pekin ducks)	For ducks, the selected doses improved hatchability when administered on day 20.	Nowaczewski *et al.* (2012)
No injection or riboflavin (60 or 600 μg)	Broilers. Evaluation of body and organ weight, as well as hatching parameters. DOI 6 d	600 μg of riboflavin provoked a tendency to reduce body weight while 60 μg reduced hatching time with higher synchronization. Blood T_4 levels were increased by riboflavin supplementation, while T_3 ones were reduced.	Trzeciak *et al.* (2014)
No injection/0.1 ml distilled water/1 mg folic acid	Broiler. Performance, blood biochemical, and muscles traits. DOI 14 d	Folic acid injection provoked better performance (BW and FCR) results, increased carcass yield, and got higher blood proteins.	Abd El-Azeem *et al.* (2014)
No injection/water/ choline 0.25 or 0.375 or 0.5 mg	Broiler. Hatchability performance, Immune response, broiler growth, and carcass trait. DOI 12 d	Choline *in ovo* injection increased chicken weight and chicken weight to egg weight ratio. 0.25 mg of choline had the lowest abdominal fat.	Gholami *et al.* (2015)
No injection/water/folic acid injection (40, 80 or 120 μg)	Broiler. Performance, carcass characteristics, and blood constituents. DOI 7 d	Folic acid injection increased feed conversion ratio, blood glucose, folic acid, and phosphorous while reducing cholesterol, triglyceride, HDL and LDL, calcium, and alkaline phosphatase.	Nouri *et al.* (2017)
No injection/saline solution/vitamin C 3 mg	Chinese yellow broilers. Antioxidant capacity and immune-related gene expression. DOI 18 d	Vitamin C enhanced antioxidant defense and immune system for newly hatched chicks.	El-Senousey *et al.* (2018)
No perforation or only perforation or water or vitamin B_6 injection (400, 600 or 800 μg)	Turkey. Hatchability, chick weight, and some blood chemical traits/ DOI 10, 17 and 24 d	Hatchability was improved by 600 and 800 μg on day 10 and 800 μg on day 17. Chicken weight was increased by B_6 injection on days 10 and 17.	Hekal *et al.* (2018)

No injection/physiological serum/0.121 mg nicotinic acid or 0.052 mg pantothenic acid or 0.007 mg of folic acid	Broiler. Performance and immune system of broilers. DOI 14 d	Pantothenic acid and nicotinic acid injection increased Newcastle virus antibodies at 18 d. SRBC were reduced by pantothenic acid at 18 d and by nicotinic acid and folic acid at 35 d. Pantothenic acid increased the lymphocyte to heterophiles ratio while folic acid reduced. Chickens supplemented with pantothenic and nicotinic acid had lower weight at the two firsts rearing weeks.	Parnian *et al.* (2019)
Normal saline or vitamin C, 3 mg	Broiler. Growth performance, antioxidation, and immune function of broilers. DOI 15 d	Hatchability, immune function, and antioxidant activity was improved by vitamin C injection.	Zhu Y.F. *et al.* (2019a)
No injection/dry punch/normal saline/folic acid 0.2 mg/folic acid 0.2 mg + glucose 125 mg	Broilers. Growth performance and blood components. Injection four days before hatching	Folic acid plus glucose increased body weight at two- and four weeks of age, increasing the dressing percentage.	Abdel-Halim *et al.* (2020)
No injection/water/vitamin B_{12} (20 or 40 µg) on D13 or D15	Broiler. Hatchability, broiler growth performance, carcass characteristics, and blood constituents. DOI 13 d and DOI 15 d	Vitamin B_{12} reduced hatchability when injected 20 or 40 µg on D13 or 20 µg on D15; increased egg glucose and protein as in a dose-dependent way; improved food conversion ratio, increasing body weight gain	Teymouri *et al.* (2020)
Normal saline or vitamin C 3 mg	Broiler. Hatchability, broiler performance, immune status, and DNA methylation-related gene expression. DOI 11 d	Improved hatchability, feed intake, daily gain, feed conversion ratio, immune status, and increased DNA methylation-related gene expression.	Zhu Y. *et al.* (2020)
No injection/saline-injected control/vitamin C (3, 6, 12 or 36 mg)	Broilers. Growth performance, carcass characteristics, plasma antioxidant capacity, and meat quality. DOI 17 d	3 to 12 mg per egg positively affected post-hatch growth, leg muscle development, and systemic antioxidant capacity. Higher dosages may improve meat quality.	Zhang Y. *et al.* (2021)
No injection/biotin (75 or 100 µg at day 0; 100 or 4,175 µg at day 18)	Broilers. Growth and embryonic development, hatchability/ DOI 0 and DOI 18	Biotin in-ovo injection changes embryonic characteristics improving hatchability, mainly with 75 µg at day 0 or 4175 at day 18.	Alkubaisy *et al.* (2021)
No injection/deionized water/vitamin C (3 or 6 mg)/vitamin E (0.5, 0.75 or 1.0 IU)	Broilers. Hatchability, growth, and carcass trait.	Vitamin C (3 mg) or vitamin E (0.75) increased hatchability.	Ghane *et al.* (2021)

Vitamin B_2 (riboflavin)

Details about current Vitamin B_2 recommendations for breeders, provided by institutional sources and genetic companies, can be found in Tables 5.2 to 5.6.

The riboflavin content in the egg increases in direct proportion to its ingestion by the hen, reaching 5 mg/kg. Not all the quantity of riboflavin contained in the fertile egg is used during embryo development. Reserves are generated in the liver and the yolk sac, covering the chick's requirements for a few days after birth. Squires and Naber (1993b) suggested a supply of riboflavin (4.4 mg/kg) above the minimum standards to increase production and hatchability and achieve around 2.5 µg of riboflavin per g of egg albumen. When breeders consume levels lower than their requirements, the riboflavin content in the egg is reduced in only 2 days, producing high mortality in the intermediary phase of incubation, accompanied by hatching problems and malformations at birth (Leeson and Summers, 1978; Flores-Garcia, 1992; Flores-Garcia and Scholtyssek, 1992; Squires and Naber, 1993b; Whitehead *et al.*, 1993b; Wilson, 1997).

Over 7 weeks, the lack of riboflavin supply in the feed caused the hens to stop laying eggs practically. When 7 mg/kg of vitamin B_2 were reintroduced over 2–3 weeks, the hatchability was restored to 95% in the fourth-week post supplementation (Leeson and Summers, 2008). These data confirm that the quantity of riboflavin in the hen's feed influences the chick embryos' vigor and survival capacity.

The minimum level proposed by the NRC in 1994 for leghorn breeder strains was 3.6 mg/kg. Some researchers indicated that the dietary levels for breeders should be triple or quadruple the levels for commercial egg hens (Whitehead and Portsmouth, 1989). Most tables published by recognized bodies recommend levels between 7 and 20 mg/kg of riboflavin for breeder feeds.

Vitamin B_6 (Pyridoxine)

Details about current Vitamin B_6 recommendations for breeders, provided by institutional sources and genetic companies, can be found in Tables 5.2 to 5.6.

For breeder birds, inadequate consumption of vitamin B_6 causes reductions in the production of eggs and their hatchability. The vitamin B_6 content in the feed is reflected in the deposition in the egg: however, the efficiency is limited, especially at high intake levels (Fuller *et al.*, 1961). The quantity of vitamin B_6 needed to obtain maximum fertility is double that for maintaining the number of eggs produced, and the safety margin is small (Fuller *et al.*, 1961).

Robel (2002) reported that when increasing levels of pyridoxine, from 12.9 to 24.4 mg/kg, were supplied in the feed for female turkey breeders, no improvement in hatchability was observed compared to the basal diet supplemented with 6.2 mg/kg of vitamin B_6 (Figure 5.12). In the same study, despite no significant differences in the number of eggs per hen detected, a slight numerical mean increase was observed in upper dosages. The lack of effect in this study could be associated with supplementation of vitamin B_6 already higher than recommended in the basal diet (3–4 mg/kg of pyridoxine).

It has been demonstrated that inoculating pyridoxine into fertile eggs increases the percentage of hatching chickens (Bhanja *et al.*, 2007) and turkeys by approximately 4.2% (Robel and Christensen, 1991). Whereas, severe deficiencies of vitamin B_6 cause involution of the genital organs both in females and males (Weiss and Scott, 1979; Scott *et al.*, 1982) and early embryo mortality (Landauer, 1967). Lu *et al.* (2021) demonstrated that supplying adequate folic

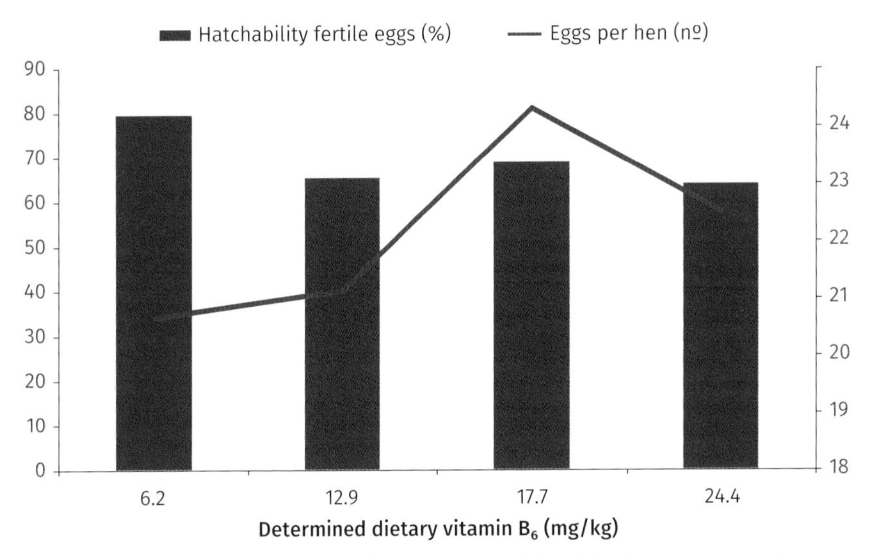

Figure 5.12 Effect of increasing levels of vitamin B_6 on hatchability of fertile eggs and number of eggs per turkey hen (adapted from Robel, 2002)

acid (1.25 mg/kg diet) and pyridoxine (5 mg/kg diet) in broiler breeder diets is necessary for chick embryonic methionine metabolism.

The recommendations for dietary supplementation of pyridoxine for broiler breeder hens stand between 3 and 6 mg/kg. Evidence in table egg layers indicated some benefits of a larger supplementation and interactions with trace minerals like zinc. Kucuk *et al.* (2008) found that zinc (30 mg of zinc/kg diet) and pyridoxine (8 mg of pyridoxine/kg diet) supplementation improved FCR, egg production, shell weight, Haugh unit scores, and plasma calcium and phosphorous concentrations in laying hens.

Vitamin B_{12} (cyanocobalamin)

Details about current Vitamin B_{12} recommendations for breeders, provided by institutional sources and genetic companies, can be found in Tables 5.2 to 5.6.

Despite vitamin B_{12} being a water-soluble vitamin, a certain degree of storage occurs, mainly in the liver. As the vitamin B_{12} content in the hen's feed increases, so does its deposition in the egg, increasing its availability for embryonic development. Chicks from breeders fed levels above the minimum vitamin B_{12} recommendations form an important vitamin reserve for their subsequent development. After 2–5 months of administering a diet with an inadequate quantity of vitamin B_{12}, it can be observed that the reserves of this vitamin in the newly hatched chick are insufficient, and the rate of mortality rises (Patel and McGinnis, 1977; Scott *et al.*, 1982).

Inadequate vitamin B_{12} is associated with low hatchability and disorders in the progeny (Olcese *et al.*, 1950; Tuite and Austic, 1974; Patel and McGinnis, 1980; Ward *et al.*, 1985). On the other hand, Squires and Naber (1992) observed that increasing the supplementation of vitamin B_{12} in broiler breeders' feeds produced a greater number of eggs, which were heavier, and with better hatchability.

Panic *et al.* (1970) observed that supplementing vitamin B_{12} at a level of 20 µg/kg produced an increase in the content of this vitamin in the egg and an increase of 20% in hatchability.

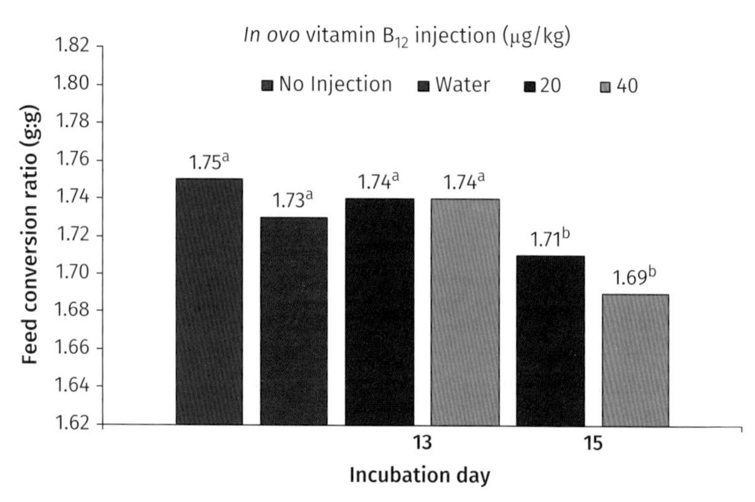

Figure 5.13 Effect of *in ovo* injection (DOI 13 and 15) of vitamin B_{12} on the FCR of heat-stressed broilers, values with no common superscripts differ significantly, $P < 0.05$; (adapted from Teymouri *et al.*, 2020)

Including 10 μg/kg of vitamin B_{12} in the hen's feed improved the live weight and growth of the progeny (Patel and McGinnis, 1977). Teymouri *et al.* (2020) have shown that *in ovo* feeding of vitamin B_{12} had positive effects on hatchability and subsequent performance in broiler chickens. Inclusions of 20 and 40 μg caused improvements in body weight gain and FCR at 42 days (Figure 5.13).

It is important to consider the interaction with other micronutrients such as riboflavin and pantothenic acid (Tuite and Austic, 1974; Balloun and Phillips, 1957). El-Husseiny *et al.* (2018) demonstrated that the supplementation of cyanocobalamin (0.15 mg/kg feed) affected the values of relative economic efficiency. But it does not significantly affect the broiler breeder's egg quality parameters or hatchability. Most published tables recommend supplementation of vitamin B_{12} in breeder feed which ranges between 20 and 70 μg/kg.

Niacin (vitamin B_3)

Details about current niacin recommendations for breeders, provided by institutional sources and genetic companies, can be found in Tables 5.2 to 5.6.

Low levels of niacin will hinder eggs' production and hatchability. During embryo development and after hatching, chicks obtain niacin by transforming the tryptophan present in the proteins, which are part of the egg yolk. As Cunha (1982a,b) indicated, it is better to supplement niacin in a bird's feed without considering its content in cereals since the bioavailability is very low. The same author highlighted that it is better to ensure the supply of niacin is adequate to prevent the essential amino acid tryptophan from being diverted into the synthesis of niacin.

Some authors indicated that supplementation between 66 and 132 mg/kg of niacin improved the quality of the eggshell (Leeson *et al.*, 1991) and lowered mortality in both the embryo (Briggs, 1946) and the breeder hen (Jackson, 1992). Harms *et al.* (1988a) observed that egg weight increased in parallel with niacin supplementation in breeders, with dosages ranging between 8.4 and 33.4 mg/kg (0.17% of tryptophan in the diet).

El-Husseiny *et al.* (2008b), in a study on dietary zinc and niacin, found no significant differences in egg weight with niacin supplementation up to 450 mg/kg. In contrast, significant differences in body weight gain were observed for hens fed the different dietary zinc and niacin levels. Hens fed diets containing 450 mg of niacin/kg recorded the highest body weight gain. It was concluded that a diet containing 30 mg of niacin/kg resulted in the best eggshell thickness and economic performance. The minimum requirements published by the NRC (1994) of 10 mg/kg appear largely insufficient. Different authors recommend levels between 25 and 70 mg/kg for broiler breeders.

Pantothenic acid (vitamin B_5)

Details about current pantothenic acid recommendations for breeders, provided by institutional sources and genetic companies, can be found in Tables 5.2 to 5.6.

There is a direct linear relationship between the pantothenic acid content in the breeder diets and the proportion of eggs hatched. Supplementation with 4 mg/kg pantothenic acid prevents losses in reproduction, and doses of 8 mg/kg increase hatchable egg production and the viability of the offspring (Beer *et al.*, 1963).

Embryo death generally occurs in the final days of incubation. The requirement for pantothenic acid to ensure viable offspring may be even greater, and Utno and Klieste (1971) have suggested a 20 mg/kg dosage. Some authors have observed that increasing dietary pantothenic acid increased the live weight of the progeny. However, this effect is observed in situations of vitamin B_{12} deficiency (Balloun and Phillips, 1957).

In a study with breeder males supplemented with 24 mg pantothenic acid/kg feed, the quantity and quality of the semen increased, and the weight of the testicles compared with animals fed deficient diets with 0.38 mg/kg pantothenic acid (Goeger and Arscott, 1984).

When feed allocation is controlled, the pantothenic acid content in the feed must be adjusted to ensure the proper level of vitamin intake. Furthermore, pantothenic acid requirements may increase when other vitamins are present at marginal levels of bioavailability. Parnian *et al.* (2019) found a positive impact of *in ovo* injection of 0.052 mg pantothenic acid on some immunological parameters of broiler chicks.

The NRC (1994) reported that pantothenic acid is a critical vitamin for reproduction and set the minimum requirements for laying breeder hens at levels 3.5 times higher than laying hens. Most tables published by recognized bodies and genetic companies recommend levels between 10 and 20 mg/kg for broiler breeder feeds and from 25 to 30 for turkey breeders.

Biotin (vitamin B_7)

Details about current biotin recommendations for breeders, provided by institutional sources and genetic companies, can be found in Tables 5.2 to 5.6.

Biotin is the only vitamin for which the NRC (1994) estimates minimum requirements for broiler breeders. That organization specified requirements of 16 µg of biotin per hen per day, which is 60% more than for laying breeder strains (10 µg/hen/day). These data are based on the results of Whitehead *et al.* (1985), and they considered that this is the minimum level that makes it possible to reach at least a biotin concentration in the egg yolk of 550 ng/g.

The level of biotin recommended by genetic companies stands between 200 and 400 µg/kg for broiler breeder hens and between 300 and 450 µg/kg for female turkey breeders, which is between 2 and 2.5 times higher than the NRC requirements (1994). There are significant differences in the metabolism and deposition of biotin between breeder hens and turkeys, which could be responsible for the different vitamin requirements for these 2 species (Whitehead, 1988a,b).

The physiologically active form of biotin is linked to enzymes of great metabolic importance like biotin carboxylase and biotin decarboxylase. Because of its functions, biotin (100–150 µg/kg) contributes to such important processes as growth, skin regeneration, bone development, and reproduction (El-Garhy *et al.,* 2019). Biotin is also necessary for normal embryonic development and hatchability (Daryabari *et al.,* 2014).

Biotin is transferred to the egg's white and yolk through the binding proteins of avidin and biotin, respectively. The biotin-binding proteins are synthesized in the hen's liver and provide biotin to the developing follicle, constituting the future yolk. The biotin in the yolk is the principal vitamin source for the developing embryo. On the other hand, albumen contains avidin, a glycoprotein secreted in the oviduct during the albumen depositing phase, and it has important antibacterial properties. Biotin bound to avidin has very low availability during the embryonic stage. However, it can be a vitamin source for the newly hatched chick.

An inadequate quantity of biotin in a breeder's feed decreases laying and hatchability, with high mortality during the last week of incubation and bone deformities in the progeny (Cravens *et al.*, 1944; Ferguson *et al.*, 1961; Robel, 1991). Supplementation of 150–252 µg/kg of biotin in the breeder feed ensured an adequate deposition of this vitamin in the egg and hatchability of 80% (Brewer and Edwards, 1972). Furthermore, these authors observed that chicks coming from breeders with higher levels of biotin were heavier at 2 weeks of age.

Whitehead *et al.* (1985) have demonstrated a correlation between the quantity of biotin in the egg yolk and the level of biotin in the plasma of the progeny, a level inversely related to hatchability, viability, and growth after hatching. High levels of biotin in the egg will permit the proper development of the embryo and allow the chick to achieve its genetic potential.

Similarly, Robel (1989) attended that when the breeder feed contained 165 µg/kg of biotin, the fertile eggs had a hatchability of 84%. When the dose of biotin was higher (440 µg/kg), hatchability reached 89%.

Alkubaisy *et al.* (2021) have demonstrated that eggs injected with a concentration of 75 µg biotin/egg at 0 and 18 days led to the best results by improving embryonic growth and reducing mortality (Figure 5.14). Consequently, this concentration increased hatchability and improved the quality of chicks and the weight of the chicks hatched.

In the case of turkey breeders, maximum hatchability was obtained by supplementing the feed with 520 µg/kg of biotin during the initial and intermediary phases of reproduction. This figure increased to 750 µg/kg of biotin in the breeder feed during weeks 50–54 of life, making it possible to increase hatchable egg production by 22% and chick hatchability by 10% (Robel, 2002). These findings suggested that commercial turkey breeder diets may warrant higher dietary biotin levels to optimize hatchability in older turkey hens. By injecting *in ovo* 87 µg of biotin into each egg, it was possible to improve hatchability by 4–5%. These data indicate that metabolic requirements for biotin increase as a breeder age.

Daryabari *et al.* (2014) used young (30–33 weeks) and old broiler breeders (53–56 weeks of age) to evaluate 2 levels of biotin in the drinking water (0.30 and 0.45 mg/L). The lower dose of biotin supplementation (0.30 mg/L) increased egg production (~6%). The biotin by age interaction revealed that biotin supplementation effectively increased egg production in young hens but not in the old hens. Supplementary biotin at 0.45 mg/L increased fertility by about 4.4% (Figure 5.15).

The results of Harms *et al.* (1979) demonstrated the relationship between supplementation with biotin in breeders and the repercussion on aspects of welfare and quality of the final

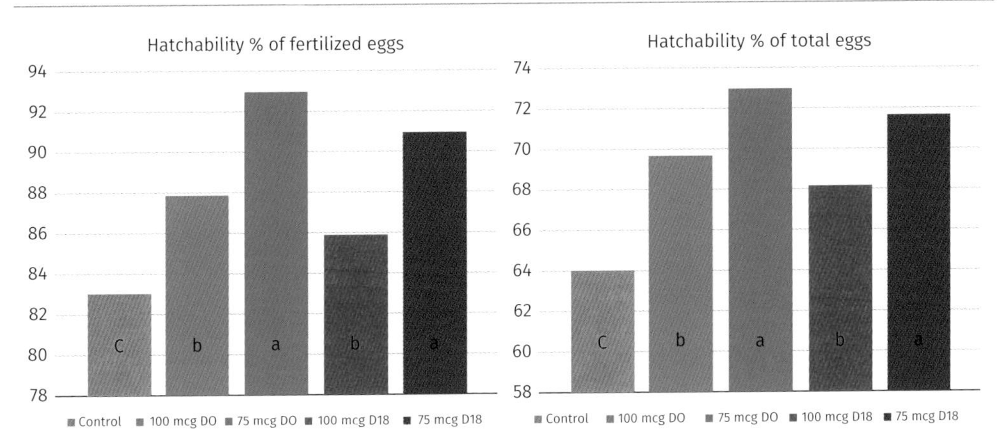

Figure 5.14 Effect of biotin *in ovo* injection (DOI 0 or 18) on hatchability of total eggs, values with no common superscripts differ significantly, $P < 0.05$ (adapted from Alkubaisy *et al.*, 2021)

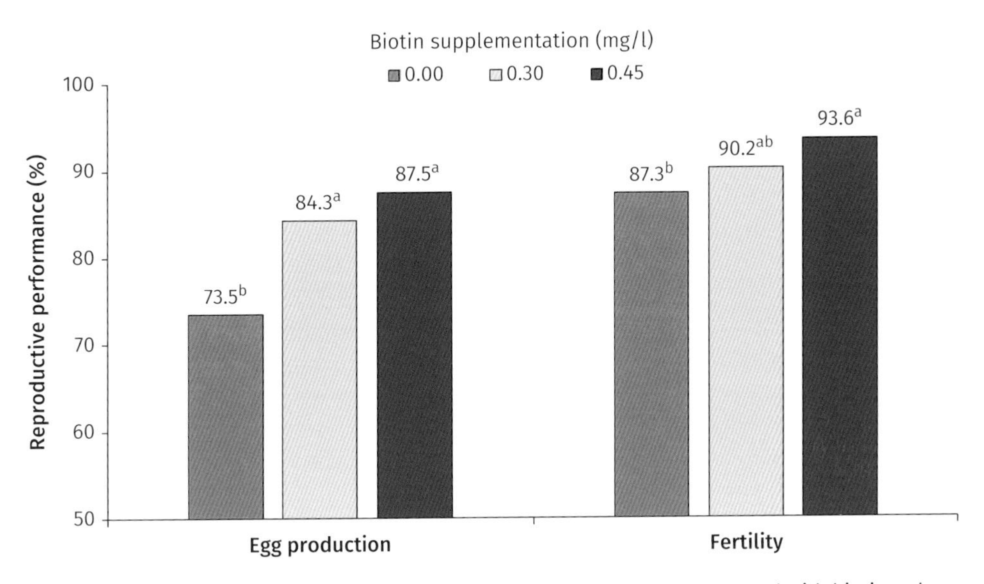

Figure 5.15 Reproductive performance in young broiler breeder hens supplemented with biotin, values with no common superscripts differ significantly, $P < 0.05$ (Daryabari *et al.*, 2014)

product. Incorporating 200 µg/kg of biotin in the hen's feeds made it possible to reduce the incidence of footpad dermatitis and breast lesions in the progeny.

In the case of turkey breeders, Robel (2002) obtained maximum hatchability by supplementing the feed with 520 µg/kg of biotin during the initial and intermediary phases of reproduction. This figure increased to 750 µg/kg of biotin in the breeder feed during weeks 50–54 of life, making it possible to increase hatchable egg production by 22% and chick hatchability by 10% (Figure 5.16). These findings suggested that commercial turkey breeder diets may warrant higher dietary biotin levels to optimize hatchability in older turkey hens. Injecting *in ovo*, 87 µg of biotin into each egg, it was possible to improve hatchability by 4–5%. These data indicate that metabolic requirements for biotin increase as a breeder gets older.

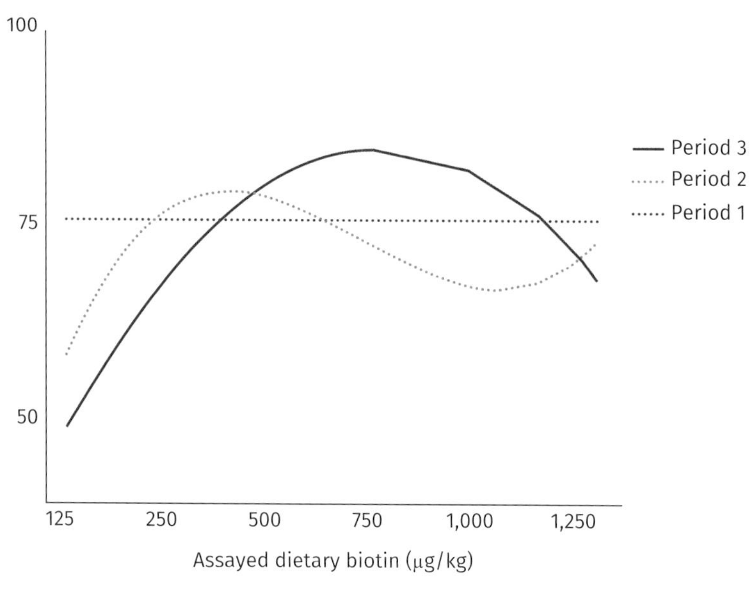

Figure 5.16 Hatchability of fertile turkey eggs at different biotin supplementation levels (adapted from Robel, 2002)

Folic acid (vitamin B_9)

Details about current folic acid recommendations for breeders, provided by institutional sources and genetic companies, can be found in Tables 5.2 to 5.6.

An inadequate supply of folic acid in hens hinders the normal development and functioning of the oviduct, accompanied by a defective deposition of albumen (Siddons, 1978). Feeds for broiler breeders tend to incorporate 1–1.5 mg/kg folic acid, while it ranges between 1 and 2 mg/kg in turkey breeders. The transfer of folacin from feed to eggs is very high.

The residual yolk is the main source of nutrients during the transitional period between the hatch and grow-out phases (Henderson *et al.*, 2008; Nouri *et al.*, 2017). Folic acid acts as a coenzyme in single-carbon transfer in the synthesis and metabolism of nucleic and amino acids (Abd El-Azeem *et al.*, 2014). Folic acid is a critical vitamin for all animals during reproduction, and its requirement for hatchability is higher than egg production (Nouri *et al.*, 2017).

Zhang *et al.* (2021) demonstrated that 5 and 10 mg/kg folic acid supplementation might reduce fat accumulation by regulating gene expression and several metabolic pathways, such as folate biosynthesis, peroxisome proliferator-activated receptor (regulating fatty acid storage and glucose metabolism) signaling, and DNA replication, among others.

It is widely accepted that the folacin requirements for hatching eggs are higher than for the production of table eggs (Taylor, 1947; Robel, 1993a; NRC, 1994). The study carried out by Robel (1993a) with breeding turkeys using a diet supplemented with 2.64 ppm and 5.51 ppm folic acid suggests that increasing the supplementation dosage above the 1 ppm established by the NRC (1994) as a minimum requirement for this species did not lead to improvements in hatchability of fertile eggs or embryo mortality. However, a positive linear response to supplementation was observed in the transfer of folic acid to the egg, specifically the yolk. The production parameters studied did show effects of supplementation with folic acid: higher egg weight and

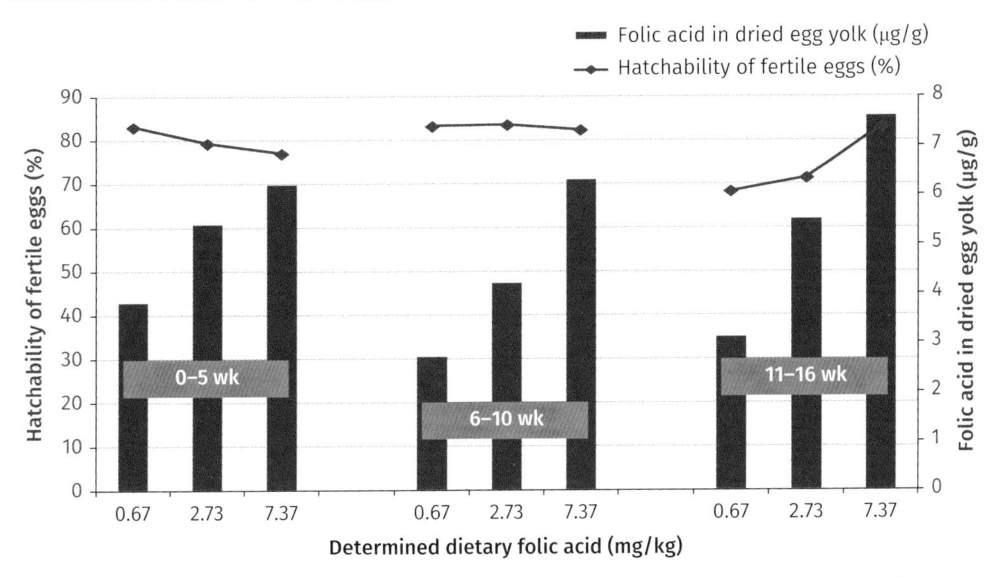

Figure 5.17 Hatchability of turkey eggs from hens fed a basal diet supplemented with folic acid (0.65, 2.73, and 7.37 mg/kg) over 3 equal periods of production (0–5; 6–10 and 11–16 weeks) and vitamin contents of egg yolk (adapted from Robel, 2002)

higher bird weight for the 16 days of the experiment with a higher level of supplementation (5.51 *vs.* 2.64 ppm), the differences in both cases being statistically significant. No differences in the number of eggs produced by the turkey were noted due to supplementation.

Robel (2002) recommends incorporating folic acid in the feed of broiler breeder hens at levels higher than 1 mg/kg, values which reach 2 mg/kg for female turkey breeders (Figure 5.17). The recommendations of the genetic companies go so far as 2–5 mg/kg for broiler breeders and 4–6 mg/kg for turkey breeders.

Vitamin C

Details about current vitamin C recommendations for breeders, provided by institutional sources and genetic companies, can be found in Tables 5.2 to 5.6.

Most results demonstrate the beneficial effect of vitamin C supplementation in feeds for hens in the laying phase – be it of eggs for consumption or incubation hatchability – and in stress situations, principally heat-induced. Several authors observed improved egg production, eggshell strength and thickness, and a higher chick survival rate (Peebles and Brake, 1985; Chung *et al.*, 2005). Birds need vitamin C for their metabolism, but owing to their capacity for endogenous synthesis, there are no recommendations for supply in the feed from the NRC (1994). However, as the biosynthesis of ascorbic acid diminishes as the bird ages, in the final phases of reproduction, endogenous synthesis may be insufficient to cover requirements (Bains, 2001).

Therefore, several authors advise supplying vitamin C in the diet (between 50 and 250 mg/kg) for various reasons. These recommendations are justified since ascorbic acid requirements increase in different circumstances, such as exposure to immunological or environmental stress, deficiencies in nutrients such as vitamin A and situations of metabolic alterations.

Additionally, ascorbic acid consumption above the strict physiological requirements benefits the animal's immune response.

There is practically no storage of vitamin C in the body, which means there is no reservoir for coverage at times of deficiency. Vitamin C is the only missing vitamin in the infertile egg, as there is no transfer from the hen. However, vitamin C is found in the developing embryo deriving from endogenous synthesis (Pardue and Thaxton, 1986; Zwaan and Lam, 1992).

During the initial phases of embryonic development, ascorbic acid is synthesized in the yolk membrane and liberated into the liver and other peripheral tissues (Surai and Speake, 2000). The antioxidant action of vitamin C is beneficial to the embryo, especially if stressful situations arise due to excess heat during the incubation process. Inoculation with 3 mg vitamin C in eggs during the last part of incubation improved the viability and hatch weight of the chicks (Zakaria and Al-Anezi, 1996).

In breeder males, vitamin C could help protect spermatozoa from the negative effects of oxidation. The concentration of ascorbic acid in the seminal fluid is higher than in the serum (Luck *et al.*, 1995). It has been demonstrated that supplementation with vitamin C benefits fertility. Supplementation of 100 mg/kg ascorbic acid increased the size of the testicles of growing males (Pardue and Thaxton, 1986). Furthermore, adding doses of ascorbic acid up to 500 mg/kg to the feeds of breeder males of broiler breeder strains in high-temperature situations produced an increase in the volume of semen, the number of spermatozoa per ejaculation, and sperm motility (Perek and Snapir, 1963; Monsi and Onitchi, 1991). Khan *et al.* (2012a) demonstrated that vitamin E (100 mg/kg feed) and C (500 mg/kg feed) or their combination were the most potent nutrients to improve semen traits and seminal biochemical characteristics in roosters after zinc-induced molting.

Recent studies confirmed that vitamin C in roosters and turkey diets improves reproductive parameters concerning semen. For example, Uzochukwu *et al.* (2020) concluded that combined supplementation of vitamins E (125 mg/kg diet) and C (400 mg/kg diet) in tom diets enhanced semen quality (Figure 5.18).

Attia *et al.* (2020a) investigated the influence of heat stress and vitamin C and vitamin E on semen quality of 32-week-old rosters, and they found that either 200 mg/kg vitamin C or 150 mg/kg vitamin E improved semen quality, fertility, seminal plasma (Figure 5.19).

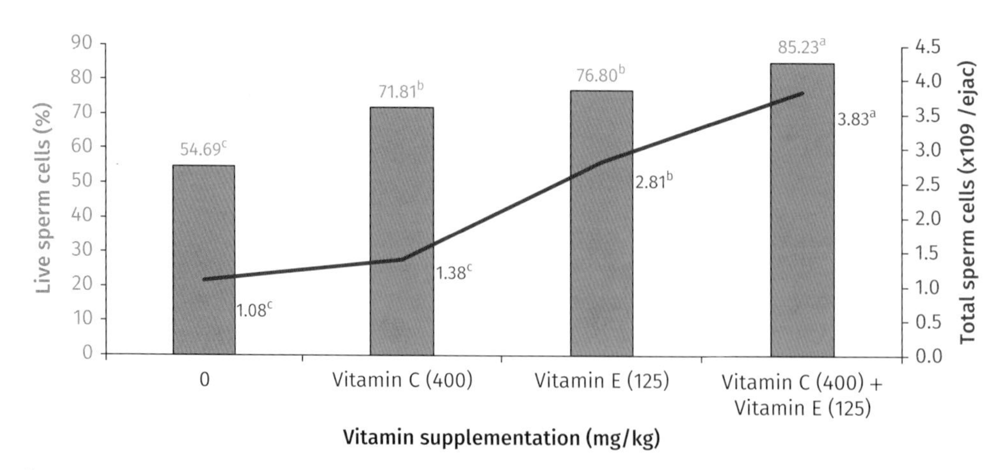

Figure 5.18 Effect of vitamin C and E supplementation on semen characteristics of turkey toms (adapted from Uzochukwu *et al.*, 2020)

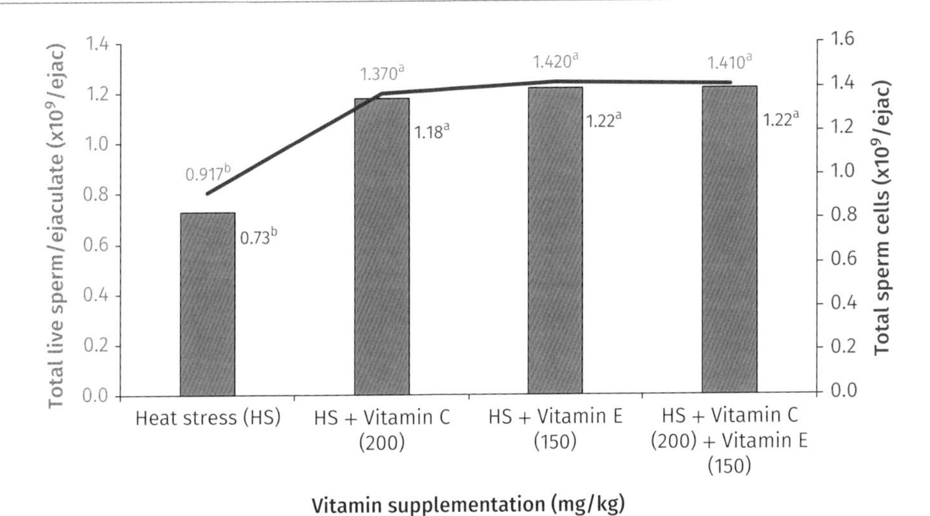

Figure 5.19 Effects of dietary vitamin C, vitamin E, and combined supplementation on semen quality and seminal plasma constituents in roosters reared under heat stress conditions (adapted from Attia *et al.*, 2020a)

Choline

Details about current choline recommendations for breeders, provided by institutional sources and genetic companies, can be found in Tables 5.2 to 5.6.

The NRC (1994) does not specify minimum requirements for choline, but several publications indicate the importance of its supplementation in feed. However, the recommendations currently range widely between 750 and 1,600 mg/kg depending on the safety margin applied, considering the variability of the ingredients and the fact that the presence of precursors may be limited.

Although choline can be synthesized in the liver from the methylation of ethanolamine, young birds are dependent on the supply of choline in the feed, as they have a less well-developed capacity for synthesizing choline from methionine or betaine (Norvell and Nesheim, 1969). It has been described that vitamin supplements influence the choline requirements of laying hens during their growth phase. Furthermore, diets with reduced choline levels during the reproduction phase affect the size of the egg, although choline deposition in the egg and embryonic development is not much affected (Klasing, 1998).

As a structural component of lecithin, choline plays an essential role in forming the very LDLs assigned to incorporating and mobilizing the triglycerides present in the liver. Lecithin deficiency is associated with an accumulation of fat in the liver (Rama-Rao *et al.*, 2001) and a decrease in the quantity of fat deposited in the egg yolk. In addition, the same authors showed a numerical reduction in the abdominal fat deposition when birds were fed increasing amounts of choline (Figure 5.20).

The content of this vitamin and other methyl donors like betaine in the egg impacts embryo development with important effects on the life post-hatch. Gholami *et al.* (2015) administered 0.25, 0.375, and 0.50 mg of either betaine and choline *in ovo* and evaluated their effects at hatch, during broiler growth, and in their carcass traits. The supplementation of betaine and

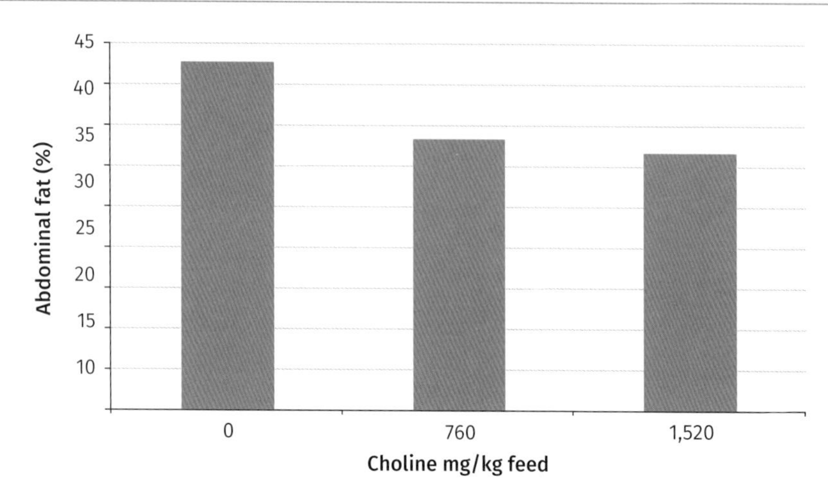

Figure 5.20 Abdominal fat deposition was reduced when high choline levels were fed to broiler breeders (adapted from Rama-Rao, 2001)

choline *in ovo* improved hatching weight, final body weight at 42 days of age, FCR, and reduced abdominal fat. No effects were observed on the carcass or cut-up parts yield or immunological parameters. After observing these experimental effects *in ovo* feeding, it is logical to think that the proper nutrition of the breeder to enrich eggs with phosphatidylcholine may also have a relevant impact on the progeny. Janist *et al.* (2019) concluded that 1,500 mg choline/kg feed is necessary to maximize phosphatidylcholine in the yolk of layers.

Chapter 6

Optimum vitamin nutrition in broilers and turkeys

INTRODUCTION

Broiler and turkey feed should be supplemented with vitamins as the main feed ingredients are deficient and, apart from vitamin C, birds are either unable to synthesize them or do so, for B group and vitamin K_2, in very limited quantities, most of which are excreted in any case.

Animals can store some vitamins – A, D_3, B_{12}, and, to a lesser extent, E and K_3 – primarily in the liver. However, all vitamins play roles in all cells, especially those critical for growth and survival. Cellular metabolic functions in bones, muscles, gut, and immune systems critically depend on multiple vitamins.

This chapter will focus on discussing OVN™ levels, the factors that may modify these optimum levels, and the recommendations for vitamin supplementation for broilers and turkeys during the grow-out phase. The information about vitamin active forms, units of quantification, conversion factors, functions, metabolism, signs of vitamin deficiencies, and general factors that influence vitamin requirements and vitamin utilization were discussed in Chapter 4 of this book. Additional information on the importance of vitamins in the feeding of broilers and turkeys can be found in the reviews by Larbier and Leclercq (1992, 1994), McDowell (2000a,b; 2004), Whitehead (2002b), Leeson and Summers (2008).

GENERAL ASPECTS OF VITAMIN SUPPLEMENTATION

There are many reasons in the broiler and turkey industries to strengthen vitamin supplementation and work with high safety margins.

Changes in the genetic make-up of broilers and turkeys

Broiler growth rates have increased by over 460% between 1957 and 2005 (Zuidhof *et al.*, 2014), with 85–90% of this increase being attributed to genetic selection and the remainder attributed to diet (Havenstein *et al.*, 2003) (Figure 6.1).

The FCR has reduced by 50% in the same period. In the past 20 years, the average market weight in many countries has increased to satisfy the increasing demand for breast and deboned meat (Maharjan *et al.*, 2021). The 2020 market share of broilers heavier than 2.73 kg was 70% in the US, and the breast yield has increased from 17.6 to 25% from 2001 to 2017 (Figure 6.2).

Turkey body weights also have been increasing in the past 20 years for all genetic lines currently used (Table 6.1).

Cerrate and Corzo (2019) discussed the trends in US broiler body composition and nutrient efficiency during the past 20 years (Figure 6.2). The broiler body (abdominal) fat has

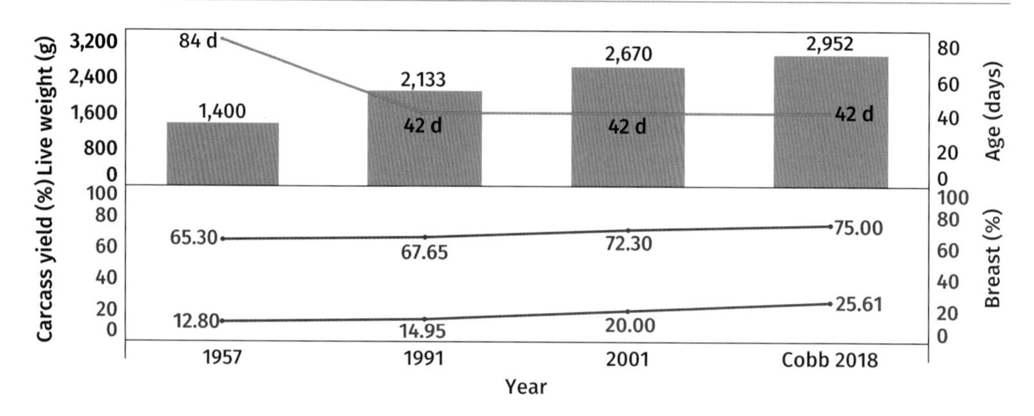

Figure 6.1 Development of live weight, age at processing, carcass, and breast yield of broilers from 1957 to 2018 (source: Havenstein *et al.*, 1994, 2003; Cobb-Vantress, 2020)

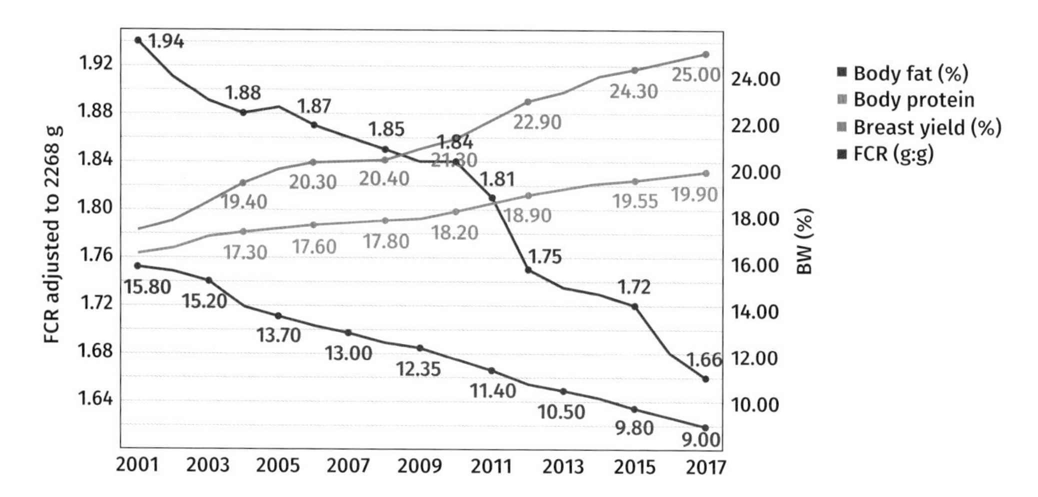

Figure 6.2 Feed conversion rate (FCR), breast yield, body protein, and body fat change in broilers over time. Breast yield and FCR adjusted to 2,268 g of body weight (adapted from Cerrate and Corzo, 2019)

reduced by 6%, while body protein has increased by 4% annually since 2000. As body protein increases, FCR has decreased from 1.91 to 1.66 in US broilers. The continuous improvement in the FCR means that current broilers consume much less feed per kilogram of weight, so their vitamin intake is proportionally significantly smaller. In 2007, Leeson had calculated that the average ingestion of vitamin E per kilogram of weight by a 2 kg chicken has decreased by 0.8% per year in the last 20 years and by 0.6% in a 14 kg turkey, leading to the suggestion that vitamin levels should be increased by 0.6 and 1% per year simply to maintain the same vitamin intake level.

Moreover, selection to achieve more rapid growth has directly or indirectly produced profound modifications in different aspects of the birds' physiology. Dunnington and Siegel (1996) summed up the results of studies carried out over 38 generations of selection to increase daily gain: modifications in appetite control and thermoregulatory mechanisms, oxygen

Table 6.1 Turkey body weights currently and in 1999 (sources: Herendy *et al.* [2004] and genetic companies' performance objectives)

Body weight (kg)	Males					Females				
	1999	Nicholas Select, 2020	BUT 6, 2020	BUT Premium, 2020	Hybrid, 2020	1999	Nicholas Select, 2020	BUT 6, 2020	BUT Premium, 2020	Hybrid, 2020
6 weeks	2.59	3.01	2.81	2.68	2,.97	1.60	2.28	2.28	2.17	2.49
10 weeks	6.72	7.96	7.60	7.24	7.67	5.24	5.48	5.71	5.44	6.33
16 weeks	13.90	16.95	16.16	15.32	16.63	10.19	11.44	11.29	10.79	11.53
20 weeks	19.14	22.66	21.50	20.35	21.92	12.62	14.86	12.79*	12.24*	–

Note: *18 weeks.

consumption, body temperature, and heat production, in the capacity to absorb nutrients and in the activity of digestive enzymes, in hormone and serum levels in general, in physical composition for broilers (Figure 6.2) and turkeys (Table 6.2), in the immune response and stress resistance.

It is now commonplace for modern broilers to have reduced levels of triiodothyronine and corticosterone hormones and altered expression of genes regulating thyroid hormone activity. This contributes to lower heat production, reduced stress response, and altered nutrient partitioning leading to more efficient feed utilization and faster growth (Vaccaro *et al.*, 2022).

Energy utilization efficiency has remained almost constant (~74%). In comparison, the lysine digestibility efficiency has improved from 61 to 76% due to a reduction in protein degradation and an increment in protein synthesis from 2001 to 2017 (Cerrate and Corzo, 2019). However, due to the decrease in feed intake, the calorie conversion has improved by 16% from 1994 to 2018 (Maharjan *et al.*, 2021) or 18% from 2001 to 2017 (Cerrate and Corzo, 2019). The intake of lysine and other amino acids has increased by almost 19% in the past 2 decades (Figure 6.3).

Table 6.2 Body composition of slow-growing turkeys and fast-growing turkeys (BUT-6) (adapted from Damaziak *et al.*, 2015)

	Males, week 21		Females, week 15	
	Slow grow	Fast grow	Slow grow	Fast grow
Body weight (g)	5.787	21.535	3.026	11.586
Breast muscle (%)	14.9	27.0	14.9	23.7
Leg muscle (%)	17.0	18.5	15.3	17.2
Wings (%)	9.1	8.2	10.0	8.6
Fat and skin (%)	7.6	8.9	5.8	10.0

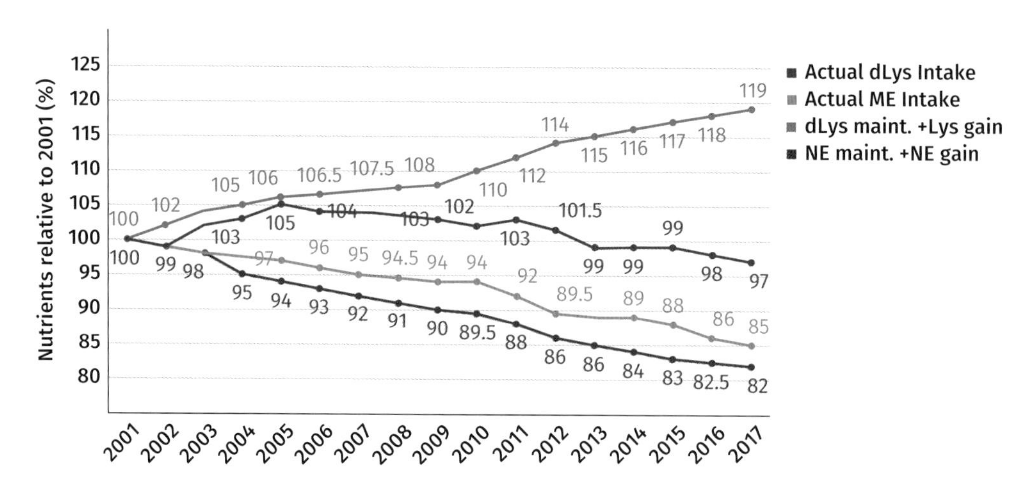

Figure 6.3 Nutrients 2017 relative to 2001 [(nutrients, 2001–2017)/(nutrients, 2001) × 100]. Nutrient intakes were obtained from the US industry reporting service AgriStats. Net energy for maintenance (NE maint.), net energy for body gain (NE gain), digestible lysine for maintenance (dLys maint.), lysine for protein gain (Lys gain), and digestible lysine (dLys) were calculated (adapted from Cerrate and Corzo, 2018)

Several vitamins are involved in these metabolic processes that improve the efficiency of energy and protein utilization. Consequently, it is logical to raise vitamin levels following the increases in body weights, meat yields, and lower feed intakes. Vitamins of the B group play an important role in energy metabolism. Higher protein and lysine and methionine levels needed to maximize breast yield increase the requirements for vitamin B_{12}, biotin, and pyridoxine.

Animal health and well-being

Intensive rearing means that birds may be exposed to a variety of stress factors, whether environmental (high density, high temperatures, damp bedding), immunological (vaccinations, infections), or nutritional (fat rancidity, fungus contamination, etc.). Modern broilers and turkeys have high productive potential but are more susceptible to infections (Bayyari *et al.*, 1997; Yunis *et al.*, 2000; Hocking, 2014; Hartcher and Lum, 2020).

Clear positive effects of general vitamin fortification against stress conditions arising from one of these factors, or a combination of several of them, have been demonstrated in both species (Ferket and Qureshi, 1992; Coelho and McNaughton, 1995; Taranu *et al.*, 1995; Deyhim and Teeter, 1996; Dunn, 1996; McKnight *et al.*, 1996a; Gouda *et al.*, 2020; Shakeri *et al.*, 2020; Ahmadian *et al.*, 2021; Yu *et al.*, 2021).

The role of vitamin C in alleviating heat stress and improving the immune response are already well established. Other vitamins, e.g., C, D_3 and its metabolites, E and most of the B group, have also shown positive effects in preventing or reducing the severity of metabolic problems, such as ascites, bone issues, footpad dermatitis, myopathies, most of which are connected to rapid growth (Whitehead, 2000a; Malan *et al.*, 2001; Leeson and Summers, 2008; Gouda *et al.*, 2020; Shakeri *et al.*, 2020; Yu *et al.*, 2021; Uribe-Diaz *et al.*, 2021).

Product quality

It is today more necessary than ever to consider product quality which was previously neglected in the requirements established by the NRC. In recent years, numerous studies have demonstrated that a higher supplementation with some vitamins, especially vitamin E, can reduce skin problems and improve the stability of meat against oxidation (Sheehy *et al.*, 1995; Jensen *et al.*, 1998; Weber, 2001). Vitamin C and E could be beneficial in reducing the severity of myopathies, but in this aspect, the results are still contested (Petracci *et al.*, 2015; Bodle *et al.*, 2018; Wang *et al.*, 2020a,b). Furthermore, the enrichment of vitamin content in poultry meat is achieved by using higher doses in feed (Hernández *et al.*, 2002; Castaing *et al.*, 2003; Pérez-Vendrell *et al.*, 2003; Michalczuk *et al.*, 2016; Pompeu *et al.*, 2018; Barnkob *et al.*, 2020) could be attractive to many consumers.

Variations in the content and bioavailability of vitamins in feed ingredients

Variations in the content and bioavailability of vitamins may be caused by many factors, such as interactions with other vitamins and nutrients, mycotoxins, etc. In Europe, poultry diets are more variable than in the US. The predominance of wheat rather than corn makes it more necessary to supplement the diet with niacin, biotin, pantothenic acid, vitamin A, and B_6 (Whitehead, 1993; Ahmadian *et al.*, 2021).

There have been changes in feed formulation worldwide, which may affect vitamin requirements, such as the ban or limitation of the use of meat and other animal proteins (formerly important sources of vitamin B_{12} and pantothenic acid), and the greater use of completely vegetarian diets, rich in unsaturated fats, which may involve higher requirements of vitamin E for its antioxidant effect. The ban on growth-promoting antibiotics in the EU and their reduced use worldwide make vitamins with immunomodulatory functions more beneficial.

Increasingly aggressive manufacturing processes, such as drying at high temperatures, other heat treatments, pelleting, extrusion, and expansion, are potentially causing vitamin losses of between 15 and 40%, which will increase if the feed is kept for any length of time or in unsuitable conditions. These and other technical aspects, such as how well vitamin sources are protected, and the composition of premixes, when these are added to the feed, may cause a significant reduction of real vitamin content in the feed compared to the expected levels (Putnam, 1983; Cooke and Raine, 1987; Putnam and Taylor, 1997; Whitehead, 2002a; Lauzon *et al.*, 2008).

Cost–benefit relationship

The cost of vitamin fortification today makes up less than 1% of the total cost of the feed. This investment is small concerning the possible improvement it may bring and the prevention of risks that may be very economically damaging. Studies carried out under practical field conditions by Coelho and McNaughton (1995) on broilers demonstrated that the group of companies that used higher supplementation levels achieved improved growth, feed conversion, and viability of birds, especially in conditions of moderate stress (Figures 6.4, 6.5 and 6.6) and improved yield at the slaughterhouse, which amply compensated for the additional cost.

The return on investment in supplementation was confirmed in similar specific investigations for vitamin E (Kennedy *et al.*, 1992; Bird and Boren, 1999) with levels of 180–240 ppm, and for some vitamins of the B group (Coelho *et al.*, 2001) supplemented at levels 4 times higher than normal in the North American poultry industry and 16 times more than the NRC level. There is no reason why these increases in vitamin content should be harmful since toxicity does become a risk until 100–1,000 times higher than the minimum requirements (NRC, 1987; Leeson and Summers, 2008), except for vitamins A and D_3, for which toxicity occurs at approximately 10 times higher than the given requirement.

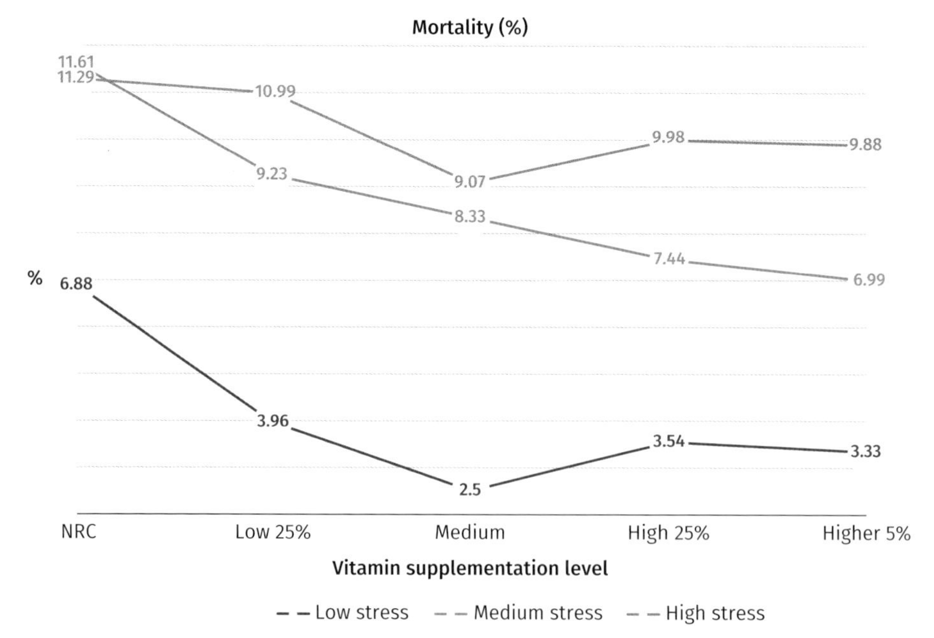

Figure 6.4 Effect of vitamin supplementation levels under various stress conditions on mortality at 42 days (source: Coelho and McNaughton, 1995)

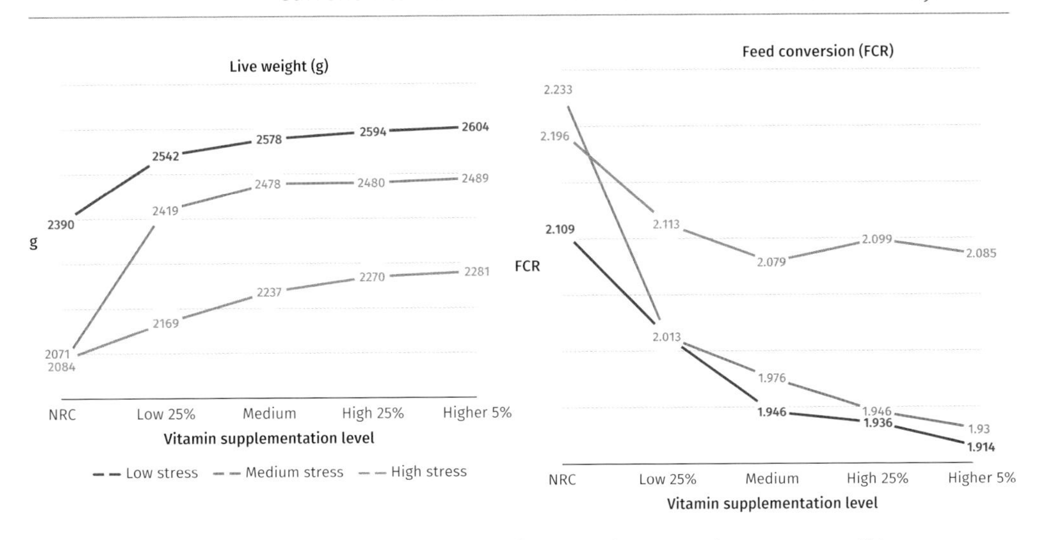

Figure 6.5 Effects of vitamin supplementation level (at 51 days) under various stress conditions on weight gain and feed conversion (source: Coelho and McNaughton, 1995)

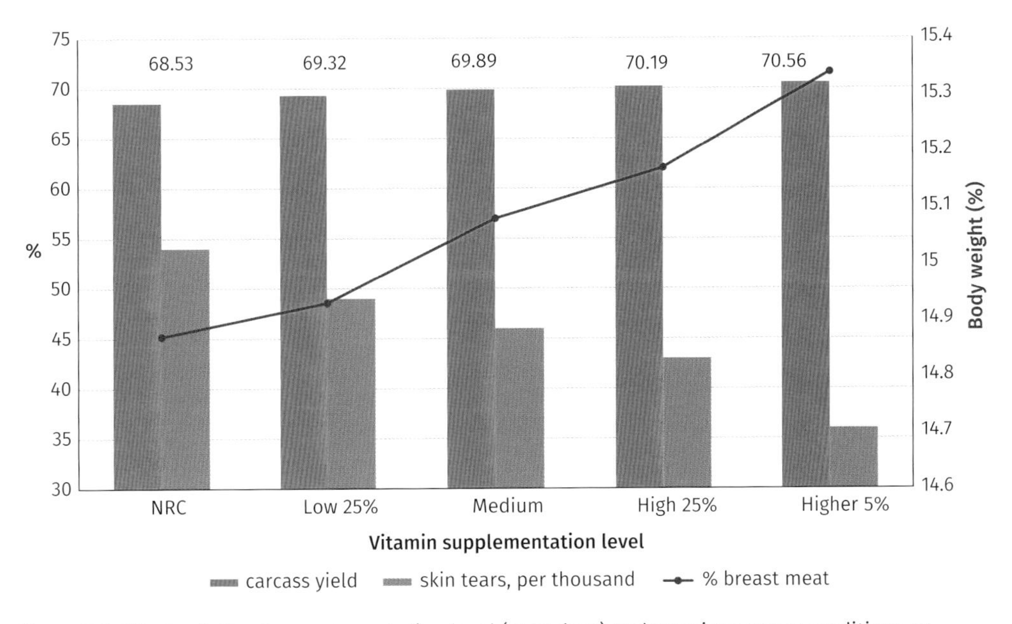

Figure 6.6 Effects of vitamin supplementation level (at 51 days) under various stress conditions on carcass quality (source: Coelho and McNaughton, 1995)

CURRENT VITAMIN RECOMMENDATIONS FOR BROILERS AND TURKEYS

The key reference of basic research related to the vitamin needs of chickens and turkeys continues to be the latest edition of the US National Research Council publication on the nutritional requirements for poultry (NRC, 1994).

In this publication, the levels were established to represent the minimum to guarantee the absence of deficiencies. Nowadays, vitamin deficiencies are infrequently detected unless due to batching and mixing errors in the factory, low-quality vitamins with lower potency than expected, or the loss of a significant amount of the vitamin activity after storage and/or feed treatment (e.g., pelleting or extrusion).

Moreover, in the NRC publication many of the studies were conducted with purified diets that were difficult to pelletize and therefore consumed in mash form, with very low growth rates, and took place under conditions of a laboratory or poultry experimental research stations (Leeson, 2007). It should also be pointed out that while the NRC (1994) expressed vitamin recommendations as total requirements, other sources of recommendations have expressed them for feed supplementation. In practice, the vitamin content of the basal feed ingredients was ignored (Whitehead, 1993; Leeson, 2007).

Another important aspect is that the levels of vitamins listed in the NRC (1994) for broilers in the starter, grower, and finisher phases and turkeys do not ensure the expression of the genetic potential of today's birds, having a significantly better FCR and body weight compared to 1994 birds. There is greater doubt about vitamin requirements in the finishing phase for heavier broilers and turkey toms produced nowadays with their greater muscle development (Cerrate and Corzo, 2019; Damaziak *et al.*, 2015).

A comparison of vitamin recommendations from the principal scientific sources, which constitute a habitual reference point for poultry nutrition specialists, are presented in Tables 6.3, 6.4, and 6.5 for broilers during the starter, grower, and finisher phases, respectively. Overall, the recommended vitamin levels correspond to the higher levels reported already 10 years ago by several sources.

The NRC (1994) values for broilers fall well below those of the other sources: the levels recommended are 3–10 times lower for vitamins A, E, K, pantothenic acid, and B_{12} and 10–20 times lower for D_3 than the ones recommended by other authors. There is less difference in the vitamins B_1, B_2, B_6, niacin, and biotin levels. These levels have not been altered in more than 40 years and are based on outdated experimental data. For choline, the NRC figures are 2–5 times higher than the other sources, but they refer to total requirements and not supplementation levels. Moreover, most of the recommendations available were formulated for corn-soybean diets only.

Looking at recommendations from other authors, we can observe how Leeson and Summers (2008) exceeded levels indicated by NRC (1994), making them closer to those reported by Foundation for the Development of Animal Nutrition (FEDNA) many years later (2018). Interestingly, French researchers Larbier and Leclercq (1992) recommended values that were already in line with those recommended by other authors 20 years later. Also, Whitehead (2002b) suggested much higher levels in comparison to NRC.

Interestingly, Rostagno *et al.* (2017) proposed a methodology to calculate an optimum level of supplementation for each vitamin according to the body weight gain. One limiting factor could be represented by the fact that this methodology does not consider the impact of vitamin supplementation on immunity, stress, and meat quality of broilers at processing time. The tables confirm the body weights at the end of each phase. The estimations provided values within the ranges recommended by others for the starter and grower phases but were slightly lower for the finisher phase. These values were estimated using a Gompertz curve, targeting different body weights in the middle point of each phase. The calculations used the daily body weight gain and feed intake per phase, estimating the daily feed intake according to the equation described by the same authors for metabolizable energy needs in kilocalorie per bird per day.

Table 6.3 Recommended vitamin levels (IU or mg/kg air-dry feed) for broilers during the starter phase by various sources

	Broilers								
	Starter								
	Unit/kg	Larbier and Lecquerq, 1992	NRC, 1994	Whitehead, 2002c	Leeson and Summers, 2005	FEFANA, 2015	Rostagno *et al.*, 2017	FEDNA, 2018	OVN™ (DSM Nutritional Products, 2022)
Vitamin A	IU	12,000	1,500	10,000–15,000	8,000	11,000–13,000	14,712	10,000	12,600–15,700
Vitamin D_3	IU	2,000	200	4,000–5,000	3,500	3,000–5,000	3,678	3,500	4,200–5,200
25OHD_3 (HyD)	mg	–	–	–	–	0.069	–	–	0.069
Vitamin E	mg	30	10	30–180	50	40–60	55.2	25	160–210
Vitamin K	mg	2.5	0.5	2–3	3	3–4	2.94	2.5	3.2–4.2
Vitamin B_1	mg	2	2	1.5–2.5	4	3–4	3.95	2	3.2–4.2
Vitamin B_2	mg	6.0	3.6	6–8	5	8–10	9.84	6.5	8.4–10.5
Vitamin B_6	mg	–	3.5	4	4	4–6	5.52	3	4.2–6.3
Vitamin B_{12}	mg	0.02	0.01	0.01–0.016	0.01	0.02–0.04	0.02	0.02	0.021–0.042
Niacin	mg	30	35	35–60	40	60–80	59.8	45	64–84
D-panthothenic acid	mg	15	10	12–18	14	15–20	19.8	12	16–21
Folic acid	mg	1.00	0.55	1.5–2.5	1	2.0–2.5	1.38	1	2.1–2.6
Biotin	mg	0.10	0.15	0.18–0.25	0.1	0.2–0.4	0.14	0.13	0.26–0.42
Vitamin C	mg	–	–	–	–	100–200	–	–	105–210
Choline	mg	600	1,300	250–350	400	400–700	598.0	1,250	420–740

Table 6.4 Recommended vitamin levels (IU or mg/kg air-dry feed) for broilers during the grower phase by various sources

	Broilers								
	Grower								
	Unit/kg	Larbier and Lecquerq, 1992	NRC, 1994	Whitehead, 2002c	Leeson and Summers, 2005	FEFANA, 2015	Rostagno *et al.*, 2017	FEDNA, 2018	OVN™ (DSM Nutritional Products, 2022)
Vitamin A	IU	12,000	1,500	10,000–15,000	8,000	10,000–12,000	10,204	9,000	10,500–13,100
Vitamin D_3	IU	2,000	200	4,000–5,000	3,500	3,000–5,000	2,551	3,000	4,200–5,200
$25OHD_3$ (HyD)	mg	–	–	–	–	0.069	–	–	0.069
Vitamin E	mg	30	10	30–180	50	20–30	38.27	25	55–105
Vitamin K	mg	2.5	0.5	2–3	3	3–4	2.04	2.2	3.2–4.2
Vitamin B_1	mg	2	2	1.5–2.5	4	2–3	2.74	1.5	2.1–3.2
Vitamin B_2	mg	6.0	3.6	6–8	5	7–9	6.82	5.5	7.4–9.5
Vitamin B_6	mg	–	3.5	4	4	4–6	3.83	2.5	4.2–6.3
Vitamin B_{12}	mg	0.02	0.01	0.01–0.016	0	0.02–0.03	0.02	0.02	0.021–0.032
Niacin	mg	30	35	35–60	40	50–80	41.46	35	63–84
D-panthothenic acid	mg	15	10	12–18	14	12–18	13.71	11	12.6–19
Folic acid	mg	1.00	0.55	1.5–2.5	1	2.0–2.5	0.96	0.8	2.1–2.6
Biotin	mg	0.10	0.15	0.18–0.25	0	0.2–0.3	0.10	0.1	0.26–0.42
Vitamin C	mg	–	–	–	–	100–200	–	–	105–210
Choline	mg	600	1,300	250–350	400	400–700	415	1,200	420–740

Table 6.5 Recommended vitamin levels (IU or mg/kg air-dry feed) for broilers during the finisher phase by various sources

	Broilers								
	Finisher								
	Unit/kg	Larbier and Lecquerq, 1992	NRC, 1994	Whitehead, 2002c	Leeson and Summers, 2005	FEFANA, 2015	Rostagno *et al.*, 2017	FEDNA, 2018	DSM Nutritional Products, 2022
Vitamin A	IU	10,000	1,500	10,000–15,000	8,000	10,000–12,000	10,204	9,000	10,500–13,100
Vitamin D_3	IU	1,500	200	4,000–5,000	3,500	3,000–5,000	2,551	3,000	4,200–5,200
25OHD_3 (HyD)	mg	–	–	–	–	0.069	–	–	0.069
Vitamin E	mg	20	10	30–180	50	20–30	38.27	25	55–105
Vitamin K	mg	2.0	0.5	2–3	3	3–4	2.04	2.2	3.2–4.2
Vitamin B_1	mg	2	2	1.5–2.5	4	2–3	2.74	1.5	2.1–3.2
Vitamin B_2	mg	4.0	3.6	6–8	5	7–9	6.82	5.5	6.3–8.4
Vitamin B_6	mg	2.5	3.5	4	4	4–6	3.83	2.5	4.2–6.3
Vitamin B_{12}	mg	0.01	0.01	0.01–0.016	0.012	0.02–0.03	0.02	0.02	0.021–0.032
Niacin	mg	20	30	35–60	40	50–80	41.46	35	53–84
D-panthothenic acid	mg	10	10	12–18	14	12–18	13.71	11	10.5–15.8
Folic acid	mg	1.00	0.55	1.5–2.5	1	2.0–2.5	0.96	0.8	2.1–2.6
Biotin	mg	0.20	0.55	0.18–0.25	0.1	0.2–0.3	0.10	0.1	0.26–0.42
Vitamin C	mg	0.05	0.15	–	–	100–200	–	–	105–210
Choline	mg	–	–	250–350	400	400–700	415	1,200	420–630

The Spanish FEDNA continues to propose more conservative recommendations than the other references examined. Vitamin E and all B complex vitamins are recommended in moderately lower levels. But choline is now recommended at 2 to 3 times higher (1,100 to 1,250 mg/kg) than the value recommended by the other sources or the previous recommendation 10 years ago.

There are some limitations to estimating the optimum vitamin levels because limited research on vitamin requirements for poultry has been carried out in recent decades, with some exceptions, such as vitamins C, $D_{3,}$ and E. The literature in poultry vitamin research indicates more interest in investigating the effects of higher vitamin supplementation and solving developmental health issues affecting livability, animal welfare, and meat quality.

In commercial poultry nutrition, the industry has tended to use vitamin supplementation levels considerably above the NRC (1994) for vitamin D, niacin, and folic acid and, to a lesser extent, for riboflavin, biotin and pantothenic acid. In most cases, the broiler industry's levels in the EU and the US 20 years ago were already 50 to 100% higher than the NRC's (1994) figures (Villamide and Fraga, 1999; Coelho, 2000). These levels varied if the cereal in the diet was wheat or corn or if the conditions where birds were raised were moderate or under heat stress. The last publication related to vitamin use in the US turkey industry was presented by Coelho (2000) 20 years ago. However, it already indicated similar trends of higher vitamin supplementation for turkeys.

Several studies evaluated levels that include 30 to 50% higher supplementation than those used commercially, except for vitamin E, which was supplemented 10 times more. In general, positive and significant responses in productivity were obtained (Hernández *et al.*, 2002; Castaing *et al.*, 2003, 2007; Pérez-Vendrell *et al.*, 2003; Moslehi *et al.*, 2004), especially under stress conditions.

In most of the experiments, increments in feed intake were observed together with the improvements in several parameters like carcass and breast meat yield, reduction in abdominal fat (Hernández *et al.*, 2002; Castaign *et al.*, 2003), oxidative stability of the meat (Pérez-Vendrell *et al.*, 2003; Pérez-Vendrell and Weber, 2007 and its vitamin content. Particularly, the content of thiamine, pantothenic acid, and vitamin E were enhanced in the meat (Castaign *et al.*, 2003; Pérez-Vendrell *et al.*, 2003). When the optimum vitamin (and mineral) premix also included the metabolite of vitamin D_3, 25-hydroxycholecalciferol (25OHD_3; commercial name Hy-D®), locomotor problems were reduced, and both the resistance and the bone ash content were increased, in both chickens and turkeys (Larroudé *et al.*, 2005; Pérez-Vendrell and Weber, 2007). Moslehi *et al.* (2004) compared 7 different levels of supplementation. They found that the optimum vitamin levels reduced mortality and feed conversion index in broilers and did not increase production costs any more than most other treatments. In fact, the highest price per kilogram of weight came from applying the NRC recommendations.

The most updated vitamin recommendations for turkeys in all feeding phases are presented in Table 6.6, 6.7 and 6.8. The situation is similar to that already described for broilers. Although, in practice, between 6 and 8 feeding phases are employed, these are grouped into 3. The levels recommended by all sources have increased somewhat, but especially during the finisher phase, due to the high value of the heavy and high meat yield toms raised to 20–21 weeks with body weights more elevated than 22 kg. Turkey diets have high inclusion levels of fats and oils; however, choline levels are lower than those used in broilers, and FEDNA recommendations are lower than other sources.

The most recent recommendations from broiler genetic selection companies are shown in Table 6.9. Cobb's vitamin levels remained like those observed 10 years ago (Cobb-Vantress, 2022). In contrast, the recommendations given by Ross increased slightly for all vitamins

Table 6.6 Recommended vitamin levels (IU or mg/kg air-dry feed) for turkeys during the starter and grower phases (0–8 weeks) by various sources

	Turkeys						
	Starter (0–8 weeks)						
	Unit/kg	Larbier and Lecquerq, 1992	NRC, 1994	Leeson and Summers, 2005	FEFANA, 2015	FEDNA, 2018	OVN™ (DSM Nutritional Products, 2022)
Vitamin A	IU	15,000	5,000	10,000	11,000–13,000	13,000	12,600–15,700
Vitamin D_3	IU	3,000	1,100	3,500	4,000–5,000	4,600	4,200–5,200
25OHD_3 (HyD)	mg	–	–	–	0.092	–	0.092
Vitamin E	mg	25	12	100	40–60	80	160–210
Vitamin K	mg	3	1.75–1.5	3	4–5	4	4.2–5.2
Vitamin B_1	mg	2.0	2.0	3.0	4.5–5.0	3.5	4.7–5.2
Vitamin B_2	mg	8	3.6–4	10	15–20	10	16–21
Vitamin B_6	mg	4.0	4.5	6.0	6–7	5.5	6.5–7.5
Vitamin B_{12}	mg	0.02	0.00	0.02	0.04–0.05	0.03	0.042–0.052
Niacin	mg	65	60	60	100–150	75	105–160
D-panthothenic acid	mg	20	10–9	18	30–35	20	32–37
Folic acid	mg	1.0	1.0	2.0	4–6	2.5	4.2–6.2
Biotin	mg	0.20	0.25–0.2	0.25	0.25–0.40	0.27	0.26–0.42
Vitamin C	mg	–	–	–	100–200	–	105–210
Choline	mg	800	1,600–1,400	800	1,000–1,200	400	1,050–1,250

Table 6.7 Recommended vitamin levels (IU or mg/kg air-dry feed) for turkeys during the grower (phase 2) and finisher phases (9–16 weeks) by various sources

	Turkeys						
	Grower (9–16 weeks)						
	Unit/kg	Larbier and Lecquerq, 1992	NRC, 1994	Leeson and Summers, 2005	FEFANA, 2015	FEDNA, 2018	OVN™ (DSM Nutritional Products, 2022)
Vitamin A	IU	10,000	5,000	10,000	10.000–12.000	10,000	10,500–12,600
Vitamin D_3	IU	2,000	1,100	3,500	3.000–5.000	4,100	3,200–5,200
$25OHD_3$ (HyD)	mg	–	–	–	0.092	–	0.092
Vitamin E	mg	20	10	100	30–50	45	65–85
Vitamin K	mg	2	1–0.75	3	3–4	3	3.2–4.2
Vitamin B_1	mg	1.0	2	3	3.0–5.0	2.5	3.2–5.2
Vitamin B_2	mg	4	3	10	10–15	7	11–16
Vitamin B_6	mg	3.0	3.5	6	5–7	4.0	5.5–7.5
Vitamin B_{12}	mg	0.01	0.03	0.02	0.03–0.04	0.02	0.032–0.042
Niacin	mg	50	50	60	80–100	70	85–105
D-panthothenic acid	mg	12	9	18	20–25	16	21–26
Folic acid	mg	1.0	0.8–0.7	2	2–3	1.5	2.1–3.1
Biotin	mg	0.10	0.125	0.25	0.25–0.30	0.25	0.26–0.32
Vitamin C	mg	–	–	–	100–200	–	105–210
Choline	mg	600	1100	800	500–1000	320	525–1,050

Table 6.8 Recommended vitamin levels (IU or mg/kg air-dry feed) for turkeys during the finisher phase (>16 weeks) by various sources

	Turkeys						
	Finisher (>16 weeks)						
	Unit/kg	Larbier and Lecquerq, 1992	NRC, 1994	Leeson and Summers, 2005	FEFANA, 2015	FEDNA, 2018	OVN™ (DSM Nutritional Products, 2022)
Vitamin A	IU	10,000	5,000	10,000	7.000–9.000	8,000	8,400–10,500
Vitamin D_3	IU	2,000	1,100	3,500	3.000–5.000	3,200	3,200–4,200
$25OHD_3$ (HyD)	mg	–	–	–	0.092	–	0.092
Vitamin E	mg	20	10	100	30–40	30	32–52
Vitamin K	mg	2	0.75–0.5	3	3–4	2	3.2–4.2
Vitamin B_1	mg	1.0	2.0	3.0	2.0–4.0	1.3	3.2–4.2
Vitamin B_2	mg	4	3	10	8–10	6	8.5–10.5
Vitamin B_6	mg	3.0	2–4	6.0	3–6	3.0	3.2–6.2
Vitamin B_{12}	mg	0.01	0.00	0.02	0.015–0.030	0.02	0.022–0.032
Niacin	mg	50	40	60	60–80	50	65–85
D-panthothenic acid	mg	12	9	18	15–20	14	16–21
Folic acid	mg	1.0	0.7	2.0	2.0–2.5	1.0	2.1–2.6
Biotin	mg	0.10	0.10	0.25	0.20–0.25	0.18	0.21–0.26
Vitamin C	mg	–	–	–	100–200	–	105–210
Choline	mg	600	950–800	800	400–600	230	420–630

Table 6.9 Current recommended vitamin levels (IU or mg/kg air-dry feed) for broiler starter, grower, and finishe dietary phases according to genetic line guidelines

	Broilers						
		Starter				Grower	
	Unit/kg	Hubbard, 2019	Aviagen, 2022	Cobb-Vantress, 2022	OVN™ (DSM Nutritional Products, 2022)	Hubbard, 2019	Aviagen, 2022
Vitamin A	IU	12,500	13,000	13,000	12,600–15,700	12,500	11,000
Vitamin D_3	IU	5,000	5,000	5,000	4,200–5,200	4,000	4,500
$25OHD_3$ (HyD)	mg	–	–	–	0.069	–	–
Vitamin E	mg	100	80	80	160–210	80	65
Vitamin K	mg	3	4	3	3.2–4.2	2	3.6
Vitamin B_1	mg	4	5	3	3.2–4.2	3	4
Vitamin B_2	mg	9	9	9	8.4–10.5	8	8
Vitamin B_6	mg	6	5	4	4.2–6.3	4	4
Vitamin B_{12}	mg	0.025	0.02	0.02	0.021–0.042	0.02	0.018
Niacin	mg	70	70	60	64–84	60	65
D-panthothenic acid	mg	15	25	15	16–21	12	20

		Finisher				
Cobb-Vantress, 2022	OVN™ (DSM Nutritional Products, 2022)	Hubbard, 2019	Aviagen, 2022	Cobb-Vantress, 2022	OVN™ (DSM Nutritional Products, 2022)	Broiler references
10,000	10,500–13,100	10,000	10,000	10,000	10,500–13,100	Savaris *et al.* (2021) 15,148 IU max weight gain 1–42 days; Shojadoost *et al.* (2021) 20,000 IU better immune response
5,000	4,200–5,200	4,000	4,000	5,000	4,200–5,200	Raza *et al.* (2021) 4,000 IU; Shojadoost *et al.* (2021) 5,000 IU better immune response
–	0.069	–	–	–	0.069	Sakkas *et al.* (2019) 0.075 mg
50	55–105	60	55	50	55–105	Niu *et al.* (2017) 200 mg; Desoky (2018); Choi *et al.* (2020); Khalifa *et al.* (2021) 100–300 mg; Ekunseitan *et al.* (2021) 400 mg immune response and performance
3	3.2–4.2	2	3.2	3	3.2–4.2	Guo *et al.* (2020) 4 mg
2	2.1–3.2	3	3	2	2.1–3.2	Wei *et al.* (2003) 2 mg performance
8	7.4–9.5	7	7	6	6.3–8.4	Jegede *et al.* (2018) 8 mg; Suckeveris *et al.* (2020) 49 mg performance 18 days
3	4.2–6.3	4	3	3	4.2–6.3	Jegede *et al.* (2018) 7 mg
0.015	0.021–0.032	0.02	0.016	0.015	0.021–0.032	Alisheilkhov *et al.* (2000) 0.035 mg; Suckeveris *et al.* (2020) 0.12 mg/kg performance 18 days
50	63–84	60	50	50	53–84	Nazir *et al.* (2017) 25 mg; Ahmadian *et al.* (2021) 33 mg; Suckeveris *et al.* (2020) 298 mg/kg performance 18 days
12	12.6–19	12	15	10	10.5–15.8	Latymer and Coates (1981) 25 mg; Suckeveris *et al.* (2020) 98 mg performance 18 days

Table 6.9 (continued)

	Broilers						
		Starter				Grower	
	Unit/kg	Hubbard, 2019	Aviagen, 2022	Cobb-Vantress, 2022	OVN™ (DSM Nutritional Products, 2022)	Hubbard, 2019	Aviagen, 2022
Folic acid	mg	2	2.5	2	2.1–2.6	2	2
Biotin	mg	0.4	0.35	0.15–0.2	0.26–0.42	0.4	0.28
Vitamin C	mg	200	–	–	105–210	200	–
Choline	mg	700	1,700	500	420–740	600	1,600

except for vitamin A, which is almost unchanged, and Vitamin D_3, which is reduced only in the grower phase to 4,500 IU/kg (Aviagen, 2022). However, the Ross recommendations are one of the highest levels observed.

The vitamin supplementation levels presently recommended by the turkey genetic companies (Table 6.10) indicate for several vitamins higher recommendations from Hybrid than from Aviagen. The levels recommended by Hybrid agree more with the other sources reviewed, and there is less variability in these values than observed 10 years ago.

As previously said, higher levels of vitamins have been used in practice for broilers and turkeys than those recommended by the NRC (1994) (Ward, 1993; Coelho and McNaughton, 1995; McKnight *et al.*, 1995a,b; Troescher and Coelho, 1996; Whitehead, 1996; Coelho, 2000).

In 2014, Nelson Ward conducted an industry survey covering approximately 65% of the US broiler industry to determine the vitamin supplementation levels used. The survey was repeated in 2022, accounting for over 90% of the US broiler industry. The results of both surveys are presented in Table 6.11. The vitamin supplementation level declines from starter to withdrawal diets. The main divergence between companies was observed in biotin, vitamin K, folic acid, vitamin D, and vitamin E levels. A narrower range of supplementation was observed for pantothenic acid riboflavin and vitamin A. The safety margins are greater for the fat-soluble vitamins (3–6 times the NRC 1994 values) than for the B group. However, the levels used for vitamin E and K are almost half of the current OVN value recommended in 2022. Similar variability had been reported by Villamide and Fraga (1999) in Spain, Coelho *et al.* (2000) in the US, and Maiorka *et al.* (2010a,b) in the Brazilian poultry industry. In many cases, what was considered a high level of vitamins in the 1990s and early 2000s for broilers (Villamide and Fraga, 1999; Coelho, 2000) is now regarded as moderate or even low.

Comparing 2014 and 2022, it is worth noting that supplementation of all vitamins has increased in the US broiler industry in the past 8 years in all grow-out phases. The increase

		Finisher				
Cobb-Vantress, 2022	OVN™ (DSM Nutritional Products, 2022)	Hubbard, 2019	Aviagen, 2022	Cobb-Vantress, 2022	OVN™ (DSM Nutritional Products, 2022)	Broiler references
2	2.1–2.6	2	1.8	1.5	2.1–2.6	Gouda *et al.* (2020) 1.5 mg in ovo feeding; Suckeveris *et al.* (2020) 6.9 mg performance 18 days
0.12–0.18	0.26–0.42	0.4	0.22	0.12–0.18	0.26–0.42	Sun *et al.* (2017) 1.5 mg
–	105–210	200	–	–	105–210	Jain *et al.* (2018) 120 mg; Tavakoli *et al.* (2021) 200 mg; Amer (2021) 200 mg performance and intestinal morphology
400	420–740	700	1,550	350	420–630	Igwe *et al.* (2015) 2,000 mg; De Lima *et al.* (2018) 1,042–1,228 mg

ranges from 25 to 30% in the starter, grower, and finisher phases. The main increments have been seen in the finisher phase, probably due to the increased yield of broilers and the high value of deboned meat and products' shelf life. In the withdrawal phase, the supplementation remained roughly unchanged.

The lower vitamin levels observed in the finisher and withdrawal diets still correspond to cost-saving strategies adopted by some poultry companies, sometimes reducing the inclusion rate of the vitamin premix and sometimes even withdrawing some vitamins (or even all) in the finisher feed or during the last 5 to 7 days before processing. The pressure to reduce feeding costs introduced this strategy in the 1990s. Withdrawing vitamin supplementation during the finisher phase still has controversial results.

Several studies, evaluating all its potential consequences, found no statistically significant effects on productivity, foot problems, or carcass quality from withdrawing the vitamin-mineral premix during 5 to 7 days and even up to 14 days (Christmas *et al.* 1995; Vo *et al.*, 1999; Khajali *et al.*, 2006; Moravej *et al.*, 2012; Mirshekar *et al.*, 2013). Deyhim and Teeter (1993) attributed the absence of statistical significance observed in these experiments to the small number of birds used, the scant replication of treatments, and the use of diets with animal by-product meal, which contains double the amount of B vitamins of soy. In their study, they found differences very close to significance for growth (–6%) and feed conversion index (–8%), carcass yield (+0.2 points), and breast meat percentage (+0.8 points) concerning the unsupplemented control group and they emphasized that these numerical differences are significant economically. Similar results were found in a subsequent experiment (Deyhim *et al.*, 1995, 1996).

Other authors observed increased locomotor problems, TD, and loss of uniformity in chicken carcasses (Skinner *et al.*, 1992; Mochamat *et al.*, 2017). These researchers suggested supplementation should continue if stress conditions prevail (heat and high humidity, mycotoxins, high

Table 6.10 Current recommended vitamin levels (IU or mg/kg air-dry feed) for turkey starter, grower, and finisher dietary phases according to genetic line guidelines

	Turkeys										
		Starter			Grower			Finisher			
	Unit/kg	Hendrix Genetics, 2016	Aviagen, 2020	OVN™ (DSM Nutritional Products, 2022)	Hendrix Genetics, 2016	Aviagen, 2020	OVN™ (DSM Nutritional Products, 2022)	Hendrix Genetics, 2016	Aviagen, 2020	OVN™ (DSM Nutritional Products, 2022)	Turkey references
Vitamin A	IU	12,500	11,000	12,600–15,700	11,500	8,000	10,500–12,600	9,500	6,000	8,400–10,500	Sklan *et al.* (1995) 17,400 IU immune response
Vitamin D_3	IU	5,000	4,000	4,200–5,200	5,000	3,000	3,200–5,200	4,800	3,000	3,200–4,200	Coelho (2000) 4,000–5,000 IU
25OHD_3 (HyD)	mg	–	–	0.092	–	–	0.092	–	–	0.092	Owens and Ledoux (2001) 0.090 mg; Shanmugasundaram *et al.* (2019) 0.101 mg immune response coccidiosis
Vitamin E	mg	100	100	160–210	70	30	65–85	50	25	32–52	Qureshi *et al.* (1993) 250 mg immunity; Heffels-Redmann *et al.* (2003) 400 mg up to 6 weeks' immunity and performance
Vitamin K	mg	5	4	4.2–5.2	3.5	2	3.2–4.2	3	2	3.2–4.2	-
Vitamin B_1	mg	4	4	4.7–5.2	2	2	3.2–5.2	2	1.5	3.2–4.2	-
Vitamin B_2	mg	15	10	16–21	10	5	11–16	8	4	8.5–10.5	Salami *et al.* (2016) 8 mg

Vitamin B_6	mg	6.5	7	6.5–7.5	4.5	4	5.5–7.5	3.5	2	3.2–6.2	Salami *et al.* (2016) 7 mg
Vitamin B_{12}	mg	0.03	0.03	0.042–0.052	0.025	0.02	0.032–0.042	0.02	0.02	0.022–0.032	-
Niacin	mg	85	80	105–160	70	55	85–105	55	45	65–85	Adebowale *et al.* (2018) 180 mg; Maurice *et al.* (1990a,b) 100–140 mg performance
D-panthothenic acid	mg	25	28	32–37	18	16	21–26	15	12	16–21	-
Folic acid	mg	3	4	4.2–6.2	2	1	2.1–3.1	1.5	1	2.1–2.6	-
Biotin	mg	0.27	0.3	0.26–0.42	0.2	0.2	0.26–0.32	0.165	0.1	0.21–0.26	Youssef *et al.* (2012) 2 mg
Vitamin C	mg	–	–	105–210	–	–	105–210	–	–	105–210	-
Choline	mg	600	1,600	1,050–1,250	550	600	525–1,050	490	400	420–630	Whitehead and Portsmouth (1989) 1,600 mg

Table 6.11 US broiler industry survey vitamin fortification levels (mg/kg) in the starter, grower, finisher and withdrawal diets (Ward, 2014, 2022)

		Broilers							
	Unit/kg	Starter		Grower		Finisher		Withdrawal	
		2014	2022	2014	2022	2014	2022	2014	2022
Vitamin A	IU	8,580	8,962	7,440	8,102	5,980	6,845	5,230	4,905
Vitamin D_3	IU	3,690	3,715	3,080	3,274	2,560	2,811	2,340	2,028
Vitamin E	mg	41	48	29	40	25	34	20	23
Vitamin K	mg	2.09	2.54	1.89	2.29	1.62	2.00	1.36	1.33
Vitamin B_1	mg	1.98	2.40	1.68	2.10	1.33	1.80	1.06	1.20
Vitamin B_2	mg	7.61	8.50	6.57	7.60	5.37	6.40	4.47	4.60
Vitamin B_6	mg	2.98	3.50	2.59	3.2	2.17	2.60	1.79	1.80
Vitamin B_{12}	mg	0.015	0.021	0.013	0.018	0.011	0.016	0.009	0.010
Niacin	mg	43	52	38	47	31	41	26	27
D-pantothenic acid	mg	12.0	13.5	10.0	12.7	9.0	10.8	7.0	7.6
Folic acid	mg	0.73	1.33	0.88	1.17	0.69	0.99	0.63	0.58
Biotin	mg	0.114	0.175	0.093	0.163	0.085	0.151	0.072	0.091

stocking density). For Whitehead (2002c), eliminating the vitamin premix from the withdrawal feed is inadvisable from the viewpoint of animal well-being since the birds would shortly have to deal with the stress of loading and transport to the slaughterhouse, and vitamins E and C are particularly important in counteracting this stress. Patel *et al.* (1997) confirmed the negative effects of the withdrawal of vitamins in 3 different strains, in particular withdrawal of riboflavin, which caused a linear reduction in growth.

Ferket and Qureshi (1992) removed the vitamin premix from 21 days of age, which resulted in a weight loss of 68 g at 43 days and a feed conversion index 7% higher than the broilers with vitamin supplementation. Furthermore, the broilers supplemented had lower mortality when heat stress was induced and exhibited more elevated IgG immunoglobulins.

Deyhim *et al.* (1994) also found a better immune status in broilers that received vitamin supplements until the end of the cycle under hot environmental conditions. Moreover, Deyhim and Teeter (1996), Patel *et al.* (1997), and Kavita *et al.* (1997) observed a 30–50% reduction in vitamin B_1 and B_2 breast content in unsupplemented birds, especially in thermal stress situations. Maiorka *et al.* (2002) withdrew supplementation during the last 4 and 7 days and obtained a worse feed conversion index and a tendency to reduce slaughtering weight. More recently, Abed *et al.* (2018) reported that the negative effects of the vitamin premix withdrawal in the finisher phase could include a reduction in both body weight gain and development of immunological organs in broilers fed wheat-based diets.

OPTIMUM VITAMIN NUTRITION FOR BROILERS AND TURKEYS

Fat-soluble vitamins

Vitamin A

Details about current vitamin A recommendations for broilers and turkeys, provided by institutional sources and genetic companies, can be found in Tables 6.3 to 6.10.

An evaluation conducted by Khoramabadi *et al.* (2014), using wheat-based diets with different vitamin A supplementation with or without xylanase inclusion, found no treatment effect on the feed intake of broilers at 21 days of age. However, vitamin A supplementation at 9,000 or 15,000 UI/kg of feed improved body weight gain and FCR compared with broilers fed diets without vitamin A supplementation. Moreover, supplementing vitamin A in a wheat-based diet may improve intestinal epithelium and reduce the erosive effect of non-starch polysaccharides, resulting in better nutrient digestibility.

Savaris *et al.* (2021) evaluated vitamin A supplementation and its interaction with the type of fat in the diet. The effects of 2 lipid sources and 5 different levels of vitamin A (0, 3,000, 6,000, 12,000, and 24,000 IU/kg of feed) were evaluated on live performance, blood parameters, fat and protein deposition, and bone growth of broilers at 21 and 42 days of age. There was no effect on lipid source, but it was possible to estimate a potential requirement for vitamin A, 15,585 IU/kg for 1 to 21 days, and 15,527 IU/kg or 15,148 IU/kg for 22 to 42 days of age (Figure 6.7).

Immunity

The optimum dosage of vitamin A for preventing or reducing certain pathologies is not the same for all diseases. In challenges with the Newcastle virus and other antigens, Seeman and Hazijah (1985) and Sklan *et al.* (1994, 1995) observed an increase in the proliferation of lymphocytes and macrophages and the numbers of specific antibodies up to a dosage of 18,999 IU/kg feed in both chickens and turkeys. In challenges by *E. coli*, the immune response improved

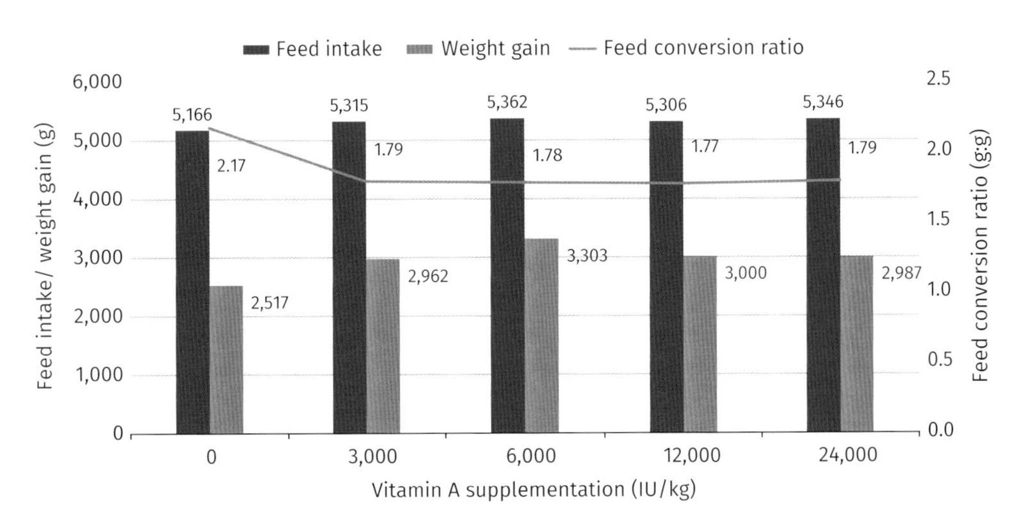

Figure 6.7 Performance results with different vitamin A levels supplementation (Savaris *et al.*, 2021)

until 60,000 IU/kg of vitamin A was reached (Tengerdy and Nockels, 1975; Tengerdy and Brown, 1977). Using 20,000 IU/kg, Sklan *et al.* (1995) observed a greater increase in specific antibodies in the face of the chicken pox and Newcastle disease viruses after vaccination than if they used 6,700 IU/kg. However, in other studies, an excess of vitamin A led to a depression of the humoral immune response (Friedman and Sklan, 1989; Friedman *et al.*, 1991; Lessard *et al.*, 1997; Shojadoost *et al.*, 2021).

A balance needs to be maintained between the fat-soluble vitamins since they compete to be absorbed, and an excess of one will alter the plasma concentrations of the others (Aburto and Britton, 1998a,b; Abawi and Sullivan, 1989). For example, in diets containing barely adequate levels of vitamins D_3, E, and K, an increase in dietary vitamin A of 4 to more times the recommended dose may cause a deficiency of one or more of the other fat-soluble vitamins. The effect could be more pronounced if one of the other fat-soluble vitamins is fed below recommendations (e.g., 20,000 IU/kg vitamin A and 500 IU/kg vitamin D_3). It can even affect the proper functioning of the lymphoid organs (She *et al.*, 1997). In turkeys, adding vitamin E (30–40 mg), vitamin A (12,000–15,000 IU), and a high level of oxidants (100–150 mEq O_2/kg) to the diet did not adversely affect health. Still, turkey vitamin E reserves diminished, as did the hepatic lactate-dehydrogenase activity. A certain predisposition to infection by the virus causing hemorrhagic enteritis was also observed (Zduńcyk *et al.*, 2002). Additionally, the existence of legal upper limits on the inclusion of vitamin A in feed in some countries has induced subsequent research directed at improving immunity by nutritional means to concentrate principally on vitamin E (Whitehead, 2002a).

Nevertheless, a synergy between vitamin A and E in birds suffering stress situations has been demonstrated using normal dosages of vitamin A. The use of 15,000 IU vitamin A in conjunction with 250 mg/kg vitamin E reduced serum and hepatic levels of MDA (a lipid oxidation indicator) in broilers subjected to thermal stress (Sahin *et al.*, 2001, 2002a,b).

Bone quality

Other investigations have studied the role of vitamin A in preventing skeletal development anomalies such as rickets and TD. But the responses obtained have been contradictory or not statistically significant (Waldenstedt, 2006). This appears to be related to the interactions between vitamins A and D_3 (Jensen *et al.*, 1983; Ballard and Edwards, 1988; Luo and Huang, 1991; Aburto *et al.*, 1998). An excess of vitamin A (more than 20,000 IU/kg) can impair the metabolism of vitamin D_3, reducing its availability when fed at low levels (500 IU/kg) (Aburto and Britton, 1998a,b). In this situation, reductions in growth and bone ash content have been observed, as well as the appearance of osteodystrophies such as rickets, especially in turkeys (Veltmann and Jensen, 1986; Britton, 1994; Aburto and Britton, 1998a,b) and swelling of the growth cartilage (Veltmann and Jensen, 1986; Tang *et al.*, 1984; Ruksomboonde and Sullivan, 1985). At vitamin A ranges likely encountered in usual commercial practice (8,000–15,000 IU/kg), Whitehead *et al.* (2004a) found no indication of interaction between dietary vitamins A and D_3 levels. Moreover, Luo and Huang (1991) showed that there are no significant effects with a high-Cl^- basal diet used to favor the appearance of TD or supplementation with 45,000 IU/kg of vitamin A on the growth performance and incidence of TD lesions in broilers. Supplementation with 1,000 IU/kg of vitamin D_3 improved the chick growth rate and reduced the incidence of TD significantly.

Meat quality

Excessive levels of vitamin A, in the range of 40,000 to 60,000 IU/kg, can have adverse effects on carcass pigmentation (Jensen *et al.*, 1981; Wyatt, 1991; Li *et al.*, 2008). Moreover, some studies have been conducted on the possible benefits of a higher dietary supplementation of vitamin A or ß-carotene to improve meat stability against oxidation, but they have proved to be much less effective than vitamin E (King *et al.*, 1995; Ruiz *et al.*, 1998). However, there appear to be no adverse interactions in this area such as those described above, as the use of 30,000 IU/kg vitamin A did not impair the antioxidant action of vitamin E at 150 ppm, although it had no protective effect against fat oxidation either (Bartov *et al.*, 1997).

Vitamin D

Details about current vitamin D recommendations for broilers and turkeys, provided by institutional sources and genetic companies, can be found in Tables 6.3 to 6.10.

The NRC (1994) indicated requirements of 200 IU/kg for broilers of any age, corresponding to 5 µg/kg (1 µg/kg = 40 IU/kg), based on studies from the 1960s and aimed at the prevention of rickets. Whitehead (2000a) already considered these figures very low, especially in the absence of ultraviolet light (in windowless sheds), which sometimes does not even fulfill their original objective. This conclusion was based on the following research. The earliest work reviewed by Pierson and Hester (1982), Ameenudin *et al.* (1985), and Soares and Lofton (1986) indicated that after testing levels up to 8,000 IU/kg, 400 IU/kg were the level considered to be the most appropriate to achieve optimum growth and calcification at any age.

Subsequently, minimum requirements for growth have been estimated at 275 IU/kg (6.9 µg/kg), 550 (13.8 µg/kg) to achieve the maximum concentration of vitamin D in blood plasma and 900 (22.6 µg/kg) to prevent rickets in (Edwards *et al.*, 1994; Edwards, 1999). Whitehead (1995b) compared the effects of using 400 or 800 IU/kg with the higher level increasing growth and the plasma concentration of $25OHD_3$. The same author indicated that 1,000–1,250 IU/kg will still not achieve total prevention of rickets nor maximum bone ash content (Whitehead, 2002b, 2003). Kasim and Edwards (2000) obtained a maximum bone ash level within this range, with 1,100 IU/kg of vitamin D. In the absence of UV light, these requirements, based on bone ash content and growth, would increase to 1,600 IU/kg (Edwards *et al.*, 1992a; Mitchell *et al.*, 1997a). Mireles (1997) compared 2,100 IU/kg in the starter phase and 1,300 IU/kg during development with levels 3 times higher, with no effects on production indices or the incidence of TD.

Applegate and Angel (2014) reported that historically, inclusion levels of vitamin D in the poultry industry exceed what is typically reported as the requirement by the NRC (1994). These higher levels are due to the uncertainty as to whether the birds are receiving an adequate quantity, given the possible presence of stress, mycotoxins, and poor absorption processes, which hamper the absorption and hydroxylation of vitamin D (Cook, 1988; Whitehead, 1991a; 2002a; Leeson and Summers, 2008; Rama-Rao *et al.*, 2007).

Allowances must also be made for the possible presence in the feed of antinutritional factors that interfere with vitamin D absorption and metabolism, as happens with raw soy and rice (Pierson and Hester, 1982) and high levels of fat in feed, which lower calcium retention and bone calcification due to soap formation.

Additional amounts should be included for the adverse effects on renal calcitriol synthesis of pathogens that affect the kidney, such as certain infectious bronchitis viruses or the Gumboro disease virus, even if they come from vaccines (Bains, 1999).

Furthermore, it has been found that the various sources of vitamin D_3 can show variable biopotency (40–134% in turkeys) (Yang *et al.*, 1973), although this variability currently appears to be lower in broilers (86–118%) (Kasim and Edwards, 2000).

Świątkiewicz *et al.* (2017) reviewed several recent studies evaluating the efficacy of different forms and levels of vitamin D_3 in the diets of broilers and laying hens. These authors concluded that to maximize mineral digestibility, performance and immunity indices, and bone health (as well as eggshell quality) is necessary to provide vitamin D at 3,000 IU/kg feed (Table 6.12).

In commercial practice, dietary inclusion levels in broiler diets range between 2,000 and 5,000 IU/kg (50–125 µg/kg) of feed. Scientific research has also investigated vitamin D levels far higher than those recommended by the NRC (1994). However, the current legal dietary limit in the EU and some other geographies (Canada, China) is 5,000 IU/kg feed. The basis for the establishment of the upper limit is rather ambiguous and does not consider bird genetic improvement. Previous studies indicated adverse effects on performance, bone ash, and renal calcification at levels of supplementation levels above 20,000 IU/kg (Baker *et al.*, 1998; Yarger *et al.*, 1995a,b; Browning and Cowieson, 2014).

The estimation of vitamin D_3 requirements can be affected by the evaluation criterion used and by genetics, chick quality, vitamin nutrition of breeders, and the calcium and phosphorus levels in the diet. These last factors present the most obvious interactions with vitamin D requirements (Huyghebaert *et al.*, 2005) and will be discussed in the section devoted to bone quality.

While most of the dietary levels for fast-growing broiler strains use levels between 4,000 and 5,000 IU/kg, slow-growing strains may require lower levels of supplementation. In China, there is a big market for slow-growing yellow-feathered chickens. The requirement for vitamin D_3 of Chinese yellow-feathered broilers (Ministry of Agriculture, People's Republic of China, 2004) was established at 1,000 IU/kg, although this is based on very few studies.

Recently, Jiang *et al.* (2015) tried to estimate the optimum vitamin D_3 supplementation for Lingnan yellow male broilers using 8 levels of vitamin D_3 (100; 200; 300; 400; 500; 600, and 700 IU/kg) for treatments 2 to 8 through the addition of vitamin D_3 to the basal mash diet which otherwise lacked detectable vitamin D_3. A linear effect of vitamin D_3 supplementation was observed on average daily gain, feed intake, tibial weight, and breaking strength. Quadratic responses were obtained on tibial length, bone density, bone ash, ash calcium and phosphorus content, and the calcium: phosphorus ratio (Figure 6.8). Adding vitamin D_3 improved meat color a* value and decreased birds' shear force and drip loss at 63 days. Considering bone characteristics and composition, the authors concluded that the vitamin D_3 requirements of Chinese, yellow-feathered broilers from 1 to 21 days for optimal tibial ash content were 464 IU/kg, 539 IU/kg from 22 to 42 days, and 500 IU/kg from 43 to 63 days. These yellow-feathered broilers only reach 3 kg after 63 days, and their FCR is over 2.3. Consequently, broilers with a higher growth rate and feed efficiency will need more vitamin D_3.

The vitamin status of chicks after hatching appears to be of importance to their subsequent vitamin D requirements (Hocking, 2007; Saunders-Blades and Korver, 2015), which is explained by the fact that at an early age, the 25-hydroxylase enzyme shows little activity (Rama-Rao *et al.*, 2007). Driver *et al.* (2006) used 250 and 2,000 IU/kg in the nutrition of broiler breeder hens. They found that the higher level reduced the incidence of TD in their offspring. However, only in the hatchings of the middle and final laying phases, possibly because when egg production fell, more vitamin D_3 was deposited in the eggs.

Atencio *et al.* (2005a) supplied breeders with vitamin D supplementation between 125 and 4,000 IU/kg and their offspring between 200 and 3,200 IU/kg. The broilers that received the higher level and that came from hens supplemented with 2,000–4,000 IU/kg were the ones that showed the best growth and highest bone ash. These results were repeated in other experiments (Atencio *et al.*, 2005b), and these chickens also responded better to low-calcium diets, exhibiting a lower degree of rickets and TD. Rama-Rao *et al.* (2007) state that if the hens' diet

Table 6.12 Effects of vitamin D_3 and $25OHD_3$ in broilers (adapted from Świątkiewicz *et al.*, 2017)

Vitamin D_3 form and dietary level	Study characteristics	Result	References
Cholecalciferol (2,000/1,500 IU/kg in starter/finisher diet) in 20, 40, 60, 80, 100% by $25OHD_3$	1–42 days. Growth performance, bone mineralization, Ca and P balance	Partial and complete substitution of $25OHD_3$ for cholecalciferol improved performance, Ca content in tibia, results of Ca and P balance.	Koreleski and Świątkiewicz (2005)
Cholecalciferol 200, 1,200, 2,400, 3,600 IU/kg of diet with suboptimal Ca and non-phytate P level	2–42 days. Growth performance, leg abnormality score, bone mineralization and mineral retention	High level cholecalciferol addition (3,600 IU/kg) positively affected growth performance, bone mineralization and mineral retention in chickens fed diet with low level of Ca (0.5%) and non-phytate P (0.25%).	Rama Rao *et al.* (2006)
Cholecalciferol 200, 1,500, 2,500, 3,500 IU/kg	1–42 days. Growth performance, bone mineralization, incidence tibial dyschondroplasia (TD), blood incidences	Positive effect of increased dietary cholecalciferol level (1,500–3,500 IU/kg) on performance, dressing percentage, breast yield, bone mineralization. Incidence and severity of TD was decreased in chickens fed diet with 3,500 IU cholecalciferol/kg.	Khan *et al.* (2010)
Cholecalciferol (2,000/1,600 IU/kg in starter/finisher diet) substituted by $25OHD_3$, $1,25(OH)_2D_3$ or $1\alpha OHD_3$	1–42 days. Growth performance, bone parameters and meat quality	No positive effects.	Garcia *et al.* (2013)
Cholecalciferol 200, 2,000, 4,000 IU/kg	1–42 days. Growth performance, tibia bone characteristics, development of footpad and hock dermatitis	Increased dietary level vitamin D_3 improved walking ability/tibia quality indices, reduced development footpad/hock dermatitis, without a clear effect on performance.	Sun *et al.* (2013)
Cholecalciferol (3,000 IU/kg) replaced by $25OHD_3$	1–35 days. Performance and immune response after liposaccharide (LPS) injection	Increased BWG, decreased the inflammatory gene IL-1β mRNA amounts in liver post-LPS injection.	Morris *et al.* (2014)
Cholecalciferol 3,500 IU/kg (C); (C) + 1,954 IU of $25OHD_3$, or (C) + 3,500 IU of cholecalciferol	1–42 days. Performance and bone characteristics	Lowest cholecalciferol supplementation (3,500 IU/kg) is enough to get better results on chicken performance and bone quality.	Colet *et al.* (2015)

Table 6.12 (continued)

Vitamin D_3 form and dietary level	Study characteristics	Result	References
Cholecalciferol 100–700 IU/kg	1–63 days. Slow-growing yellow feathered Chinese chickens. Performance, bone characteristics, meat quality and serum biochemistry	Increasing level vitamin D_3 produced linear positive response in growth performance, bone breaking strength, density and mineralization, serum cones Ca, P, $25OHD_3$, osteocalcin, calcitonin, meat quality indices.	Jiang *et al.* (2015)
Cholecalciferol (2,760 or 5,520 IU/kg), or $25OHD_3$ (5,520 IU/kg)	1–42 days Performance, breast muscle yield and protein synthesis	$25OHD_3$ produced better results on breast yield and protein synthesis rate.	Vignale *et al.* (2015)

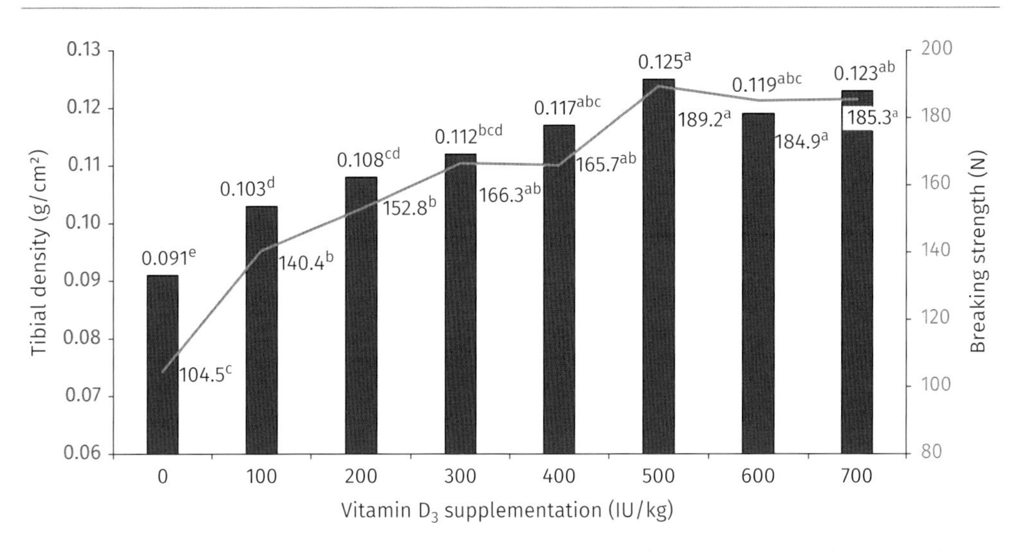

Figure 6.8 Effects of vitamin D_3 supplementation on bone characteristics for slow-growing male Chinese yellow-feathered chickens with approximately 1,950 kg of final average body weight at 63 days of age (31 g/day), values with no common superscripts differ significantly, $P < 0.05$ (Jiang *et al.*, 2015)

contains insufficient vitamin D, the progeny will have leg problems whatever their supplementation level.

Various studies have revealed the action of ultraviolet light emitted by fluorescent lighting but not by incandescent lamps. If a broiler diet contains 200 to 2,000 IU/kg of vitamin D_3 or is supplemented with 1,25$(OH)_2D_3$, there is a limited incidence of TD if the calcium level is correct. However, TD is observed even with 2,000 IU/kg without UV light. Where there is UV light, TD starts to decrease with 1,100 IU/kg of vitamin D_3 except in genetic strains with a high incidence of the problem, which requires much higher supplementation (Edwards *et al.*, 1992a, 1994; Elliot and Edwards, 1997; Mitchell *et al.*, 1997a; Leach and Monsonego-Ornan, 2007). TD is more prevalent with infections and vaccinations with the bronchitis virus (Mireles, 1997; Bains *et al.*, 1998; Huang *et al.*, 2019).

Clear differences in vitamin D metabolism have been found between genetic strains with a high or low predisposition to TD. Those prone to TD respond better to higher vitamin D levels (Shafey *et al.*, 1990; Whitehead, 1995b; Mitchell *et al.*, 1997b; Shirley *et al.*, 2003). During the first 2 weeks, the growth rate strongly affects the incidence of TD and requirements for vitamin D and its metabolites; both are reduced if birds gain weight more slowly in this period (Thorp, 1994; Elliot and Edwards, 1994; Leach and Monsonego-Ornan, 2007; Huang *et al.*, 2019).

The vitamin D requirements of turkeys are higher than chickens, although few studies have been published as with the other vitamins. The situation is somewhat different since turkeys may suffer from rickets due to vitamin D_3 deficiency in commercial production. The NRC (1994) recommended 1,100 IU/kg for all ages, but the North American industry has been using 4 and up to 5 times more on average in the starter phase (4,000–5,000 IU/kg) and 2 to 4 times more after that (Coelho, 2000).

Rickets sometimes appears in the field at these levels, whether due to the interference of mycotoxins with vitamin D_3 functions. This species is sensitive to poor absorption processes, interactions with other minerals, or imbalances of calcium and phosphorus (Riddell, 2000). Bar *et al.* (1987) reported 22 cases of rickets that occurred in Israel. There were clear signs of vitamin D_3 deficiency like low plasma concentrations of calcium, $25OHD_3$, and the calcium carrier protein. The diet included 4,440 IU/kg (111 µg/kg), i.e., 4 times the level indicated by the NRC (1994). They could not identify the cause, but, significantly, the process was not repeated on an experimental farm, even using the same feed that had caused the problems in the field. Rickets could be due to many nutritional imbalances; vitamin D deficiency is often cited but is not always the cause of the problem (Dinev, 2012a,b).

Rickets develops more readily in turkeys than in chickens and is more persistent (Perry *et al.*, 1991). For this reason, vitamin D_3 supplementation must always be raised above the level recommended by the NRC (1994). A minimum level of 1,200 IU/kg was already being recommended in 1980 (Whitehead and Portsmouth, 1989), and in 1991 Sanders and Edwards showed that at 21 days, no less than 2,700 IU/kg were required to prevent rickets induced by low-calcium diets and that continuing supplementation at this level improved growth up to 14 weeks of age.

Bone health

As previously indicated, the effects of vitamin D and its metabolites depend on calcium and phosphorus levels in the diet. If concentrations of these minerals are adequate, 1,400 to 2,000 IU/kg (35–50 µg/kg) of vitamin D_3 are enough to achieve good cortical bone quality (Waldenstedt, 2006), and 1,600 to 1,800 IU/kg (40–45 µg/kg) to prevent rickets completely (Ledwaba and Roberson, 2003). Although other researchers have assessed this requirement to be as high as 3,100 IU/kg (77.5 µg/kg) (Elliot and Edwards, 1997), 1,000 to 3,000 IU/kg (25–75 µg/kg) have generally been used to prevent TD, with poor results. Whitehead *et al.* (2004a) considered these levels ineffective, and according to their results, 125–250 µg/kg are needed for this purpose.

Baker *et al.* (1998) investigated the effects of various mineral combinations: adequate levels of calcium and phosphorus, marginal deficiency in calcium, and deficiency in both minerals. The latter 2 cases found the most effective level to be 1,600 mg/kg, or 8 times higher than the NRC (1994). Still, where diets were deficient in phosphorus, supplementation at 5,000 IU/kg, i.e., 25 times higher than the NRC, increased bone ash with no negative effect on growth or feed conversion. They deduced that chickens have a high tolerance to higher levels of vitamin D if their diets are deficient in phosphorus.

Subsequently, Rama-Rao *et al.* (2006) found that to improve ash content and feed conversion index with diets low in calcium and phosphorus, a minimum of 3,600 IU/kg of vitamin D_3 was needed in the starter phase. In another experiment using up to 9,600 IU/kg with diets both low and adequate in calcium and phosphorus, they observed improvements like those published by Whitehead *et al.* (2004a). However, the improvement in growth was not as great as that which can be achieved with the correct levels of calcium and phosphorus (Rama-Rao *et al.*, 2008).

It was already noticed that there are clear differences in vitamin D metabolism between genetic strains with a high or low predisposition to TD (Whitehead *et al.*, 1994). Overall, there are discrepancies in the literature on the efficacy of vitamin D in preventing TD. Most studies induced the condition with diets unbalanced in calcium and phosphorus and used between 1,000 and 3,000 IU/kg of vitamin D_3. Sometimes no positive responses were achieved under these conditions (Edwards, 1989; Rennie *et al.*, 1993; Mitchell *et al.*, 1997a; Whitehead, 2000b), but in other papers, significant reductions were obtained with 2,000–4,000 IU/kg vitamin D_3 (Edwards *et al.*, 1992a; Xu *et al.*, 1997; Fritts and Waldroup, 2003).

In some experiments, TD increased with the same dosages (Edwards *et al.*, 1992a). Edwards *et al.* (2002) suggested that when studying this vitamin, there are inevitably factors, nutritional or otherwise, which vary between experiments (and even more so in the field), which may give rise to results that are hard to explain as a group, but which appear clear within one experiment. Whitehead (1995b) stated that at available levels of 1.2% and 0.6% calcium and phosphorus, respectively, 1,000 mg/kg (25 μg/kg) vitamin D_3 are enough to prevent TD. Still, the same dose is ineffective if the diet has an unbalanced calcium: phosphorus ratio. Rama-Rao *et al.* (2007) indicated a fall of 1–2% in the incidence of TD for every additional 400 IU vitamin D_3 up to 2,800 IU/kg under these conditions. Saxena (1996) considered that under practical conditions and with normal mineral levels (calcium, 1%; available phosphorus 0.45%), broilers needed 4,000 IU/kg (20 times NRC) and demonstrated that the NRC levels increased the incidence of TD.

It has been confirmed that much higher vitamin D_3 levels are needed to eliminate TD or reduce it to minimum levels. McCormack *et al.* (2002) and Whitehead *et al.* (2004a) compared 200 to 10,000 IU/kg levels in starter feeds and found a linear increase in ash content and tibia strength, better growth, and total absence of TD. These improvements were achieved with 5,000 IU/kg in diets balanced in Ca and P but with 10,000 IU/kg if they were unbalanced. Whitehead *et al.* (2004b) concluded that current broiler vitamin D requirements to prevent TD might be above the maximum limit permitted in the EU (5,000 IU/kg or 125 μg/kg).

In turkeys Huff *et al.* (2000) investigated the effects of vitamin D_3 on preventing turkey osteomyelitis complex, a disease involving *E. coli* and *S. aureus*. Using turkeys immunodepleted with dexamethasone and inoculated with *E. coli* and 2,064 or 4,128 IU/l of drinking water, they found a reduction in losses, airsacculitis, and the lesions typical of this complex, and a lower heterophil: lymphocyte ratio.

As mentioned before, the EU legislation imposes a maximum of 5,000 IU/kg vitamin D_3 in feed for both broilers and turkeys (Directive 85/429), and some other countries have stricter standards with lower levels. This limit of 5,000 IU/kg vitamin D_3 does not appear to be justified as bird tolerance to high doses of vitamin D_3 seems very high, with a safety margin of at least 10 times the normal commercial supplementation.

Immune system modulation

Macrophages, dendritic cells, T and B lymphocytes express VDR and 1-α-hydroxylase, leading to local production of the active $1,25(OH)_2D_3$ from serum $25OHD_3$. The overall impact of vitamin D immune actions may be in establishing immune homeostasis and playing an immunomodulatory role (Rodriguez-Lecompte *et al.*, 2016).

Vitamin D supports the innate immune system and avoids the overactivation of the adaptive immune response and its potentially damaging effects. Vitamin D regulates the growth, maturation, and activity of immune cells, which are involved in recognizing and killing off pathogens. It acts on macrophages and dendritic cells, which plays an anti-inflammatory effect by downregulating activity (decreasing IL-8 and IL-1β expression). It also activates T-cells increasing the host cell ability to express TLR-2 and TLR-4, leading to an increase in antimicrobial peptide expression (cathelicidin), increasing IL-10 and decreasing IFN-γ, IL-2, and IL-17 expression, and increasing Treg cells (regulatory activity). As the use of the vitamin D_3 metabolite $25OHD_3$ has been proven to be more effective in modulating the immune system, more details are provided in the paragraph dealing with this metabolite.

Interactions with other nutrients and phytase

High levels of vitamins A and E may reduce the status of vitamin D (Aburto and Britton, 1998a,b). Vitamin A at very high dosages of 45,000 IU/kg was harmful to bone health, increasing TD. This negative effect was already apparent at practical levels, from 1,500 to 15,000 IU/kg, if the vitamin D concentration was low (500 IU/kg) since growth and bone ash were reduced and the requirement of vitamin D to overcome these negative effects was 3 times greater. The adverse effect of vitamin D, in contrast, took place at levels of 10,000 IU/kg.

The possible synergy between ascorbic acid and vitamin D_3 and its metabolite $1,25(OH)_2D_3$, based on the first role in the biosynthesis of the second, is dealt with in more detail in the section related to vitamin C. In some trials, the combination of vitamins C and D has reduced rickets (Roberson and Edwards, 1994) and increased bone strength (Weiser *et al.*, 1990; Lohakare *et al.*, 2005a). Whitehead and Keller (2003) indicate that combined supplementation of $1,25(OH)_2D_3$ and vitamin C has a potential application in reducing TD. However, Edwards (2000) and Waldenstedt (2006) considered that the current experiments offer no conclusive results. The metabolism of vitamin D_3 may also be related to electrolyte balance. In cases of acidosis, generally induced by an excess of chlorine and low sodium and potassium levels, calcitriol biosynthesis falls by 50% (Leeson and Summers, 2008).

The need for vitamin D_3 could be affected by including exogenous phytase since this enzyme improves the digestibility of phosphorus, calcium, trace minerals, and other nutrients. Recently an experiment conducted by Raza *et al.* (2021) demonstrated that supplementation of 4,000 IU/kg improved body weight gain and the FCR of broilers raised to 35 days. Still, this effect was bigger when 400 FTU/kg was included. The data indicates that the best tibia ash percentage was obtained with 8,000 IU/kg vitamin D_3 and additional phytase only slightly increased this value (Figure 6.9).

Vitamin D_3 metabolites

Research and commercial practice have focused on increasing supplies of vitamin D_3 by including some of its metabolites in feed. In particular, the discovery that vitamin D metabolites may reduce TD (Edwards, 1989; Rennie *et al.*, 1993) opened a new field of research on their role in broiler nutrition, bone, and health problems. The most studied and effective are:

- 25-hydroxycholecalciferol ($25OHD_3$) or calcidiol
- 1α-hydroxy calciferol ($1\alpha OHD_3$), a synthetic metabolite
- 1,25-dihydroxycholecalciferol ($1,25(OH)_2D_3$) or calcitriol

It must be noted that $25OHD_3$ is the only metabolite authorized as a feed additive and commercially available (as HyD®), having a safety margin very similar to that of vitamin D_3.

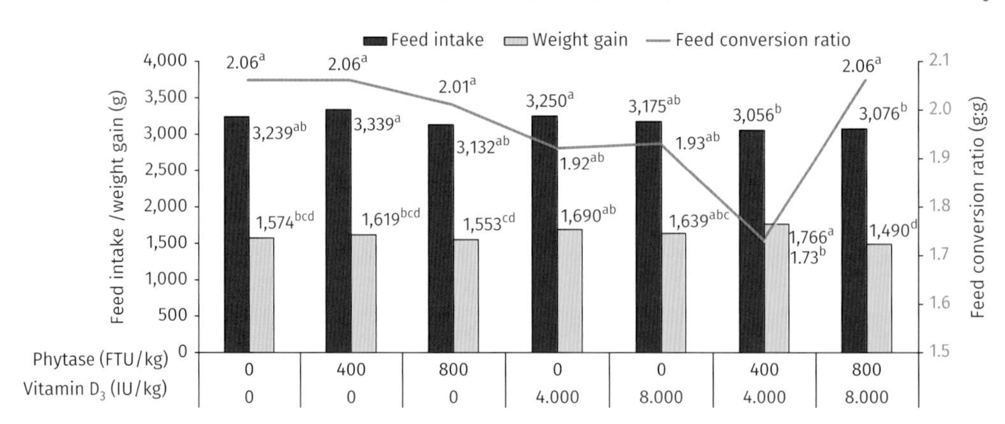

Figure 6.9 Effects of vitamin D_3 supplementation (0, 4,000, and 8,000 IU/kg) and exogenous phytase (400 FTU/kg or 800 FTU/kg) on broiler performance at 35 days, values with no common superscripts differ significantly, $P < 0.05$ (Raza *et al.*, 2021)

The other metabolites have, on the contrary, a very narrow safety margin and, as such, are much more harmful to being used by the feed industry.

25-hydroxycholecalciferol [25OHD$_3$] or calcidiol

The metabolite 25OHD$_3$ is, as said, the only metabolite of vitamin D$_3$ authorized as a feed additive. Its safety margin has been evaluated, as for vitamin D$_3$, at 10 times the recommended dose (Yarger *et al.*, 1995b; Rennie and Whitehead, 1996), giving it a safe application in feed. The 25OHD$_3$ is the first metabolite in the conversion of cholecalciferol to calcitriol, the active form, and it is the "storage" form of vitamin D$_3$ in the body (blood). In fact, the assessment of the vitamin D$_3$ nutritional status is made by measuring the 25OHD$_3$, in blood.

By feeding, it has been proven that the circulating level of this metabolite in the blood is increased more rapidly and efficiently than with a corresponding dose of vitamin D$_3$, mostly due to its more efficient absorption mechanism: 90% compared to 70–75% for vitamin D$_3$ (Bar *et al.*, 1980; Han *et al.*, 2016). Being fed to birds, the higher circulating level of 25OHD$_3$ makes available a higher amount of this metabolite to be used for both classical and non-classical functions of vitamin D$_3$, the former related to calcium and phosphorus metabolism and bone modeling and the latter those connected to immune modulation and cell differentiation, particularly muscle cell growth. The following sections will discuss the benefits of adding 25OHD$_3$ on live production parameters, muscle cell growth, bone health, immune response, and utilization of phytic phosphorus in broilers and turkeys.

Effects of 25OHD$_3$ on live production parameters

Recent experiments have confirmed the benefits of 25OHD$_3$ on production indices and product quality (Świątkiewicz *et al.*, 2017). Saunders-Blades and Korver (2006), using the 25OHD$_3$ commercial product (HyD®), increased the rate of growth at all ages, the carcass yield, and the weight and proportion of legs and breast. The plasma concentration of 25OHD$_3$ did not fall between 0 and 10 days of age, something observed with vitamin D$_3$; consequently, the mineral density and strength of the femur increased.

Santos and Soto-Salanova (2005) conducted a commercial trial in 4 sheds of 20,000 broilers to compare the effects of using 3,000 IU/kg of vitamin D$_3$ and additionally including 37.5 µg/kg of 25OHD$_3$. This last treatment improved live weight by 53 g (1.7%), reduced the feed conversion index by 56 g (–2.6%), increased bone strength by 9%, and reduced drip shrinkage in the carcass (20–40%) and breast (25–50%), with these improvements, they calculated a benefit of €60,000 for every million broilers reared under these conditions.

In some studies, vitamin D$_3$ has been totally replaced by 25OHD$_3$ with no adverse effects (Rennie and Whitehead, 1996). Mireles (1997) used 69 µg/kg without vitamin D supplementation from day 1 or day 7 of the chickens' life. In both cases, a greater reduction in TD was achieved than with the control diet, with adequate vitamin D supplements. In the first case, growth increased compared to the control diet, but the result was reversed in the second, suggesting that the first week of life is critical for response to this metabolite.

Lately, Sakkas *et al.* (2019) evaluated the vitamin D requirements of 2 modern growing modern broiler genotypes that offered calcium and phosphorus adequate diets. They used day-old chicks of each of the Ross 308 and 708 genotypes, randomly allocated to 1 of 4 dietary treatments: a diet offering low levels of vitamin D$_3$ (1,000 IU/kg), which aimed at inducing a marginal vitamin D deficiency, a diet offering a medium level of vitamin D$_3$, close to what is used in commercial practice (MD, 4,000 IU/kg), a diet offering high levels of vitamin D$_3$, which is above the EU legal limit of 5,000 IU/kg (7,000 IU/kg D$_3$) and a diet offering the medium level of vitamin D$_3$, where the majority of D$_3$ was substituted by 25OHD$_3$ (25MD; 1,000 IU/kg D$_3$ + 75 µg/kg

25OHD$_3$). The authors concluded that although dietary treatment effects on performance were absent, offering a diet that included 25OHD$_3$ led to consistent improvements in bone mineralization. These were seen as improvements in femur and tibia ash content (per unit of BW) and reduced black bone syndrome. At the end of the grower period (~25 days of age), the effects were more obvious than at the starter and finisher periods. The impact of the high vitamin D$_3$ on bone mineralization was less consistent and not statistically different from either the effects of MD or 25MD.

Parkinson and Cransberg (2004) reduced TD and increased body weight up to 14 days in a diet containing 69 µg/kg of 25OHD$_3$ on top of 3,000 IU/kg of vitamin D$_3$. Other experiments showed that 25OHD$_3$ was more effective than vitamin D$_3$ in increasing bone ash content and that the advantages of using this metabolite are greater when working with low dosages of vitamin D$_3$ (500 IU/kg), but that the benefits diminish at higher levels (2,000–4,000 IU/kg).

Philips *et al.* (2005) presented data with dosages between 35 and 560 µg/kg in diets without vitamin D supplementation. The weight of the broilers increased linearly up to 280 µg/kg, the feed conversion index fell by 5% from 140 µg/kg, and the plasma concentration of 25OHD$_3$ increased with the inclusion level. Koreleski and Świątkiewicz (2005) tried substituting 50–60% vitamin D$_3$ with equivalent quantities of 25OHD$_3$ and improved bone strength and production indices, while Papesova *et al.* (2008) reported synergy between vitamin D$_3$ and its metabolite, as they obtained better weight gain and calcium and phosphorus in the bones with 2,500 IU/kg vitamin D$_3$ and 50 µg/kg 25OHD$_3$ than with only 5,000 IU/kg vitamin D$_3$. It, therefore, seems possible, as Huyghebaert *et al.* (2005) indicated, that the 2 substances perform specific and complementary actions.

Effects of 25OHD$_3$ on muscle cells growth

It has been shown that improving vitamin D status in broiler chickens by feeding 25OHD$_3$ can result in enhanced BW gain (Bar *et al.*, 2003; Fritts and Waldroup, 2003), feed efficiency, and breast meat yield (Cantor and Bacon, 1978; Yarger *et al.*, 1995a) but information regarding the mechanism by which 25OHD$_3$ influences skeletal muscle hypertrophic growth is limited.

Berri *et al.* (2013) observed a positive effect of dietary 25OHD$_3$ on the expression of the VDR in skeletal muscle. This overexpression is likely the result of the increased availability of active 1,25(OH)$_2$D$_3$ at the level of the target tissues. It has also been observed the induction of 2 myogenic factors, MyoD and Pax7, suggests an increased proportion of proliferative satellite cells in the muscle of 7-day-old chicks fed 25OHD$_3$ instead of vitamin D$_3$. These observations are consistent with the last transition between embryonic and neonatal myosin heavy chain isoforms observed in the *Pectoralis major* (PM) muscle of 25OHD$_3$ chicks at day 7, with results obtained *in vitro*.

To further elucidate the mechanism, Hutton *et al.* (2014) investigated if an improvement of broiler chicken vitamin D status because of replacing a significant proportion of dietary vitamin D$_3$ with 25OHD$_3$ could influence satellite cells (SC) activity and skeletal muscle growth characteristics in 2 different skeletal muscles, the PM and *biceps femoris*. The control diet contained 5,000 IU/kg of vitamin D$_{3,}$ whereas the experimental diet contained 2,240 IU vitamin D$_3$/kg diet + 69 µg (2,760 IU) of 25OHD$_3$/kg of diet. Improved vitamin D status as a result of feeding 25OHD$_3$ increased the number of mitotically active (Pax7+; BrdU+) SC (P = 0.01) and tended to increase the density of Pax7+ SC (P = 0.07) in the PM muscles of broilers on d 21 and 35, respectively. Broiler chickens fed 25OHD$_3$ also tended to have greater Myf-5+ SC density (P = 0.09) on day 14, greater total nuclear density (P = 0.05) on d 28, and a greater muscle fiber cross-sectional area (P = 0.09) on day 49 in their PM muscles compared with control birds. Collectively, these results suggest that improvement of vitamin D status by replacing the majority of D$_3$ in the diet with

$25OHD_3$ can stimulate SC activity in the predominantly fast-twitch PM muscle and provide evidence toward understanding the mechanism behind previously observed increases in breast meat yield in $25OHD_3$-fed commercial broiler chickens.

Another study aimed to elucidate the mechanism by which $25OHD_3$ influences skeletal muscle hypertrophic growth was conducted by Vignale *et al.* (2015). More precisely, the objective was to determine the effect of $25OHD_3$ on broiler growth performances, breast meat yield, and protein synthesis and whether this effect is mediated through the rapamycin (mTOR) signaling pathway or not. mTOR is a protein kinase mostly controlling protein synthesis.

In this trial, a total of 1,440 1-day-old male Cobb 500 broilers have been used, and 4 vitamin D supplementation strategies have been confronted: (1) normal vitamin D_3 2,760 IU/kg feed for 42 days (control); (2) high level of vitamin D_3 5,520 IU/kg feed for 42 days (VD3); (3) a diet with 62.5 mg/kg of $25OHD_3$ on top of 5,520 IU/kg feed of vitamin D_3 for 42 days (HyD-42); (4) diet 3 up to day 21 and then the control feed from day 21 to day 42 (HyD-21). The HyD-42 group had significantly increased breast meat yield compared with the control and cholecalciferol supplemented groups. The HyD-21 group, however, had moderately increased the breast meat yield at 42 days compared with the control and VD3 groups, but the effect was not statistically discernable (P = 0.06). The HyD-42 group had an induced expression of vitamin D receptor (VDR) protein and a phosphorylated concentration of mTOR compared with the control group (P <0.05), as well as a significantly upregulated expression of mTOR and Rps6k genes. The upregulation of VDR expression *in vivo* (and *in vitro*) after $25OHD_3$ treatment indicates that VDR is capable of mediating a direct effect of $25OHD_3$. Moreover, this study also measured an increased concentration of muscle protein Fractional Synthesis Rate through $25OHD_3$ supplementation, indicating that protein synthesis machinery was switched on, additionally explaining the improved breast meat yield.

Effects of $25OHD_3$ on bone health

$25OHD_3$ is more effective in preventing TD than vitamin D_3 (Fritts and Waldroup, 2003). Although these supplements do not eliminate TD, they do reduce clinical lameness and improve production results in proportion to dosage (Ward, 1995; Yarger *et al.*, 1995a; Rennie and Whitehead, 1996) and time of administration (Mireles *et al.*, 1999; Mireles, 1997).

Early tests showed some variability (Edwards, 2000), and in stress-free situations, supplementation was often ineffective (Roberson, 1999). In more practical conditions, marked and progressive improvements have generally been achieved, reducing the incidence and severity of TD at $25OHD_3$ dosages between 70 and 250 µg/kg (Rennie and Whitehead, 1996; Mitchell *et al.*, 1997a; Zhang *et al.*, 1997).

The effect is clearer if diets are low in calcium or their calcium: phosphorus ratio is unbalanced (Rennie and Whitehead, 1996; Ledwaba and Roberson, 2003). Results also vary according to the birds' predisposition to TD (Mireles *et al.*, 1999): if this is low, the improvement is slight (Roberson *et al.*, 2005), but if it is very high, then higher doses are needed (Mitchell *et al.*, 1997a). Ledwaba and Roberson (2003) published a series of 5 experiments conceived to try and elucidate the question. In the diets designed to induce TD, supplementation with 40 or 70 µg/kg $25OHD_3$ reduced the incidence and severity of this disorder, especially if calcium was low and no vitamin D_3 was supplemented. However, the TD was decreased even more when 1,100 IU vitamin D_3 was added together with 10 µg/kg $25OHD_3$.

To prevent rickets in turkeys, vitamin D and its metabolites have been used (Perry *et al.*, 1991; Sanders and Edwards, 1991; Atia *et al.*, 1994; Owens and Ledoux, 2000; Owens and Ledoux, 2001). At 90 µg/kg, $25OHD_3$ produced effects like the inclusion of 3,650 IU/kg of vitamin D_3 in combination with phytases (Owens and Ledoux, 2001). However, the response depends on the strain of turkey and the type of diet (Mireles *et al.*, 1999), and these effects were small or non-existent when feed was very deficient in calcium and phosphorus (Owens and Ledoux, 2000).

There has been no appreciable effect of vitamin D_3 metabolites on TD in turkeys (Sanders and Edwards, 1991; Nixey, 2005). Although the characteristics of the lesion are like those in broilers, it is less severe, does not cause deformities or poor gait and tends to heal with age (Whitehead, 2005). Unlike in broilers, TD in turkeys appears to have no relation to calcium or phosphorus levels (Hocking *et al.*, 2002). Nixey (2005) proposed that the etiology of this disorder may be different in chickens and turkeys. In the latter, it may be due to the lack of some trace element at an early age, possibly copper, given that TD may be induced by the *Fusarium* fungus, and some fungicides respond well to treatments with copper. Pines *et al.* (2005) indicate that the 2 species show differences in the regulation of angiogenesis in the growth plate, which means that TD prevention would have to be accomplished by different strategies.

Other papers indicate the existence of a relationship between the vitamin nutrition of breeders and the efficacy of $25OHD_3$ in their offspring (Atencio *et al.*, 2005b,c; Saunders-Blades and Korver, 2015). The initial work combined vitamin D_3 up to 2,000 IU/kg and 12.5 µg/kg $25OHD_3$ in the feed of breeder hens, and subsequently, the chicks received 27.5 µg/kg $25OHD_3$. Live weight and tibia ash content increased by over 20% if the hens had received supplementation very low in vitamin D_3 (125 IU/kg). Still, with 500 IU/kg, there was already little difference from the controls. The best results in all evaluated parameters were achieved if the breeders received 2,000 IU/kg vitamin D_3 in feed. Rickets and TD increased in broilers whose mothers received only 3.1 or 12.5 µg/kg $25OHD_3$, which indicates that these quantities are severely deficient (Atencio *et al.*, 2005b).

Another series of experiments with higher levels of $25OHD_3$ and vitamin D_3 (Atencio *et al.*, 2005c) revealed that chickens that received unbalanced calcium and phosphorus diets supplemented with 40 µg/kg $25OHD_3$ had a lower incidence of TD and rickets, gained more weight and had a higher level of calcium in bones and serum. These advantages were also achieved by including 4,000 IU/kg in the breeder's feed. Still, the best results came from broilers whose mothers received this high level of vitamin D and an adequate calcium level, including 40 µg/kg $25OHD_3$.

Bozkurt *et al.* (2017) showed that enhancing vitamin D status by $25OHD_3$ supplementation, alone or in combination with calcium and available phosphorus (aP), may improve sternum structure and mineral accretion.

$25OHD_3$ also seems to be useful in preventing another bone problem in broilers known as black bone syndrome (BBS), which is characterized by the blackening of the leg bones, more usually in the tibia but sometimes also in the femur of the broiler, and with the discoloration extending to the adjacent meat, especially after cooking (Lyon and Lyon, 2002; Saunders-Blades and Korver, 2006). This problem now appears more widespread than previously appreciated. It seems to be linked with the diffusion of bone marrow from the medulla through the bone structure, particularly when deboned cuts are frozen. Cooking can exacerbate the defect, as well as blacken the marrow. The problem is already impacting the market (Kam *et al.*, 2007).

The cause of BBS appears to be a disruption of intramembranous ossification because the structure of the cortical bone is more porous in modern broilers (Rath *et al.*, 2000; Whitehead, 2005). Saunders-Blades and Korver (2006) demonstrated that improving bone mineral density and including $25OHD_3$ in the feed can reduce marrow diffusion and discoloration and enhance acceptance of poultry meat by consumers.

Effects of 25OHD$_3$ on the immune response

Many studies on humans and laboratory animals link vitamin D$_3$ with immune status (DeLuca and Zierold, 1998; Lal *et al.*, 1999; Huff *et al.*, 2000; Praslickova *et al.*, 2008; Shojadoost *et al.*, 2021). At the same time, there is still little information on birds. The results point to a relationship with cell-meditated immunity since it is needed for the maturation and functioning of macrophages, especially in the first 2 weeks of a chicken's life (Garlich *et al.*, 1992; Rama-Rao *et al.*, 2007; Saunders-Blades and Korver, 2008).

Aslam *et al.* (1998) found a reduced immune response at the cellular level and a reduction in thymus weight if there was a vitamin D$_3$ deficiency, which did not appear with supplementation of 800 IU/kg. Still, Fritts and Waldroup (2004) found no improvement with 2,000 and 4,000 IU/kg of vitamin D$_3$. Praslickova *et al.* (2008) demonstrated that resistance to Marek's disease is connected to a marker in the vitamin D receptor gene, with the vitamin inducing a change in T lymphocyte response favorable to combating this virus.

These actions seem to be more effective if the metabolite 25OHD$_3$ is used. Saunders-Blades and Korver (2008) infected chicks for 1 and 4 days with *E. coli* and *Salmonella typhimurium* from hens that received 2,760 IU vitamin D$_3$ or 60 µg/kg 25OHD$_3$ in their diet. They observed that the latter treatment improved the maturation of the macrophages and increased the proportion of bacteria destroyed by the phagocytes.

Positive effects of using the metabolite 25OHD$_3$ on humoral immunity in the face of certain pathologies have also been published. Mireles (1997) reported a better immune response after vaccinating against Newcastle disease with the inclusion of 69 µg/kg of this metabolite in feed, and other experiments established an increase in the titer of infectious bronchitis antibodies and a general increase in the titers of antibodies in the presence of coccidiosis (Mireles *et al.*, 1999).

Gill (2002) published the results of a trial in which broilers were infected with the virus causing malabsorption syndrome. Adding 37.5 µg/kg 25OHD$_3$ to the feed and greatly increasing the concentration of this metabolite in blood plasma also reduced mortality and resulted in better growth and feed conversion than 1,500 or 2,200 IU/kg of vitamin D$_3$. Saunders-Blades and Korver (2015) concluded that maternal supplementation with 25OHD$_3$ increased *in vitro* chick immunity toward *E. coli*.

Morris and Selvaraj (2014) conducted *in vitro* trials in chicken monocytes and a chicken macrophage cell line (HD11) to study the effects of supplementing with 25OHD$_3$ on nitrite production and mRNA amounts of interleukin (IL)-β, IL-10, 1α-hydroxylase and 24-hydroxylase post-lipopolysaccharide (LPS) challenge. Results indicated that 25OHD$_3$ improved all aspects investigated. Further, they demonstrated the capability of HD11 cells for local production of active vitamin D by the induction of the 1α-hydroxylase enzyme after an LPS challenge.

Three experiments were conducted to study the effects of 25OHD$_3$ supplementation on BW gain, IL-1β, and 1α-hydroxylase mRNA expression in different organs of broiler chickens following a lipopolysaccharide (LPS) injection (Morris *et al.*, 2015). In experiments 1 and 3, 3,000 IU/kg vitamin D$_3$ or 69 µg/kg 25OHD$_3$ were used. In experiment 2, 6.25, 25, and 50 µg/kg of feed of 25OHD$_3$ or vitamin D$_3$ at 250 IU/kg of feed was used. Overall, 25OHD$_3$ supplementation improved growth performance and decreased inflammatory gene IL-1β mRNA amounts in the liver post-LPS injection. In particular, in experiment 2, improvements have been obtained with 2 and 50 µg/kg of 25OHD$_3$ but not with the low dose.

Vazquez *et al.* (2018) evaluated the effects on performance and immunity of 25OHD$_3$ to broiler diets in a 2 × 2 factorial design with 2 dosages of vitamin D$_3$ (200 and 5,000 IU/kg) and 2 levels of 25OHD$_3$ (0 and 69 mg/kg). The results showed significantly increased growth and tibia ash ($P < 0.05$) in the birds fed 5,000 IU vitamin D$_3$/kg + 25OHD$_3$. Additionally, the cellular immune response increased significantly ($P < 0.05$) in both treatments with added 25OHD$_3$.

In turkeys, Huff *et al.* (2002) investigating the effects of the inclusion in the feed of 99 µg/kg 25OHD$_3$ or 10 µg/kg 1,25OHD$_3$, were able to suppress colibacillosis lesions. However, 1,25OHD$_3$ resulted in higher mortality and lower live weight in the turkeys than 25OHD$_3$.

Effects of 25OHD$_3$ on the utilization of phytic phosphorus

Interest in the metabolites of vitamin D$_3$ has also increased in the US, Europe, and other parts of the world due to strict regulations on using bedding as fertilizer according to its phosphorus concentration. The vitamin D metabolites liberate phytic phosphorus used separately or with phytases (McNaughton and Murray, 1990; Soares *et al.*, 1995), which reduces the inorganic phosphorus supply in the diet and its excretion. According to Applegate *et al.* (2003), the likely mechanism is not a direct influence on the activity of intestinal phytases but rather an intestinal calcium absorption, reducing its chelation with the phytin molecule and its solubility, which would make it more accessible to phytase action.

In the 1990s, several trials were conducted to assess the possibilities of reducing the available phosphorus in the diet by using different vitamin D metabolites in feed. Using 1,25(OH)$_2$D$_3$ at 5 µg/kg allowed the available phosphorus to be reduced by 0.030–0.059% (Edwards, 1993, 1995b, 1999); with 1αOHD$_3$, at 5 µg/kg, between 0.025 and 0.03%, and 0.06% at 20 µg/kg (Biehl and Baker, 1997); and with 25OHD$_3$ there were no significant effects at 5 µg/kg (Edwards, 1995a,b, 1999), but with 35–70 µg/kg a reduction of 0.03–0.035% was demonstrated (Angel *et al.*, 2001a,b).

Angel *et al.* (2001a) conducted 2 experiments directed at improving phosphorus utilization by broilers housed in cages and receiving a diet with low levels of calcium and phosphorus, comparing the efficacy of 200–500 units of phytase, 35–70 µg/kg 25OHD$_3$, 3% citric acid and all combinations thereof. The percentage of bone ash improved in all cases. The combination of the 3 additives saved 0.116–0.126% of available phosphorus in the formulation 25OHD$_3$, 0.037%, and 500 units of phytase 0.065%. The 2 last treatments combined reduced requirements for available phosphorus by between 0.067% and 0.092%.

Subsequently, in another trial, 3 flocks of broilers were reared on bedding and fed lower in phosphorus than the NRC recommendations. Angel *et al.* (2005, 2006) demonstrated that it was possible to reduce the cumulative available phosphorus consumption per bird from 18.2 to 8.65–11 g at the same time as reducing the total content of phosphorus in the bedding by 60% with the use of 25OHD$_3$, and the quantity of soluble phosphorus by another 60%. Despite using diets low in phosphorus, these treatments influenced neither growth nor bone fractures at slaughter.

More clarification is needed on the specific conditions under which available phosphorus can be reduced and by how much in the context of supplementation with 25OHD$_3$ and/or phytases since there are some contradictory data. Ledwaba and Robeson (2003) found a linear increase in the retention of phytic phosphorus in low-calcium diets when adding 27.5 µg/kg 25OHD$_3$ and incremental dosages of vitamin D$_3$ (up to 2,800 IU/kg). This retention also increased with higher 25OHD$_3$ supplementation levels (40 and 70 µg/kg) in diets lower in vitamin D$_3$, but the difference diminished when higher vitamin D concentrations were used.

With caged broilers that received no vitamin D supplementation, Philips *et al.* (2005) tried levels of 25OHD$_3$ between 35 and 560 µg/kg. They found improvements in phosphorus utilization of 49 and 51% at the highest dosages of 25OHD$_3$. Calcium utilization improved by around 40% with all levels of 25OHD$_3$ supplementation.

Subsequently, Philips *et al.* (2008) assessed the effects of 69 µg/kg $25OHD_3$ and 750 units of phytase in diets with 3 levels of vitamin D (200, 500, and 2,000 IU/kg). With the lower vitamin D concentrations, the combination of phytase and $25OHD_3$ improved production results, tibia bone strength, ash content, and the utilization of calcium and phosphorus. Phosphorous utilization improved even further if the feed included 2,000 IU vitamin D, in contrast to the experiments of Ledwaba and Robeson (2003).

Angel *et al.* (2001b) reported 3 experiments in cages with turkeys with the same objectives as broilers. When used alone at dosages from 35 to 105 mg/kg provided aP savings of 0.033 to 0.046 g/kg and from 0.032 to 0.049 when fed at 35 to 70 mg/kg. When 35 or 70 mg/kg of $25OHD_3$ were associated with 600 or 300 units of phytase, the aP savings were 0.106 and 0.074 g/kg.

In another trial with 2 flocks of turkeys reared in floor pens, the same researchers compared the efficacy of 600 units of phytase and/or 50 µg/kg $25OHD_3$ in diets with the phosphate levels recommended by the NRC (1994) or the higher levels used by the North American industry. They estimated savings of 0.03% available phosphorus, practically the same as with the cages trials. Phytase and $25OHD_3$ reduced the concentration of phosphorus in bedding when used both in combination and separately. Growth was not affected by these treatments.

Bar *et al.* (2003), however, conducted a series of experiments with different levels of $25OHD_3$, concluding that the benefits were more evident in diets low in calcium or phosphorus but only up to 20–30 µg/kg and that at 75 µg/kg there was a decline in growth. Nevertheless, the results from different trials are not comparable. In most of them, the vitamin D_3 supplements were below 3,000 IU/kg in the starter phase when the current recommendation is 4,000–5,000 IU/kg.

Some studies on broilers and turkeys have revealed that supplementation with 69 µg/kg $25OHD_3$ was linked to using a higher level of all the vitamins in general. With this treatment, which included 90 µg/kg $25OHD_3$ up to week 6 and 50 µg/kg subsequently, Philips *et al.* (2005) were able to delay locomotor problems in turkeys until 15 weeks of age and improve productivity and breast yield compared to the standard vitamin levels in France, with or without the addition of $25OHD_3$.

Pérez-Vendrell and Weber (2007) conducted a similar trial with broilers using 62.5 µg/kg $25OHD_3$ throughout the cycle, compared to the vitamin levels typically used in Spain and without supplementing $25OHD_3$. Vitamin D_3 (2,500 IU/kg) was used throughout both treatments. The higher vitamin levels, combined with the $25OHD_3$ supplementation, resulted in better growth and FCR in the starter phase, better meat quality, higher breast proportion, and improved lipid oxidative stability.

1,25 dihydroxycholecalciferol [$1,25(OH)_2D_3$] or calcitriol

Initially, all the studies focused on evaluating the efficacy of this metabolite as it is the hormonal form since its concentration in the blood plasma of birds with TD is low (Vaiano *et al.*, 1994). It has often been confirmed that supplementing it in feed can improve calcium and phosphorus metabolism (Snow *et al.*, 2004) and increase bone ash content (Edwards, 2000).

Using 5 µg/kg of calcitriol reduces TD significantly (Rennie and Whitehead, 1996; Roberson and Edwards, 1996; Mitchell *et al.*, 1997b); at 10 µg/kg, the effect disappears completely (Edwards *et al.*, 1992a). It was originally suggested that this supplementation be limited to the first weeks of life, given that at this age, chicks have a lower capacity for producing it (Vaiano *et al.*, 1994). Still, this strategy was ineffective in reducing TD (Rennie *et al.*, 1993). This metabolite has proven much more effective than vitamin D levels, even 10 times higher (2,000 IU/kg) than those recommended in 1994 by the NRC (Rennie, 1994; Elliot and Edwards, 1997; Świątkiewicz *et al.*, 2017).

Using $1,25(OH)_2D_3$ reduces TD with a dosage-dependent response (Edwards, 1989, 1990; Rennie *et al.*, 1993), but its efficacy, as with other metabolites, depends on the incidence of this disorder (Rennie and Whitehead, 1996). In genetic strains with a higher predisposition to TD, higher supplementation is needed, from 10 to 15 µg/kg (Thorp *et al.*, 1993; Whitehead, 1995a; Mitchell *et al.*, 1997b; Xu *et al.*, 1997). A practical strategy could be to combine it with ascorbic acid since there appears to be synergy between the 2 substances (Völker and Fenster, 1991; Rennie, 1995). This aspect is discussed in more detail in the section on vitamin C.

Besides its high cost and limited availability, the major constraint to using 1,25$(OH)_2D_3$ is its toxic effects. Since endogenous production of 1,25$(OH)_2D_3$ from 25OHD_3 is tightly regulated according to metabolic needs, the provision of dietary 1,25$(OH)_2D_3$ has the potential to override normal production and produce unwanted effects.

The calcitriol form extracted from *Solanum glaucophyllum* (Bachmann *et al.*, 2013) is in glycoside form: the presence of the glycosidic bond, to be cleaved in the intestine, can mitigate potential toxicity. The safety margin remains extremely narrow and critical for feed application. Toxicity can be worsened by high calcium diets (> 0.9–1% Ca): hypercalcemia and reduced growth have been observed already at 5 µg/kg and are marked at 10 µg/kg (Elliot *et al.*, 1995; Rennie *et al.*, 1995; Roberson and Edwards, 1996; Elliot and Edwards, 1997; Mitchell *et al.*, 1997a). However, if calcium levels are low or the calcium: phosphorus ratio is unbalanced, the birds' tolerance is higher, and their growth is not impaired (Edwards *et al.*, 1992a; Rennie *et al.*, 1993, 1995; Whitehead, 1995a; Roberson and Edwards, 1996). The safe limit appears to be 3.5 µg/kg at normal calcium concentrations. Still, even under these conditions, the safety margin between effective and toxic dosages is narrow, making its commercial application problematic (Whitehead, 2000a).

1α-hydroxycholecalciferol (1αOHD_3)

1α-hydroxycholecalciferol (1αOHD_3) is a synthetic form, not a natural metabolite of vitamin D_3. Nevertheless, it is hydroxylated rapidly to 1,25$(OH)_2D_3$: its metabolic activity thus seems to be largely, if not exclusively, attributable to its conversion to 1,25$(OH)_2D_3$. It promotes a faster absorption and mobilization of calcium (Edwards *et al.*, 2002) and appears to be about as effective as 1,25$(OH)_2D_3$.

In experiments with vitamin D_3 levels between 0 and 1,600 IU/kg (40 µg/kg) and dosages of 1αOHD_3 from 0.635 to 10 µg/kg, the bioavailability of the metabolite was 1.9 to 21.2 times higher than that of vitamin D_3 (Kasim and Edwards, 2000). The percentage of bone ash was increased by 35% with the maximum level of vitamin D_3 and by 40% with 10 µg/kg 1αOHD_3.

Rennie and Whitehead (1996) reduced TD at 21 days to minimal figures (5%) using this metabolite. Biehl and Baker (1997) observed no negative effects when using up to 40 µg/kg in a low-calcium diet. Edwards *et al.* (2004) used 5–10 µg/kg 1αOHD_3 and obtained good results for weight at 16 days. Bone ash, and plasma calcium concentration, both in high- and low-calcium diets still observed rickets where the calcium level was low. On the other hand, at a normal calcium level, 20 µg/kg of 1αOHD_3 produced hypercalcemia and reduced growth, indicating that calcium level must be reduced when this metabolite is used.

Compared with 1,25$(OH)_2D_3$, 1αOHD_3 improves phosphorus retention synergistically or additively with phytases (Edwards, 1993; Mitchell and Edwards, 1996; Biehl and Baker, 1997). This allows calcium and phosphorus to be saved in diets (Roberson and Edwards, 1994; Biehl *et al.*, 1995). Driver *et al.* (2005) evaluated the efficacy of 5 µg/kg 1αOHD_3 and 1,000 units of phytase in diets very low in calcium and phosphorus during the starter (0.60% calcium and 0.47% total phosphorus) and grower (0.30% calcium and 0.37% total phosphorus) phases. The birds that had not been given the supplements presented many cases of twisted legs (*valgus-varus*), and those supplemented showed growth rates and leg conditions like those from diets with normal calcium and phosphorus. However, there were differences between the 2 experiments for unknown reasons, which the authors attributed to a different quality of the day-old chicks. This influence has been demonstrated by Shim *et al.* (2008), who found that the age of breeders had a significant effect on the presence of rickets when feeding their offspring with low-phosphorus diets. Using 5 µg/kg of 1αOHD$_3$ increased the live weight of broilers, but this increase was lower in those originating from young hens. This metabolite reduced mortality and rickets caused by low phosphorus and increased phosphorus retention and bone ash content.

Recently, San Martin Diaz (2019) and Warren *et al.* (2020) confirmed all these effects in a study on Ross 708 male broiler chicks to evaluate a supplementation of 5 µg 1αOHD$_3$/kg in starter and grower broiler diets containing phytase with different calcium inclusion levels (0.80, 0.95, 1.10, 1.25, and 1.40%). These authors concluded that the inclusion of 1αOHD$_3$ was beneficial to increasing calcium absorption and bone mineralization during the starter phase only when calcium levels were below 0.95%. No significant effects of 1αOHD$_3$ were observed in the grower phase when the starter diet contained 1αOHD$_3$. The authors observed that dietary calcium levels should be reduced to avoid potential calcium toxicity or antagonism while using 1αOHD$_3$ during the starter and grower phases.

Finally, the safety margin of this metabolite is, as observed for 1,25(OH)$_2$D$_3$, quite low. For example, Pesti and Shivaprasad (2010) carried out an experiment in which a control diet was used containing 1,100 IU D$_3$/kg. This was then supplemented with 0, 5, 15, or 25 µg 1αOHD$_3$/kg, and the diets were fed to male and female broilers from day-old to 42 days. The authors only emphasized growth impairment at 25 µg 1αOHD$_3$/kg based on the significance of the difference between treatments. However, impairment of growth, and certainly uniformity, was apparent already with 15 µg 1αOHD$_3$/kg. Potentially toxic effects of this concentration were confirmed by increased kidney mineralization observed in histology samples. It might even be considered surprising that the diet supplemented with 5 µg/kg did not give better growth than the basal diet containing only 1,100 IU/kg, a concentration that might be considered inadequate. Perhaps even 5 µg 1αOHD$_3$/kg was thus having an inhibiting effect on performance. The narrow safety margin did not allow this metabolite to be so far as authorized as a feed additive in animal nutrition.

Vitamin E

Details about current vitamin E recommendations for broilers and turkeys, provided by institutional sources and genetic companies, can be found in Tables 6.3 to 6.10.

The relative biological activity of vitamin E is expressed in international units (IU), 1 IU corresponding to the activity of 1 mg of (all-rac)-α-tocopheryl acetate. The NRC (1994) minimum requirement to prevent encephalomalacia and exudative diathesis, the typical signs of vitamin E deficiency, was set at 10 mg/kg based on studies from the 1950s and 1960s. But already by the 1990s it was common to fortify broiler and turkey diets with 20–30 mg/kg (Ward, 1993). It has been calculated that broiler selected for increased lean tissue has requirements 50% higher using the vitamin E plasma concentration as a criterion (Whitehead, 1991b).

The use of much higher levels (150–400 ppm) has not led to improvements in production indicators on a practical level, either in chickens (Blum *et al.*, 1990; Bartov and Frigg, 1992; Macklin *et al.*, 2000; Coetzee and Hoffman, 2001) or in turkeys (Applegate and Sell, 1996; Sell *et al.*, 1995, 1997; Kalbfleisch *et al.*, 2000) but are associated with benefits in other criteria, such as immunity and resistance to stress and meat quality.

The long-recognized relationship between vitamin E and selenium has been further reinforced by recent experiments. Thus, improvements have been found in production parameters

(Okolelova *et al.*, 2006), the immune status of birds (Singh *et al.*, 2006), and the oxidative stability of the product (Özkan *et al.*, 2007; Ryu *et al.*, 2005).

These aspects have been studied extensively over the last 20 years. Pompeu *et al.* (2018) reviewed the effects of vitamin E supplementation on the growth performance, meat quality, and immune responses of male broiler chickens using a meta-analysis methodology. Vitamin E supplementation increased muscle content, decreasing the lipid peroxidation and improving immune response to multiple challenge agents. Consequently, these effects will be discussed in the following sections.

Nevertheless, some reports show improvements in live performance due to vitamin E supplementation. Ognik and Wertelecki (2012) evaluated all-rac-α-tocopherol acetate and RRR-D-α-tocopherol in turkey hens from 1 to 16 weeks of age. Six-hundred turkey hens of the Big 6 line were divided into 5 groups. From 1 to 9 weeks all-rac-tocopherol acetate was given at 50, 100, and 150 mg/kg feed and RRR-D-α-tocopherol at 25 and 50 mg/kg feed. From 10 to 16 weeks, the levels were reduced, respectively, to 45, 90, and 135 mg/kg for all-rac-α-tocopherol acetate and 22.5 and 45 mg/kg for RRR-D-α-tocopherol. The turkey hens fed the synthetic dl-α-tocopherol acetate at the medium and highest dose were characterized by significantly higher performance than the control birds yet were comparable with the groups provided the natural form of RRR-d-α-tocopherol additive. The RRR-D-α-tocopherol had a better dressing percentage, lower abdominal fat, and antioxidant status. The economic evaluation indicated that duplicating the level of tocopherol was most recommendable.

In the same way, broilers under heat or other stresses like higher stocking density have received benefits from vitamin E supplementation (Desoky, 2018; Khalifa *et al.*, 2021). Under high stocking density, Desoky (2018) observed that vitamin E supplementation (100 and 200 mg/kg) improved body weight from 2,392 g in the non-supplemented group to 2,511 and 2,615 g in the 2 supplemented groups and feed conversion from 1.72 to 1.60 g:g (Table 6.13).

Effect of vitamin E on the resistance to stress

There are signs that vitamin E requirements increase under conditions of stress. In chickens subjected to excessive temperatures, positive physiological responses with vitamin E supplementation have been shown, such as a smaller rise in body temperature, reduced mortality, and a large increase of the hormone triiodothyronine in plasma (Kan *et al.*, 1993; Qureshi *et al.*, 2000). Sahin *et al.* (2002a,b), using a combination of vitamins E and A, obtained a 50% reduction of the concentration of malondialdehyde in the liver and serum of broilers subjected to heat stress.

More recent experiments have gone deeper into the physiological effects of vitamin E in stress situations. Maini *et al.* (2007) found that supplementing starter feed with 200 mg/kg of

Table 6.13 Effect of vitamin E supplementation (mg/kg) in broilers under 2 stocking densities (Desoky, 2018)

Density (birds/m²)	Vitamin E (mg/kg)	Bodyweight (g)	Feed consumption (g/bird/day)	Feed conversion ratio (g:g)
10	0	2,676[a]	100.85[a]	1.61[b]
12	0	2,392[c]	94.71[c]	1.72[a]
12	100	2,511[b]	94.04[c]	1.60[b]
12	200	2,615[a]	98.12[b]	1.60[b]
P-value		<0.01	<0.01	<0.01

vitamin E reduced the peroxidation of erythrocytes and in various tissues at 3 and 5 weeks of age in chickens subjected to heat stress.

A field trial with 1.5 million chickens, using 33 or 240 mg/kg vitamin E, Boren and Bond (1996) obtained the following improvements: feed conversion index, −2.3%; live weight, +0.7%; viability, +0.1%; downgrading, −34%; septicemia-toxemia, −25%; inflammatory processes, −61%.

Subsequently, other studies (Bird and Boren, 1999; Siegel *et al.*, 2000) with this same level improved all production parameters. The large-scale trial run by Bird and Boren (1999) also confirmed an increase in breast yield and a reduction in both downgrading and the proportion of defects in the carcass and its cuts. Results of this type have led some researchers to state that "the only valid scientific method to study optimum vitamin requirements is by evaluation in field tests using a large number of birds, provided that these be controlled in a precise and uniform manner" (Rice and McIlroy, 1988, quoted by Kennedy *et al.*, 1992).

Effect of vitamin E on the immune response

The role of vitamin E in the functioning of the immune system has been studied in depth over the last few years by several research groups, although there remains much to be learned (Klasing, 2007; Khan *et al.*, 2012c; Shojadoost *et al.*, 2021).

It is believed that this action is based on the function of vitamin E as a lipophilic antioxidant capable of preventing lipid peroxidation in membranes caused by free radicals. Disease is an important factor in producing free radicals, either during prostanoid synthesis or as a consequence of macrophage function (Panda and Cherian, 2014).

The relationship between vitamin E and immunity first came to light in 1975, when researchers, using 300 mg/kg of vitamin E, improved immune response and reduced mortality in birds facing an *E. coli* challenge (Tengerdy and Nockels, 1975; Tengerdy and Brown, 1977).

Subsequent studies have found similar effects with dosages between 100 and 300 mg/kg in cases of colibacillosis (Siegel *et al.*, 2000), coccidiosis (Colnago *et al.*, 1984), and listeriosis in turkeys (Zhu *et al.*, 2003), in the immune response to vaccinations against Newcastle disease (Franchini *et al.*, 1986; Hesabi, 2007) and bronchitis (Klasing, 1998, Hesabi, 2007). Erf *et al.* (2000) recorded an increase in vitamin E concentration in the principal immune organs when using 150 mg/kg. They related to the greater immune response elicited following vaccinations for Newcastle disease and hemorrhagic enteritis.

It has been shown that vitamin E promotes the phagocytic activity of macrophages, especially at the thymus level (Konjufca *et al.*, 2004), and in other immune mechanisms mediated by cells (Chang *et al.*, 1990; Erf *et al.*, 1998; Leshchinsky and Klasing, 2001, 2003; Konjufca *et al.*, 2004).

Abdukalykova *et al.* (2006, 2008) assessed the improvement in the cell response to challenges from vaccination against infectious bronchitis and in the humoral response to Sheep Red Blood Cells (SRBC) inoculation. Levels of vitamin E of 80, 200, and 400 mg/kg were combined with 2 levels of arginine, 1.2 and 1.5%. The highest doses of vitamin E did not result in improvements compared to 80 mg/kg suggesting that the latter can be considered adequate if combined with arginine and that the 2 substances have positive effects on immune function and health prevention of broilers.

However, contradictory results can be found in scientific literature. Allen and Fetterer (2002) did not find improvements in live weight or lesion prevalence after *Eimeria maxima* infection. Friedman *et al.* (1998) found the humoral immune response impaired with 30 mg/kg rather than 10 mg/kg of vitamin E following colibacillosis infection and vaccination against Newcastle disease, while for Leshchinsky and Klasing (2001), levels of 25–50 ppm vitamin E are immunomodulatory in broilers. They concluded that supplements of 100 and 200 mg/kg were less effective in increasing the production of antibodies following bronchitis vaccination.

Various hypotheses have been proposed to explain these discrepancies. First, the effect of vitamin E on humoral response appears to differ according to the antigen under consideration. Hesabi (2007) indicated that 50 mg/kg was needed to improve the number of antibodies in the face of Newcastle disease, 75 mg/kg for better protection against bronchitis, and up to 100 mg/kg to increase defenses against mycotoxins. On the other hand, in certain pathological processes, the humoral immune response is the most relevant. In others, such as bronchitis, immunity is mediated by special important cells. An anti-inflammatory role has also been indicated for this vitamin since it inhibits the production of certain cytokines dose dependent (Leshchinsky and Klasing, 2003). Silva *et al.* (2011) significantly improved the cellular immune response of broilers vaccinated against coccidiosis supplemented with 65 mg/kg vitamin E, attributing the effect to its antioxidant and immunomodulating properties.

Whitehead (2002c) considers that more virulent strains of the Gumboro virus vaccine are currently used in many countries and entail greater immunological stress, which may increase the benefits of using a higher vitamin E supplementation in feed. Other authors report that the magnitude of the response differs according to the degree of the pathogen challenge, which appears to vary between the different experiments.

It is thought that the relationship between vitamin E and immunity can be altered by various factors such as genetic selection (Boa-Amponsem *et al.*, 2006; Siegel *et al.*, 2006) and the strain of birds used since some studies have found different responses depending on the strain under consideration (Maurice *et al.*, 1993; Siegel *et al.*, 2000; Boa-Amponsem *et al.*, 2001). However, Yang *et al.* (2000) found no clear relationship between vitamin E supplementation and the production of antibodies in the face of the SRBC antigen or of a challenge from *E. coli* in chickens from strains selected for low or high production of antibodies against SRBC.

In turkeys, Qureshi *et al.* (1993) showed that it takes 250 mg/kg vitamin E to induce an increase in IgG (confirmed by Ferket and Qureshi, 1999) and stimulate the proliferation of T-lymphocytes with these levels. Heffels-Redman *et al.* (2000, 2001) also observed this phenomenon, although 400–800 mg/kg vitamin E did not improve the rate of hemagglutination-inhibiting antibodies following vaccination against Newcastle disease. The same was found in the experiment in poults by Kalbfleisch *et al.* (2000), who did, however, confirm an improved humoral response to vaccination against hemorrhagic enteritis. Vitamin E may act on immunity by several mechanisms, and it would be worth conducting similar studies to those previously indicated for broilers.

Maternal immunity still active at the time of the outbreak may also influence (Leshchinsky and Klasing, 2001), as may the vitamin status of the day-old chick, which is related to the vitamin E supplementation level in breeders. These factors determine the efficiency of the chick's antioxidant systems in the embryonic and early postnatal periods (Surai *et al.*, 1997b, 1999a,b; Surai, 2000). The concentration of vitamin E in the chick's tissues depends on the hen's diet and its consequent accumulation in the egg yolk. Thus, if breeders receive 365 mg/kg vitamin E instead of 150 mg/kg, the vitamin E content in the yolk sac membrane, liver, brain, and lung were, respectively, 5.0, 4.3, 1.7, and 5.6 times greater for those derived from the hens on the high vitamin E diet compared with those from the control group (Surai *et al.*, 1999a,b).

After hatching, vitamin E concentration falls rapidly in the yolk sac: in only 9 days from 566 to 26.7 µg/kg in broilers and from 156 to only 0.1 µg/kg in turkeys (Surai *et al.*, 1997b; Surai, 2000). Suppose the breeder and starter feed of broilers contain high levels of unsaturated fats, the high levels of higher PUFA adversely affect the vitamin status of chickens and turkeys after hatching (Cherian and Sim, 1997, 2003).

Haq *et al.* (1996) showed that chicks from hens that received supplementation of 300 mg/kg vitamin E presented better humoral immunity and more active lymphocytes. This finding was confirmed by Rebel *et al.* (2004): they showed that broilers infected with the virus causing malabsorption syndrome suffered less damage and recovered sooner if the breeders had received a higher vitamin E supplementation. Hossain *et al.* (1998) found that increasing vitamin E to 75 mg/kg in the diet of breeders increased its concentration in the egg yolk and improved the antibody titers of their offspring after vaccination against Newcastle disease.

The decline after hatch in young poults is more pronounced in young turkeys than in broilers. Within 7–10 days post-hatch, there is a marked drop in its levels in the liver, from 144 to only 0.5 µg/g, and its plasma concentration between 7 and 21 days, and these remain low until 21 days (Soto-Salanova and Sell, 1995) and similar data have been found by other authors (Soto-Salanova *et al.*, 1991, 1993; Soto-Salanova and Sell, 1996; Waibel *et al.*, 1994; Surai *et al.*, 1997b). This phenomenon occurs, albeit to a lesser degree, even when the vitamin E level in starter feed is raised to 150 ppm (Applegate and Sell, 1996) or when the diet of breeding turkeys is fortified. However, Surai *et al.* (1999a,b) found that using 365 ppm in breeder feed raised the concentration of vitamin E in the liver, brain, and lungs of the offspring between 3 and 5 times, which reduced the susceptibility of these organs to oxidation.

In conclusion, it is not easy to indicate with precision the optimum levels and period of vitamin E supplementation needed to improve the immunity of broilers and turkeys since the degree of protection necessary will depend on the type and degree of immunological pressure induced by different vaccination programs, nutritional and environmental conditions as well as by potential exposure to different pathogens. Concerning vitamin E, the focus should be on improving its metabolic status rather than merely preventing its deficiency.

One example of this approach is the study by Gore and Qureshi (1997), who injected 0, 10, 20, or 30 mg of vitamin E into the amniotic fluid of turkey embryos 3 days before hatching. Levels above 10 mg led to a drop in hatchability. Still, they observed more antibodies at this dosage than in the control groups and a greater proportion of macrophages in a post-hatch challenge with SRBC. The same occurred with chicken embryos. In broilers, Hossain *et al.* (1998) obtained similar results, improving titers against Newcastle disease and significant improvements in weight at 42 days, viability, and the feed conversion index. This may offer a promising way of improving the immune status of birds.

In a study with turkeys, poults were supplemented with either 40 or 400 mg/kg vitamin E during the initial 6 weeks of age (Heffels-Redmann *et al.*, 2003). The higher level of vitamin E was beneficial for the development and maturation of the thymus and bursa of Fabricius at an earlier age, indicating a more rapid onset of immunocompetence. The higher level of vitamin E also led to a significantly higher lymphocyte proliferation rate. Although the 400 mg/kg vitamin E level was fed until only 6 weeks of age, significant increases in body weights of toms and hens were still present at processing (Heffels-Redmann *et al.*, 2003).

Recently, Desoky (2018) evaluated the supplementation of vitamin E at 100 and 200 mg/kg in broilers under 2 stocking densities (10 or 12 broilers/m^2) as a stress model for broilers. Several serological parameters and bone calcium and phosphors content were improved. The total intestinal bacterial count was reduced, especially *E. coli* and *Clostridium*. Finally, it was remarkable the improvement in antibody titers against Newcastle disease, Infectious bronchitis, and avian influenza (Figure 6.10).

Another immunomodulatory action of vitamin E recently explored with culture and molecular methods is the influence on gut microbiota composition presented by Desoky (2018) but better discussed by Choi *et al.* (2020). They demonstrated that vitamin E intake affects the ratio of *Firmicutes* to *Bacteroidetes* in mice. Generally, the dosages of vitamin E proposed for

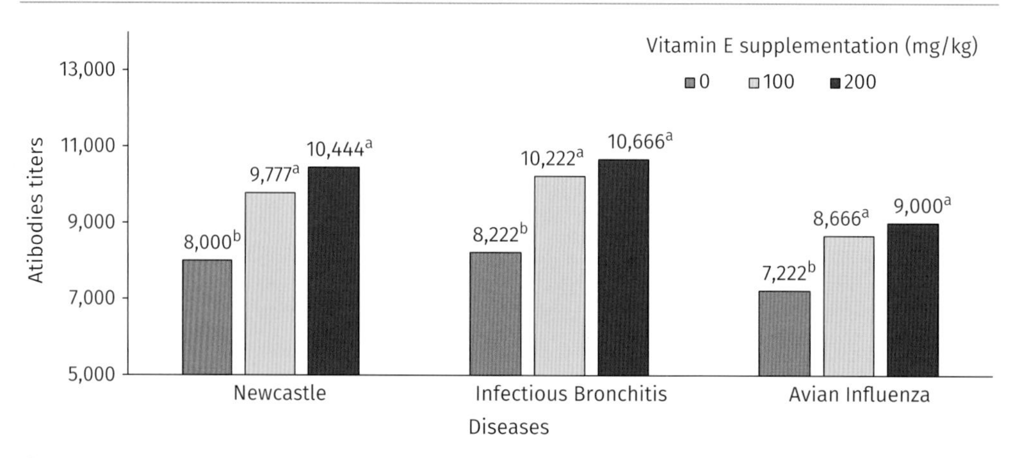

Figure 6.10 Vitamin E supplementation affects the immune response of broilers placed under high stocking density, 12 broilers/m^2, values with no common superscripts differ significantly, $P < 0.05$ (Desoky, 2018)

improving immune status are much greater (100 to 300 mg/kg) than those for growth, which means they represent an important extra cost. This raises the subject of their cost/benefit relationship, which has been assessed in some studies.

Kennedy *et al.* (1992) reported net income as a comparative index of broiler performance. He reported that broiler flocks fed a 180 mg/kg vitamin E diet had a 1.3% significantly heavier ($P < 0.05$) weight bird and a 0.84% better ($P < 0.05$) feed efficiency than controls fed 44 mg/kg vitamin E. Net income for the flock on high vitamin E was 2.7% more than for the control flocks.

McIlroy *et al.* (1993) supervised 79 flocks in Northern Ireland during a Gumboro epidemic, administering either 48 or 178 mg/kg of vitamin E. Clinical symptoms were not detected because all the birds were vaccinated. Still, in 43 flocks, the subclinical infectious bursal disease was diagnosed with bursal lesions. With 48 ppm vitamin E, there was a reduction of 28% in the net income; however, 128 mg/kg improved by 10%. In healthy chickens, a much lower improvement of 2% was obtained.

Effect of vitamin E on disease prevention

The antioxidant action of vitamin E has led to many studies on its relationship with hypoxic syndrome or ascites, which is still causing significant economic losses, although less so than in previous years. In 1986, Dale and Villacres (1986) analyzed the first studies to note a possible relationship, and later Malan *et al.* (2001) and Baghbanzadeh and Decuypère (2008) have reviewed the published evidence. Ascitic chickens exhibit a high production of ROS and a reduction in ascorbic acid and vitamin E levels in the liver and lungs and consequently signs of lipid peroxidation in these organs (Iqbal *et al.*, 2001, 2002). Bottje and Wideman (1995) and Bottje *et al.* (1995) demonstrated that mortality from ascites was reduced when vitamin E was given, released at 15 mg/head/day from pellets implanted under the skin through a small incision in the back of the neck.

However, tests using higher feed levels of vitamin E, mainly in starter feed (100–500 mg/kg), with or without the addition of selenium (whose synergies with this vitamin are well known), have only been partially successful or have not reduced the incidence of ascites (Bottje *et al.*, 1997, 1998; Stanley *et al.*, 1997; Roch *et al.*, 2000a,b; Villar-Patino *et al.*, 2002; Panda and Cherian, 2014). Belay *et al.* (1996) observed no reduction in mortality with a supplement of antioxidant vitamins 25% higher than the levels used commercially at the time. However, the birds were significantly heavier without this entailing a higher incidence of ascites. More recently, supplementation with vitamin E, on its own or in combination with arginine, did not improve pulmonary relaxation following epinephrine challenge or bioavailability of the nitric oxide synthetase enzyme. However, vitamin E levels of the order of 400 mg/kg were associated with long periods of recovery from arteriopulmonary pressure (Lorenzoni and Ruiz-Feria, 2006).

Whitehead (2002c) indicated that nutrition is not the root cause of the hypoxic syndrome, so it is doubtful whether changes in diet composition can prevent it. Broz and Ward (2007) considered that since ascites are a condition of multifactorial origin, it is necessary to conduct more research under practical conditions to confirm whether either vitamin E or vitamin C can have a protective effect against this pathology.

Another line of research relates to "cellulitis," a subcutaneous infection, generally by *E. coli*, a problem becoming the primary cause of downgrading in broiler slaughterhouses. The results have been inconsistent, although certain improvements have been noticed in some experiments, particularly if the vitamin E supplement (50–100 mg/kg) is linked with zinc complexes (Downs *et al.*, 1999, 2000; Macklin *et al.*, 2000). In broilers intoxicated with ochratoxins, the combination of 500 mg/kg vitamin E and 0.1 mg/kg selenium improved growth and allowed the birds to recover better (Kurkure *et al.*, 2004).

The scientific literature mentions a possible role of vitamin E in reducing skeletal problems, given that its deficiency increases the incidence of twisted feet, with deviations of the distal portion of the tibia or the tarsus at the proximal level (Summers *et al.*, 1984). However, vitamin E at levels 5–10 times higher than normal can affect the utilization of vitamin D_3 if this is at marginal levels (500 IU/kg) and thus adversely affect ossification (Aburto and Britton, 1998a,b).

Rehman *et al.* (2018) recently concluded that since Newcastle disease virus causes oxidative stress and histopathological changes in duodenum and jejunum in broiler chickens, vitamin E supplementation at 50 mg/day/kg of body weight in challenged birds could partially or fully ameliorate these effects of the virus.

On the other hand, Khalifa *et al.* (2021) investigated the impact of vitamin E (100 mg/kg) and/or selenium (0.3 mg sodium selenite/kg diet) on the production performance, serum biochemistry, and expression of some growth-related genes in the liver tissue of broilers. They concluded that dietary supplementation of vitamin E and/or selenium improved the production parameters and upregulated the growth-related genes (GHR and insulin-like growth factor 1) without affecting the general health status of the broilers.

In turkeys, particular attention has been paid to vitamin E's efficacy in improving health. It is usually added to the diets at levels at least 3 to 4 times higher than those recommended by NRC (1994) to prevent deficiencies. In fact, cases of encephalomalacia at 3–4 weeks used to appear with some frequency (Klein *et al.*, 1994), as does so-called "fatigue syndrome," where a significant reduction in the plasma concentration of vitamin E has been found in affected turkeys (Meldrum *et al.*, 2000), which respond well to vitamin E supplementation in drinking water (Sell, 1996). Using rancid fats and the consequent production of oxidation products can severely reduce the vitamin E level in plasma (Csallany *et al.*, 1988; Soto-Salanova and Sell, 1995).

Effect of vitamin E on meat quality

The beneficial effects of including high dosages of vitamin E in poultry feed have been extensively researched, particularly concerning its impact on oxidative meat stability, its sensory quality, and the possibility of enriching poultry meat with vitamin E.

Oxidative stability

In poultry, meat shelf life is lower than for beef or pork due to its higher PUFA content (Rhee *et al.*, 1996). Oxidation processes are responsible for unpleasant smells and flavors, changes in the nutritional value (reduction in the meat's PUFA and fat-soluble vitamin content), and even for the appearance of potentially harmful components of health, such as cholesterol oxides. Oxidative processes can affect the ability of the membranes to function as a semi-permeable barrier and may contribute to fluid leakage or drip loss.

The risk of oxidation increases if meat undergoes prolonged defrosting and when restructured and pre-cooked meat products are manufactured since salt application and cooking accelerate oxidation processes. The problem is greater if the fat in the meat contains a high level of PUFA, which are highly valued nowadays from a nutritional perspective but also very susceptible to oxidation (Barroeta, 2007).

The determination of thiobarbituric acid reactive substances (TBARS), the most important of which is malondialdehyde, has mainly been used to assess these effects. Although the TBARS method has often been criticized for not being sufficiently specific, it is the one that has been used in the great majority of studies conducted on chickens and turkeys.

A significant negative correlation has been found between the TBARS values obtained and vitamin E ingestion (Bartov and Frigg, 1992; Sheehy *et al.*, 1993, 1995, 1997; Sheldon *et al.*, 1997; Guo *et al.*, 2003; Cortinas *et al.*, 2005; Pesut *et al.*, 2005; Sárraga *et al.*, 2006, 2008; Koreleski and Świątkiewicz, 2006), as well as its content in meat (Gatellier *et al.*, 1998; Ruiz *et al.*, 1999; Hsieh *et al.*, 2002; Bou *et al.*, 2004; Yan *et al.*, 2006) and liver, and plasma concentration *in vivo* (Guo *et al.*, 2001).

It has been established that higher levels of vitamin E in feed reduce the concentration of secondary oxidation products (aldehydes and ketones) by around 50%, especially hexanal (De Wynne and Dirinck, 1996; Wen *et al.*, 1996; García-Regueiro *et al.*, 1998). Vitamin E supplementation in feed is much more effective in maintaining oxidative stability than adding it to meat postmortem since it is not incorporated in cellular membranes (Vara-Ubol and Bowers, 2001).

The reduction of TBARS in fresh chicken meat normally ranges from 40 to 90% and from 39 to 66% in processed and/or pre-cooked products (Jensen *et al.*, 1998). This wide range of variation suggests many factors affect the levels, such as the composition of the feed (principally, its lipid fraction), storage and packaging conditions, type of product derived, and, of course, the dosage and administration time of α-tocopherol acetate.

Barroeta (2007), in a trial carried out on broilers, showed that 200 mg of vitamin E/kg of feed reduced the development of TBARS – a by-product of lipid peroxidation – by between 84 and 88%. The production of oxidized cholesterol compounds in chicken meat was also reduced by 50%.

Gao *et al.* (2010) studied the effects of long-term exogenous glucocorticoids (dexamethasone; DEX) administration, which is used to induce oxidative stress and dietary supplementation of α-tocopheryl acetate on the induction of lipid peroxidation and meat quality aspects in skeletal muscle. Supplementation of 200 mg/kg dietary vitamin E recovered the growth reduction induced by DEX and suppressed the formation of lipid peroxidation in both plasma and skeletal muscle tissues.

Zdanowska-Sąsiadek *et al.* (2016a,b) evaluated the effects of supplementing a broiler diet that contained 44 mg/kg of vitamin E with an additional 200 mg/kg. In this case, a Polish experimental slow-growing line was used with a final weight at slaughtering of 2.18 kg at 63 days. The results confirmed the benefits of vitamin E supplementation: carcass yield improved from 68.5 to 69.8% ($P < 0.01$), and abdominal fat was reduced from 3.3 to 2.88 ($P < 0.05$). The breast muscle pH 24 hours post-slaughter was increased from 5.90 to 6.08, the cooking loss reduced from 14.9 to 11.8%, and the water holding capacity increased. The meat of chickens from the experimental group was darker, more saturated with red color, and less saturated with yellow color. A sensor panel categorized the cooked breast fillets from vitamin E supplemented chickens as more tender and with better juiciness than those from non-supplemented broilers. Decreased lipid peroxidation and changes in the histological parameters in the muscles were observed. The effects of vitamin E at 200 mg/kg, reducing shear force, and improving color were confirmed by Niu *et al.* (2017) in fast-growing broilers.

Ekunseitan *et al.* (2021) conducted one experiment to establish the effect of vitamin E and selenium on chicken meat quality, hematological indices, and oxidative stability. They concluded that to ensure good chicken performance and improve the oxidative stability of meat in a hot climate it is recommended to feed broilers with 400 mg/kg feed of vitamin E and 0.2 mg/kg of selenium.

In addition to the reduction in TBARS, other favorable effects of vitamin E have been shown, such as the reduction in protein oxidation in turkey meat (Mercier *et al.*, 2001; Batifoulier *et al.*, 2002; Gatellier *et al.*, 2003) and the decrease in the content of oxidized cholesterol compounds in chicken meat – an aspect of great nutritional interest, since these are substances which have been linked to the risk of cardiovascular disease. Generally, the compounds are found in meat after 6–12 days and increase with time, showing a positive correlation with the TBARS index. Supplementation with 200 ppm vitamin E reduces oxidized cholesterol compounds in chicken meat by 50%, and with 800 ppm, a 70–75% reduction is possible (Galvin *et al.*, 1998; Grau *et al.*, 2001b).

An important aspect to consider is that it is necessary to include high levels of fat in the diets of broilers and turkeys to satisfy their high energy requirements and achieve maximum growth with the lowest possible feed conversion indices. This makes it necessary to include vegetable oils in the formulation of feed, mainly soy and sunflower oil, whose proportions in the diet are increasing, given the tendency to avoid fats of animal origin. This may increase the likelihood of meat becoming rancid since the lipid composition of fat in birds greatly reflects that in the diet, and these oils are abundant in PUFA. It is now well known that the optimum level of vitamin E supplementation to protect the meat from fat oxidation depends on the lipid composition of the diet (Ahn *et al.*, 1995; Cortinas *et al.*, 2001; Barroeta, 2007).

The consensus is that if the most unsaturated ones are used, vitamin E at 200 ppm needs to be added for several weeks to maintain the oxidative stability of chicken meat (Malczyk *et al.*, 1999; Sárraga and García-Regueiro, 1999; Grau *et al.*, 2000, 2001b; Cortinas *et al.*, 2001; Villaverde *et al.*, 2004b; Rebole *et al.*, 2006). Less vitamin E is necessary if tallow or olive oil is used – not economically viable today – but improvements can be observed nevertheless (Lauridsen *et al.*, 1997; O'Neill *et al.*, 1998a). Supplementation with high levels of vitamin E is even more important if the fat incorporated in the feed is altered by oxidation or by heat, which is more likely if soy, sunflower, or linseed oil is used (Sweeney *et al.*, 1992; Sheehy *et al.*, 1993; Engberg *et al.*, 1996; Galvin *et al.*, 1997; Jensen *et al.*, 1997).

An increase in the dosage of vitamin E is required if the aim is to raise the concentration of omega-3 PUFA in meat, which are of great nutritional interest, but also the most easily oxidized: the strategy thus entails a potential risk of abnormal flavors occurring, e.g., rancidity and fish. Incorporating fish and linseed oil in feed has been tried to achieve this objective.

To prevent rancidity and its undesirable effects, a minimum of 100 ppm α-tocopherol acetate is required if the degree of enrichment is moderate (<2%) (Lin *et al.*, 1989a,b; Huang and Miller, 1994; Zanini *et al.*, 2003a,b) but this dosage should be raised to 250–300 mg/kg if these oils are included at a level of 2% or more (Gualtieri *et al.*, 1993; Khattak *et al.*, 1996; Nam *et al.*, 1997), especially if the meat is to be stored for long periods (Miller and Huang, 1993). On the other hand, supplementation with vitamin E or mixtures of tocopherols permits a greater degree of enrichment with omega-3 PUFAs, especially in thigh meat (Ajuyah *et al.*, 1993; Ahn *et al.*, 1995; Surai and Sparks, 2001b). Furthermore, the benefits of the vitamin E antioxidant properties have also been observed in the breast muscle or serum of 42-day-old broilers fed corn-soybean diets with corn oil (Niu *et al.*, 2017). The total antioxidant capacity, total superoxide dismutase, and glutathione peroxidase were increased linearly as vitamin E concentration was augmented in the diet (Figure 6.11).

In a similar way to that indicated above for the muscle content of vitamin E, the protective effect is lower in fresh meat or in meat refrigerated for a very short time than in the meat stored for 7–12 days and frozen meat, in which dosages around 200 mg/kg have been successful in preventing signs of rancidity in chicken carcasses (abnormal smell, discoloration), even after 9 months of freezing (Brandon *et al.*, 1993; Coetzee and Hoffman, 2001; Bou *et al.*, 2004, 2006; Fellenberg and Speisky, 2006). In turkeys, supplementation with 150 ppm throughout the fattening period maintains frozen meat in good condition for up to 108 days (Bartov and Kanner, 1996) and 300 ppm for up to 12 months (Higgins *et al.*, 1998b).

Manufacturing processes also increase the risk of oxidation, such as mincing (Pikul *et al.*, 1997), adding salt (O'Neill *et al.*, 1999), or cooking (Grau *et al.*, 2000). In these studies, the dosages of vitamin E were effective in preventing the occurrence of bad flavor in pre-cooked products (warmed-over flavor), already detectable after being refrigerated for 48 hours (Mielche and Bertelsen, 1994; Weber, 2001). These positive effects were confirmed in raw and cooked turkey burgers, either refrigerated or frozen (Wen *et al.*, 1996; Nam *et al.*, 2003) and in minced and frozen chicken meat (Pikul *et al.*, 1997).

Reduction in TBARS normally ranges between 39 and 66% in processed and/or pre-cooked chicken products and between 50 and 77% in turkey products (Jensen *et al.*, 1998; Higgins *et al.*, 1999). The effect is more evident in products packaged normally than in vacuum-packed products, a procedure with its protective effect against oxidation (Ahn *et al.*, 1995; Higgins *et al.*, 1998a; Ruiz *et al.*, 1999).

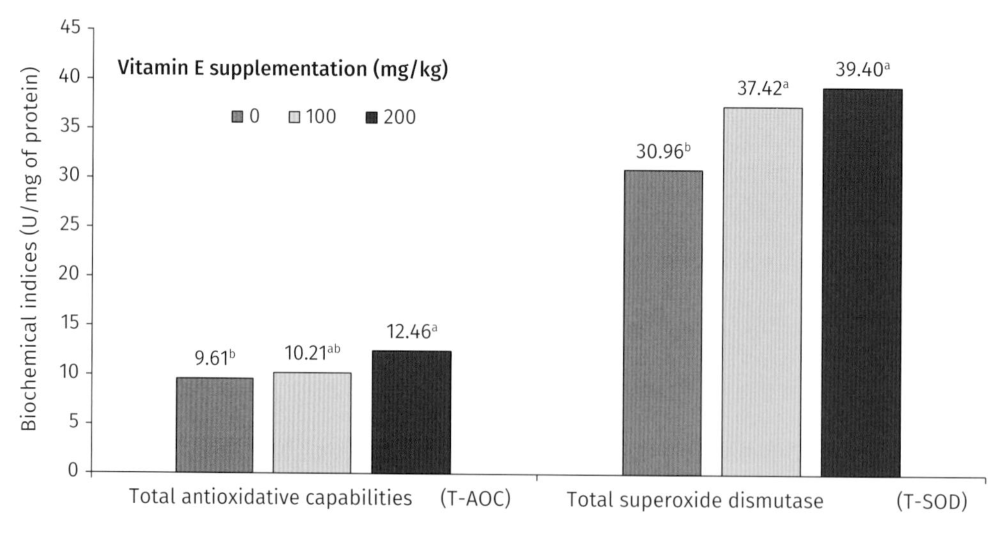

Figure 6.11 Biochemical indices of total antioxidative capabilities and total superoxide dismutase on breast muscle of broilers fed corn-soybean meal diets with the inclusion of corn oil and 2 levels of vitamin E supplementation, values with no common superscripts differ significantly, $P < 0.05$ (Niu *et al.*, 2017)

On the other hand, supplementation with 600 ppm in turkey feed for 147 days removed the need to use nitrites as meat preservers, maintaining oxidation indexes and color stability (Walsh *et al.*, 1998). Meat irradiation, a decontaminating process legal in the US, reduces its vitamin E content and accelerates oxidation, which is already intense in just 3 days (Lakritz and Thayer, 1994), particularly in turkey meat (Lakritz *et al.*, 1995; Ahn *et al.*, 1997). Fortification with 200 ppm vitamin E in the last 2 weeks did not succeed in counteracting this effect (Eslick *et al.*, 1997), which is better overcome with continuous supplementation of 100 ppm, followed by 400–600 ppm in the last 14 days of fattening, provided that the meat is vacuum-packed (Ahn *et al.*, 1998; Nam and Ahn, 2003). Similar conclusions were reached by Yan *et al.* (2006) following an experiment in which they also included conjugated linoleic acid to stabilize the final product.

The interrelationships between vitamin E and other vitamins also impact the oxidative stability of meat. Carreras *et al.* (2004) confirmed that α-tocopherol acetate increased the levels of vitamin E in the raw breast. Still, the presence of 1.5 ppm ß-carotene reduced its deposition and resulted in TBARS values no different from those of the control. Similar results were obtained by Sárraga *et al.* (2006). Both vitamin E and ß-carotene decreased rancidity in meat; the combination of both of them modified the texture in terms of pastiness and firmness.

Finally, it is worth discussing the work seeking alternatives to the use of vitamin E. It seems evident that the protective effect of α-tocopherol acetate is superior to that of other vitamins or provitamins with antioxidant action, such as vitamin A (Bartov *et al.*, 1997; Smallmann *et al.*, 1998), ß-carotene (Barroeta and King, 1991; King *et al.*, 1993; Ruiz *et al.*, 1999), or vitamin C (Bou *et al.*, 2001; Grau *et al.*, 2001a,b).

King *et al.* (1995) found an improvement in TBARS values and the meat's sensory quality with a 150 mg/kg dosage throughout the fattening period, while ß-carotene, at 25 mg/kg, or 0.15% vitamin C in drinking water did not have positive effects. Nevertheless, in heat stress situations, the combination of 250 ppm vitamin C and 280 ppm vitamin E significantly increased the oxidative stability of meat during storage (Gheisari *et al.*, 2004).

Some studies have also compared the effectiveness of vitamin E with that of essential oils of aromatic plants, such as rosemary and sage (López-Bote *et al.*, 1998b), oregano (Botsoglou *et al.*, 2002; Young *et al.*, 2003; Basmacioğlu *et al.*, 2004; Messikommer *et al.*, 2005; Smet *et al.*, 2005), grape skins and seeds (Mielnik and Skrede, 2003; Goñi *et al.*, 2007; Brenes *et al.*, 2008), mustard (Khattak *et al.*, 1996), sesame (Yoshida and Takagi, 1999; Du and Ahn, 2002), mint (Maini *et al.*, 2007), and tea catechins (Tang *et al.*, 2001; Gheisari *et al.*, 2006). However, all these ingredients succeeded in reducing TBARS values and cholesterol oxide, but vitamin E activity at a dosage of 200 ppm was superior on average by 30 to 50% (Table 6.14).

Other trials assessed the results of using feed with high levels of oats, but while there was an important reduction in TBARS values and cholesterol oxide (López-Bote *et al.*, 1998a), the effect of vitamin E again proved to be much higher. Furthermore, broiler weight gain and feed intake reduce linearly in response to the increase in the oat content of the diet (Valaja *et al.*, 2001). The incorporation of 1.5% carnosine (a natural muscular dipeptide) in feed has also been investigated; in this case, a more comparable antioxidant effect was found, which was additive to vitamin E (O'Neill *et al.*, 1998b, 1999). However, it may have potential as more than just a feed additive, as it may be added to meat during processing, together with vitamin E (Morrissey *et al.*, 1998).

Finally, all these results demonstrate the difficulty of establishing recommendations for vitamin E supplementation, which apply to all situations, since many factors may affect optimum dosages, starting with the desired outcomes; and, as has been pointed out, the polyunsaturated

Table 6.14 Comparative effects of vitamin E and other antioxidants on the oxidative stability of chicken thighs

Reference	Antioxidant and dosage	Type of sample	TBARS (mg/kg)
King *et al.* (1995)	Vitamin E, 150 mg/kg	Cooked meat	0.29
	ß-carotene, 30 mg/kg		1.85
Khattak *et al.* (1996)	Mustard oil, 4%	Fresh meat	0.67
	Vitamin E, 10 mg/kg		0.51
López-Bote *et al.* (1998a)	Vitamin E, 200 mg/kg	Refrigerated meat, 9 days	0.19
	Oat, 20%		0.37
López-Bote *et al.* (1998b)	Vitamin E, 200 mg/kg	Cooked meat, 4 days	2.71
	Rosemary oil, 500 mg/kg		4.58
	Sage oil, 500 mg/kg		6.28
Tang *et al.* (2001)	Vitamin E, 200 mg/kg	Frozen meat, 1 month	0.15
	Tea catechins, 100 mg/kg		1.10
Botsoglou *et al.* (2002)	Vitamin E, 200 mg/kg	Fresh meat	0.42
	Oregano oil, 50 mg/kg		0.25
	Oregano oil, 100 mg/kg		0.10
Goñi *et al.* (2007)	Vitamin E, 200 mg/kg	Refrigerated meat, 7 days	0.28
	Grape residues, 3%		0.35
Grau *et al.* (2001b)	Vitamin E, 225 mg/kg	Cooked meat	2.91
	Vitamin C, 110 mg/kg		4.08

fatty acid content of the feed is decisive. However, it is clear that the efficacy of vitamin E supplementation increases in line with the dosage and the period of administration.

Bartov and Frigg had already demonstrated in 1992 that increased supplementation to broilers 2 weeks before slaughter gave meat moderate protection against oxidation. However, this protection was improved if the higher level was applied throughout the fattening cycle.

Brandon *et al.* (1993) advised supplementing broiler diets with 150–200 mg/kg α-tocopherol acetate for 4–5 weeks. These findings were confirmed by subsequent research (Morrissey *et al.*, 1997; Grau *et al.*, 2000). The latter authors believe that using 225 ppm for 3 weeks before slaughter is equivalent to 150 ppm in the last 32 days, which may be more economical. For turkeys, Morrissey *et al.* (1998) calculate the minimum supplementation needed as 300 ppm for 13 weeks, based on the results of Wen *et al.* (1997b) and Sheldon *et al.* (1997).

Organoleptic quality

Some studies have more directly evaluated the effects of high levels of vitamin E on the sensory quality of meat, using objective methods and/or panels of trained tasters. Olivo *et al.* (2007) found a smaller drop in postmortem pH, which indicates a potential use in preventing pale, soft, and exudative (PSE) meat syndrome. Drip losses diminish (O'Neill *et al.*, 1998a; Olivo *et al.*, 2007), even when supplements are given only in the last 2–3 weeks of fattening (McKnight *et al.*, 1996b; Malczyk *et al.*, 1999).

Sheehy *et al.* (1995) found an improvement in meat taste using 160 mg/kg vitamin E compared to the usual level of 20 ppm. An improvement in flavor was detected with just 80 ppm (Ristic and Lidner, 1992), which continued up to 160 ppm (Blum *et al.*, 1990). De Wynne and Dirinck (1996) and Janssens *et al.* (1999) found that continuous use of 200 ppm vitamin E instead of 50 ppm significantly improved perceptions of texture, succulence, flavor, abnormal flavors, and general acceptability and that evaluation of flavor corresponded with the lowest concentration of aldehydes, especially hexanal.

These effects are less pronounced in very fresh meat after 1–4 days (Ruiz *et al.*, 2001) but are clearly evident with longer storage times of 7–12 days (Blum *et al.*, 1990; Janssens *et al.*, 1999). If the diet is fortified only in the last week of fattening the effects are undetectable as there is too little time for the fortification to have an effect (Thomas *et al.*, 1988). An improvement in the color stability of meat may also be expected by preventing the oxidation of myoglobin to metmyoglobin. This has been demonstrated in other species, although the meat of birds, especially breast meat, has a lower pigment content (Jensen *et al.*, 1998).

In the literature on this topic some papers did not confirm the effect of vitamin E on meat quality. For example, in one study published by Vieira *et al.* (2021), the impact of different doses of dietary vitamin E on breast meat quality of broiler chickens in the finishing period was evaluated. Five doses of vitamin E were used (30, 90, 150, 210, and 270 mg/kg feed) in broiler diets from 42 to 54 days of age. The diets supplemented with vitamin E doses had little effect on qualitative characteristics of broiler breast meat, as it only affected meat brightness. Probably the lack of response has been caused by the late and short period of vitamin E application. It must be considered that the part of the effect of vitamin E is based on its deposition in muscle cell membranes. Therefore, supplementation must be at high dosages (150 to 200 mg/kg feed) for at least 3 weeks before slaughtering. Increasing the dose and feeding it for a shorter period is not recommended as the high dose could impair vitamin E absorption.

More data on the subject is available for turkey meat, but using higher levels of supplementation, between 250 and 600 ppm. *In vitro* studies have shown that myoglobin oxidation is reduced (Yin and Cheng, 1997; Lynch *et al.*, 1998), which has also been confirmed on a practical level (Santé *et al.*, 1992), together with an improvement in the red (a*) value by spectrophotometry (Santé and Lacourt, 1994; Higgins *et al.*, 1998b), and subjective color evaluation (Sheldon *et al.*, 1997; Janssens *et al.*, 1999).

A reduction has been observed in the frequency of PSE-type meat (Ferket and Allen, 1994), a problem that is now more prevalent in turkeys than chickens. Significant differences have also been demonstrated in tasting tests: the frequency of "typical flavor" assessments increases, those of "abnormal flavors" decrease (Sheldon *et al.*, 1997), and assessments of texture, succulence, flavor, and general appreciation improve (Janssens *et al.*, 1999).

The poultry industry has been facing problems for several years with particular myopathies, namely wooden breast, white stripping, and "spaghetti meat" (Petracci *et al.*, 2019; Prisco *et al.*, 2021; Baldi *et al.*, 2021). Several nutritional strategies have been evaluated to reduce their incidence and severity. Indeed, even though white striping has some similarities to nutritional muscular dystrophy, which is related to vitamin E deficiency, it was found that dietary inclusion of different vitamin E levels had no or little effect on the incidence of white striping (Guetchom *et al.*, 2012; Kuttappan *et al.*, 2012b).

Recently, Wang *et al.* (2020a) evaluated the effects of supplementation of 200 mg/kg of vitamin E and omega-3 (n-6 : n-3 ratio of 3 : 1) fatty acids independently or in combination when fed during the starter phase (0–10 days) or grower phase (11–24 days) to Ross-708 male

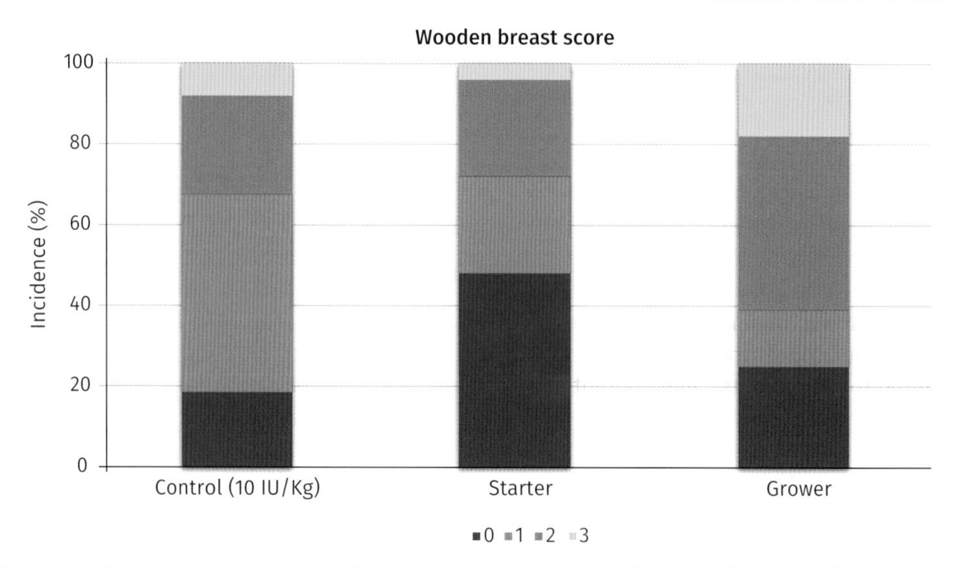

Figure 6.12 Vitamin E supplementation (200 IU/kg) during the starter (0–10 days) or grower (11–24 days) phase on wooden breast score (Wang *et al.*, 2020a)

broilers. The results indicated that only vitamin E during the starter phase halved the mild wooden breast score (score 1), increasing by 2.6 times the number of fillets without myopathies (score 0) and reducing the fat content and sheer force of meat (Figure 6.12). The authors attributed these effects to the potent antioxidant effect of vitamin E during the first week of life with the highest mitotic activity of satellite cells, which minimizes the myofiber degeneration causing the myopathies.

Content of vitamin E in meat

The most immediate effect of supplementing vitamin E above the levels recommended by the NRC (1994) is the enrichment of poultry meat with this vitamin (Marusich *et al.*, 1974; Hsieh *et al.*, 2002; Koreleski and Swiatkiewicz, 2006; Villaverde *et al.*, 2008), which improved the nutritional content of the meat, although transfer efficiency is lower than in the egg (Flachowsky *et al.*, 2001).

The increase is more rapid in the liver and kidney tissue than in muscle and fat (Sheehy *et al.*, 1991; Surai *et al.*,1993; Flachowsky *et al.*, 2001) and greater in the darker muscles of the thigh and leg, which have higher fat content and are rich in type I and II oxidative metabolism fibers, than in glycolytic metabolism fibers, such as breast (*pectoralis*) (Brandon *et al.*, 1993; Jensen *et al.*, 1998; Malczyk *et al.*, 1999), in which the vitamin E concentration also diminishes more rapidly (Sheldon *et al.*, 1997).

Vitamin E is deposited in cellular membranes, where oxidation begins (Asghar *et al.*, 1990), and in subcellular organelles, such as mitochondria and microsomes (Lauridsen *et al.*, 1997; Mercier *et al.*, 1998a,b). The enrichment of meat with vitamin E is directly proportional to its levels in the diet and the length of the supplementation period (Sheehy *et al.*, 1991; Bartov and Frigg, 1992). However, a plateau was reached above 500 ppm (Jakobsen *et al.*, 1995; Flachowsky *et al.*, 2001).

Using a standard feed supplemented with 200 mg/kg of vitamin E over 4–5 weeks, it has been possible to increase the vitamin E content in chicken meat by 4–6 times, from 3.5 to 14–20 mg/kg (Brandon *et al.*, 1993; De Wynne and Dirinck, 1996; Maraschiello *et al.*, 1999; Niu *et al.*, 2017). This means that a portion of chicken would provide up to 10–15% of the recommended daily intake in human nutrition (10 mg/day). Bou *et al.* (2004) found that in diets with high levels of fish oil, this percentage can vary between 14 and 19% if levels of 70–140 ppm vitamin E are used.

It has, however, been demonstrated that the lipid composition of feed modifies the deposition of vitamin E. Cortinas *et al.* (2003, 2005) and Villaverde *et al.* (2004b) demonstrated that the extent of enrichment varies in inverse proportion to the PUFA content in the diet and that with an increase of 32 g/kg PUFA, the α-tocopherol content of meat was reduced by 52% when 100 mg/kg vitamin E was added to feed. If the feed has a high PUFA content (45–61 g/kg), the vitamin E in the thigh rises by 0.6 mg/kg for every 10 mg/kg increase of its dose in feed, while with a lower concentration (15–34 g/kg PUFA) this increase rises to 1.14 g/kg. The vitamin E required to maintain its thigh content at a constant level increases between 2.5 and 3.7 mg/kg for every gram of PUFA in the diet, and this makes supplementation of 200 mg/kg necessary for broiler diets containing 30 g/kg PUFA or more (Barroeta, 2007).

Nobakht *et al.* (2011) observed that the highest concentration of breast muscle was obtained when chickens were fed diets that contained a mixture of sunflower, canola, and soybean oil instead of 3 times the concentration of each oil. Authors determined that fatty acid balance may influence vitamin E deposition in the breast muscle.

This concept was recently evaluated by Leskovec *et al.* (2019), who supplemented with vitamin E (200 mg/kg feed), C (250 mg vitamin C/kg feed), and selenium (0.2 mg Se/kg feed) broiler diets with high levels of omega-3 PUFA from linseed oil. Their results indicated that vitamin E alone combined with selenium and vitamin C increased breast muscle tocopherol concentration and protected against lipid peroxidation in fresh, frozen stored, cooked fresh, and frozen stored meat.

Supplementing feed with organic selenium can also increase vitamin E content in the liver and muscles. Skřivan *et al.* (2008) found that in diets with 50 mg/kg vitamin E, the vitamin E content of breast and thighs increased by about 25% when 0.3 mg/kg organic selenium was included in the diet. Konieczka *et al.* (2017) also found that supplementation of 150 mg/kg vitamin E increased the concentration of the vitamin and the oxidative stability of frozen stored breast and thigh meat, but in this experiment, no additional benefit was observed in feeding 0.7 mg/kg yeast selenium in combination with vitamin E.

The capacity of turkeys for depositing vitamin E in their tissue is 4–5 times lower than that of broilers, even where the lipid composition of their meat is similar (Marusich *et al.*, 1974, Sheldon, 1984; Surai *et al.*, 1993). This has been explained by reduced intestinal absorption and greater tocopherol catabolism in this species of poultry (Sklan *et al.*, 1982; Viau *et al.*, 1998). The concentrations of vitamin E achieved fall with some rapidity in frozen meat, although if turkeys have received extra supplementation, the speed of the process is slowed to half (Wen *et al.*, 1996; Higgins *et al.*, 1998a). Using supplementation levels twice as high as the NRC's, the vitamin E content of muscle falls rapidly in the first 3 weeks and remains low subsequently. Even with 600 ppm vitamin E in feed, its deposition is slow, equivalent to 0.3 μg/week (Wen *et al.*, 1997b). The concentration also depends on the muscle under consideration (Higgins *et al.*, 1998b; Viau *et al.*, 1998). Including oxidized fats in the diet considerably reduced hepatic reserves of vitamin E in turkeys (Zdunczyk *et al.*, 2002).

Turkeys, therefore, require a higher and continuous vitamin E supply than broilers to achieve the same effects (Sklan *et al.*, 1982; Morrissey *et al.*, 1997). It takes 13 weeks to reach the accumulation plateau in the thigh muscle (Wen *et al.*, 1997b). The vitamin E content in turkey meat rose with an increase in its level in feed to 275 ppm only between 16 and 18 weeks of age, but the improvement is minimal, from 0.1 to 0.5 mg/kg (Sheldon, 1984). Using 200 ppm over 6 weeks is also insufficient, especially if soy oil is used in the feed, and using 400 mg/kg between 11 and 16 weeks of age, the vitamin E content in meat is less than that in chickens that received 200 ppm over 5 weeks (Genot *et al.*, 1998; Viau *et al.*, 1998). It took a minimum of 300 ppm for 13 weeks or 200 ppm for 16 weeks to increase the vitamin E content of turkey meat by 6 times (Wen *et al.*, 1997b; Mercier *et al.*, 1998a,b).

Vitamin K

Details about current vitamin K recommendations for broilers and turkeys, provided by institutional sources and genetic companies, can be found in Tables 6.3 to 6.10.

The minimum requirement set by NRC (1994) was 0.5 mg/kg feed for broilers and from 1.75 to 0.5 mg in turkeys from starter to finisher phases. In contrast, industry levels are 2 to 4 times higher than NRC (1994), aligned with recommendations provided by genetic companies.

Portsmouth (1996) indicated that the values recommended by the NRC (1994), based on work carried out more than 50 years ago, might be too low for current conditions and the stress produced by illness. Still, there is no confirmation of this because no studies have been published recently. Jin and Sell (2001) estimated the vitamin K_1 requirements in turkeys between 7 and 14 days of age using the concentration of prothrombin in the plasma and the coagulation time as an indicator. The estimated requirements range between 0.079 and 0.13 mg/kg.

Vitamin K, a coenzyme for γ-carboxylase, plays an important role in bone formation and mineralization (Hamidi *et al.*, 2013). It was reported that the broiler starter period (weeks 0 to 3) is an important phase for improving bone quality. Zhang *et al.* (2003) evaluated the effects of increasing vitamin K_3 on bone development, and they obtained the best results with 8 mg/kg in the starter phase and 2 mg/kg in the grower and finisher phases. However, the importance of vitamin K for skeletal development under practical conditions has not been sufficiently studied (Whitehead, 2002b; Waldenstedt, 2006).

Recently, Guo *et al.* (2020) conducted a study investigating the interactive effects between vitamin K_3 with probiotics, using 3 levels of dietary vitamin K_3 (0, 0.5, and 4.0 mg/kg) and *Bacillus subtilis* PB6, on the growth performance and tibia quality of broiler chickens. The authors concluded that vitamin K_3 and *B. subtilis* PB6 improved the growth performance of broiler chickens in starter and grower phases, respectively. Vitamin K and the probiotic synergistically promoted tibias' physical and chemical traits, especially during the grower phase, by regulating the metabolism of calcium and phosphorus and osteogenic gene expression (Figure 6.13).

Trials conducted with dicumarol (a vitamin K antagonist) found higher shrinkage from bleeding and, therefore, a lower carcass yield (Marion *et al.*, 1985), which led the authors to suggest that under field conditions, the same could happen where there is a vitamin K deficiency. Scott *et al.* (1982) attributed the capillary fragility and the presence of muscular hematomas and petechiae to marginal deficiencies in vitamin K. Still, there is no clear evidence that this is the cause of such defects, which are now quite common in carcasses.

Water-soluble vitamins

The principal functions of the B group vitamins are connected with metabolizing energy from carbohydrates, fatty acids, and proteins. Except in organs with high metabolic requirements, such as the heart, the liver, and the kidneys, birds lack reserves of these vitamins. In contrast, even in these organs, the reserve is very small after hatching, which means a continuous supply is needed. The presence of aflatoxins in feed if their concentration reaches

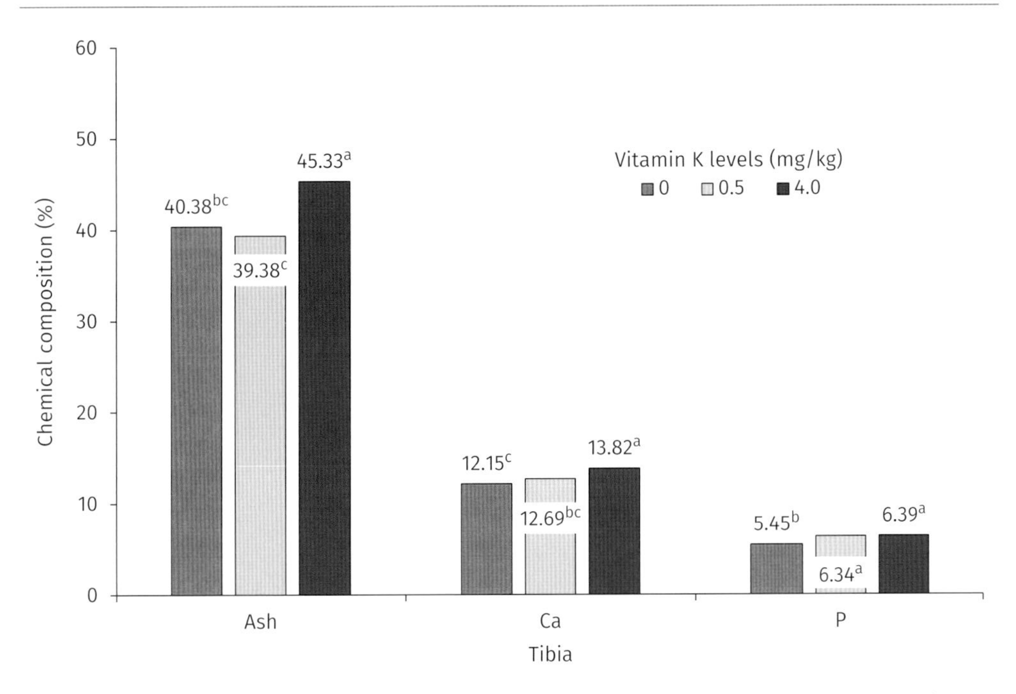

Figure 6.13 Tibia chemical composition of broilers with different levels of vitamin K_3 supplementation and *Bacillus subtilis* PB6, values with no common superscripts differ significantly, $P < 0.05$ (Guo *et al.*, 2020)

5 mg/kg feed reduces the level of most of these vitamins in plasma and the liver by 50 and 20%, respectively (Bains, 2001). Furthermore, a greater supply of these vitamins reduces the adverse effects of mycotoxins by favoring their breakdown and detoxification in the liver.

Stress conditions increase energy requirements and reduce feed consumption, and a supplementation of these vitamins at a higher level, even over short periods, helps birds to overcome the consequences of stress prejudicial to their productivity and immune status. Thus, Ferket and Qureshi (1992), who administered a combination of water-soluble vitamins and electrolytes in the drinking water of broilers, which they intermittently subjected to heat stress for 4–5 days, for 24 hours before and during the entire period of stress, obtained better growth rates and feed conversion and a higher level of IgG immunoglobulins, which were, in fact, comparable to those obtained with a complete vitamin shock also including vitamins A, D_3, and E.

In an experiment under practical conditions, Coelho *et al.* (2001) compared different degrees and conditions of stress (population density, new or permanent bedding, *E. coli,* coccidia infection, etc.). The effects of multiplying by various factors (1×, 2×, 4×, 8×, and 16×) the levels indicated by the NRC (1994) for riboflavin, niacin, folic acid, pantothenic acid, and vitamin B_{12}. These vitamins were chosen specifically for their role in protein deposition, which has increased in modern strains with high breast yields. Under extreme stress conditions, the increased levels could not compensate fully for the reduction in performance, but the most favorable results came with dosages higher than fourfold. The live weight, viability, and feed conversion index improved in proportion to the supplementation level in the groups subjected to a low or moderate stress level. The sixteenfold level produced the maximum benefits (+16.4% live weight and −6.6% in feed conversion compared to the NRC level). Carcass and breast yield and the percentage of abdominal fat also improved significantly. At fourfold inclusion, the profits per bird were US$0.17 and 16 times the dose of US$0.30 and returns on investment were calculated as 4.2% and 1.5%, respectively.

Suckeveris *et al.* (2020) conducted 2 trials on chicks from 1 to 18 days old to evaluate the effects of supranutritional levels of selected B vitamins in different diets on broiler performance. In experiment I, the chicks were fed a corn and soybean meal-based diet; in experiment II, a diet containing oxidized animal by-product meals and soybean oil was used. Both experiments followed a completely randomized design in a 3 × 2 factorial arrangement, consisting of the factors: (1) supplementation levels of selected B vitamins (control, 3× or 6× the control level of the vitamins riboflavin, pantothenic acid, niacin, folic acid, and vitamin B_{12}); (2) dietary nutritional density (low or high), totaling 6 treatments and 8 replicates of 6 birds each (3 male and 3 female). The control level of vitamins was the one indicated in the Brazilian tables (Rostagno *et al.*, 2017). Experiment I chicks showed higher weight gain (741.1 *vs.* 697.3 g) and feed intake (920.2 *vs.* 878.5 g) when fed a low-nutritional density diet with supranutritional vitamin level 6× higher than the control. However, this effect was not found in the performance of chickens fed a high-nutritional density diet, despite the poor quality of the ingredients used in experiment II, no statistical effect was shown using vitamin super-dose in rations with different dietary nutrient densities. It is known that all vegetable diets are more aggressive to the intestinal mucosa of birds than diets containing animal by-product meals. Therefore, the results obtained in this study concluded that when we use low-nutritional density in corn-soybean meal-based diets, supranutritional levels of vitamin supplementation may be needed for the birds to reach their maximum production potential (Figure 6.14).

Other researchers have looked at the effects on product quality. Swierczewska *et al.* (2005) evaluated the chemical and sensory composition of the breast and leg of chickens fed with vitamins B_2, B_6, B_{12}, and folic acid at a double level than those recommended by the NRC (1994). Analysis of the muscle composition revealed more protein and less fat than the birds in the control group. The cholesterol level, which very much depends on the type of muscle

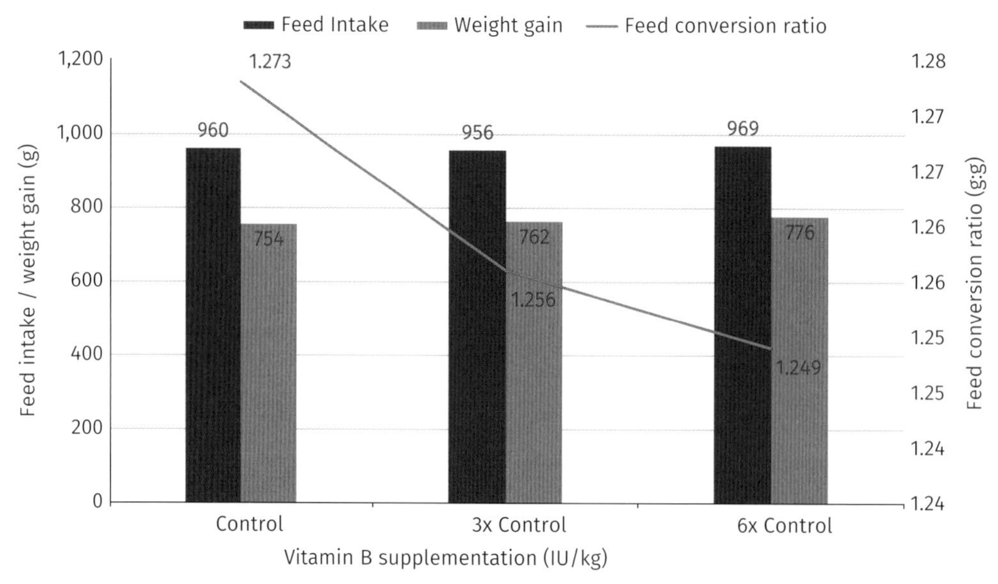

Figure 6.14 Effects of supplementation of B vitamins (control = 3.28 mg/kg thiamine, 8.17 mg/kg riboflavin, 16.42 mg/kg pantothenic acid, 49.6 mg/kg niacin, 1.145 mg/kg folic acid, and 0.019 mg/kg vitamin B_{12}) on broiler performance at 18 days (Suckeveris *et al.*, 2020)

considered, was higher in the legs of the birds which received a supplement and any level of vitamins, probably because of the fat contained in the supplement. The smallest amount of collagen was found in the diets, including a standard vitamin level. There were no effects on the sensory quality of the meat.

Vitamin B-group deficiencies are rare nowadays (Whitehead, 2002c). However, an inadequate supply of these vitamins with important roles in the regulatory processes of bone growth usually manifests itself in disorders of the epiphyseal growth plate, with the reduction in the proliferation of chondrocytes, which results in shortened and twisted bones and deformity of the condyles of the tibiotarsal articulation, which rotates 90–180°, causing displacement of the gastrocnemius tendon (slipped tendon), an abnormal condition known as chondrodystrophy or perosis (Rama-Rao *et al.*, 2003; Waldenstedt, 2006). This problem can also be caused indirectly by mycoplasma since they reduce the supply of nutrients the growth plate receives (Whitehead, 2005). Of particular importance in preventing the condition are pyridoxine and folic acid (especially if the diet is high in protein), riboflavin, niacin, biotin, and choline, and in the initial phases, birds respond well to extra supplementation with vitamins of the B group (Klein-Hessling, 2006).

Vitamin B_1 (thiamine)

Details about current vitamin B_1 recommendations for broilers and turkeys, provided by institutional sources and genetic companies, can be found in Tables 6.3 to 6.10.

The NRC (1994) recommends a supplementation in broiler feed of 1.8 ppm, based on studies carried out in the 1960s. Thiamine requirements have been investigated very little in the last 60 years, but they appear to be higher than those indicated by the NRC (Portsmouth, 1996).

Thiamine is one of the vitamins most likely to be deficient for poultry. Diet composition can dramatically influence thiamine requirements, and diets based on grains and plant protein sources are often borderline to deficient in riboflavin. Since thiamine is specifically involved in carbohydrate metabolism, the level of dietary carbohydrate relative to other energy-supplying components affects thiamine requirement. The need for thiamine increases as the consumption of carbohydrates increases (McDowell, 2000b; Elmadfa *et al.*, 2001).

Olkowski and Classen (1996) found that with 2–4 ppm, the plasma content of B_1 decreased with age but was higher and more constant at 8 ppm and increased continuously with 16 and 32 ppm. Leeson and Summers (2008) and genetic companies suggest levels 2–3 times higher than the NRC's (1994), especially in hot climates since it is known that at 32°C, the requirements for preventing polyneuritis are triple than those appropriate at 21°C (Whitehead and Portsmouth, 1989). In turkeys, the difference is 50%.

Other factors which affect optimum thiamine levels are the hen's nutrition, which influences the reserves and metabolism of her progeny (Olkowski and Classen, 1999), and the existence of pathological processes.

Fusarium moniliforme and *F. proliferatum* produce a thiaminase that could destroy vitamin B_1, and its deficiency in affected chicks could be prevented by adding more vitamin B_1 to the diet by autoclaving the moldy substrate or by injecting the chicks with thiamine hydrochloride (Fritz *et al.*, 1973). In feeds contaminated with *F. proliferatum*, vitamin B_1 supplementation at levels of 20–90 mg/kg depending on the contamination level, improved weight gain in the starter phase and effectively prevented immunosuppression and other toxicity signs induced by *Fusarium* (Nagaraj *et al.*, 1994; Yang and Wu, 1997). Thiaminases are also present in fish, but heat treatment destroys them.

Disease conditions also result in increased thiamine requirements. When dietary thiamine is marginal, typical deficiency signs of thiamine are more likely to develop in infected animals than in normal animals. Endoparasites, such as nematodes and coccidia, compete with the birds for this vitamin. It has been shown that experimental infection with coccidia results in a considerable reduction in thiamine blood levels. Thiamine levels found were directly correlated to infection severity (McManus and Judith, 1972). Likewise, conditions, such as diarrhea and malabsorption, increase the requirement. Deyhim *et al.* (1996) withdrew vitamin and trace minerals for 21 days in broiler diets, during heat stress, in the finisher phases, and found 23% less thiamine in the *PM* muscle.

Vitamin B_2 (riboflavin)

Details about current vitamin B_2 recommendations for broilers and turkeys, provided by institutional sources and genetic companies, can be found in Tables 6.3 to 6.10.

The levels recommended by the NRC are based on studies carried out over 33 years ago. Riboflavin is an important cofactor for multiple flavin enzymes. Deficiency in broilers results in decreased growth and diminished appetite due to mucosa inflammations and epithelial irritations (Ogunmodede, 1977; Chung and Baker, 1990; Lambertz *et al.*, 2020).

Ruiz and Harms (1988a) showed that broiler starter diets containing 2.6 mg/kg vitamin B_2 caused reduced growth rates, severe paralysis, and high mortality and that 3.6 mg/kg was needed to achieve maximum productivity and 4.6 ppm to prevent foot problems. Rutz *et al.* (1989) obtained optimum performance by supplementing 2 mg/kg riboflavin, above that there was no further improvement.

Subsequent studies with more replicates raised the optimum dosage to 5.0–7.2 (Deyhim *et al.*, 1990, 1991; Olkowski and Classen, 1998). Deyhim *et al.* (1991) used a vitamin B_2 concentration 2 times higher than that recommended by the NRC (1994) and achieved an increase of 6% in live weight; when broilers were subjected to cyclical heat stress (24–35–24°C), the improvement was maintained at 5%, while the feed conversion index and mortality fell by 2% and 6%, respectively, compared to the control. In contrast, Deyhim *et al.* (1996) withdrew vitamins and trace minerals for 21 days in broiler diets during heat stress and found 37% less riboflavin in the *PM* muscle.

Whitehead (1999) induced chronic heat stress in chickens from 7 to 21 days of age and supplemented with 2.8, 3.3, 7, and 15 ppm. Heat stress reduced the growth rate by an average of 10%. No significant effects on the riboflavin level were detected, but curved claws were observed even at 7 mg/kg. At normal temperatures, 3.3 mg/kg was sufficient. Under tropical conditions, positive responses were found at 5.1–10 ppm (Ogunmodede, 1977; Ibrahim, 1998).

Whitehead (1999) pointed out that riboflavin requirements for growth, expressed as a percentage of the diet, had not changed despite the considerable genetic progress in broiler productivity, but that if the well-being of the birds was adopted as an additional criterion, requirements could be doubled under stress conditions. The recommendations of the principal genetic selection companies tend in this direction. Leeson and Summers (2008) and most North American companies (Coelho, 2000) used appreciably higher supplementation levels.

Jegede *et al.* (2018) concluded that the NRC (1994) recommendation of 4 mg/kg riboflavin (and 3.5 mg/kg pyridoxine, see next paragraph) might be no longer valid for modern broiler production. An upward review of up to 8 mg/kg riboflavin (and 7 mg/kg pyridoxine) to improve broiler body weight gain, crude protein retention, and health status of the modern broiler chickens was recommended (Figure 6.15, and see Chapter 7).

Recently, Biagi *et al.* (2021) analyzed the effects of vitamin B_2 supplementation on the ileum, caeca, and litter microbiota of Ross 308 broilers and the metabolic profile of the caecal content. Sequencing of the 16S rRNA V3–V4 region and metabolomics were used to explore microbiota composition and the concentration of metabolites of interest, including short-chain fatty acids. They found that vitamin B_2 supplementation significantly modulated caeca microbiota, with the highest dosage being more effective in increasing the abundance of health-promoting bacterial groups, including *Bifidobacterium*, resulting in boosted production of butyrate, a well-known health-promoting metabolite, in the caeca environment.

In turkeys, the most recent studies on riboflavin requirements were conducted by Lee (1982), who proposed 4 mg/kg as the most suitable level, and by Ruiz and Harms (1988a, 1989a), on whose results the current NRC recommendations are based. In young turkeys of 0–21 days, it was estimated that a total provision of 3.5 mg/kg was enough to achieve maximum production. However, to prevent paralysis and curved claws, it was necessary to increase it to 4.6 ppm. The same investigators determined that to maximize the live weight of males of 4–8 and 9–11 weeks, the optimum dietary levels were 3.6 and 2.5 mg/kg, respectively.

Salami *et al.* (2016) measured the bioavailability of copper, zinc, and magnesium from a commercial mineral chelate and corresponding inorganic salts in feed containing supplemental riboflavin and pyridoxine at 8 mg/kg or 7 mg/kg, respectively, in turkeys. Riboflavin supplementation improved the bioavailability of trace mineral chelates or inorganic salts. This may indicate that the optimum riboflavin level for turkeys could be close to 8 mg/kg.

Vitamin B_6 (pyridoxine)

Details about current vitamin B_6 recommendations for broilers and turkeys, provided by institutional sources and genetic companies, can be found in Tables 6.3 to 6.10.

Vitamin B_6 is one of the B vitamins that often receives the least attention when formulating poultry rations. Owing to its wide distribution in feedstuffs, nutritionists generally expect adequate levels in typical poultry diets. However, it must be considered that, on average, only 50% of pyridoxine contained in feedstuffs is bioavailable and that the optimum requirements of pyridoxine are related to the levels of protein and amino acids in the diet (Daghir and Shah, 1973). Consequently, as amino acid levels have increased in the past years (Cerrate and Corzo, 2019), pyridoxine requirement would increase by 25% (Portsmouth, 1996) or more.

The NRC (1994) position is based on studies from the early 1970s, and it proposes 3.5 mg/kg feed for broilers and turkeys from 8 weeks onwards and 4.5 mg/kg for turkeys in the first 8 weeks. Different studies estimate a requirement of 6 mg/kg both for turkeys (Waldroup *et al.*, 1985) and broilers (Leeson and Summers, 2008; Bains, 1999). However, recent evaluations under heat-stress conditions suggest higher supplementations.

Tagar (2005) evaluated pyridoxine supplementation in broilers at the rates of 10, 15, 20, and 25 mg/kg feed observing that the 20 mg/kg dose improved weight gain, feed efficiency, carcass weight, and reduced mortality maximum net profit/bird. Jegede *et al.* (2018) fed diets supplemented with pyridoxine at rates of 3, 5, 7, and 10,5 mg/kg feed to Marshall broiler chickens and observed the best final body weight and protein retention in diets with 7 mg/kg (Figure 6.15).

Owing to the properties of pyridoxine, such as associated with lipid peroxidation, stimulating activity of the glutathione-dependent enzyme, among others, Khakpour *et al.* (2015)

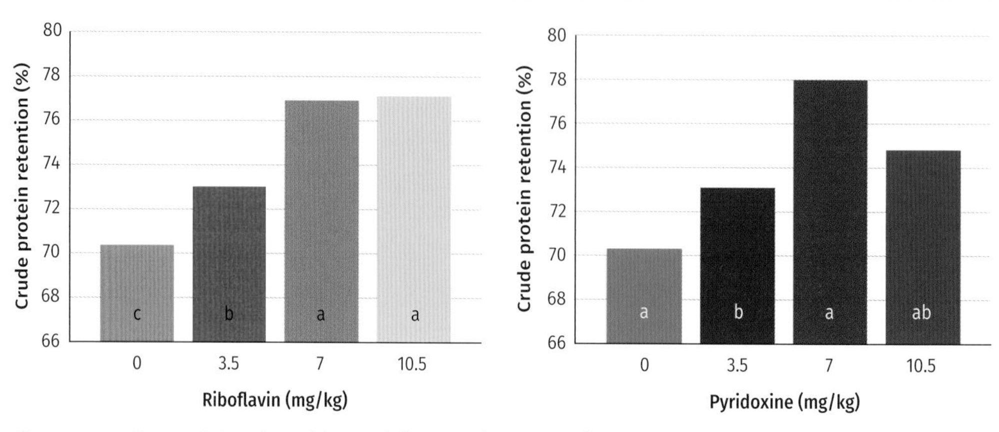

Figure 6.15 Effects of vitamin B_2 (riboflavin) and B_6 (pyridoxine) on protein retention in broilers, values with no common superscripts differ significantly, $P < 0.05$ (source: Jegede *et al.*, 2018)

investigated the effect of dietary lysine and pyridoxine on broilers during heat stress. They concluded that 3 mg/kg of pyridoxine is sufficient to support the antioxidant status and performance of the birds, and that feeding higher amounts of this vitamin alone or along with lysine has no additional effect on the antioxidant status.

Vitamin B_6 at a very high dose is significant for animal well-being. It has been shown that high pyridoxine levels (500–1,000 mg/kg) can reduce fear reactions in broilers, as assessed by the duration of the tonic immobility reaction (Schwean and Classen, 1995). These high doses had a negative effect on weight gain but improved the conversion index. Supplementing with 3 ppm pyridoxine was found beneficial, either on its own or in combination with 60 ppm L-carnitine, under thermal stress conditions (Celik *et al.*, 2006). This combination improved weight gain, feed intake, and carcass weight not observed when pyridoxine alone was used. This synergy may be attributable to the potential of both substances to regulate energy metabolism and modulate oxidative stress.

Attention has also been given to the ability of vitamin B_6 to reduce the incidence of leg problems (Cope *et al.*, 1979; Beirne and Jensen, 1981). According to Sauveur (1984), pyridoxine is involved in forming picolinic acid (derived from tryptophan), which is linked to the intestinal absorption of zinc, and all of them would act synergically in preventing leg problems. Massé *et al.* (1994, 1996) demonstrated that a marginal deficiency of vitamin B_6 leads to incomplete collagen development and an anarchic invasion of the bone growth plate by irregular blood vessels and long bone deviation. These problems could be reduced with higher supplementation of vitamin B_6. They considered this vitamin essential for the integrity of the conjunctive tissue matrix and the development of the skeleton.

The dietary needs of pyridoxine can be affected by the bioavailability of Cu, Zn, and Mn, which act as cofactors in many biochemical reactions where pyridoxine is involved. In growing turkeys, Salami *et al.* (2016) measured the bioavailability of copper, zinc, and magnesium from a commercial mineral chelate and corresponding inorganic salts in feed containing supplemental riboflavin and pyridoxine at 8 mg/kg or 7 mg/kg, respectively. The bioavailability of the trace mineral chelates or inorganic salts was improved by pyridoxine supplementation. This may indicate that the optimum pyridoxine level for turkeys could be close to 7 mg/kg.

Vitamin B_{12} (cyanocobalamin)

Details about current vitamin B_{12} recommendations for broilers and turkeys, provided by institutional sources and genetic companies, can be found in Tables 6.3 to 6.10.

Vitamin B_{12} requirements are very small (measured in micrograms per kilograms feed), but it is the only vitamin stored in the large quantities, mainly in the liver. Requirements were estimated to be 12 μg/kg in the 1970s (Whitehead and Portsmouth, 1989), and Portsmouth (1996) considered that its level should be increased by about 20% in diets without animal by-product meal.

Alisheilkhov *et al.* (2000) evaluated the combination of 35 μg/kg vitamin B_{12} and 103 mg/kg vitamin C observing increased live weight by 7.5% and energy use by 6.7% compared to the control group. Halle *et al.* (2011) compared broiler diets without supplementation with 40 μg/kg, and similar effects in feed intake and improvements in body weights were observed. Recently Teymouri *et al.* (2020) conducted an experiment to determine the effect of *in ovo* feeding 20 and 40 μg/kg vitamin B_{12} on hatchability, growth performance, and blood constituents in broilers. These results suggest *in ovo* feeding of vitamin B_{12} had positive effects on hatchability as well as on subsequent performance in broiler chicken.

Niacin (vitamin B_3)

Details about current niacin recommendations for broilers and turkeys, provided by institutional sources and genetic companies, can be found in Tables 6.3 to 6.10.

The requirements for niacin are uncertain since its availability varies depending on cereal type and the influence of tryptophan levels. Much niacin in common plant sources is in a bound form not available to animals. Therefore, niacin values for corn and other cereal grains and their by-product should be largely disregarded in formulating poultry diets. It is best to assume that these feeds provide no available niacin for the chick or pig (Cunha, 1982a,b). Moreover, most poultry diets, particularly corn-based diets, do not contain large excesses of tryptophan available to be converted into niacin.

The most critical time for supplementation is during early growth, when requirements are the highest. It is assumed that requirements have increased in correlation to the improvement in growth rate, but very little research has been carried out in the last 25 years. Whitehead and Portsmouth (1989) proposed a level of 70 mg/kg, 2 times higher than the NRC's (1994) recommendation of 35 ppm in broilers. Later Whitehead (1993) estimated requirements at 50–55 mg/kg. Waldenstedt (2006) points out that the proportion of birds with foot defects is higher in birds whose diet is low in this vitamin.

North American studies, based on corn-soy diets, are somewhat contradictory. Waldroup *et al.* (1985), in a series of 4 experiments with broilers raised to 42 days, used supplements of 33–66 mg/kg to a basal diet with 33 mg/kg and observed significant improvements in live weight (with a greater response in males) and some cases in the feed conversion index. However, Ruiz and Harms (1988c, 1990) found no significant differences when feeding supplemental niacin above 35 mg/kg on top of 22 mg/kg in the basal diet.

Ahmadian *et al.* (2021) wrote one of the most complete reviews of the effects of niacin in broilers (Table 6.15). Most studies indicated that 33 mg/kg of nicotinic acid could maintain optimum growth, carcass quality, and immune system. However, 150 mg/kg of nicotinic acid

Table 6.15 Summary of the effect of niacin and its available forms (nicotinic acid and nicotinamide) on the performance, carcass characteristics, and meat quality of broilers (Ahmadian *et al.*, 2021)

Reference	Niacin dietary level (mg/kg)	Summary of findings
Briggs *et al.* (1942)	1.5, 2, 2.5, 5, and 10 mg/kg nicotinic acid	Increased weight gain of chickens
Scott *et al.* (1946)	2 mg/kg nicotinic acid	Increased weight gain of chickens
Christian *et al.* (1971)	5, 10, and 15 mg/kg niacin	Increased weight gain
Yen *et al.* (1977)	20 mg/kg niacin	Increased weight gain and feed intake
Ang *et al.* (1984)	75% of the vitamins niacin, riboflavin and B_6	Increased live weight gain, feed intake and feed conversion ratio
Ang *et al.* (1984)	10, 75, and 125% of B vitamins	Lack of significant effect on nutrients, moisture, protein; fat and ash of breast meat
Waldroup *et al.* (1985)	33, 66, and 99 mg/kg niacin	Increased weight gain of chickens at 35 days of age
	99 mg/kg niacin + 6.25% fat	Increase feed intake
Ruiz and Harms (1988c)	3, 6, 12, and 33 mg/kg nicotinic acid and nicotinamide	Increased live weight gain and feed intake; no significant effect on feed conversion ratio
Ruiz and Harms (1990)	3, 6, 12, 24, and 36 mg/kg niacin	Lack of significant effect on feed intake, body weight and feed conversion ratio
Chen *et al.* (1996)	3, 6, and 9 mg/kg niacin + 0.16, 0.18, and 0.20% tryptophan	Increased live weight gain; increased feed efficiency; reduced fatality
Oloyo (2000)	22.5, 30, 37.5, 45, 52.5, and 60 mg/kg niacin	Increased weight gain, feed intake and lack of significant effect on feed efficiency
Oloyo (2000)	37.5, 45, 52.5, and 60 mg/kg niacin	Increased carcass weight; reduced abdominal fat
	37.5, 45 and 52.5 mg/kg niacin	Increased carcass percentage
	37.5 mg/kg niacin	Producing the highest amount of edible meat
Roth-Maier and Paulicks (2002)	Less than standard amounts of the vitamins niacin, riboflavin, pantothenic acid, B_{12}, biotin, folic acid, and choline	Reduction of fatalities; improved live weight, feed intake and feed conversion ratio
Celik *et al.* (2003)	50 mg/l niacin + 50 mg/l L-carnitine	Increased live weight gain
Celik *et al.* (2003)	50 mg/l niacin + 50 mg/l L-carnitine	Increased feed intake
	50 mg/l niacin and L-carnitine	Lack of significant effect on feed conversion ratio

Table 6.15 (continued)

Reference	Niacin dietary level (mg/kg)	Summary of findings
Javed *et al.* (2010)	8 g/kg chromium chloride + 150 mg/kg nicotinic acid + 200 mg/kg copper sulphate	Increased meat cholesterol at 15 days of age
	2 g/kg chromium chloride + 150 mg/kg nicotinic acid + 0 mg/kg copper sulphate	Lowering breast meat, increased cholesterol at 29 days of age
	2 g/kg chromium chloride + 150 mg/kg nicotinic acid + 200 mg/kg copper sulphate	Increased thigh muscle cholesterol at 15 days of age
	2 g/kg chromium chloride + 150 mg/kg nicotinic acid + 400 mg/kg copper sulphate	Decreased thigh muscle cholesterol at 29 days of age
	2 and 8 g/kg chromium chloride + 150 mg/kg nicotinic acid + 200 and 400 mg/kg copper sulphate	Reduction of crude breast muscle fat at 15 and 29 days of age; reduction of crude fat in the thigh muscle; lack of significant effect on crude protein, moisture content, and ash percentage of breast and thigh meat
Jiang *et al.* (2011)	30, 60, and 120 mg/kg nicotinic acid	Increased daily weight, feed intake and feed conversion ratio
Jiang *et al.* (2011)	30, 60, and 120 mg/kg nicotinic acid	Increased percentage of empty carcass; lack of significant effect on the thickness of subcutaneous fat; Lack of significant effect on the width of the intermuscular fat band; reduced muscle fat
	60 mg/kg nicotinic acid	Significant increase in breast muscle percentage
	30 and 60 mg/kg nicotinic acid	Increase in the percentage of abdominal fat
Jiang *et al.* (2011)	30, 60, and 120 mg/kg nicotinic acid	Lack of significant effect on pH of *Pectoralis minor*; reduction of drip loss and reduction of meat shear force; decreased breast redness
	60 mg/kg nicotinic acid	Increased lightness of meat
	30 and 120 mg/kg nicotinic acid	Decreased meat yellowness
Nazir *et al.* (2017)	6.5 mg/kg of the antibiotic Lincomycin + 25 mg/kg of niacin	Lack of significant effect on feed intake, water intake, live weight and mortality rate; decreased feed conversion ratio compared to separate uses of niacin and antibiotics
Nazir *et al.* (2017)	25 mg/kg niacin + 6.5 mg/kg antibiotic lincomycin	Lack of significant effect on carcass and liver weight; increased weight of the heart and gizzard

combined with chromium and copper sulfate effectively reduced cholesterol in broiler breast and thigh muscles.

The data for turkeys is also inconsistent. Ruiz and Harms (1990b) worked with 0, 3, 6, 12, 24 and 36 mg/kg niacin supplement to a corn-soybean meal diet containing 22 mg/kg niacin and 0.23% tryptophan and concluded that niacin supplementation in poults from 3 to 7 weeks of age not necessary.

The same authors tried supplementation levels up to 88 ppm in young turkeys of 0–21 days old (Ruiz and Harms, 1988a). They concluded that a minimum of 44 mg/kg was sufficient to maximize productive results and reduce the incidence and severity of foot problems.

Furthermore, Maurice *et al.* (1990a) obtained significant improvements in live weight at 8 weeks with diets containing 140 mg/kg, more than twice as much as proposed by the NRC (1994), an improvement maintained to a lesser extent under stress conditions from damp bedding. In a subsequent investigation, the same authors (Maurice *et al.*, 1990b) found that in turkeys older than 8–12 weeks, niacinamide at 100 mg/kg counteracted the reduction in growth caused by high population density and tended to increase carcass protein (+2.4%) and decrease carcass fat (−4.0%). On the other hand, in respiratory infections from *Bordetella*, positive effects were obtained from adding niacin to drinking water (Yersin *et al.*, 1989).

Whitehead (2001) proposed adding 70 mg/kg of niacin to feeds for up to 12 weeks but considered these levels inadequate for wheat diets and growth rates. He conducted and published 2 experiments. The best results for live weight and conversion at 3 and 6 weeks were obtained with 80–100 mg/kg. Under heat-stress conditions, the niacin requirement for maximum growth dropped to 50 mg/kg due to the lower weight gain caused by the high temperatures.

Adebowale *et al.* (2018) investigated the influence of dietary high or recommended nicotinic acid on various parameters of growing turkeys. They compared a control diet with the basal level of 26.7 mg/kg niacin, a diet supplemented with 60 mg/kg niacin termed as recommended niacin supplementation, and a diet supplemented with 180 mg/kg niacin termed as high niacin supplementation. Collectively, high dietary supplementation of niacin (180 mg/kg) improved production performances, reduced serum and meat fat content, and improved indicators of stress resistance ability in growing turkeys.

Pantothenic acid (vitamin B_5)

Details about current pantothenic acid recommendations for broilers and turkeys, provided by institutional sources and genetic companies, can be found in Tables 6.3 to 6.10.

The established requirements of pantothenic acid for chickens (10 mg/kg feed) are based on studies from the late 1970s. There are few more recent experimental datasets, although contrary to the situation with other vitamins, they tend to confirm earlier findings. Deyhim *et al.* (1992) tried concentrations 2 and 4 times higher than normal in broilers without improving their growth rate or energy balance. Harms and Nelson (1992) tried supplementation levels of up to 14.4 mg/kg in chicks (0–21 days) without finding significant differences in growth rate or feed conversion index compared to the levels currently established by the NRC (1994).

However, the current recommended levels for commercial strains are 2–3 times higher, probably because of the role of pantothenic acid in general resistance to stress and the prevention of skin lesions (Bains, 1999). The study by Deyhim *et al.* (1992) offers another interesting aspect: the possibility of enriching pantothenic acid content in poultry meat. At the dosages of 30 and 50 mg/kg pantothenic acid in breast meat significantly increased by 35–74% ($P < 0.05$).

Parnian *et al.* (2019) found a positive effect of *in ovo* injection of pantothenic acid on some immunological parameters of broiler chicks, influencing the broilers' final weight.

Studies in turkeys have produced similar results, both in the starter period (Ruiz and Harms, 1989b) and between 4 and 12 weeks, where the use of levels lower than those of the NRC (4–8 mg/kg) in corn-soy diets did not entail significant changes in these parameters (Harms and Bootwalla, 1992). Latymer and Coates (1981) feeding broilers a diet with a semi-purified diet containing pantothenic acid at various doses from 0 and 25 mg/kg and copper sulfate ($CuSO_4$) at 250 mg/kg showed that when the doses of pantothenic acid were marginally adequate or less the copper sulfate supplementation induced severe signs of pantothenic acid deficiency, suggesting that high dietary supplements of copper sulfate cause pantothenic acid deficiency through interference in the biosynthesis of coenzyme A.

Biotin (vitamin B_7)

Details about current biotin recommendations for broilers and turkeys, provided by institutional sources and genetic companies, can be found in Tables 6.3 to 6.10.

The study of this vitamin received much attention to the appearance in the 1970s of a serious metabolic problem in broilers known as FLKS, described in detail by Whitehead *et al.* (1976a,b), Whitehead (1977, 1985, 1988a) and Bryden (1991). The imbalance between 2 enzymes dependent on biotin prevents the hepatic gluconeogenesis from re-establishing glycemia levels in cases of greater demand due to fasting or heat stress. Mobilizing lipid reserves to obtain glucose fails, leading to fatty infiltration of the organs and death by acidosis. Whitehead *et al.* (1976a,b) demonstrated clearly that FLKS occurs in response to insufficient biotin in the diet. This pathology was seen in particular when broiler diets were relatively low in fat and protein, but in 2000 Whitehead (2000a,b) indicated that the problem was again being found in the UK.

Moreover, we must consider that biotin is poorly supplied by cereals and present in both bound and free forms. The amount bound either to protein or lysine is unavailable to the animal. For poultry, and presumably other species, often less than one-half of the microbiologically determined biotin in a feedstuff is biologically available (Scott, 1981; Whitehead *et al.*, 1982; Frigg, 1984, 1987).

Studies carried out more than 40 years ago (Whitehead and Bannister, 1980) established a level of 170 µg/kg as the biotin requirement for growth in broilers. However, based on older data, the NRC (1994) maintained its recommendation at 150 µg/kg. Other authors (Misir and Blair, 1984; Watkins and Kratzer, 1987a,b,c; Oloyo, 1991, 1994; Chee and Chang, 1995) found linear responses up to 200 µg/kg. Whitehead (1988a) indicated that the biotin requirement could increase under conditions of nutritional or environmental stress and that diets slightly low in fat or protein and providing 250–300 µg/kg biotin might be necessary to minimize mortality.

Oloyo (1991, 1994) specified a requirement of 200 µg/kg to prevent FLKS, pododermatitis, and foot deformities completely, a level rather higher than that required to achieve optimum live weight and feed conversion. Some diets with unshelled sunflower seeds required up to 240 µg/kg biotin to achieve the same results.

In subsequent investigations, responses have been obtained to even higher values. Balios and Poupulis (1992) brought significant improvements in live weight and feed conversion with 550 µg/kg when the proportion of fat added to the feed was 1.5% instead of 6.5%. Brufau *et al.* (1995) significantly increased the growth rate and feed conversion efficiency by adding 200 µg/kg to diets with 50% wheat, and Jian *et al.* (1996), with wheat-based diets, obtained an increase in live weight at 21 days by using up to 300 µg/kg. With feeds based on wheat and 6 supplementation levels – between 0 and 250 µg/kg of biotin available – Whitehead (2000b) obtained 100 g more live weight at 40 days with the maximum level of 300 µg/kg of total biotin and a numerical improvement of the feed conversion index.

Quarantelli *et al.* (2007) observed similar results reporting improved growth rates when supplementing biotin at dosages of 200, 300, and 400 mg/kg. The response was quadratic, with a maximum improvement in body weight gain when supplementing biotin at 200 µg/kg. Biotin improved broiler standing and walking ability, and femur and tibiotarsus bone mineral density were also enhanced by biotin supplementation at 200 and 400 µg/kg.

Biotin is also related to other aspects of animal health and well-being. It has been observed that sudden death syndrome tends to decrease when higher levels of biotin are used (Hulan *et al.*, 1980; Whitehead and Randall, 1982), although the etiology of this condition remains unclear. A significant reduction in lesions from reovirus infection like tenosynovitis and twisted feet has also been found when the biotin concentration in the diet was 200% higher than that indicated by the NRC (Cook *et al.*, 1984a,b).

Another health issue that has been linked to biotin is plantar pododermatitis. Various studies have established a relationship between biotin deficiency and digital and plantar lesions (Harms and Simpson, 1975; Harms *et al.*, 1977; McIlroy *et al.*, 1987). The incidence of footpad lesions has increased over recent years (Ekstrand *et al.*, 1997; Martrenchar *et al.*, 2002; Folegatti *et al.*, 2006; Pagazaurtundúa and Warris, 2006), and there is pressure in the EU to reduce incidence for animal welfare reasons. The causes are known to be multifactorial, including genetic susceptibility. Kjaer *et al.* (2006) investigated the degree of inheritance foot pad dermatitis (FPD) and hock burn (HB) in broilers. A total of 2,118 birds from 2 strains were allocated to 12 groups of 93–100 birds, each in 2 time-separated replicates. The development of FPD and HB were recorded weekly from day 8 to slaughter on a set sample of live animals (7 per group). The relatively high heritability of FPD and the low genetic correlation to body weight suggested that genetic selection against susceptibility to FPD should be possible without negative effects on body weight gain.

The primary cause of pododermatitis stems from rearing poultry on excessively damp bedding (Haslam *et al.*, 2007; Mayne *et al.*, 2007a) and certain types of bedding and their depth (Martrenchar *et al.*, 2002; Haslam *et al.*, 2007). It can also be caused by an insufficient ventilation flow (Folegatti *et al.*, 2006), an excessive population density (Ekstrand *et al.*, 1997), or through the influence of certain ingredients or nutritional imbalances, which lead to wet droppings (Oloyo, 1991, 1994; Bilgili *et al.*, 2005; Eichner *et al.*, 2007).

High stocking density affects the performance and well-being of broilers through litter-independent and litter-dependent mechanisms. Increasing supplemental biotin favors growth performance and improves footpad and hock health in both dry- or wet-litter conditions. However, no nutritional intervention may effectively prevent the lesions when moisture levels are too high.

The effects of biotin on footpad dermatitis have been controversial, but the level of inclusion and interactions with minerals may play a role in its efficacy. Abd El-Wahab *et al.* (2013) tested the prophylactic effects of higher dietary biotin (2,000 µg/kg diet, a normal level would be 300 µg/kg diet) and zinc levels for broilers exposed to litter with high moisture (35% water) on the development of footpad dermatitis. Their results suggest combining the maximum levels of zinc (especially of zinc-methionine) and high levels of biotin when clinically relevant alterations in the footpad occur.

In broilers, Sun *et al.* (2017) evaluated the responses to stocking density, dietary biotin concentration, and litter condition on Ross 308 male broilers from day 22 to day 42, with 2 levels of

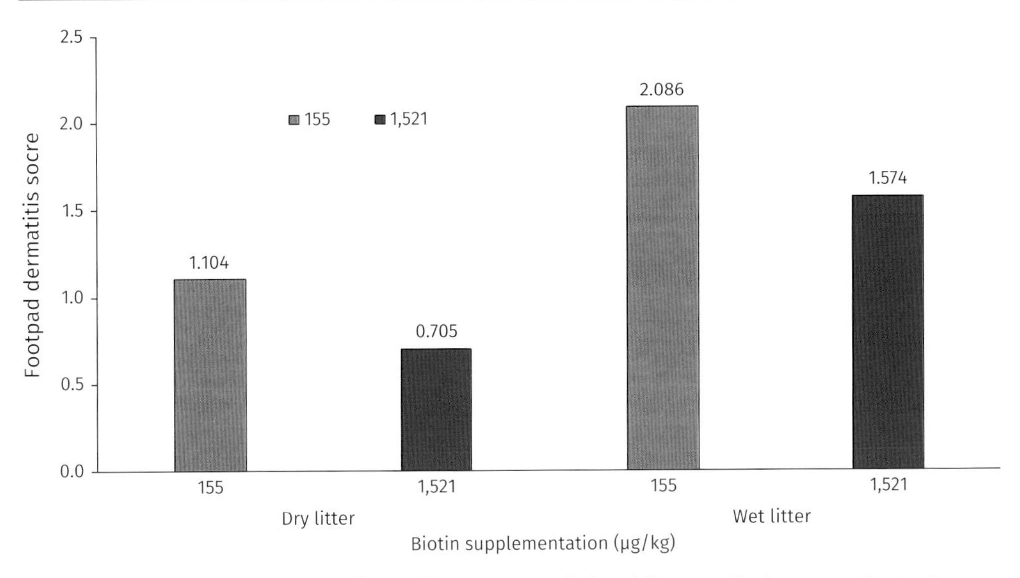

Figure 6.16 Biotin supplementation (155 µg/kg *vs.* 1,521 µg/kg) and litter quality impact on footpad dermatitis score at a high stock density (Sun *et al.*, 2017)

biotin, normal 155 µg/kg, and high 1,521 µg/kg. Results indicated that increasing supplemental biotin has a favorable effect on growth performance and footpad and hock health of high stocking density broilers under either dry- or wet-litter conditions (Figure 6.16). These findings provide a basis for a new approach to preventing dermatitis and the resulting production problems.

In turkeys under commercial conditions, the characteristic signs of biotin deficiency (dermatitis, perosis) have been observed more frequently than in broilers (Whitehead, 1988b; Waldenstedt, 2006), and turkeys, especially the males, are more prone than females to plantar pododermatitis, which causes pain and impaired mobility. Therefore, turkey biotin requirements are especially high (Whitehead, 1977; Mayne, 2007b). In early studies, 300 µg/kg feed levels were needed to reverse plantar lesions (Dobson, 1970; Whitehead, 1977). Around 1970 the biotin requirement of fattening turkeys was estimated at some 250 µg/kg feed, and the subsequent literature recommended levels of 200–325 µg/kg in the starter phase (Misir and Blair, 1988; Whitehead and Portsmouth, 1989), although male turkeys needed 50 µg/kg more than females. Biotin requirements fall with age but increase if there is a high proportion of soy in the ration and/or the bedding is damp.

Today's recommended biotin dosage might be higher, considering the genetic improvement achieved in the last 50 years (Clark *et al.*, 2002). Buda (2000) reported that very high inclusion rates of dietary biotin (2,000 µg/kg) in the turkey diet reduced the severity of footpad lesions. However, Mayne *et al.* (2007a) could not observe any effect of biotin levels in turkey diets – 0, 200, 800, and 1,600 µg/kg – on macroscopic and histopathology of footpads dermatitis under wet-litter conditions (45% moisture). Whitehead (2002c) and Mayne *et al.* (2007b) consider it highly advisable to increase biotin levels in such a case. No effects on growth or other parameters were observed in that experiment.

Youssef *et al.* (2012) mentioned that a high concentration of biotin of 2,000 µg/kg and zinc of 50 mg/kg of turkey diet reduced the development and severity of footpad dermatitis on fresh dry litter (25% moisture) but not on very wet new litter (73% moisture). FLKS rarely appears in turkeys, although it can be induced experimentally with low biotin diets and an 18 hour fast (Whitehead and Siller, 1983). There is little information about the possible effects of biotin on meat quality. Oloyo (1991) indicated that 200 μg/kg was necessary to maximize muscle percentage and the meat-to-bone relationship. At the same time, 160 μg/kg was sufficient to achieve maximum weight and carcass yield. Balios and Poupulis (1992) compared diets with 1.5 and 6.5% fat and 120–150 *vs.* 550 μg/kg of biotin. With the higher dosage, they observed a tendency to reduce abdominal fat and a significant increase in its degree of saturation.

Mahmood and Ahmed (2017) studied the effect of adding biotin to the diet of broilers submitted to oxidative stress on some broiler performance traits. The authors concluded that adding biotin 350 and 450 μg/kg could reduce the harmful effect of oxidative stress. Shekhu *et al.* (2019) evaluated the effects of biotin levels on live performance, protein and fat apparent digestibility, and carcass characteristics. The treatments were a control diet without additives and 3 levels of biotins which were 1,000, 1,500, and 2,000 mg/10 l drinking water, respectively, during the whole grow-out period. Results indicated that supplemental biotin in the drinking water had a favorable effect on body weight gain and FCR. However, biotin did not affect carcass characteristics and relative organs weight.

Folic acid (vitamin B_9)

Details about current folic acid recommendations for broilers and turkeys, provided by institutional sources and genetic companies, can be found in Tables 6.3 to 6.10.

The NRC (1994) recommendation was 0.55 mg/kg, and few recent studies have been published. Still, these have generally found improved responses at higher dosages, and the industry levels are actually 4 times higher. Folic acid requirements vary according to the composition of the diet. They increase if the protein level is high since it is required to synthesize uric acid (Creek and Vasaitis, 1963). The need for folic acid is also influenced by the metabolism of certain amino acids (methionine, glycine, serine) and other vitamins. Folic acid needs to increase if B_{12} and especially choline are deficient.

Pesti *et al.* (1991) demonstrated that corn-soy diets with theoretical content of 1.5 ppm of folic acid produced clear signs of folic acid deficiency because their actual concentration was 3 times lower. Other authors found positive growth and feed conversion responses with 1.8–2 mg/kg (Pesti and Rowland, 1989; Ryu and Pesti, 1993; Ryu *et al.*, 1994).

Ryu *et al.* (1995) considered existing requirements to be poorly established due to inadequacies of the analytical methods, the widespread belief that soy-based diets do not require supplementation, and the fact that many nutritional factors may modify their requirements. They estimated the total requirements at 1.45 mg/kg and recommended adding 1.2–1.3 mg/kg depending on the choline levels in the diet.

With choline and methionine levels close to those recommended by the NRC, 1.2 mg/kg supplements have been suggested (Pesti *et al.*, 1991; Ryu *et al.*, 1995). However, Whitehead *et al.* (1995) did not observe this supposed dependence on choline levels, suggesting that methionine deficiency may be more significant for folic acid requirements. In their experiments, maximum growth and feed conversion results were obtained with a total content in the starter diet as the meal of 1.7–2.0 mg/kg, thus, requiring supplementation with an estimated 1.5 mg/kg. The authors recommend a supplement of 2.5 to 3 mg/kg for pellet feeds.

Along the same lines, El-Husseiny *et al.* (2007) presented a study that evaluated the efficacy of folic acid and betaine in situations where methionine was adequate or limiting. In both cases, improvements were obtained in production parameters, digestibility of nutrients, and carcass yield with levels of both folic acid and betaine of 0.5–0.75 or 1 mg/kg.

Folic acid appears to be effective in preventing certain pathological disorders and improving immunity. In the case of *reovirus* infection, lesions decreased if the concentration of folic acid in diets was 2 times higher than that proposed by the NRC (Cook *et al.*, 1984b).

In cellular *in vitro* studies, Uribe-Diaz *et al.* (2021) demonstrated that folic acid supplementation modulated B lymphocyte responses and improved innate immune proinflammatory and antiviral responses.

Some authors showed that low levels of folic acid in high-protein diets increase foot problems (Ryu *et al.*, 1995; Waldenstedt, 2006). A trial using thiram (tetramethyl thiuram disulfide) to induce TD in chickens (Rath *et al.*, 2006) evaluated the protective capacity of various vitamins (A, D, B_6, and folic acid) against this condition. They concluded that folic acid levels 5 times higher than those recommended by the NRC (1994) were the most effective for this purpose.

Gouda *et al.* (2020) investigated the impact of supplemental L-ascorbic acid (200 mg/kg) and folic acid (1.5 mg/kg) on broiler chickens. The combination of ascorbic acid and folic acid improved body weight gain, feed intake, and FCR (Table 6.16) and increased the antioxidant status, thyroid hormone levels, insulin growth factor 1 (IGF-1), blood hemoglobin, total protein, albumin, globulin, heat shock protein 70, catalase enzyme activity, superoxide dismutase enzyme activity, antibody titers against Newcastle disease virus and decreased heterophil/lymphocyte ratios (Figure 6.17). Folic acid was more effective in improving the great majority of these parameters than vitamin C.

McCann *et al.* (2004) showed that adding 2 mg/kg of folic acid to the non-supplemented diet resulted in a 57% increase in breast meat folate level (15.9 *vs.* 10.1 µg/100 g). Adewole *et al.* (2021) conducted a trial to assess folic acid's impact on white striping. Broilers were allocated to 8 treatments consisting of 2 energy levels: normal and high, and 4 folic acid levels: 2, 2.5, 10, and 15 mg/kg feed. Birds fed high energy diets had reduced ($P<0.05$) feed intake and FCR than those on normal energy diets. With increasing folic acid levels, there was a reduced ($P<0.05$) white striping score and increased ($P<0.05$) normal breast fillet percentage in female chickens but not in the males. White striping scores were higher ($P<0.01$) in male chickens than in females.

Table 6.16 Effect of dietary supplementation of ascorbic acid and/or folic acid on the growth performance (adapted from Gouda *et al.*, 2020)

Vitamin C (mg/kg)	Folic acid (mg/kg)	Feed intake (g)	Bodyweight (g)	Feed conversion ratio (g:g)
0	0	2,614[d]	1,502[d]	1.8[a]
200	0	2,684[c]	1,682[c]	1.6[b]
0	1.5	2,710[b]	1,733[b]	1.6[bc]
200	1.5	2,793[a]	1,811[a]	1.6[c]

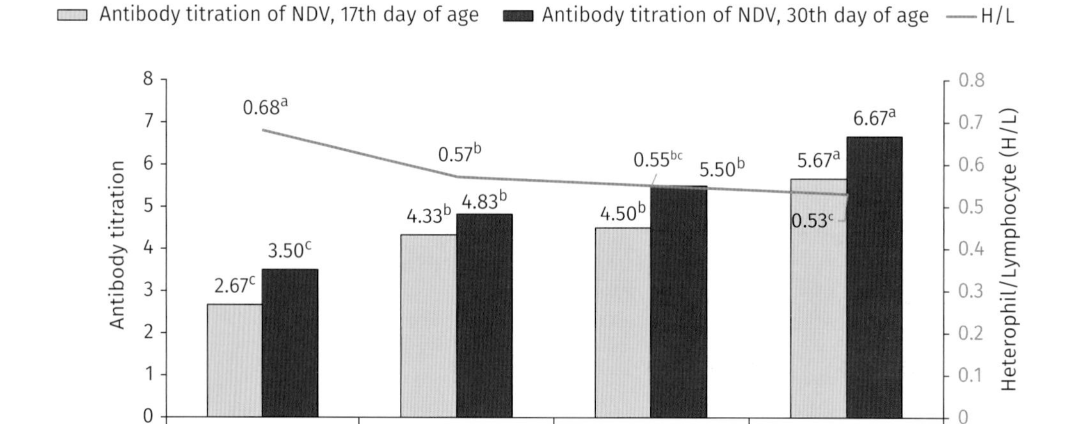

Figure 6.17 Effect of dietary supplementation of ascorbic acid and/or folic acid on the stress and immune response, values with no common superscripts differ significantly, $P < 0.05$ (adapted from Gouda *et al.*, 2020)

Vitamin C

Details about current vitamin C recommendations for broilers and turkeys, provided by institutional sources and genetic companies, can be found in Tables 6.3 to 6.10.

Under normal conditions, poultry can synthesize vitamin C in the kidney from carbohydrate precursors, thus assuming that they do not require dietary sources of the vitamin. However, the ability to do this is reduced in the first week of life, especially in males. Moreover, vitamin C synthesis also falls during stress (Pardue and Thaxton, 1986; Pardue, 1989; Hooper *et al.*, 1989; Seemann, 1991; Jones, 1996; Jones and Satterlee, 1997), increasing the probability of vitamin C deficiency.

Several factors may explain the variability in response to vitamin C supplementation: its low stability in feed, which has been improved in encapsulated forms (Whitehead and Keller, 2003), and also in drinking water, especially if alkaline and/or unchlorinated (Krautmann, 1989); the level and the duration of the administration, the age of the birds (van Niekerk *et al.*, 1989); and the intensity and the combination of stress factors (McKee and Harrison, 1995, 1996; McKee *et al.*, 1997; Teeter and Belay, 1996; Balnave, 2004). Therefore, it is important to closely consider the conditions in which trials have been carried out to assess the merits of vitamin C in poultry nutrition. In the next paragraphs, we will review the effects of vitamin C on some specific aspects.

Resistance to stress

In experiments carried out under excellent operating conditions, the response to adding ascorbic acid to feed tended to be statistically insignificant (Kafri *et al.*, 1988; Kutlu and Forbes, 1994; Marron *et al.*, 2001), although other researchers have found positive responses in weight gain, digestibility of nutrients and carcass yield with diets supplemented with 200 ppm (Lohakare *et al.*, 2005b).

Jain and Pandey (2018) studied vitamin C's effects on broiler growth performance. Four groups were given ascorbic acid of 30, 60, 90, and 120 mg/kg feed, respectively, as a supplement in feed.

They found that increased body weight, body weight gain, and feed intake were observed in the groups supplemented compared with control, especially at higher levels of supplementation. It may be concluded that vitamin C supplementation was beneficial for body weight gain and feed intake. In contrast, the FCR remained similar to the control treatment. From the economic point of view, diets supplemented with vitamin C at 120 mg/kg feed had the best return on investment.

Positive return on investment also has been reported when authors evaluated higher supplementation levels. Tavakoli *et al.* (2021) reported that treatment with vitamin C at 200 mg/kg feed had the lowest feed cost per kilogram of live weight when evaluating both 200 and 400 mg/kg additions in Ross 308 broilers up to 42 days under heat stress. In this experiment, remarkable improvements were observed in body weight, feed intake, FCR, and European production factor (Figure 6.18), carcass, and cut-up parts (Figure 6.19).

The situation changes when stress is induced (Pardue and Thaxton, 1982; Pardue *et al.*, 1984; McKee and Harrison, 1995; Mahmoud *et al.*, 2004) or if trials are conducted under commercial conditions, although in these cases, too, the responses vary depending on the degree of stress (Balnave, 2004). It has been established that vitamin C supplementation in feed or drinking water reduces the plasma levels of adrenocorticotropic hormone and corticosterone (Sahin and Sahin, 2002), triiodothyronine (T_3) and thyroxine (T_4) (Sahin *et al.*, 2003), and the respiratory quotient of birds (McKee *et al.*, 1997). All this helps limit metabolic stress symptoms and alleviate their consequences, which improves the birds' productivity and immunocompetence (Whitehead and Keller, 2003).

Supplementing ascorbic acid at normal temperatures appears to offer few advantages (Gous and Morris, 2005; Abidin and Khatoon, 2013), but the situation changes at high temperatures, the stress factor that, in practice, most frequently affects particularly finishing birds, inducing oxidative stress: ascorbic acid, one of the most important organic antioxidants, can help counteract. Some studies did not find a significant impact on production parameters when using vitamin C levels between 125 and 1,000 mg/kg (Stilborn *et al.*, 1988; Orban *et al.*, 1993; Puron *et al.*, 1994; Teeter and Belay, 1996; Rose and Peter, 2000; Abidin and Khatoon, 2013), however, in many others (Ogbuinya, 1991; Daghir, 1996; Abidin and Khatoon, 2013) significantly better

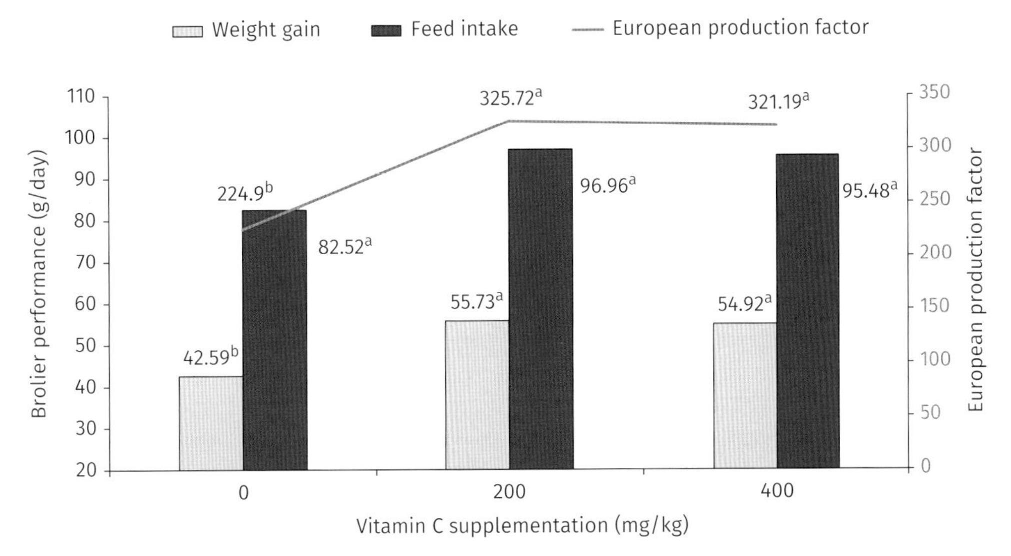

Figure 6.18 Effects of dietary vitamin C supplementation on performance parameters of broilers chickens, values with no common superscripts differ significantly, $P < 0.05$ (Tavakoli *et al.*, 2021)

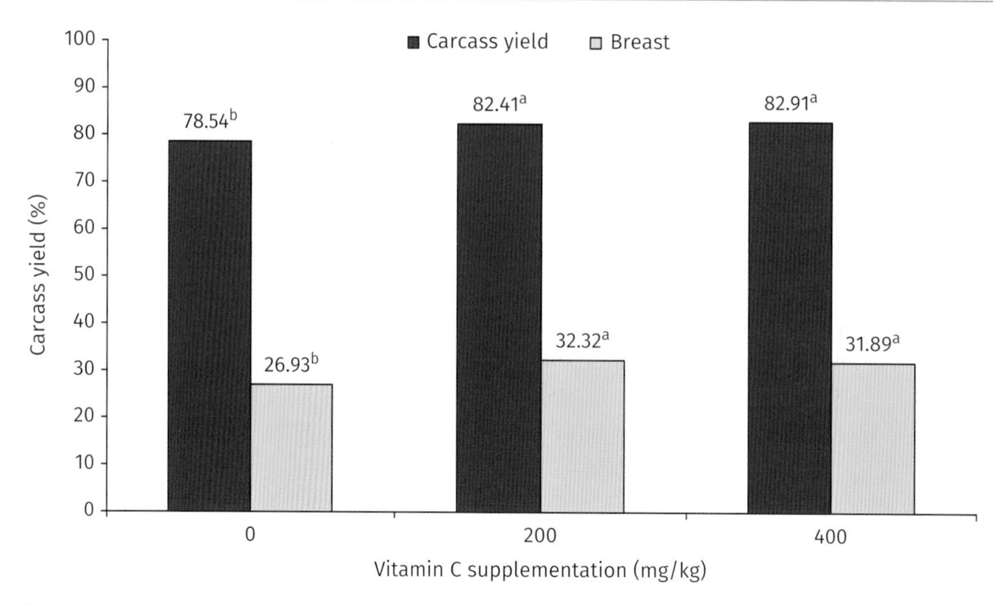

Figure 6.19 Effects of dietary vitamin C supplementation on carcass and breast meat yields of broilers chickens, values with no common superscripts differ significantly, $P < 0.05$ (Tavakoli *et al.*, 2021)

results have been found, with increased feed consumption, live weight, immunity and reduced mortality, oxidative stress, rectal and body temperature, carcass weight, and improved FCR. Notably, these include nearly all the trials carried out in hot countries, where supplementation with this vitamin is normal commercial practice.

Qureshi *et al.* (2000) obtained positive responses by adding vitamin C to the feed when, at the same time, electrolytes were added to the drinking water, suggesting that this could be a factor explaining the discrepancies observed. Horváth and Babinszky (2018), in a comprehensive review, concluded that the application of antioxidant vitamins like vitamin A (9,000–15,000 IU/kg diet), E (150–500 mg/kg diet), and C (150–500 mg/kg diet) is more effective when combined with zinc (30/60 mg/kg diet) and selenium (0.1–1 mg/kg diet).

In general, the dosages considered optimum are from 200–250 mg/kg, although in extreme conditions, further improvements have been confirmed at 500 and 1,000 ppm (Kafri and Cherry, 1984; Njoku, 1984, 1986; Pardue *et al.*, 1985; Kovar *et al.*, 1990; Cier *et al.*, 1992; Rajmane and Ranade, 1992; Daghir, 1995, 1996; Hussein, 1995; Dzhambulatov *et al.*, 1996; Díaz-Cruz *et al.*, 2001; Abidin and Khatoon, 2013). Curça *et al.* (2006) concluded that 2,000 ppm improved the weight of broilers kept at high temperatures by 12% at 4 weeks. Benefits are more evident when other stress factors, such as coccidiosis, or beak trimming in turkeys, are present (McKee and Harrison, 1995; Seokand and Singh, 1996). Satterlee *et al.* (1989) observed a reduced duration of the tonic immobility reaction in birds supplemented with vitamin C, indicating a situation of less fear.

Experiments with choice-feeding under heat stress indicated that broilers chose to eat the feed supplemented with 200 ppm vitamin C, increasing their intake in 3–5 days (Kutlu and Forbes, 1994). Moreover, levels of ascorbic acid in a feed show a negative correlation with those of heat shock protein (HSP 70) (Mahmoud *et al.*, 2004). Bottje *et al.* (1998) observed a reduction of vitamin C concentration in the pulmonary fluid under low-temperature conditions; this is possibly why similar dosages of vitamin C have also had positive results in the face of cold stress (Gross, 1988). Adding 1,000 ppm to the drinking water of day-old chicks that had suffered prolonged transportation significantly reduced mortality (Vo *et al.*, 1996).

Immunity

Vitamin C is known for its capacity to improve the immune response of chickens facing particular diseases and the consequent drop in growth or production and finally reduce mortality. There are many papers reviewed by Pardue (1989), Latshaw (1991), Chew (1996), Klasing (1998), Ferket and Qureshi (1992, 1999), Whitehead and Keller (2003), and Bahram *et al.* (2021) indicating the positive effects of vitamin C on poultry immune system. To this end, it has been recommended that before and during a pathogen threat, vitamin C levels of 300–330 mg/kg be used: in severe cases, up to 1,000 mg/kg have been used, although some researchers report that efficacy was lower with dosages above 400 ppm (Gross *et al.*, 1988; Davelaar and Van den Bos, 1992; Wen *et al.*, 1997). The most commonly observed effects are the significant reduction in mortality and lesions, the improvement in cellular immunity, and the amounts of specific antibodies (Gross, 1992). Also important is its antioxidant effect, which allows the stability of cellular membranes to be maintained (Dimanov *et al.*, 1994; van Dyck and Adams, 2003) and important organs such as the liver to be protected from oxidation (Hayashi *et al.*, 2004).

Favorable immune responses, frequently accompanied by decreases in morbidity and mortality, have been observed in various pathologies: coccidiosis (McKee and Harrison, 1995; Crevieu-Gabriel and Naciri, 2001), Newcastle disease (Edrise *et al.*, 1986; Franchini *et al.*, 1994; Gross *et al.*, 1988; Lohakare *et al.*, 2005b), infectious bronchitis (Davelaar and van den Bos, 1992; Okoye *et al.*, 2000), Gumboro disease (Wu *et al.*, 2000; Amakye-Anim *et al.*, 2000; Hayashi *et al.*, 2004; Lohakare *et al.*, 2005b), colibacillosis (Gross *et al.*, 1988; van Niekerk *et al.*, 1989), Marek's disease (Yotova *et al.*, 1990), aflatoxicosis and other intoxications (Pardue *et al.*, 1987; Maynard *et al.*, 1979; Tudor and Bunaciu, 2001) and ascites (Decuypère *et al.*, 1994; Bottje and Wideman, 1995a, 1998; Ladmakhi *et al.*, 1997; Díaz-Cruz *et al.*, 2001; Walton *et al.*, 2001; Xiang *et al.*, 2002). Nevertheless, vitamin C supplementation alone is not enough to prevent or cure all these diseases.

Bone quality and interactions with vitamin D

Other investigations have been directed at discovering the possible role of vitamin C in preventing leg and bone problems. Ascorbic acid stimulates the renal synthesis of the active form of vitamin D_3, calcitriol or $1{,}25(OH)_2D_3$, acting as a cofactor of the enzyme 1α-hydroxylase. Ascorbic acid at a level of 250 ppm, combined with calcitriol in the feed, can reduce rickets (Roberson and Edwards, 1994; Rennie, 1995). Vitamin C at 2,000 mg/kg improved femur bone strength by 16% (Orban *et al.*, 1993), although the combination of 200 mg/kg of vitamin C and 200 IU of vitamin D was enough to improve bone strength (Lohakare *et al.*, 2005a). Weiser *et al.* (1990) also demonstrated greater bone strength with 100 mg/kg and variable vitamin D levels in the diet. Whitehead (2002b, 2005) stated these benefits are greater in hot environments.

Vitamin C has also been used to prevent TD. Initial studies in which very high levels were tried (500–1,000 mg/kg) did not show positive effects. Rather, they were inconclusive since improvements were found in some experiments but not repeated in others (Edwards, 1989; Roberson and Edwards, 1994). The only consistent finding was a reduction of bone ash (Leach and Burdette, 1985; Edwards, 1989), which by contrast, increased when lower dosages were applied, both when vitamin C alone was used (Whitehead, 1995a) and when it was combined with higher calcium levels (Doan, 2000). Rennie (1995) indicated that 250–500 mg/kg feed were only effective with normal calcium levels.

According to Whitehead (2000a), adding 250 mg/kg vitamin C and 10 µg/kg calcitriol to feed completely prevents TD and counteracts the reduction in growth rate usually provoked by calcitriol. This synergy, considered dubious by Edwards (2000), would be due not only to the stimulation of $1{,}25(OH)_2D_3$ production but also to the fact that vitamin C promotes an increase in receptors for vitamin D and collagen biosynthesis and therefore stimulates bone matrix production (Farqhuarson *et al.*, 1998). This is why Whitehead and Keller (2003) concluded in their review that the combination of ascorbic acid and calcitriol is potentially useful for preventing TD. Petek *et al.* (2005) published positive results by adding 150 mg/l to drinking water.

Meat quality

The relationship between vitamin C and meat quality has also been widely studied. The addition of 0.1% ascorbic acid to the drinking water of chickens 24–36 hours before their collection and transport to the slaughterhouse significantly increased the carcass yield (on average by 1%) in practically all of the conducted tests, and frequently also, the breast percentage (Farr *et al.*, 1988; Quarles and Adrian, 1989; Fletcher and Cason, 1991; Krautmann *et al.*, 1991; Völker and Fenster, 1991; Grashorn and Völker, 1993).

Although some variation can be seen in the responses, and these effects are, as expected, more pronounced the more stressful are the conditions of these operations. Vitamin C supplementation reduced the levels of different stress indicators (Satterlee *et al.*, 1991).

Kutlu (2001) found that supplementing with 250 mg/kg reduced the lipid content in the carcass and increased carcass yield in broilers exposed to 35–37°C for 8 hours a day. The improvement in yield is based on the reduction of shrinkage during transport and increased water retention (Grashorn and Völker, 1993; McKnight *et al.*, 1996b). The latter may be because, in treated birds, less change has been found in the plasma concentration of aldosterone and the sodium/potassium ratio (Pardue *et al.*, 1985; Satterlee *et al.*, 1991).

Yin *et al.* (1993) demonstrated *in vitro* the vitamin C antioxidant activity on myoglobin, which could improve the color stability of the meat. Lohakare *et al.* (2005a) found an improvement in color stability at 200 mg/kg. Leeson *et al.* (1995) cited sources from the turkey industry that indicated positive effects of vitamin C on the prevention of PSE meat, which are known to be linked to stress situations suffered before the slaughter of the birds.

Vitamin C has an antioxidant effect *in vivo* by reducing the radical tocopheroxyl and thus restoring the antioxidant activity of vitamin E. It was therefore supposed that supplementing with it might favor the oxidative stability of meat fat. However, Morrisey *et al.* (1998) concluded in their review that this effect was small or non-existent. Neither the addition of 1,000 mg vitamin C to drinking water 24 hours before slaughtering (King *et al.*, 1993 and 1995) nor the supplementation of feed with 110 mg/kg ascorbic acid (Grau *et al.*, 2001a,b; Bou *et al.*, 2001) proved to have a protective effect against fat oxidation (measured by TBARS values), and they did not improve the organoleptic quality of the meat (Bou *et al.*, 2001). In contrast, McKnight *et al.* (1996b) found that in stress situations, the TBARS concentrations in the breast were reduced if a level of 200–300 mg/kg was used during the 3 weeks before slaughter.

Young *et al.* (2003) obtained similar results when supplementing 1,000 mg/kg vitamin C for 6 weeks together with 200 mg/kg vitamin E. These effects of protecting against oxidation and the synergic action of the 2 vitamins were also confirmed in the experiments by Gheisari *et al.* (2004) and Leskovec *et al.* (2019) using vitamin C at 240 mg/kg feed.

Skřivan *et al.* (2012) supplemented broiler diets with vitamin C at 280 and 560 mg/kg of diet, and selenium (sodium selenite or selenized yeast) at 0.3 mg/kg for 5 weeks. Vitamin C or selenium increased the protein concentration of the meat at the expense of fat. Vitamin C supplementation increased the vitamin C content of the meat in a dose-dependent manner and decreased the vitamin A concentration in the meat regardless of the selenium supplement. Vitamin C reduced the lipid oxidation in meat stored for 5 days. No sparing effect of vitamin C was observed on vitamin E in the meat.

Vitamin C supplementation also affects the fatty acid profile of breast meat in broilers. Tavakoli *et al.* (2020) evaluated 200 and 400 mg/kg vitamin C supplementation in Ross 308 broilers.

Table 6.17 Effect of vitamin C supplementation on the fatty acid profile of Ross 308 broiler breast meat at 42 days of age (adapted from Tavakoli *et al.*, 2020)

Breast meat fatty acids (%)	Vitamin C (mg/kg)		
	0	200	400
Myristic Acid Methyl Ester C14:0	2.02	0.61	1.85
Palmitic Acid Methyl Ester C16:0	37.48	35.17	36.04
Palmitoleic Acid Methyl Ester C16:1c	3.14	2.92	4.15
Stearic Acid Methyl Ester C18:0	11.4	9.4	10.11
Oleic Acid Methyl Ester C18:1n9c	22.57	23.69	28.76
Linoleic Acid Methyl Ester C18:2n6c	17.65	21.91	14.28
Linolenic Acid Methyl Ester C18:3n3	0.5	0.54	0.68
cis-11,14- Eicosadienoic Acid Methyl Ester C20:2c	0.38	0.62	0.29
cis-8,11,14- Eicosatrienoic AcidMethyl Ester C20:3n6c	0.67	0.55	0.84
cis-11,14,17- Eicosatrienoic Acid Methyl Ester C20:3	4.18	4.59	3

The authors observed that 200 mg/kg vitamin C was sufficient to reduce the concentration of saturated fatty acids such as myristic, palmitic, and stearic acid. In contrast, the amount of unsaturated fatty acids linoleic acid, cis-11,14-eicosadienoic acid, and cis-11,14,17-eicosatrienoic acid increased (Table 6.17). Vitamin C participates in the creation of dehydroascorbic acid through rapid oxidation; this compound protects the cell membrane against free radicals.

Interactions with other nutrients

The interactions of vitamin C with other substances have been studied. Vitamin C combined with citric acid and phytase improved life weight and conversion index. There have also been reports of 27% increases in apparent metabolizable energy digestibility in diets low in calcium and phosphorus compared to values obtained using phytase alone (Afsarmaneh *et al.*, 2004). In a later study, Afsarmaneh *et al.* (2005) added vitamin D_3 to this diet, increasing live weight and protein digestibility by 18 and 60%, respectively. Both feed consumption and feed conversion also improved compared to low phosphorus diets.

Under heat-stress conditions, vitamin C used at 250 ppm combined with chromium supplemented at 400 ppm improved live weight, feed intake, and FCR, demonstrating the 2 substances' synergic action (Sahin *et al.*, 2003). The serum concentrations of insulin, T_3, T_4, vitamin E, and vitamin C also increased while plasma levels of corticosterone, glucose, cholesterol, and MDA fell. These researchers indicated that the synergism between the 2 nutrients might be due to the increased insulin synthesis induced by the chromium. Since the hormone contributes to the transport of vitamin C to the red cell, vitamin C, used in conjunction with acetylsalicylic acid, boosted the immune response, increasing the weight of the bursa of Fabricius, thymus, and spleen and the serum levels of antibodies, even if the birds were subjected to high temperatures (Naseem *et al.*, 2005). The combined use of acetylsalicylic acid, sodium bicarbonate, and potassium chloride in drinking water improved production parameters in heat-stress situations (Roussan *et al.*, 2008).

In similar conditions of heat stress, combinations with other antioxidants have proven to have several benefits. Attia *et al.* (2017) evaluated the supplementation of vitamin C (200 mg/kg diet), combined with vitamin E (100 mg/kg diet) and probiotics (*Saccharomyces cerevisiae* and *Lactobacillus acidophilus* at 2 g/kg diet) in broilers under heat stress. The heat stress corresponded to 7 hours/day at 36 ± 2°C and 75–85% relative humidity from 25 to 42 days of age, compared with a thermoneutral group. Vitamins E and C were equally potent in alleviating the negative effects of heat stress observed on live performance, blood parameters, and phagocytic activity. But combining the 2 vitamins and the probiotic was even more effective. Vitamin C increases the immunological response.

A combination of vitamin C (200 mg/kg) with FA (1.5 mg/kg) also has been proven to have beneficial effects in heat-stressed broilers (Gouda *et al.*, 2020). Both vitamins also improved the antioxidant status, hematological and serum biochemical parameters, heat shock protein 70 (HSP70) expression, and immunological responses.

Choline

Details about current choline recommendations for broilers and turkeys, provided by institutional sources and genetic companies, can be found in Tables 6.3 to 6.10.

Choline requirements are very high in the starter phase, the most studied, and they diminish as the synthesizing capacity of the birds increases with age. Choline needs are also lower in slower-growing genotypes. Quillin *et al.* (1961) determined that 1 g of choline could substitute 2.3–2.4 g of methionine as a methyl group donor, a ratio that falls to 2: 1 in the work of Wang *et al.* (1987). Whitehead *et al.* (1992) calculated that using a total level of 1,250 mg of choline between 0 and 3 weeks of age could substitute for 0.13 g/kg methionine. This relationship depends on the concentrations of the 2 nutrients. Recently, Mahmoudi *et al.* (2018) reported that choline supplementation at 280 mg/kg reduced methionine requirements of heat-stressed chickens by 20%.

Low protein diets are becoming common for reducing the cost of the diet, the nitrogen environmental impact, and enhancing sustainability. Under these conditions, choline and threonine can be precursors of glycine. Choline can be transformed, if l-homocysteine is available, via the reactions:

choline → betaine aldehyde → betaine → dimethylglycine → sarcosine → glycine

Siegert *et al.* (2015) reported that choline intake in broilers influences the required intake of glycine and serine or glycine equivalent. One mass unit of choline may replace up to 0.54 mass units of glycine, and interactions can be observed with the level of threonine intake. However, this response is variable, and broilers' regulatory mechanisms are under investigation (Hofmann *et al.*, 2020).

Choline requirements increase if the diet is relatively low in sulfur amino acids and, at these levels, productive responses to the supplementation of choline were observed (Pillai *et al.*, 2006a,b). The growth reduction caused by a lack of methionine is aggravated if there is also a choline deficiency (Whitehead and Portsmouth, 1989). When methionine is very deficient it becomes the major limiting factor, and extra supplies of choline have no effect (Whitehead *et al.*, 1992), as also happens if there is excessive methionine (Miles *et al.*, 1987).

However, Whitehead *et al.* (1992) found no positive effect in broilers 3 to 6 weeks old when supplementing choline at 500 mg/kg (total dietary content 1,120 mg/kg) with 6 different levels of methionine. In more recent experiments conducted under controlled conditions (Pillai *et al.*, 2006a,b), choline only had positive effects on growth and hepatic remethylation of homocysteine in diets unsupplemented by methionine. These improvements were no longer significant if methionine levels were adequate or slightly deficient. There is no advantage in working with diets deficient in choline since, in such cases, its requirements will be covered partly through methionine, one of the most limiting nutrients in poultry diets from the economic viewpoint.

Several experiments have verified that the addition of choline produces significant improvements in growth, feed consumption, and FCR and that the dose-response relationship was linear on the levels evaluated (Tillman and Pesti, 1985; García *et al.*, 1999), although in some cases this was only found in the starter phase (Bond *et al.*, 1985). The estimated optimum supplementation levels in corn-soy diets (whose theoretical content is some 1,350 mg/kg) vary widely, between 120 and 1,000 ppm, due to differences in the feed composition. Emmert and Baker (1997) ascertained an almost linear growth response from 10–22 days up to 1,115 mg/kg supplementation levels and observed further improvements up to 2,000 mg/kg. A supplement of 800 ppm (total dietary content 1,900 ppm) was sufficient to optimize feed conversion, and these values are much higher than those proposed by the NRC. Based on this work and other INRA trials, Workel *et al.* (1998, 1999) recommended a feed supplement of 500–800 mg/kg for older broilers, depending on the growing phase.

In a more recent evaluation, Farina *et al.* (2017) determined the choline requirements for body weight gain as 778, 632, and 645 mg/kg for the phases of 1–7, 1–35, and 1–42 days of age, respectively. In the same experiment, 2 sources of choline, phosphatidylcholine and choline chloride, were evaluated (Figure 6.20). Both choline supplements linearly improved FCR between 15 and 28 d, and the phosphatidylcholine source was equivalent to 2.52 units of choline supplied as choline chloride.

De Lima *et al.* (2018) re-evaluated the choline requirements of male broiler chickens from 1 to 21 days of age in 2 studies using choline chloride and at 2 levels of digestible methionine: 0.59% in study 1 and 0.44% in study 2. Five levels of choline were tested: 715, 1,040, 1,365, 1,690, and 2,015 mg/kg. The results showed that the diet with the 25% reduction in methionine limited the maximum weight gain by approximately 10%. The ideal choline intake was estimated in study 1 to be 1,228; 1,111, and 1,042 mg/kg diet (27, 44.5, and 62.5 mg/bird day) with 0.59% digestible methionine and in study 2 1,276, 1,046, and 1,010 mg/kg diet (26.8, 41.8, and 56.6 mg/bird day) with 0.44% digestible methionine.

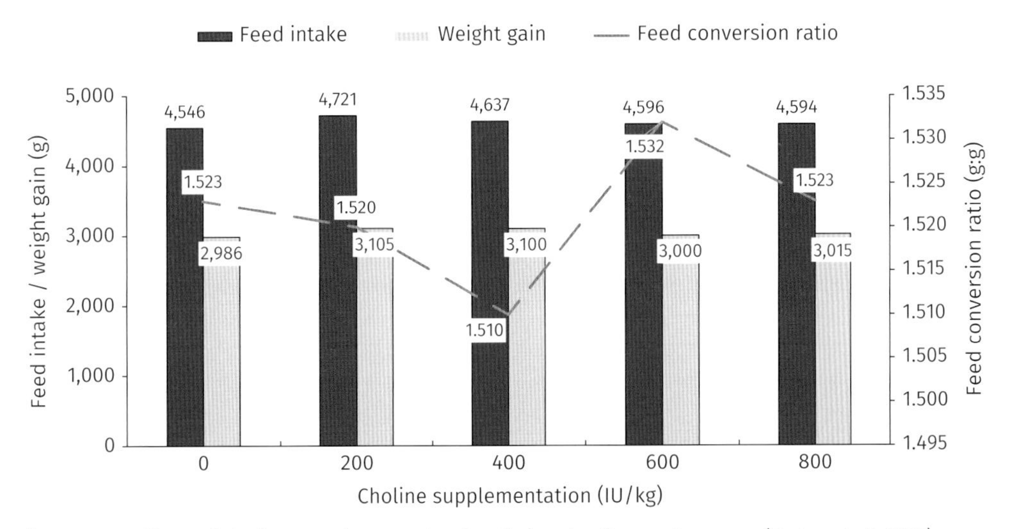

Figure 6.20 Effects of choline supplementation (mg/kg) on broiler performance (Farina *et al.*, 2017)

Another aspect that has been investigated is whether it might be possible to substitute betaine for choline as a methyl group donor in broiler diets since it is known that 55–62% of choline converts to betaine in the liver after oxidization (Kettunen *et al.*, 1999). This is possible only to a limited extent. Lowry *et al.* (1987) showed that 75% of choline requirements must be provided by choline itself. In experiments by Emmert and Baker (1997), adding 500 ppm betaine to diets with a total of 600 mg choline produced no effect, while performance improved linearly with the addition of choline. In studies by Pillai *et al.* (2006a, b), an increase in the choline level improved the liver's capacity for homocysteine remethylation in methionine-deficient diets.

This was also achieved with betaine, but to a lesser extent and less consistently. On the other hand, Waldroup *et al.* (2006) found the addition of 1,000 mg/kg of betaine or choline from the first day of life, or a combination of each of them at 500 mg/kg, improved the feed conversion index and breast yield at 35 and 42 days, and this independently of methionine levels. In contrast, Waldroup and Fritts (2005) studied the effects of betaine or choline, alone or in combination, in threat situations from coccidiosis and found few or no benefits in terms of weight gain and feed conversion or mortality. The improvements in carcass and breast yield at 42 days of age resulted from betaine supplementation instead of choline supplementation. However, this was no longer the case at 49 days.

Maghoul *et al.* (2009) also studied the efficacy of substituting betaine for choline. The results were unclear since the live weight and conversion index improved from 0 to 21 days and 22 to 42 days, but not between 42 and 49 days. There was also an increase in breast yield and a decrease in abdominal fat percentage. The results of both investigations suggested that the age of the broilers may be an important factor in the efficacy of the combination of these 2 substances. Maghoul *et al.* (2009) also evaluated betaine supplementation as a replacement for choline on broiler performance and carcass characteristics. Only reduction of abdominal fat and increased breast meat yield were observed.

In slower-growing chickens, a significant drop in the proportion of abdominal fat has also been observed with betaine and choline supplements (Hassan *et al.*, 2005). The different combinations used improved weight gain, feed conversion index, and levels of serum proteins. Adding 0.072% and 0.144% betaine to feed led to improvements similar to those obtained using 1,170 and 1,470 ppm choline. Choline at 1,170 mg/kg produced a reduction of 8.7% in abdominal fat, regardless of the betaine level. Surprisingly at 1,470 ppm choline the results for this parameter were no different from those obtained with the basal diet. On the other hand, they were increasing the betaine level linearly reduced the levels of abdominal fat, regardless of choline level. The conclusion was that a choline level of 1,170 mg/kg is adequate for the growth of this type of chicken, but it can be reduced to 870 mg/kg if 0.72% betaine is added to the diet.

A study conducted by Igwe *et al.* (2015) investigated the effects of graded levels of choline on the growth performance, carcass yield, internal organs, and hematological parameters of broiler chickens. Based on the findings of this work, it was concluded that choline should be included at 2,000 mg/kg feed.

The majority of estimates for choline requirements of turkeys are based on research published decades ago. Christmas and Harms (1988, 1989) observed that supplementing choline improved growth between 8 and 12 weeks, especially if methionine levels were relatively low, but this was not the case between 4 and 8 weeks. On the other hand, Ferket *et al.* (1993) obtained maximum growth at 16 days with supplements of 750 ppm and 9 days with 1,000 mg/kg, and they indicated that betaine could replace choline at this age by up to 50%. According to Whitehead and Portsmouth (1989), the diet of young turkeys must provide a total of 1,600 mg/kg from 0 to 4 weeks.

Chapter 7

Optimum vitamin nutrition in laying hens

INTRODUCTION

The egg industry worldwide seeks to extend the persistence of lay in a long-life layer capable of producing 500 eggs in a laying cycle of 100 weeks (Bain *et al.*, 2016; Preisinger, 2018; Underwood *et al.*, 2021). To achieve this goal is necessary to understand the physiology and nutritional needs that may vary depending on bird age and management system.

Vitamin nutrition plays a critical role in achieving this goal. This chapter will focus on data relating to the beneficial effects of OVN™ levels to maximize egg production while supporting the welfare, health, and sustainability of table egg production. Lastly, it shows the average nutritional composition of eggs produced in the US and various countries of the EU.

The information about vitamin active forms, units of quantification, conversion factors, functions, metabolism, signs of vitamin deficiencies, and general factors that influence vitamin requirements and utilization were discussed in Chapter 4.

Additional information about the importance of vitamin nutrition in layers can also be found in Bains (1999), Klasing (1998), Leeson (2007), McDowell (1989a, 2000a), NRC (1987), World Poultry-Elsevier (2001), Weber (2009), and Ward (2017).

GENERAL ASPECTS OF VITAMIN SUPPLEMENTATION

Early studies on vitamins were principally directed toward avoiding symptoms of deficiency. However, there has been an awakening of interest in the important metabolic functions of this group of nutrients in recent years. Understanding the roles of vitamins in bone development to guarantee bone health and eggshell quality in an older hen is necessary to achieve these goals. Current research also looks for optimum vitamin levels to cope with stressful conditions and to modulate immunity and microflora to maintain welfare, health, and food safety. Finally, many researchers focus on vitamin levels that enrich the egg to make it a more nutritious product.

These factors bring us to consider OVN™ and set the basis for the line of argument on the factors that justify increasing the vitamin supply in poultry diets. Calculations of the requirements of poultry were carried out under experimental conditions many years ago. Moreover, in many instances, they were estimated or extrapolated from other species and in no case using the current strains. This situation is particularly evident in the case of laying hens, where the data, especially for some vitamins, are scarce and derived from old studies that bear little relation to the type of hens and systems used today.

Current commercial egg-laying strains have changed a great deal in a few years. Birds have changed in size, sexual maturity has advanced, feed consumption has decreased, and, above all, egg production has improved in quantity and size. Logically, these changes should call for increased nutritional requirements in general and, in particular, increased vitamin requirements. Several important factors call for revisiting vitamin supplementation levels of layers.

- Feed consumption is a key factor in fulfilling the animals' nutritional requirements. Current egg-laying strains have a better nutrient conversion ratio, resulting from a lower voluntary intake. It is estimated that the progressive decrease in the FCR results in a reduction of vitamin intake in laying hens of 1% per year (Leeson, 2007). Furthermore, stress situations, especially high temperatures, reduce feed consumption. Most nutritionists formulate feeds for commercial laying hens based on feed intake; logically, as feed intake decreases, they balance the energy level and proportionally increase the supply of calcium and essential amino acids. The supply of vitamins should also be adjusted to consumption to ensure an appropriate daily vitamin intake. In these hens with high yields, the vitamins involved in energy, protein metabolism, and the immune system are doubly important.
- Despite the technical nature of poultry systems today, practical operating conditions are usually poorer than those in experiments, implying the need for greater vitamin allowances to obtain the same results.
- Stressful situations and pathological processes should be borne in mind. These can lead to lower absorption efficiency through the intestinal wall, a higher metabolic rate, or a reduction in the microbial synthesis of vitamins.
- The vitamin content and its availability in ingredients are not precisely known. Furthermore, the requirements do not account for losses in activity through processing or storage conditions (McDowell and Ward, 2008).
- Requirements have been established based on studies that did not consider the many interactions between vitamins and other compounds, which may distort or impede their use. There are no studies, such as those conducted on amino acids, to discover whether there is an order of priority or a relationship between the limiting vitamins similar to the ideal protein concept. This is more complicated for vitamins as they are metabolic substances, not structural components as are amino acids. The consequence is that vitamin dosage lacks the same accuracy.
- More detailed studies demonstrate that intake of particular vitamins at levels higher than the minimum established requirements may allow birds to achieve their genetic potential. Under commercial production conditions, the great metabolic effort required of birds in production increases the nutritional needs for the immune response, with clear repercussions for vitamin allowances. New vitamin requirements must be established considering objectives beyond those related solely to production, such as prevention and defense against certain diseases through improving the immune status.
- The increased importance of egg quality and its repercussions on nutrition and consumer health. These points support the idea that optimum vitamin supplementation, over and above the established minimum requirements and adapted to specific conditions, will improve the health and well-being of the birds and maximize their productive potential and quality.

CURRENT VITAMIN RECOMMENDATIONS FOR LAYERS

Current vitamin recommendations from diverse research groups (FEFANA, 2015; Rostagno *et al.*, 2017; FEDNA, 2018) and the minimum requirement values for layers established by the NRC (1994) are shown in Table 7.1 for the rearing phase and in Table 7.2 for the laying phase.

The NRC indicated that these figures do not allow for a safety margin and their purpose was only to avoid deficiency symptoms. The NRC (1994) established minimum requirements for rearing pullets and hens in the laying phase for white leghorn and brown strains. The NRC (1994) requirements or levels needed for brown layers in production were estimated to be 10% higher than those of leghorn layers producing white eggs based on greater body weight, higher feed intake, and greater egg volume. However, it is curious that the vitamin requirements for brown pullets during rearing were less than for white leghorn pullets, probably due to slightly higher feed intake. However, for a bigger body weight during the whole life, total vitamin requirements for brown pullets could also be higher.

Based on the limited research results and experience available, diverse research groups have recommended vitamin levels several-fold higher than the NRC (1994). During the rearing phase (Table 7.1), vitamin A recommended levels are 4 to 5 times higher, vitamin D_3 10 to 13 times higher, vitamin E 8 to 12 times more, vitamin K 4 to 10 times higher, and complex B vitamins at least twice of the levels listed by the NRC (1994). In the laying phase (Table 7.2), levels are very similar and still 3 to 4 times more than NRC (1994) for vitamin A, 8 to 12 times higher for vitamin D, 4 to 6 times higher for vitamin E, 4 to 10 times higher than vitamin K and 2 to 8 times higher for vitamins of complex B. Choline is the only vitamin recommended at lower levels than NRC (1994). However, the recent literature (Dong *et al.*, 2019; Janist *et al.*, 2019; Moghadam *et al.*, 2021) showed more benefits for 1,500 mg choline/kg feed, almost 50% higher than NRC (1994), established more than 30 years ago. Any group makes no recommendations for vitamin C; still, the literature has enough evidence of the positive effects of ascorbic acid between 250 and 500 mg/kg in hens under heat stress and even thermoneutral conditions (Reyes *et al.*, 2021; Rajabi and Torki, 2021).

Experimental findings are still limited, and most studies in the past 20 years were not designed to estimate requirements. The long-term effects of vitamin supplementation during rearing and early lay on aging hens 40 to 60 weeks later are not well established. The current tendency is to keep hens in production for 90 to 100 weeks, and this requires stronger pullets and healthier hens during the first 20 to 40 weeks of production. Available literature demonstrates some positive effects of vitamin D_3, $25OHD_3$, and biotin in pullets that can be observed in the late laying phase (Bar *et al.*, 1999; Panda *et al.*, 2006; Taniguchi and Watanabe, 2007; Souza *et al.*, 2016; Chen *et al.*, 2020a,b).

The current vitamin recommendations from the genetic companies are presented in Table 7.3. These values are similar to or higher than the other recommendations in the rearing and laying phases. The increments in vitamin supplementation in the past years correspond to the higher needs of more productive hens, with bigger average egg weight, larger egg mass production, longer cycles, and producing in more challenging environments like the furnished cages, aviaries, and free-range systems (Bain *et al.*, 2016; Preisinger, 2018; Underwood *et al.*, 2021).

Multivitamin fortification has improved eggs' productive parameters, welfare, and quality traits (Hatta et al., 2009; Zang *et al.*, 2011). Recently, Gan *et al.* (2020) evaluated the supplementation of 72–85-week-old layer diets with twice the level of liposoluble vitamins (LV), water-soluble vitamins (WV), or a combination of both (BV) compared to control according to the levels described in Table 7.4. After 13 weeks of the feeding trial, the hens in the WV group had higher yellowness of yolk color, and the LV group had an increased laying rate (82.93%) compared with the control (73.83%). Compared with the control treatment, WV and BV had better liver antioxidant stability and increased secretory immunoglobulin A concentrations in the jejunum. Finally, higher vitamin supplementation altered the intestinal microbiota composition with increased abundance of ileal *Lactobacillus* and reduced richness of ileal *Romboutsia*,

Table 7.1 Current recommended vitamin levels (IU or mg/kg air-dry feed) during the rearing period established by various sources

	Commercial layers										
		Starter – grower (0–10 week)					Pre-laying (10 week – 2% Lay)				
	Unit/kg	NRC, 1994	FEFANA, 2015	Rostagno et al., 2017	FEDNA, 2018	OVN™ (DSM Nutritional Products, 2022)	NRC, 1994	FEFANA, 2015	Rostagno et al., 2017	FEDNA, 2018	OVN™ (DSM Nutritional Products, 2022)
Vitamin A	IU	1,500	8,000–12,000	12,216	10,000	12,600–14,000	1,500	8,000–12,000	9,637	8,000	10,500–13,000
Vitamin D_3	IU	200–300	3,000–4,000	3,054	2,800	3,200–4,200	200–300	3,000–4,000	2,409	2,500	3,200–4,200
$25OHD_3$ (HyD)	mg	–	0.069	–	–	0.069	–	0.069	–	–	0.069
Vitamin E	mg	5	20–30	45.80	19	55–100	5	20–30	36.10	15	35–100
Vitamin K	mg	0.5	5–7	2.44	2.7	3.2–6	0.5	5–7	1.93	2	3.2–6
Vitamin B_1	mg	0.8	2.5–3.0	3.28	1.5	2.1–2.6	0.8	2.5–3.0	2.59	1.1	2.1–2.6
Vitamin B_2	mg	2.50	5–7	8.17	5	7–10	2.50	5–7	6.44	4.2	5.5–6.5
Vitamin B_6	mg	3	3.5–5.5	4.58	2.3	4.7–6	3	3.5–5.5	3.61	1.8	3.2–5.5
Vitamin B_{12}	mg	0.004	0.015–0.025	0.02	0.02	0.026–0.032	0.004	0.015–0.025	0.02	0.01	0.025–0.030
Niacin	mg	10	50–60	49.60	30	52–65	10	50–60	39.20	22	35–65
D-panthothenic acid	mg	2.2	15–25	16.42	9	16–18	2.2	15–25	12.95	7	12.6–15.7
Folic acid	mg	0.25	1.0–1.5	1.15	0.60	1.5–2.0	0.25	1.0–1.5	0.90	0.3	1.5–2.0
Biotin	mg	0.10	0.1–0.15	0.11	0.08	0.16–0.21	0.10	0.1–0.15	0.09	0.04	0.12–0.20
Vitamin C	mg	–	100–200	–	–	105–160	–	100–200	–	–	105–160
Choline	mg	1,050	300–500	496	240	210–420	1,050	300–500	392	100	210–420

Table 7.2 Current recommended vitamin levels (IU or mg/kg air-dry feed) during the laying phase established by various sources

	Commercial layers					
	Laying period					
	Unit/kg	NRC, 1994	FEFANA, 2015	Rostagno et al., 2017	FEDNA, 2018	OVN™ (DSM Nutritional Products, 2022)
Vitamin A	IU	1,500	8,000–12,000	9,000	9,000	8,500–13,000
Vitamin D_3	IU	200–300	3,000–4,000	2,400	3,000	3,200–4,200
25OHD_3 (HyD)	mg	–	0.069	–	–	0.069
Vitamin E	mg	5	20–30	12	13	25–50
Vitamin K	mg	0.5	5–7	2.16	1.7	3–6
Vitamin B_1	mg	0.8	2.5–3.0	1.8	1	2.6–3.2
Vitamin B_2	mg	2.5	5–7	4.8	4	5.5–7.5
Vitamin B_6	mg	3	3.5–5.5	2.1	1.8	4–5.5
Vitamin B_{12}	mg	0.004	0.015–0.025	0.02	10	0.02–0.03
Niacin	mg	10	50–60	30	20	35–55
D-panthothenic acid	mg	2.2	15–25	12	8	8.5–12.5
Folic acid	mg	0.25	1.0–1.5	0.6	0.30	1.5–2.5
Biotin	mg	0.1	0.1–0.15	0.06	0.05	0.12–0.2
Vitamin C	mg	–	100–200	–	–	105–210
Choline	mg	1,050	300–500	270	200	320–520

Table 7.3 Recommended vitamin levels (IU or mg kg air-dry feed) for laying hens by genetic companies

	Commercial layers							
		Starter – grower (0–10 week)				Rearing (10 week – 2% lay)		
	Unit/kg	Hendrix Genetics, 2020	Hy-Line, 2021	Novogen, 2020	OVN™ (DSM Nutritional Products, 2022)	Hendrix Genetics, 2020	Hy-Line, 2021	Novoge 2020
Vitamin A	IU	13,000	10,000	12,000	12,600–14,000	10,000	10,000	12,000
Vitamin D_3	IU	3,250	3,300	3,200	3,200–4,200	2,500	3,300	3,200
25OHD$_3$ (HyD)	mg	–	–	–	0.069	–	–	–
Vitamin E	mg	100	25	60–100	55–100	75	25	60–10
Vitamin K	mg	3	3.5	5	3.2–6	3	3.5	5
Vitamin B_1	mg	2.5	2.2	3	2.1–2.6	2.5	2.2	3
Vitamin B_2	mg	10	6.6	10	7–10	5	6.6	10
Vitamin B_6	mg	5	4.5	5	4.7–6	5	4.5	5
Vitamin B_{12}	mg	0.03	0.023	0.03	0.026–0.032	0.020	0.023	0.03
Niacin	mg	60	40	45	52–65	30	40	45
D-panthothenic acid	mg	15	10	16	16–18	10	10	16
Folic acid	mg	1	1	2.5	1.5–2.0	1.0	1.0	2.
Biotin	mg	0.20	0.10	0.25	0.16–0.21	0.20	0.10	0.2
Vitamin C	mg	150 (heat stress)	–	–	105–160	150 (heat stress)	–	–
Choline	mg	1,000	180	500	210–420	500	180	5

	Laying				
VN™ (DSM Nutritional Products, 2022)	Hendrix Genetics, 2020	Hy-Line, 2021	Novogen, 2020	OVN™ (DSM Nutritional Products, 2022)	Layers references
,500–13,000	12,000	8,000	12,000	8,500–13,000	Abd El-Hack *et al.* (2017) 24000 IU better FCR, egg production, heat stress and immunity
,200–4,200	3,500	3,300	3,200	3,200–4,200	Mattila (2004) 6,000–15,000 IU improved bone strength
0.069	–	–	–	0.069	Wang *et al.* (2021b); Zhao *et al.* (2021) 0.069 mg; Chen *et al.* (2020), 0.069 mg bone mineralization; Wang *et al.* (2020) 0.069 mg less broken eggs
35–100	50	20	60–100	25–50	Panda *et al.* (2008) 125 mg FCR, egg production; Ajakaiye *et al.* (2010) 150 mg egg weight, heat stress and immunity; Jiang *et al.* (2013) 100 mg; Zhao *et al.* (2021) 200 mg
3.2–6	3	2.5	5	3–6	Fares *et al.* (2018) 14 mg egg weight, egg production, shell strength; O'Sullivan *et al.* (2020) 25 mg
2.1–2.6	2.5	2.5	3	2.6–3.2	NRC (1994) min 0.7 mg
5.5–6.5	6.5	5.5	10	5.5–7.5	Squires (1998) 8.8 mg improved egg production, reduced blood spots; Leiber *et al.* (2020) 7.5 mg
3.2–5.5	5	4.0	5	4–5.5	Weiser *et al.* (1991) 6 mg prevention bone deformities; Kucuk, *et al.* (2008) 8 mg
25–0.030	0.03	0.023	0.03	0.02–0.03	Akhmedkanova (1987) 0.036 mg egg production in heat stress; El-Husseiny *et al.* (2008a) 0.02 mg
35–65	40	30	45	35–55	Baghban-Kanani *et al.* (2019) 225–275 mg; Dikicioglu *et al.* (2000) 250–1,550 mg shell quality, FCR, less cholesterol in yolk
2.6–15.7	10	8	16	8.5–12.5	Zang *et al.* (2011) 11.30 mg
.5–2.0	1	0.9	2.5	1.5–2.5	Munyaka *et al.* (2012) 4 mg immune modulation; Jing *et al.* (2014) egg weight; Nofal *et al.* (2018) 10–20 mg egg number, shell thickness
12–0.20	0.20	0.075	0.25	0.12–0.2	El-Garhy *et al.* (2019) 0.15 mg; Manson *et al.* (2019) 0.15 mg
5–160	150 (heat stress)	–	–	105–210	Gan *et al.* (2018) 250 mg antioxidant status; Panda *et al.* (2008) 200 mg FCR, egg production, heat stress and immunity; Rajabi and Torki (2021) 240 mg
0–420	1,000	180	500	320–520	Mendoca *et al.* (1989) 1,500–2,000 mg reduced fat deposition in liver; Dong *et al.* (2019) 1,700 mg

Table 7.4 Vitamin levels evaluated by Gan *et al.* (2020)

Composition	Treatments			
	CON	LV	WV	BV
Vitamin A, IU/kg	10	20	10	20
Vitamin D_3, IU/kg	3	6	3	6
Vitamin E, IU/kg	40	80	40	80
Viitamin K_3, mg/kg	2	4	2	4
Thiamine, mg/kg	2	2	4	4
Riboflavin, mg/kg	6.4	6.4	12.8	12.8
Pantothenic acid, mg/kg	10	10	20	20
Niacin, mg/kg	30	30	60	60
Vitamin B_6, mg/kg	3	3	6	6
Biotin, mg/kg	0.1	0.1	0.2	0.2
Folic acid, mg/kg	1	1	2	2
Vitamin B_{12}, mg/kg	0.02	0.02	0.04	0.04
Vitamin C, mg/kg	0	0	250	250

Notes: CON: control; LV: liposoluble vitamins; WV: water-soluble vitamins; BV: a combination of both vitamins

Turicibacter, and cecal *Faecalibacterium* in the WV group, and increased cecal *Megasphaera* and *Phascolarctobacterium* in the LV group compared to the control. This globally means more beneficial microbiota in the intestine. Higher levels of antioxidant vitamins are considered a potent modulator of gut microbial communities (Riaz Rajoka *et al.*, 2021). No significant differences were observed in FCR, but the values were 1.95, 1.93, and 1.99 g: g for LV, WV, and BV, respectively, while the control had 2.05.

Increased vitamin supplementation is based on the specific reasons already outlined above, of which the following are key factors.

- Vitamin requirements suggested by the NRC were established based on criteria far from the current situation. They have not been re-evaluated for more than 40 years and have not been adapted for present strains, methods of production, or qualitative demands of the market.
- Production conditions are not homogeneous, and vitamin supplies in feed should be adapted to the different management conditions, keeping a safety margin that ensures their availability to the animal. Several factors may alter animals' vitamin requirements and the supply of vitamins from the feed.
- Strains of laying hens evolve through genetic selection and growth rates, conformation, voluntary intake, and production change. This has repercussions on metabolic activity and the bird's immune response. Hence, vitamin requirements should be updated.
- Environmental situations such as high temperatures, infectious agents, and other stressful situations may make it difficult to achieve adequate vitamin intake as the requirements increase and the birds eat less.

- Information on the vitamin content of ingredients is limited and inexact and depends on availability. The processes to which feed is currently subjected, such as pelleting and extrusion, destroy vitamins, usually to a greater degree. During the pelleting process, the loss in vitamin activity is greatest for vitamins A, E, B_1, and C, but it may also be significant for other vitamins (Schulde, 1986).
- Finally, the minimum requirements do not consider objectives such as the well-being of birds, preventing the occurrence and development of pathological disorders, or improving the quality of eggs.

There are sufficient studies for breeding hens and broilers to indicate that increasing the vitamin level has beneficial effects, which warrants consideration of an increase in vitamin requirements. However, for commercial egg layers, the body of literature is smaller.

It is still difficult to determine optimum levels for each vitamin since evaluations take longer than broilers, and there is an age-dependent response. Still, it provides enough evidence to demonstrate that vitamin supplementation is necessary for long-term egg production, quality, and enrichment of egg vitamin content.

Some evidence (Inal *et al.*, 2001) showed that withdrawing vitamins and trace minerals from layer diets only decreased costs by 1 to 1.5% but, as a consequence, with reductions in egg production between 8 and 3% and egg weight by almost 2 g.

In contrast, Nobakht (2014) observed improvements in egg production and egg mass when vitamin and trace mineral premix were increased up to 0.45% of the control while reducing feed cost per kilogram of eggs produced.

OPTIMUM VITAMIN NUTRITION FOR LAYERS

Fat-soluble vitamins

Vitamin A

Details about current vitamin A recommendations for layers, provided by institutional sources and genetic companies, can be found in Tables 7.1 to 7.3.

The minimum requirement recommended by the NRC (1994) is 3,000 IU/kg, based on studies from 1961 and 1965. As early as 1961, Hill *et al.* indicated that 2,640 IU/kg was the minimum amount necessary to ensure maximum egg production. To minimize blood spots in the egg it was necessary to supplement 3,520 IU/kg feed, because vitamin A plays an important role in epithelial tissue integrity, particularly in the oviduct. Other studies indicate that vitamin A affects the ovary more than the magnum since variations in dosage are reflected in parameters relating to the yolk and ovulation rather than the formation of albumen, which takes place in the magnum of the oviduct (Bermudez *et al.*, 1993).

Among the more recent studies on vitamin A levels in laying hen diets, those carried out by Richter's team in Germany stand out. The team conducted various experiments using increasing dosages of vitamin A in chick starters and chick growers (Richter *et al.*, 1989 and 1996a) and layers (Richter *et al.*, 1990, 1996b,c). The authors compared different levels of supplementation between 0 and 18,000 IU/kg and focused on the effects on production parameters and vitamin A levels in the liver and, in some studies, immunity parameters. The results indicated that a minimum level of 2,500 IU/kg is necessary to prevent a drop in production. The different dosages used did not affect egg quality and feed conversion parameters. Therefore, the authors indicated a linear relationship between dietary dosages used and vitamin A levels in the liver but did not observe changes in immunity parameters. This fact agrees with the study by Coskun *et al.* (1998). After analyzing the different results, the authors noted that optimum allowances to achieve liver stores that permit maximum production are 4,000 IU/kg for pullet starters, 2,000 IU/kg for pullet growers, and 6,000 IU/kg for layers. As for the importance of liver stores, Squires and Naber (1993a) noted that in layers ingesting appropriate quantities of vitamin A, liver deposition is higher when forming eggs than during an unproductive phase.

Other studies have concentrated on increasing the levels of vitamin A in the egg (e.g., Naber, 1993; Mori *et al.*, 2003). The results indicated that as the dietary dose of vitamin A increases, the levels in the egg and liver also increase. Although it is not the principal objective of these studies, the authors analyze the effect of supplementation with vitamin A on the production and quality of eggs in parallel.

Squires and Naber (1993a) observed rising improvements in the laying percentage when supplementing vitamin A at 4,000, 8,000, and 9,000 IU/kg. In the study by Mori *et al.* (2003), no changes were observed in the weight and quality of eggs produced with a dose of 30,000 IU/kg, although the conversion ratio deteriorates above 15,000 IU/kg. These studies also noted that the content of vitamin A in plasma and yolk are not good indicators of nutritional status.

Regarding the effect of vitamin A on immune status, it has been firmly established that vitamin A plays a regulatory role in immune response in chicks and that a deficiency or excess of this nutrient leads to a reduction in their resistance to infections (*E. coli*) (Friedman and Sklan, 1989; Friedman *et al.*, 1991). Similarly, Sklan *et al.* (1994) found that the maximum immune response in broilers was obtained with doses of vitamin A higher than the minimum established by the NRC (1994). However, the study by Coskun *et al.* (1998) conducted on laying hens shows no significant effect on immunity parameters when vitamin A supplementation levels are increased to 24,000 IU/kg.

Lin *et al.* (2002) suggested that hens that suffer thermal stress immediately after vaccination need higher levels of vitamin A, up to 12,000 IU/kg, to achieve the maximum production of antibodies. They also demonstrated that supplementation of vitamin A at levels above the NRC (1994) recommendations was beneficial for the proportion of peripheral T-cells. This effect was maintained with different thermal stress periods and vaccination times. Because of this, the authors indicated that supplementation of high levels of vitamin A (9,000 IU/kg) improved egg production in hens under stress conditions. Relatedly, Lin *et al.* (2002) showed that the ingestion of vitamin A alleviates the oxidative damage caused by thermal stress and immune challenge.

Recently, Abd El-Hack *et al.* (2017) concluded that diets supplemented with vitamin A and selenium, either individually or together, alleviate the adverse effects of heat stress on production and health indices. Their results confirm the efficacy of vitamin A (16,000 IU/kg diet) in improving the productive performance parameters and internal egg quality (Figure 7.1). However, combined supplementary concentrations of vitamin A (16,000 IU/kg) and selenium (0.25 mg/kg) might be needed for better production and health of laying hens reared in hot weather.

Conversely, Abd El-Hack *et al.* (2019) concluded that layer diets supplemented with vitamin A (8,000 and 16,000 IU/kg feed) or in combination with vitamin E alleviated the harmful impacts of ambient summer temperature on different aspects of health indices and productive performance (Table 7.5 and Figure 7.2). The combination of vitamin A (16,000 IU/kg diet) plus E (500 mg/kg diet) had the best results for egg production of laying hens under hot summer conditions.

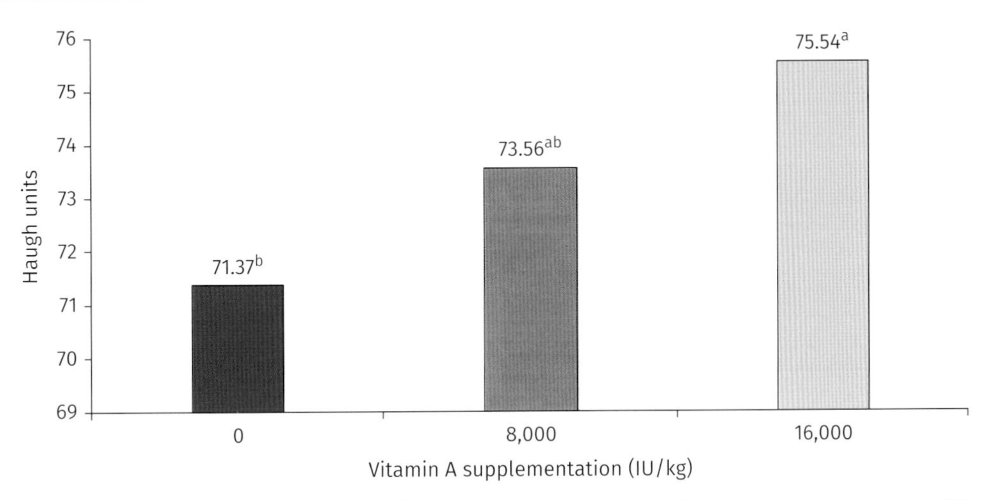

Figure 7.1 Effect of vitamin A supplementation on Haugh units, values with no common superscripts differ significantly, $P < 0.05$ (adapted from Abd El-Hack *et al.*, 2017)

Table 7.5 Effect of vitamin A and E on layer FCR and blood parameters during heat stress, values with no common superscripts differ significantly, $P < 0.05$ (adapted from Abd El-Hack *et al.*, 2019)

Vitamin A (IU/kg)	Vitamin E (mg/kg)	FCR (g feed: g egg)	Hemoglobin (mg/100 ml)	Packed cell volume (PCV,%)	Lymphocytes	Monocytes
0	0	2.67 ± 0.058[a]	9.99 ± 0.24[b]	36.94 ± 1.53[b]	73.47 ± 2.36[b]	3.54 ± 0.43[bc]
	250	2.53 ± 0.025[c]	10.26 ± 0.27[ab]	39.02 ± 0.42[ab]	70.14 ± 2.32[cd]	4.22 ± 0.57[ab]
	500	2.60 ± 0.075[b]	10.33 ± 0.31[a]	40.09 ± 1.05[a]	70.89 ± 2.24[cd]	3.96 ± 0.14[b]
8	0	2.50 ± 0.049[c]	9.84 ± 0.18[b]	35.37 ± 1.28[c]	70.52 ± 2.34[cd]	3.43 ± 0.25[c]
	250	2.45 ± 0.031[d]	10.20 ± 0.09[ab]	31.91 ± 1.50[d]	76.60 ± 2.11[a]	4.03 ± 0.46[b]
	500	2.51 ± 0.053[c]	9.88 ± 0.35[b]	37.20 ± 1.65[b]	69.89 ± 3.96[d]	4.47 ± 0.41[ab]
16	0	2.60 ± 0.021[b]	10.34 ± 0.27[a]	38.19 ± 1.23[ab]	71.53 ± 1.58[c]	4.57 ± 0.34[a]
	250	2.52 ± 0.045[c]	10.03 ± 0.24[ab]	36.98 ± 1.67[b]	73.17 ± 1.31[b]	2.97 ± 0.27d
	500	2.35 ± 0.012[e]	9.39 ± 0.29[c]	34.07 ± 1.13[c]	70.49 ± 4.34[cd]	4.69 ± 0.86[a]
P-value Interaction		< 0.01	< 0.01	< 0.01	< 0.05	< 0.01

However, it is important to point out that there is a negative interaction in the absorption level between vitamin A and the other fat-soluble vitamins and possible interactions with other nutrients, e.g., carotenoids. This is dealt with in the studies by Jiang *et al.* (1994) and Mori *et al.* (2003), which demonstrate a clear interaction between vitamin E and vitamin A in the deposition of both. Another example is the study by Kaya *et al.* (2001), which investigated the interaction between vitamin A supplementation (0 and 10,000 IU/kg) and zinc supplementation (from 0 to 200 ppm) since a connection has been shown between both nutrients for absorption, transport, and utilization. No interaction was observed for production in this study. The authors observed increased blood phosphorus and triglyceride levels related to high levels of vitamin A supplementation and supplies of zinc.

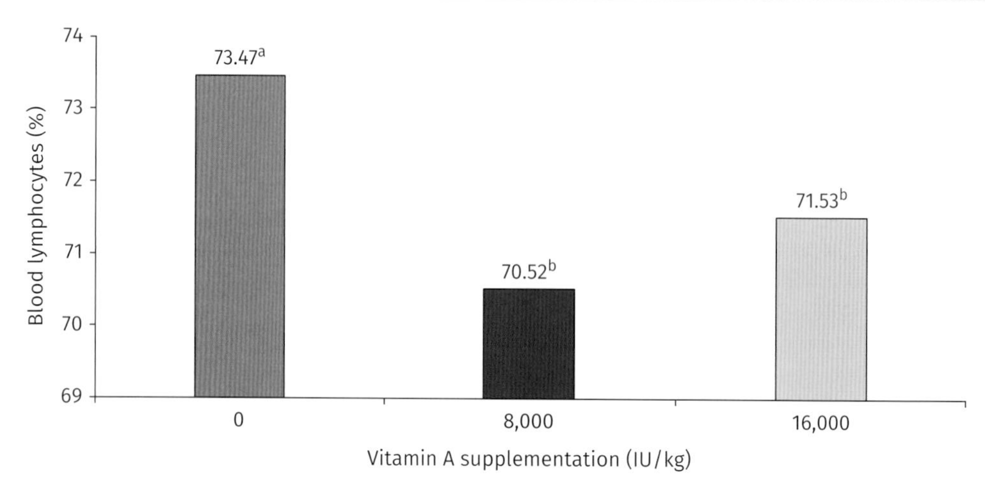

Figure 7.2 The effects of supplemental vitamin A levels on blood blood lymphocytes of laying hens at 54 weeks of age, values with no common superscripts differ significantly, $P < 0.05$ (adapted from Abd El-Hack *et al.*, 2019)

Recently, Guo *et al.* (2021) evaluated the interactive effects of supplemental levels of vitamin A (0, 7,000, and 14,000 IU/kg) and K_3 (0, 2, and 4 mg/kg) on laying performance, egg and tibia quality, and antioxidative status of 87-week-old Roman Pink laying hens. The supplemental levels were added to a basal diet containing 1,320 IU/kg vitamin A and 0.5 mg/kg vitamin K_3. Dietary treatments did not affect egg production, egg weight, or feed efficiency but supplementation of vitamins improved eggshell quality, yolk color, and the antioxidative status in the eggshell gland. The best albumen height was observed with 14,000 IU/kg vitamin A and 2 mg/kg vitamin K_3. The highest yolk color score and eggshell strength were obtained with 7,000 IU/kg vitamin A and 2 mg/kg vitamin K_3.

Eggs can be enriched with vitamin A as the concentration in the yolk is directly related to its inclusion in the hen diets. The concentration in a 60 g egg can increase from 59 to 75 μg as more vitamin A is added to the diet. The bioavailability of preformed vitamin A in the egg ranges from 90 to 100% and can account for 15% of human daily recommended dietary intake (Lima and Souza, 2018).

A minimum vitamin A requirement of 3,000 IU for layers was established solely to maintain production parameters (NRC, 1994). It is limited by interactions with other fat-soluble vitamins, such as vitamin E, and the need to stay within the tolerance level. In the light of studies, supplementation at a higher level would increase production. Furthermore, recent studies note that higher levels of vitamin A improved the immune response of the birds in stress situations (including thermal and vaccination stress), contributing to greater comfort for the animals and allowing improvements in the production of commercial eggs (Akinyemi and Adewole, 2021). It would be very useful to investigate whether positive effects accompany these improvements in egg quality.

Vitamin D

Details about current vitamin D recommendations for layers, provided by institutional sources and genetic companies, can be found in Tables 7.1 to 7.3.

The minimum requirement established by the NRC (1994) is 300 IU/kg (7.5 μg/kg) vitamin D_3. In principle, laying hens have specific calcium needs. In addition to requirements purely for the maintenance and development of bone tissue, they require calcium for shell formation and to ensure medullary bone reserves. Bearing in mind the relationship of vitamin D with calcium, it is logical in practice to use levels above the minimum requirements.

Keshavarz (1996) and Keshavarz and Nakajima (1993) studied the effect of vitamin D_3 supplementation levels from 250 to 4,400 IU/kg on different production parameters. The percentage of broken eggs ($P < 0.05$) improved with levels of 2,000 IU/kg compared with 250 IU/kg, indicating that this latter level is marginal for metabolism. Despite finding no significant differences in the other factors studied, they point out that the requirements established by the NRC (1994) are marginal and that those set out previously (500 IU/kg; NRC, 1984) are more in line with the real needs of the layer. Therefore, they suggested the application of a safety margin in the dosage of this vitamin. These results agree with Shen *et al.* (1981) reports, which indicate a minimum of 500 IU vitamin D_3/kg diet for optimum eggshell formation.

The supply of vitamin D is essential for skeletal integrity mainenance, with clear implications for bird well-being. Most studies demonstrated that doses above the NRC's (1994) recommendations are necessary to promote good bone structure and prevent fractures. Geng *et al.* (2018) also showed that the best egg production parameters, FCR, and egg quality was observed when layers were fed diets supplemented with 1,500 IU D_3/kg feed. This research group also evaluated the impact of vitamin D_3 on immunological responses using lipopolysaccharide (LPS) injection, but only at 3,000 IU vitamin D_3/kg. This supplementation repressed immune-inflammatory responses caused by LPS administration, affecting reproductive hormone secretion and regulating the nuclear factor kappa (NF-κB; a protein complex that controls transcription of deoxyribonucleic acid DNA, cytokine production, and cell survival) signaling pathway.

Wen *et al.* (2019) reported that layers had better tibia bone mineral content when fed diets with 68,348 IU/kg feed vitamin D_3 than when fed the control diets containing 8,348 or 18,348 IU vitamin D_3 after 68 weeks of age (Figure 7.3). However, these authors suggested that supplementation of dietary vitamin D_3 up to 35,014 IU/kg feed maintained if not increased laying hen performance and enhanced pullet and laying hen skeletal integrity, yolk vitamin D_3 content, and eggshell quality. Feeding pullets at a higher level of 68,348 IU/kg resulted in reduced growth and ultimately decreased the performance of laying hens from 19 to 68 weeks of age.

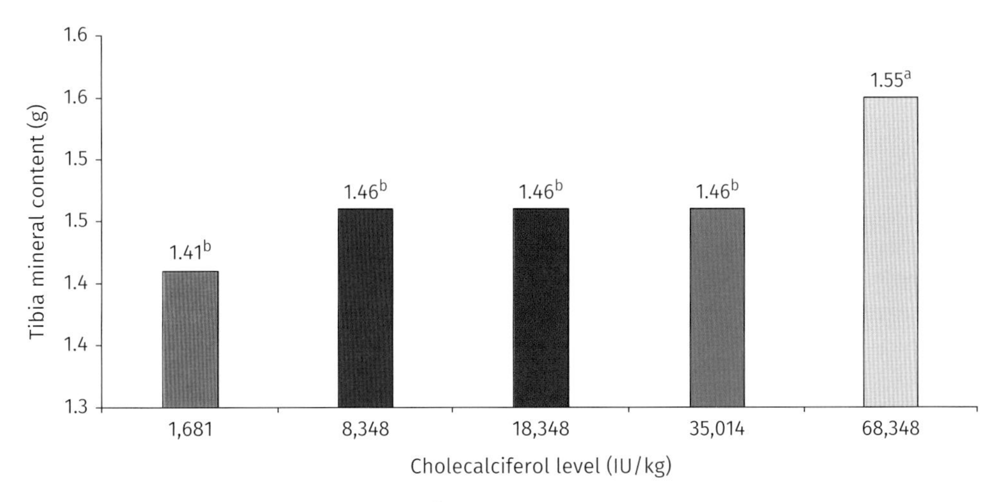

Figure 7.3 Bone quality (tibia mineral content) of hens fed diets containing 1,681, 8,348, 18,348, 35,014, or 68,348 IU vitamin D_3/kg diet, values with no common superscripts differ significantly, $P < 0.05$ (adapted from Wen *et al.*, 2019)

The difference in results between the current and previous experiments suggests that the bone development and skeletal status of pullets may play a more important role in maintaining skeleton bone health of layer hens than supplying higher dietary vitamin D_3 during the egg production phase.

The optimum level of vitamin D_3 for layer hens may depend on the dietary calcium concentrations. Attia *et al.* (2020b) evaluated the effects of calcium (3.5, 4.0, and 4.5%) and vitamin D_3 (800, 1,000, and 1,200 IU/kg) on performance, egg quality, blood biochemistry, and immunity of 60-week-old H&N brown layers. The best combination of calcium and vitamin D_3 changed slightly depending on the parameter, but the 4.0% calcium and 1,000 IU vitamin D_3/kg had the most positive effects overall.

Frost *et al.* (1990) studied vitamin D_3 supplements between 500 and 1,500 IU/kg. The results indicated that, as D_3 levels increase, so do egg production, consumption of feed, egg-specific gravity, the percentage and weight of the shell, and shell strength, which agree with the results of Faria *et al.* (1999), using from 2,500 to 3,500 IU D_3/kg. Likewise, Mattila *et al.* (2004) observed that when supplementing the diet with 6,000 and 15,000 IU/kg of vitamin D_2 (ergocalciferol) or vitamin D_3 (cholecalciferol) compared with 2,500 IU/kg of vitamin D_3, vitamin D_3 improved the resistance of bones to fracture and did not cause undesirable calcium deposits in vital organs and soft tissues and no changes were observed in the productive parameters of laying hens.

Keshavartz and Nakajima (1993) observed that both tibia weight and tibia breaking strength increased by increasing vitamin D_3 from 2,220 to 4,400 IU/kg, although no differences in tibia ash content were observed. These authors indicated that the latter observation is not a sensitive method of detecting changes in bone mineralization. The dose quadratically increased serum calcium and phosphorus levels during oviposition. Using a more precise methodology, Newbrey *et al.* (1992) demonstrated that supplementing 1,25-dihydroxycholecalciferol [$1,25(OH)_2D_3$] or calcitriol stimulates bone formation and mineral retention in the medullary bone matrix during oviposition.

The improvements in the quality of the shell observed when available phosphorus was reduced from 0.5 to 0.3% appear to be due to a stimulation of the $1,25(OH)_2D_3$ (Frost *et al.*, 1991). Consequently, feeding preformed metabolites directly, especially $25OHD_3$, and thus not depending on the organism's capacity for conversion to the active compound has been used in the past years. Some early studies indicated that the addition of vitamin D metabolites together with vitamin D_3 (above the requirements of >2,000 IU/kg) improved eggshell quality and the levels of calcium and phosphorus in blood returned to normal phosphorus levels available in the diet (Harms *et al.*, 1990a). Chennaiah *et al.* (2004), Tsang (1992), Tsang *et al.* (1990a,b), and Tsang and Grunder (1993) demonstrated that layer diets supplemented with calcitriol give rise to fewer egg breakages during classification and washing than diets with normal levels of vitamin D_3. These results agree with those of Seemann (1992) and those of Neri (2000), who observed improvements in production and bone mineralization when supplementing with $1,25(OH)_2D_3$.

However, several authors indicated that, when there is an adequate intake of vitamin D_3, supplementation of different metabolites has a reduced effect on resistance to bone breakage and production parameters (Harms *et al.*, 1988b, 1990a; Tsang and Daghir, 1990; Newman and Leeson, 1999; Keshavarz, 2003a; Käppeli *et al.*, 2011). Frost *et al.* (1990) concluded that the hen could obtain enough $1,25(OH)_2D_3$ from dietary vitamin D_3 to maintain production and eggshell quality. However, this metabolite is not produced at sufficient levels to support the desired weight and strength of the tibia, particularly in older birds. A few selected publications with research on vitamin D metabolites are summarized in Table 7.6.

Table 7.6 Summary of recent studies on vitamin D and its metabolites

Vitamin D_3 form/dietary/level	Study characteristics	Results	References
Cholecalciferol (2,200; 9,700; 17,200; 24,700; 102,200 IU/kg)	19–58 week. Laying performance, egg quality	Very high levels of dietary cholecalciferol can be used for fortification of eggs with vitamin D_3, had no detrimental influence on performance indices and quality	Persia *et al.* (2013)
Cholecalciferol (2,200; 9,700; 17,200; 24,700; 102,200 IU/kg)	19–58 week. Yolk vitamin D_3, egg quality	Content vitamin D_3 in egg yolk increased linearly as dietary vitamin D_3 increased content up to 24,700 IU vitamin D3/kg Egg quality was not affected	Yao *et al.* (2013)
Cholecalciferol (2,000 IU/kg) substituted by $25OHD_3$ or $1,25(OH)_2D_3$ in diets varying in Ca levels	80–94 week. Laying performance, eggshell quality, bone-breaking strength, serum Ca	$25OHD_3$ improved FCR. Egg production was lower and FCR worse with a $1,25\text{-}(OH)_2D_3$ supplementation compared to $25OHD_3$	Nascimento *et al.* (2014)
Cholecalciferol (2,500 and 5,000 IU/kg)	99–111 week. Laying performance, egg/shell quality, balance indices, tibia mineralization	Higher dietary level of cholecalciferol increased egg weight and Apparent Metabolizable Energy (AME) of the diet, without positive effect on other parameters	Browning and Cowieson (2014)
Cholecalciferol (2,500 and 6,000 IU/kg)	98–106 week. Laying performance, egg and eggshell quality, Ca digestibility, vitamin D3 content in the eggs	Improved eggshell quality, increased vitamin D3 concentration in yolks of hens fed a diet containing 6,000 IU vitamin D_3/kg, without differences between the treatments in performance and Ca digestibility	Plaimast *et al.* (2015)
$25OHD_3$ (6.25, 25, 50, 100 µg/kg)	Layer pullets 21 days challenge live coccidia oocyst	$25OHD_3$ at 100 µg/kg had the best BW gain and immunological response among challenged birds	Morris *et al.* (2015)
2,760 IU/kg vitamin D_3, 5,520 IU/kg vitamin D_3, and vitamin D_3 2,760 IU/kg + 69 mg/kg of $25OHD_3$	Long term use 0–90 week on bone development and performance	Positive effects on skeletal development for life and on FCR 39 to 48 wk, and egg production compared to 5,520 IU vitamin D_3/kg	Chen *et al.* (2020a, b)
$25OHD_3$ (69 mg/kg) in two stocking densities (338 and 506 cm2/hen)	45-week-old Lohmann laying hens, 16-week study. Evaluated gut health parameters	$25OHD_3$ elevated gut health through the improvement of intestinal barrier function, antioxidant capacity, and cecal microbiota composition in hens with high stocking density	Wang *et al.* (2021b)
$25OHD_3$ (69 mg/kg) and essential oil	12-week study in 48-week-old Lohmann layers	Improved eggshell ultrastructure and antioxidant capacity of the uterus	Zhao *et al.* (2021)

Nascimento *et al.* (2014) could not observe the effects of different vitamin sources on bone strength – cholecalciferol, 25OHD$_3$, or 1,25(OH)$_2$D$_3$ – when all sources provided the equivalent of 2,000 IU vitamin D. However, the amounts added were different and confirmed the higher biopotency of 25OHD$_3$ in 80-week-old-hens. On the other hand, Kakhki *et al.* (2019) found an interaction effect between calcium levels (3.0, 3.5, 4.0, and 4.5%) and levels of 25OHD$_3$ (0, 69, and 138 µg/kg) fed on top of 3,300 IU/kg vitamin D$_3$. The 25OHD$_3$ supplementation increased the femur and tibia medullary bone ash content and ash concentration, reducing these parameters in these bones' cortical area. They also observed that medullary bone starts to be formed at sexual maturity and continues to develop over the lay cycle. Nonetheless, the cortical bone loses mineral content and even increased dietary calcium or 25OHD$_3$ over 69 µg/kg cannot prevent or slow down erosion. Therefore, nutritional strategies aiming at minimizing osteoporosis should not focus on the late phase of the lay cycle or when there is a high risk of osteoporosis but instead on the early stages of skeletal development.

These effects on layer bone development have been clarified recently by Chen *et al.* (2020a). They evaluated the effect of long-term application of dietary 25OHD$_3$ on pullet and egg-laying hen (0–95 weeks) bone 3-dimensional structural development using micro-CT for 3D structural analysis and dual-energy X ray absorptiometry. The 3 dietary treatments consisted of vitamin D$_3$ at 2,760 IU/kg, vitamin D$_3$ at 5,520 IU/kg, and vitamin D$_3$ at 2,760 IU/kg plus 69 µg/kg of 25OHD$_{3,}$ which is equivalent to 2,760 IU/kg. 25OHD$_3$ increased bone growth rate at 10–12 weeks and cortical tissue volume and bone marrow at 17 weeks (Figures 7.4a and 7.4b). But 25OHD$_3$ created more pores in cortical bone, resulting in lower cortical bone mineral density but without altering bone mineral content. This effect allowed more space for bone mineral deposition during the egg-laying period. At 60 weeks, hens fed 25OHD$_3$ diets have greater bone mineral density and content, cortical volume, and trabecular bone connectivity. At 95 weeks, this treatment has higher cortical bone and lower porosity. Hens in this treatment also had higher bone mineral density and medullary bone volume but lower bone mineral content and volume of

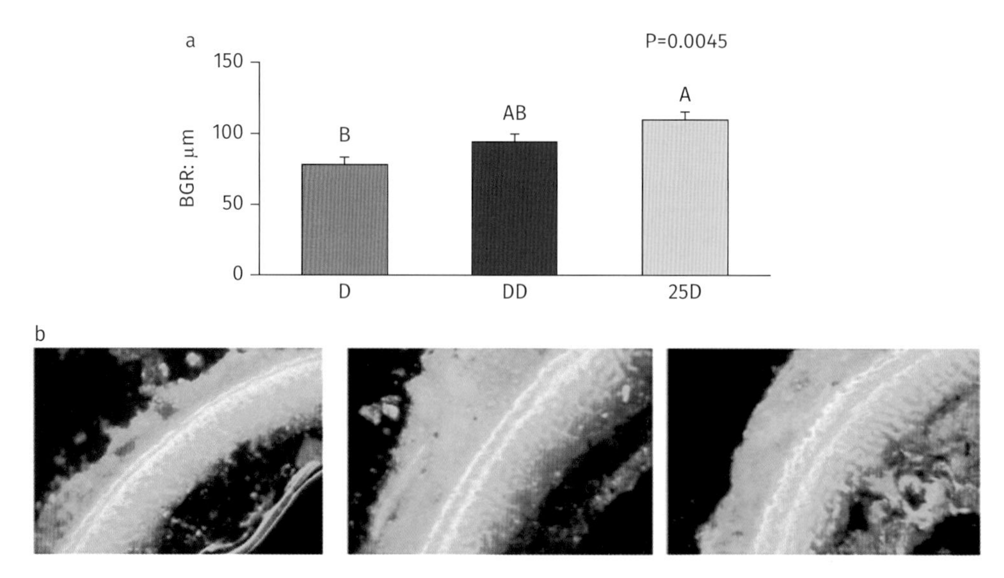

Figure 7.4a Effects of dietary supplementation of 25OHD$_3$ on pullet bone growth rate from 10 to 12 weeks. Treatments: (D) vitamin D$_3$ at 2,760 IU/kg; (DD) vitamin D$_3$ at 5,220 IU/kg; (25D) vitamin D$_3$ at 2,760 IU/kg plus 25OHD$_3$ at 69 µg/kg (2,760 IU/kg) (Chen *et al.*, 2020a)

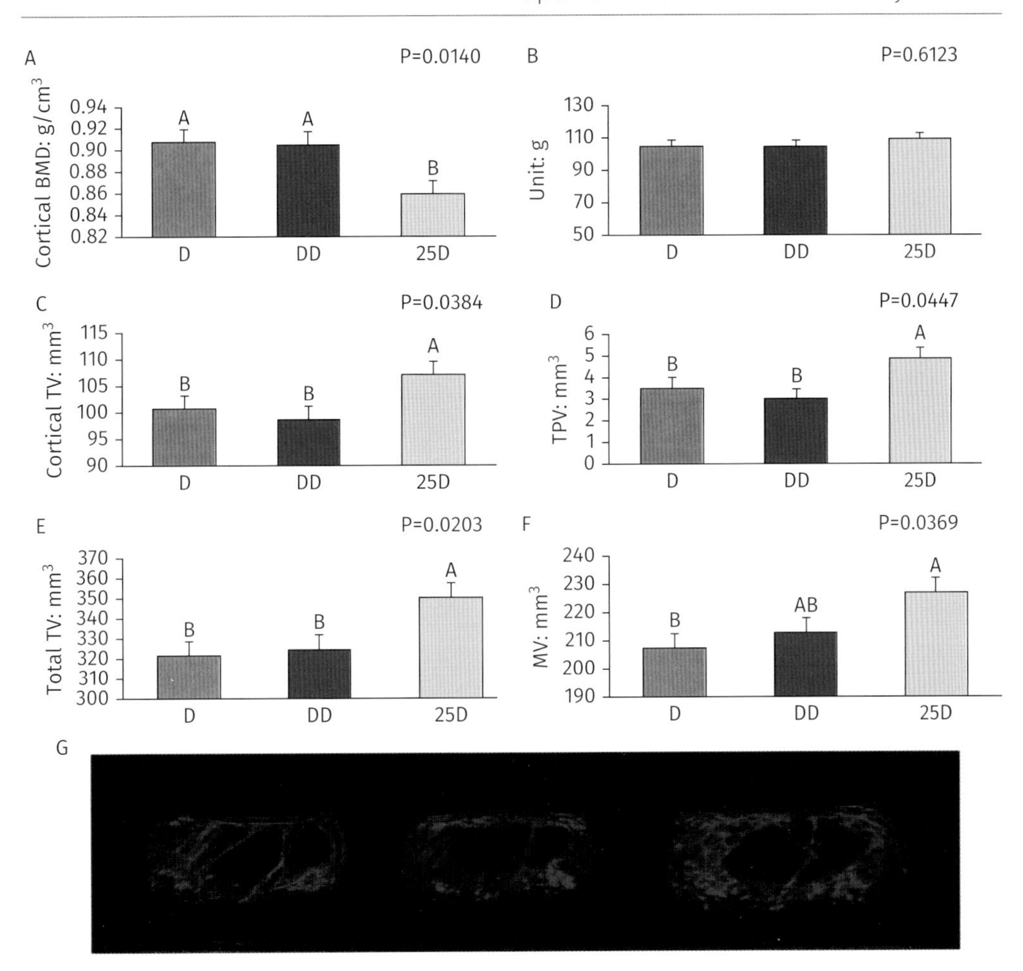

Figure 7.4b Effects of dietary supplementation of $25OHD_3$ on pullet bone development at week 17: (A) cortical bone mineral density (BMD); (B) cortical bone mineral content; (C) cortical bone volume; (D) cortical bone total volume of pore space; (E) total bone tissue volume (TV); (F) medullary volume; (G) pictures showed the cortical bone total volume of pore space from each treatment. The red color represents the pores. MV, medullary cavity volume; TPV, total pore volume. Treatments: (D) vitamin D_3 at 2,760 IU/kg; (DD) vitamin D_3 at 5,220 IU/kg; (25D) vitamin D_3 at 2,760 IU/kg plus $25OHD_3$ at 69 µg/kg (2,760 IU/kg) (Chen *et al.*, 2020a)

trabecular bone than the other 2 treatments with cholecalciferol. These results indicated the positive effects of $25OHD_3$ to stimulate bone volume to provide space for mineral mobilization during egg production.

In the same experiment, Chen *et al.* (2020b) evaluated growth performance, egg production, and quality. During the first 17 weeks, vitamin D_3 levels or sources did not affect growth. Hens fed vitamin D_3 at 5,520 IU/kg had a lower feed intake from 39 to 48 weeks but a higher intake between weeks 49 and 60 and lower hen day production (HDP) from 22 to 48 weeks than with the other treatments. During the same period, hens in the 5,520 IU vitamin D_3/kg treatment laid smaller eggs with higher specific gravity and shell thickness than with the other treatments. In contrast, layers fed diets with $25OHD_3$ had a better FCR (1.33 g feed/dozen eggs) between 39 and 48 weeks and higher overall (between 22 and 60 weeks) HDP (91.29%) compared with

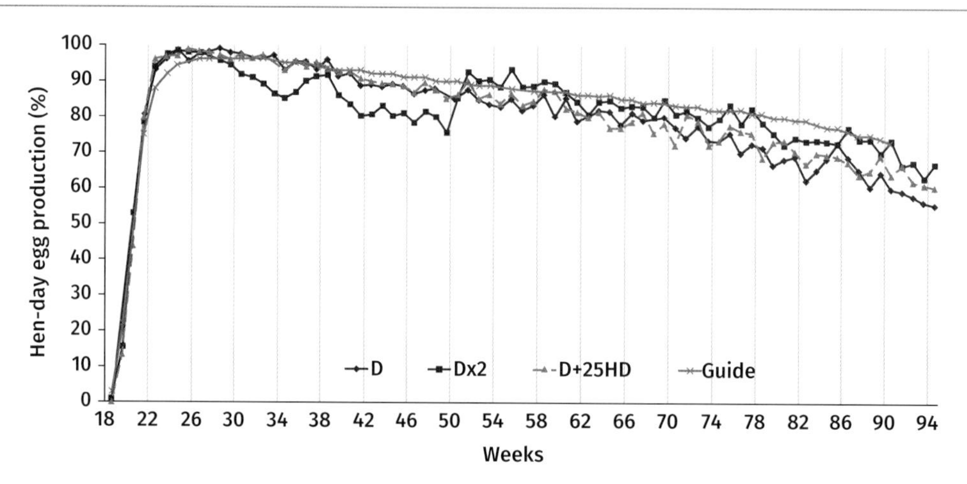

Figure 7.5 Effects of dietary supplementation of 25OHD$_3$ on HDP from 18 to 90 weeks. From the optimal production data from the Hy-Line (2021) W36 guide. Treatments: (D) vitamin D$_3$ at 2,760 IU/kg; (DD) vitamin D$_3$ at 5,220 IU/kg; (25D) vitamin D$_3$ at 2,760 IU/kg plus 25OHD$_3$ at 69 µg/kg (2,760 IU/kg) (Chen *et al.*, 2020b)

5,520 IU vitamin D$_3$/kg (1.40 g feed/dozen eggs; 88.53% HDP) (Figure 7.5). Eggs laid by hens fed 5,520 IU vitamin D$_3$/kg and 25OHD$_3$ diets between 25 and 33 weeks had higher Haugh unit than vitamin D$_3$ at 2,760 IU/kg. However, 25OHD$_3$ had no effects on eggshell quality during the entire production period and no beneficial effects on egg production after 60 weeks of age.

A few studies have evaluated the comparative biopotency of vitamin D metabolites. Nascimento *et al.* (2014) fed 80-week-old Hy-Line W36 layers, in their second cycle of egg production, diets containing cholecalciferol, 25OHD$_3$ (5 mg), and 1,25(OH)$_2$D$_3$ to obtain 2,000 IU of vitamin D$_3$ in a factorial design with 4 levels of calcium (2.85, 3.65, 4.45, and 5.25%). This research group observed lower egg production (70.17 ± 1.04 *vs.* 73.27 ± 0.58%), egg weight (68.95 ± 0.26 *vs.* 69.77 ± 0.21 g), and Haugh units (96.96 ± 0.20 *vs.* 97.64 ± 0.22) in hens supplemented with 1,25(OH)$_2$D$_3$ than in hens fed cholecalciferol. The best FCR was observed in hens fed diets supplemented with 25OHD$_3$, which were better than those fed 1,25(OH)$_2$D$_3$ (2.092 *vs.* 2.215 kg feed/kg egg and 1.781 *vs.* 1.894 kg/dozen of eggs). In contrast, birds fed cholecalciferol had intermediate results.

Kakhki *et al.* (2019) observed linear improvements in egg weight of 74- to 81-week-old Lohman LSL-lite layers when 25OHD$_3$ was added at 69 or 13 µg/kg to diets containing 3.0, 3.5, 4.0, or 4.5% calcium. No other significant effects of 25OHD$_3$ were observed in this experiment.

The optimum levels of vitamin D$_3$ and the biopotency of 25OHD$_3$ during the rearing period from 1 to 20 weeks were evaluated recently by Li *et al.* (2021) on an egg production cycle from 18 to 72 weeks. A factorial experiment evaluated 2 levels of vitamin D$_3$ (300 and 2,800 IU/kg) and 2 levels of 25OHD$_3$ (0 or 56 g/kg). Dietary treatments during rearing did not affect egg production or eggshell quality. However, vitamin D$_3$ at 2,800 IU/kg or 25OHD$_3$ increased serum calcium concentration, keel length, tibia ash, tibia calcium content, and calcification during rearing and tended to increase tibia mineralization at 72 weeks of age. Consequently, higher vitamin D$_3$ or 25OHD$_3$ during rearing mainly affects bone metabolism.

Eggshell quality is an important factor in marketing. Disease, stress, hen age, mycotoxins, toxicosis, nutrient imbalance, and management conditions influence eggshell quality. Vitamin D can alleviate some of these negative effects. However, problems with pimpling, a calcification defect in the egg, have a direct relationship with management, and there is an interrelationship with various nutrients. Goodson-Williams *et al.* (1986) showed that as age increases, high levels of vitamin D_3 worsen incidences of pimpling.

In contrast, Koreleski and Świątkiewicz (2005) demonstrated that substituting 25% (vitamin D_3 over 1,500 IU/kg) with 25OHD$_3$ improved eggshell density, thickness, and resistance to breakage, particularly of those produced at the end of laying. Wang *et al.* (2020c) showed that high stocking density reduced feed intake, egg-laying rate, egg weight, eggshell quality, and tibia strength. But when dietary 25OHD$_3$ was supplemented, skeletal strength improved, and the number of broken eggs were reduced by more in the hens under high stocking density than those under low stocking density (Figure 7.6).

The mechanisms involved in the improvements observed in eggshell quality with 25OHD$_3$ supplementation were partially explained by Zhao *et al.* (2021). They evaluated the supplementation of 69 µg/kg of 25OHD$_3$ combined with an essential oil containing 200 mg/kg thymol and 50 mg/kg carvacrol (HDV+EO) for 12 weeks in 48-week-old Lohmann layers. The HDV+EO supplementation was added to a basal diet that contained 1,000 IU/kg vitamin D_3. This HDV+EO treatment improved egg production (96.45 *vs.* 93.67%), feed efficiency (1.96 *vs.* 2.10 g: g), and eggshell strength measured as the number of broken eggs (0.45 *vs.* 2.57%) or the force required to break the eggs (4.695 *vs.* 4.387 kg/cm^3) and decreased the translucent egg score.

The improvements in eggshell quality were explained by changes in the ultrastructure of the eggshell (Figure 7.7). Eggs from hens supplemented with HDV+EO had thinner mammillary knob (74.3 *vs.* 87.6 µm), mammillary layer (72.4 *vs.* 91.3 µm), and less proportion of mammillary thickness (19.62 *vs.* 25.65%), and an increased ratio of eggshell effective thickness (80.38 *vs.* 74.35%) and total thickness (283 *vs.* 266 µm) compared to the control. Additionally, HDV+EO improved the antioxidant capacity in the uterus.

The efficacy of vitamin D_3 or its metabolites in improving eggshell traits could be enhanced by other nutrients such as microminerals and antioxidants, including other vitamins. Dos Santos *et al.* (2021) evaluated the effects of including organic zinc-methionine (32 mg/kg) and manganese (26 mg/kg), together with 25OHD$_3$ (37.5 µg/kg = 1,500 IU/kg) in 86-week-old Dekalb White laying hens. The only effect observed was an improvement in eggshell thickness using trace minerals and 25OHD$_3$.

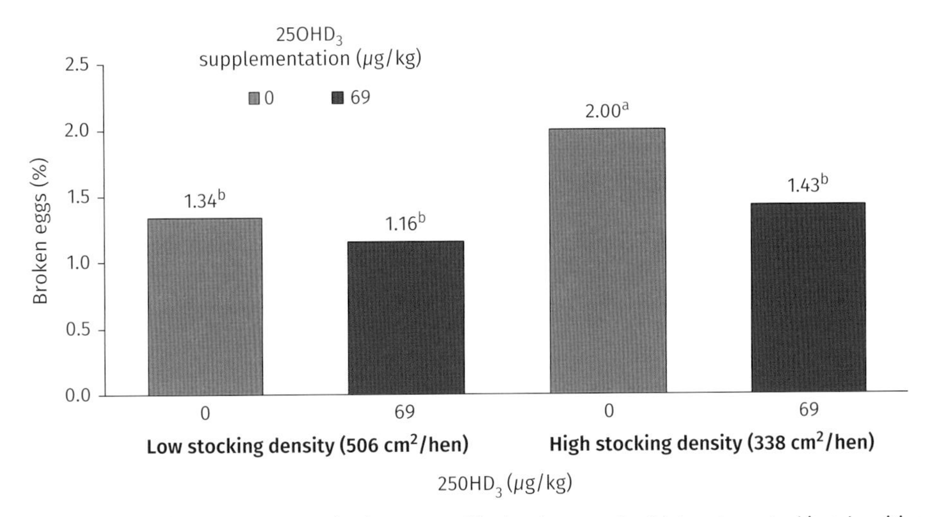

Figure 7.6 Effect of dietary 25OHD$_3$ on broken eggs of laying hens under high or low stocking densities (1–16 weeks), values with no common superscripts differ significantly, $P < 0.05$ (adapted from Wang *et al.*, 2020c)

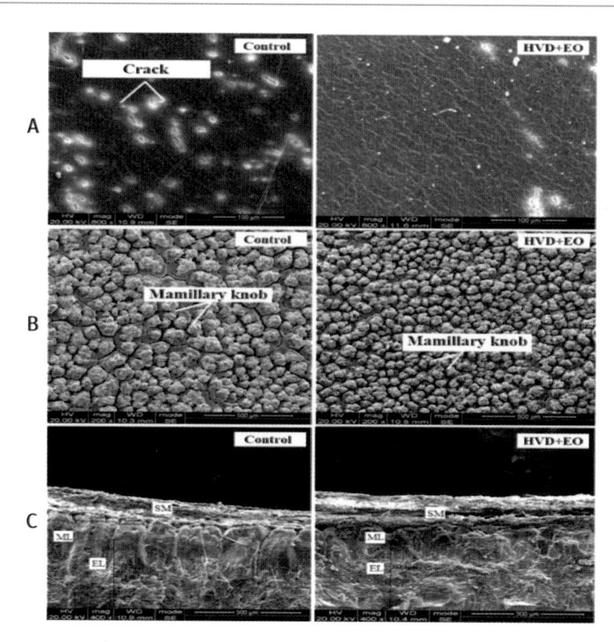

Figure 7.7 Scanning electron microscope images of the eggshell ultrastructure for Lohmann laying hens after feeding HDV and EO from 48 to 60 weeks of age. (A) Eggshell appearance. (B) Mammillary knobs of the eggshell. (C) Thickness and width of the mammillary knobs and the effective thickness of the eggshell. Control: basal diet with 1,000 IU vitamin D_3/kg; HDV+EO: control diet + 69 µg/kg HDV+EO. Scale bar: 200 µm. Abbreviations: EL, effective layer; EO, 200 mg/kg thymol + 50 mg/kg carvacrol; HVD, 25OHD$_3$; ML, mammillary layer; SM, shell membrane (Zhao *et al.*, 2021)

When examining the enrichment of the eggs with vitamin D, Mattila *et al.* (1999) found a high and positive correlation between the cholecalciferol content of the feed and the cholecalciferol (r = 0.995) and 25OHD$_3$ (r = 0.941) content of the egg yolk. Eggs enriched with vitamin D can potentially provide the full suggested requirement that a person needs and substantial quantities of 25OHD$_3$ with greater biological activity than that of cholecalciferol (Ward, 2017).

Barnkob *et al.* (2020) reviewed enhancing eggs with vitamin D naturally and concluded that it is possible to enrich eggs with vitamin D_3 and 25OHD$_3$. A maximum of 20 µg/100 g yolk can be obtained with 617.5 µg/kg feed. These authors estimated the following equation based on a literature review: vitamin D_3 in eggs (µg/100 g) = 0.033 × vitamin D_3 in feed (µg/kg) – 0.58. But the content of 25OHD$_3$ in the eggs in the function of vitamin D_3 in the feed is better expressed with a logarithmic function indicating lower incorporation in the yolk. The transfer efficiency increases as the dietary concentration increases. However, the maximum permitted dosage for vitamin D in feed for layers in the EU, China, and Canada is 80 µg/kg. When feeding vitamin D_3 the content of both D_3 and 25OHD$_3$ in the egg will increase; however, using 25OHD$_3$ alone will not increase the vitamin D_3 content of the egg (Browning and Cowieson, 2014). The avian binding protein for vitamin D_3 in the plasma requires between 8 to 21 days to reach the peak of yolk vitamin D accumulation after hen dietary supplementation is started. Hen age does not affect the transfer of vitamin D_3 in the diet, but the variability is high (coefficient of variance of 24%).

Finally, vitamin D supplementation may also play a role in intestinal health. Morris *et al.* (2015) concluded that supplementing birds with 25OHD$_3$ 100 µg/kg could be a nutritional strategy to reduce the production losses post-coccidia challenge in layer hens. This level of supplementation aid in maintaining body weight gain only 4% below the controls, while other treatments had a reduction of 15% post-coccidia challenge. Wang *et al.* (2021b) also observed that under high stocking density, 45-week-old Lohmann layers could benefit from $25OHD_3$ (69 μg/kg) supplementation by improving several gut health indicators such as intestinal barrier function, antioxidant capacity, and cecal microbiota composition. In layers stocked at a high-density (338 cm^2/hen), $25OHD_3$ decreased the enrichment of *Bacteroidetes* (phylum) and increased *Firmicutes* (phylum) and the *Firmicutes*/*Bacteroidetes* ratio.

Layer vitamin D_3 requirements have not been re-evaluated in recent decades. In current practice, vitamin D_3 metabolites are being used, and much research is being carried out to observe other benefits in the nutrition of layers. However, the optimum application levels remain to be determined since diverse groups tested give several benefits.

Vitamin E

Details about current vitamin E recommendations for layers, provided by institutional sources and genetic companies, can be found in Tables 7.1 to 7.3.

The main function of vitamin E, as discussed extensively in Chapter 4, is to act as an antioxidant on a cellular level, specifically protecting the phospholipids in the membranes from lipid oxidation. On a cellular level, vitamin E is integrated into cellular membranes where it neutralizes free radicals, effectively preventing the development of oxidation. The greater the degree of unsaturation of the lipids, the greater their susceptibility to oxidation.

In the case of layers, oxidative destruction of ovarian follicles reduces egg production and, consequently, a deterioration in the conversion ratio. Furthermore, there is evidence that vitamin E facilitates the release of vitellogenin, the precursor of yolk, from the liver and therefore increases circulation of the compounds necessary for yolk formation.

In the immune system, vitamin E avoids oxidative destruction or alteration of macrophages, representing the first line of defense against infections. It also improves the immune response, increasing the production of antibodies. Vitamin E also enhances immune function by inhibiting the production of immunosuppressive prostaglandins. In current systems of table egg production, vaccination is a routine and frequent practice. Vaccination induces immunological stress, which may be aggravated by other environmental situations, such as heat stress.

Numerous conclusive studies have demonstrated the beneficial effect of vitamin E supplementation on alleviating stress situations, particularly heat stress. Bollengier-Lee *et al.* (1998) observed that 500 mg/kg feed of vitamin E successfully alleviates the negative effects of chronic heat stress on production (improvements of between 7 and 22%), egg volume, and FCR of the hens. Previous studies had been directed toward determining optimum dosage and time of administration. The same authors (Bollengier-Lee *et al.*, 1999) deduced from a later experiment that supplementation of 250 mg/kg vitamin E in the layer diets before, during, and after heat stress prevented the reduction in laying. It is important to point out that supplementation must occur not only after but also before and during the period of stress.

These data agree with those of other authors who indicated that vitamin E supplementation before and during heat stress prevents negative effects on production (Utomo *et al.*, 1994; Whitehead, 1998; Kirunda *et al.*, 2001). The team of Scheideler at the University of Nebraska (Puthpongsiriporn *et al.*, 2001, and Scheideler and Froning, 1996) also observed beneficial effects with moderate doses (50–65 mg/kg). Likewise, Bartov *et al.* (1991) demonstrated that vitamin E supplementation between 125 and 300 mg/kg mitigated the negative impact on egg production, feed efficiency, and eggshell density caused by heat stress and illnesses. The studies by Kucuk *et al.* (2003b) and Panda *et al.* (2008) detected improvements that vitamin E and C had on production parameters and the antioxidant status of layers subjected to thermal stress (low temperatures 6°C or tropical summer conditions) with an additive effect of the 2 vitamins.

Vitamin E can protect from some of the damage caused by mycotoxins when hens are exposed to low contamination levels. Khan *et al.* (2010) fed 30-week-old white leghorn layer breeders hens with diets containing 100, 500, 2,500, 5,000, and 10,000 μg/kg aflatoxin B_1 with and without supplementation of vitamin E (100 mg/kg). This group observed that vitamin E prevented histopathological damages caused by mycotoxins up to 500 μg/kg aflatoxin B_1. A similar effect was observed in reducing immunotoxin effects observed in their progeny (Khan *et al.*, 2014).

Some authors have studied the effect of supplementation with vitamin E on the production and quality of the shell (Fan *et al.*, 1998). Scheideler and Froning (1996) found that adding 50 IU of vitamin E slightly improved egg production (96.1 *vs.* 94.3%). However, other researchers (Richter *et al.*, 1985, 1986, 1987; Botsoglou *et al.*, 2005; Florou-Paneri *et al.*, 2006) found no differences in production parameters with an increased dietary content of vitamin E in layer feeds. Still, the studies were nearly always carried out under optimum experimental conditions, far from current commercial practice.

Vitamin E supplementation at 45, 65, and 85 mg/kg diet had no significant effects on feed intake; however, 85 mg/kg improved egg production (Figure 7.8), feed efficiency, and Haugh unit in laying hens (Erhan and Bölükbaşi, 2011). However, supplementation of 85 IU vitamin E and 100 mg vitamin C per liter of drinking water increased feed conversion and egg production.

Interesting observations by Froning (2001) indicated that supplementation with 120 mg/kg vitamin E improved the functional properties of the egg, specifically the percentage of solids. Likewise, Kirunda *et al.* (2001) supplemented 60 mg vitamin E in the diets of hens exposed to high temperatures and found positive effects on the thickness of the vitelline membrane, yolk, and albumen solids foaming properties, among other parameters. These data agree with other authors who indicated that supplementation with 250 mg/kg vitamin E does not affect egg size but does affect egg volume by its effect on the yolk (Bollengier-Lee *et al.*, 1999). These authors suggested that the antioxidant action of vitamin E counteracts the negative impact of heat stress. An extra supply results in higher vitellogenin levels in the plasma, which permits greater yolk development.

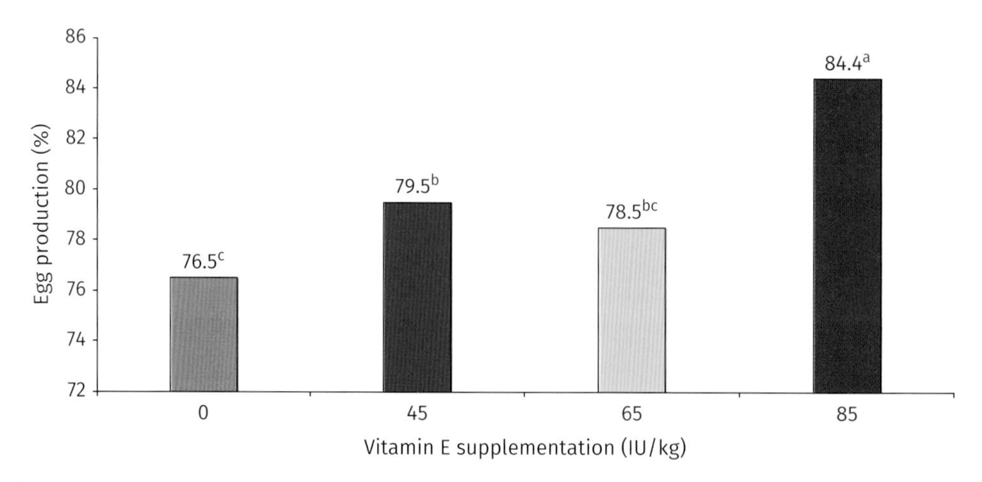

Figure 7.8 Effect of dietary vitamin E on performance in laying hens exposed to heat stress, values with no common superscripts differ significantly, $P < 0.05$ (adapted from Erhan and Bölükbaşi, 2011)

Vitamin E supplementation could minimize quality and egg contamination problems, which occur more frequently during the summer months due to high temperatures and relative humidity and bring significant economic losses for egg processing companies. The effect of vitamin E along with selenium supplementation has been studied by Aljamal *et al.* (2008). They found that including 100 mg/kg vitamin E in the diet of laying hens enhances the quality of eggs. Concerning selenium, egg production, feed intake, and specific gravity were increased dramatically as the dietary selenium level increased to 0.25 and 0.50 ppm.

The addition of incremental dosages of vitamin E in hen feed (from 0 to 320 mg α-tocopheryl acetate) does not appear to affect yolk color (Frigg *et al.*, 1992; Botsoglou *et al.*, 2005; Florou-Paneri *et al.*, 2006), although the study by Angela *et al.* (1999) found changes in yolk carotenoid concentrations when 2% vitamin E was added to the basal diet. The oxidative stability of the egg is influenced by its fatty acid composition and the method of processing to which it is subjected. In recent years, there has been a tendency to enrich these products with unsaturated fatty acids, specifically from the omega-3 family. However, it has been shown that this greater degree of unsaturation in eggs leads to increased susceptibility to lipid oxidation (Cherian *et al.*, 1996a,b; Li *et al.*, 1996; Grashorn and Steinhilber, 1999; Galobart *et al.*, 2001a). Lipid oxidation reduces the nutritional and organoleptic value of the egg. Furthermore, consuming products derived from lipid oxidation has been linked to developing various pathologies, such as cardiovascular disease, aging, and cancer.

Many studies have shown how dietary supplementation with increased levels of vitamin E prevents or reduces the oxidation levels associated with enriching eggs with PUFAs and subjected to various heat processes (Wahle *et al.*, 1993; Cherian *et al.*, 1996a,b; Li *et al.*, 1996; Qi and Sim, 1998; Cortinas *et al.*, 2001; Galobart *et al.*, 2001a,b,c; Botsoglou *et al.*, 2005). Oxidation levels of fresh eggs are very low, but oxidation values increase 10 to 12 times the values observed in fresh eggs when they are atomized for whole egg powder production. However, oxidation levels decrease considerably by supplementing the hen's diet with different levels of α-tocopheryl acetate (50, 100, and 200 mg/kg). Increasing vitamin E levels in the ration reduced thiobarbituric acid values, but these differences were only significant between 50 and 200 mg/kg. In other words, the reduction in oxidation values due to vitamin E decreases as its concentration in the diet increases. This shows that it would be necessary to adjust dietary supplementation of this compound according to the egg processing and storage conditions or for foods of animal origin. The greatest protective effect on the producer may be achieved at the lowest economic cost.

A study realized by Botsoglou *et al.* (2005) evaluated the effects of feeding a basal diet supplemented with antioxidants like α-tocopheryl acetate (200 mg/kg), rosemary (5 g/kg), oregano (5 g/kg), or saffron (20 mg/kg) on hen performance, egg quality, oxidative stability of refrigerated stored shell eggs and liquid yolks. They found that α-tocopheryl acetate had the lowest oxidation rate of all treatments during the storage time (Figure 7.9). In addition, incorporating tocopherols into eggs might also provide a source of tocopherols for the human diet.

Jiang *et al.* (2013) evaluated a similar antioxidant effect in layer diets with high levels of distillers dried grains with solubles (10 and 20% of inclusion). These diets decreased saturated fatty acids and increased unsaturated fatty acids in the egg yolk. Hy-Line Brown hens were supplemented with vitamin E at 200 mg/kg reducing malondialdehyde (MDA) and increased glutathione peroxidase and total superoxide dismutase concentrations in the yolk and serum. It was demonstrated once again the potent antioxidant effects of vitamin E. Another study by Hayat *et al.* (2010) from flax-fed hens showed that α-tocopherols 50, 100, and 150 mg/kg are a good option, like antioxidants, and their supplementation is necessary to maintain long-chain fatty content and stability and protect PUFA during storage.

Moreover, maximum α-tocopherol concentration was observed in the eggs from hens fed flax + 150 mg/kg of α-tocopherol. Storage led to reductions in α-tocopherol content in the α-tocopherol-supplemented groups (Figure 7.10).

The α-tocopherol content of the egg maintains a linear relationship with its level of supplementation in layer feed. Thus, an egg produced by a hen given 200 mg/kg α-tocopheryl acetate contains around 6–8 mg vitamin E (Galobart *et al.*, 2001c). Recommended consumption of vitamin E (recommended daily amount, RDA) for humans is approximately 10 mg. Therefore, an egg enriched with vitamin E can provide 60–80% of the RDA for this vitamin. Similar observations have been described by several authors who have investigated the possibility of increasing the vitamin E content of the egg (Frigg *et al.*, 1992; Jiang *et al.*, 1994; Surai *et al.*, 1995; Chen *et al.*, 1998; Qi and Sim, 1998; Meluzzi *et al.*, 1999; Grobas *et al.*, 2002; Mori *et al.*, 2003).

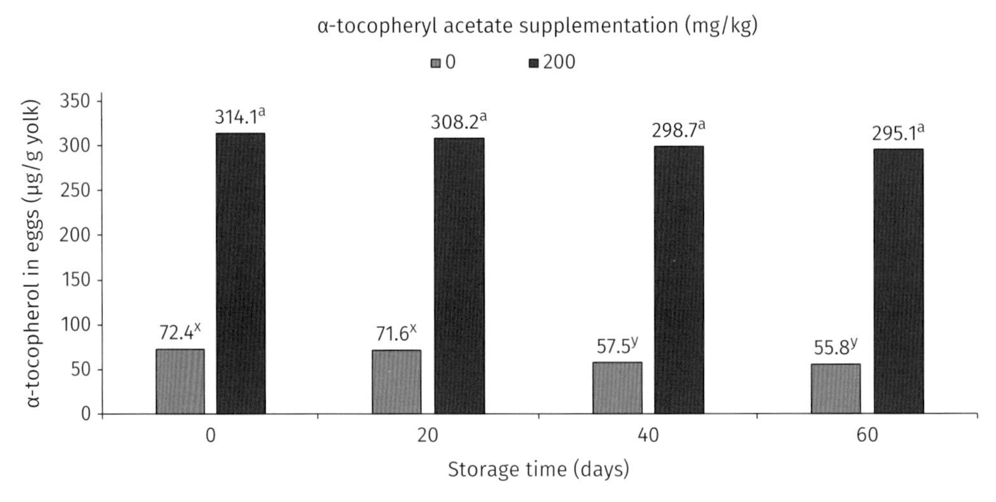

Figure 7.9 Effect of dietary antioxidants on α-tocopherol content of omega-3 enriched eggs during refrigerated storage, values with no common superscripts differ significantly, $P < 0.05$ (adapted from Botsoglou *et al.*, 2005)

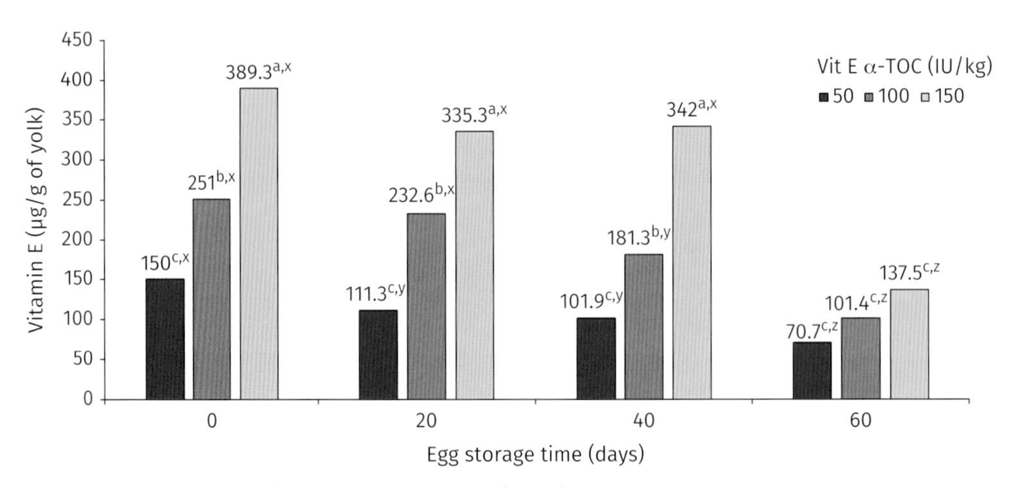

Figure 7.10 Effect of feeding flax with α-tocopherols (α-TOC) like antioxidants on vitamin E content of eggs during storage, values with no common superscripts differ significantly, $P < 0.05$ (adapted from Hayat *et al.*, 2010)

As mentioned in the section on vitamin A, the interrelation between the 2 vitamins A and E is very important, as they are involved in its absorption and subsequent deposition in the egg. Yolk α-tocopherol decreased as supplemental vitamin A increased (15,000 and 30,000 IU/kg), indicating the adverse effect of dietary vitamin A on yolk tocopherol deposition (Mori *et al.*, 2003).

The dietary supplementation with 200 mg/kg vitamin E improved egg production and quality. It enhanced the antioxidant capacity of laying hens (40 to 63 weeks of age) (Jiang *et al.*, 2013). Recently, Zhao *et al.* (2021) concluded that vitamin E supplementation enhanced laying hens' performance. Therefore, supplementing natural vitamin E could have a good effect on the laying performance of hens, and natural vitamin E at a dosage of 100 mg/kg was recommended.

Vitamin E supplementation above the minimum requirements is very beneficial in the face of routine stress situations resulting from vaccinations, beak trimming, heat, and transport. Based on all this information, it is logical to conclude that the dosage of vitamin E in layer feeds should be adjusted according to the unsaturated fatty acid content of the feed and according to the processing and storage to which the eggs will be subjected.

Vitamin K

Details about current vitamin K recommendations for layers, provided by institutional sources and genetic companies, can be found in Tables 7.1 to 7.3.

Requirements for vitamin K by layers have not been established, with the NRC giving a minimum requirement of 0.5 mg/kg in 1994, based on a study from 1964. However, the Agricultural Research Council (ARC) had already in 1975 suggested a higher minimum of 1 mg/kg and recommended level of 2 mg/kg.

The main function of vitamin K is to regulate the formation of various factors involved in blood clotting. Prothrombin is produced in the liver and used continuously by the body. Continual intake of vitamin K is necessary to activate prothrombin, which is of great importance in layers for the following specific reasons.

- When ovulation occurs, if the follicular sac does not rupture along the stigma line, an area with few blood vessels, blood spots in the yolk may result, which could be avoided with effective blood clotting.
- Layers have a propensity to nervousness, with pecking and even cannibalism. If birds are injured, for example, following uterine prolapse at oviposition, a longer blood-clotting period may trigger cannibalism.
- Beak trimming is a normal practice in the management of layers. A delay in the clotting period may delay healing.

The principal bone proteins, such as osteocalcin, also depend on vitamin K. Osteocalcin is important in calcium metabolism and is found in bone, the uterus, and eggshells. Low osteocalcin and bone matrix proteins may impede the mineralization process during skeletal development and eggshell formation (Whitehead, 2004b). Some studies relating to vitamin K in layers focus on bone metabolism. Lavelle *et al.* (1994) fed breeding leghorn hens with a diet deficient in vitamin K to study the effect on bone metabolism of layers, embryo development, and chick growth. While egg production, shell thickness, and other production parameters were not significantly affected, vitamin K deficiency reduced the concentration of coagulation and osteocalcin factors, which did not affect the initial skeletal development of chicks. Rennie *et al.* (1997) found no changes in the volume of trabecular bone in the hens on supplementing feed during laying with 20 mg/kg vitamin K. These authors did not consider whether vitamin K stimulated bone development during the whole growth period of the chicks.

With this objective in mind, Fleming *et al.* (1998) carried out a study that led them to conclude that supplementation of 10 mg/kg vitamin K_3 to a basal diet, containing already 2 mg/kg vitamin K_3, resulted in a greater volume of cancellous bone in the tarsal-metatarsal bone after 25 weeks of life. The authors noted that vitamin K could prolong the modeling period of bone formation or inhibit medullary bone loss during the first phases of laying. In a subsequent study, Fleming *et al.* (2003) confirmed these results, observing that combined supplementation of additional sources of vitamin K_3, calcium carbonate particles, and fluoride improved the quality and resistance of bones at the end of laying, with an improvement of between 12 and 20% in bone characteristics related to osteoporosis. Their results indicated that these improvements are mainly due to the extra granulated calcium supply. They also demonstrated that vitamin K_3 supplementation increased the volume of medullary bone in the tarsal-metatarsal both during the starter and grower phase and during laying up to 70 weeks. However, it was impossible to explain this effect since the concentration of plasma osteocalcin was not affected by the dietary vitamin K dose during growth.

Fernandes *et al.* (2009) using four levels of vitamin K_3 (0, 2, 8, and 32 mg/kg diet) evaluated vitamin K_3 supplementation in 67-week-old Hy-Line W-36 hens. Linear effects were observed on egg weight, percent hen-day, and feed conversion (kilogram feed/dozen eggs). A quadratic effect was observed on bone ash content but not eggshell quality. This study confirmed the importance of vitamin K on bone mineralization.

A study realized by Souza *et al.* (2016) evaluated the influence of graded levels of calcium and vitamin K_3 in laying hen diets during the rearing phase and their effects on the laying phase. The authors concluded that the dietary addition of 1.4% calcium and graded levels of vitamin K_3 (2, 8, 16, and 32 mg/kg) improved blood calcium levels, Seedor index of bone strength (bone weight/bone length) (Figure 7.11), total bone calcium, and the percentage of medullary bone in the tibiotarsus of pullets during the growing phase (Figure 7.12), while maintaining the amount

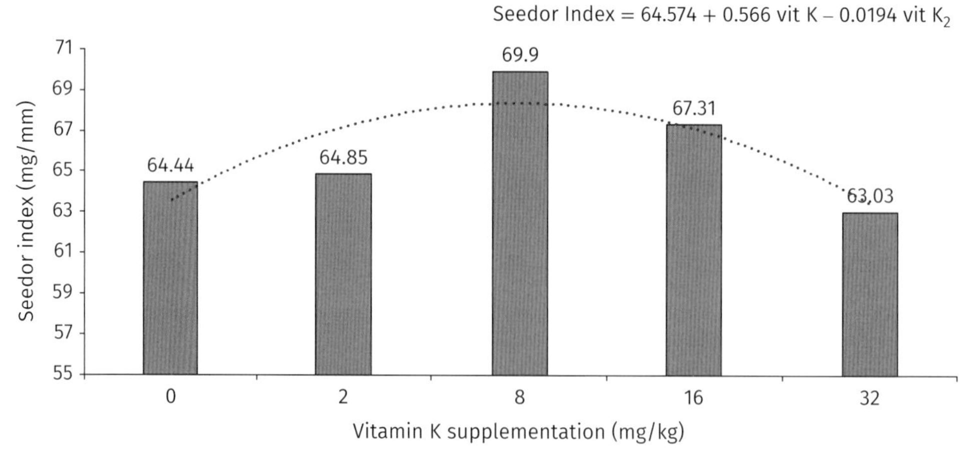

Figure 7.11 Effect of vitamin K supplementation on layer diets with 1.4% calcium on bone Seedor index in pullets at 18 weeks (adapted from Souza *et al.*, 2016)

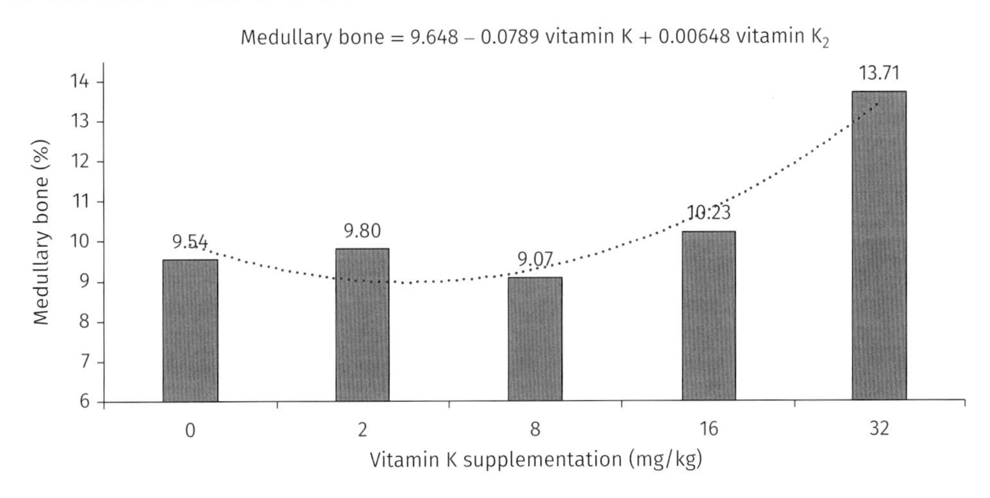

Figure 7.12 Effect of vitamin K supplementation on layer diets with 1.4% calcium on tibiotarsus medullary bone of laying hens at 32-weeks-age (adapted from Souza *et al.*, 2016)

of medullary bone during the laying phase. When the goal is to improve bone condition it is important to consider the levels of calcium and vitamin K because both synergize to enhance bone quality.

These data demonstrate that the extra vitamin K supplementation improves the formation of trabecular calcium during the growth period and prevents osteoporosis in laying hens. However, it would be useful to carry out more studies on the role of vitamin K in the development and maintenance of the skeleton in laying hens to understand the mechanisms involved. Likewise, data is needed on vitamin K activity in common stress situations in which vitamin synthesis and/or absorption are diminished.

Regarding the possibility of fortifying eggs with vitamin K, the experiment by Suzuki and Okamoto (1997) demonstrated that vitamin K_1 or phylloquinone supplementation between 10 and 100 mg/kg produces eggs with a content of 104–1,908 µg vitamin K_1 and 67–192 µg menaquinone or K_2/100 g yolk. Supplementation with vitamin K_3 or menadione (10–1,000 mg/kg) resulted in eggs fortified with menaquinone at a level of 115–240 µg/100 g yolk and with menadione at a level of only 1 µg/100 g yolk. No differences were observed in egg production related to the dosage of vitamin K.

O'Sullivan *et al.* (2020) recently evaluated the efficacy of vitamin K supplementation (3, 12.9, 23.7, and 45.7 mg/kg feed) in improving egg vitamin K content. Vitamin K was evaluated as menadione nicotinamide disulfate in Hy-Line hens. In the eggs, menaquinone-4 was the most abundant form (91–98%). Dietary supplementation increased menaquinone in the eggs to 46–51 µg/100 g, the yellowness of egg yolk, eggshell weight, and thickness. Consequently, dietary vitamin K can double the total content of vitamin K in eggs.

Water-soluble vitamins

The principal functions of the B group vitamins are connected with energy metabolism from carbohydrates, fatty acids, and proteins. Except in organs with high metabolic requirements, such as the heart, the liver, and the kidneys, birds lack reserves of these vitamins. In contrast, even in these organs, the reserve is very small after hatching, so a continuous supply is needed. The presence of aflatoxins in feed reduces the level of most of these vitamins in plasma and liver by 50 and 20%, respectively, if their concentration reaches 5 mg/kg of feed

(Bains, 2001). Furthermore, a greater supply of these vitamins reduces the adverse effects of mycotoxins by favoring their breakdown and detoxification in the liver.

Stress conditions increase energy requirements and reduce feed consumption. A higher supplement of these vitamins, even over short periods, helps birds overcome the consequences of stress prejudicial to their productivity and immune status.

Vitamin B_1 (thiamine)

Details about current vitamin B_1 recommendations for layers, provided by institutional sources and genetic companies, can be found in Tables 7.1 to 7.3.

The minimum value recommended by the NRC in 1994 was 0.7 mg/kg. In 1975 the ARC already suggested minimum requirements of 1.25 mg/kg and 1.5 mg/kg as practical requirements. Padhi and Combs (1965) conducted a study using different levels of vitamin B_1, from 0 to 1.67 mg/kg. The best productive yields were obtained with a supplementation level of 1.25 mg/kg. When dosages lower than or equal to 0.35 ppm were used, egg production ceased after 12 days of feeding, and the same occurred after 20 days of the experiment with supplementation levels of up to 0.55 mg/kg. After 27 days of intake of 0.55 mg/kg or less, symptoms of polyneuritis appeared, which could be alleviated with parenteral injections of thiamine. Accordingly, the units of activity of red blood cell transketolase increased proportionally with the level of supplementation, which stimulated the synthesis of the thiamine pyrophosphate (TPP) dependent enzyme transketolase.

Vitamin B_2 (riboflavin)

Details about current vitamin B_2 recommendations for layers, provided by institutional sources and genetic companies, can be found in Tables 7.1 to 7.3.

For birds to maintain the high metabolic demand necessary for optimum egg production sufficient riboflavin must be present. It provides the energy required to support various physiological functions, including reproductive functions. Riboflavin deficiency can negatively impact feather keratin expression (Cogburn *et al.*, 2018). The level of 2.5 mg/kg recommended by the NRC in 1994 is 13.7% higher than the 2.2 mg/kg they recommended in 1984.

In a study on breeding hens in a humid tropical environment researchers administered supplements from 2.5 to 12.5 mg/kg. Of the various production parameters analyzed, the only one for which a response was obtained was in the production of eggs, which improved significantly when the level of riboflavin was increased to 8.5 mg/kg (Arijeniwa *et al.*, 1996).

Previously, Kirichenko (1991) had found that egg production increased when riboflavin was supplemented at a level 25% higher than that recommended, while in a study carried out by Flores-Garcia and Scholtyssek (1992), where it was supplemented at levels from 1.7 to 9.7 mg/kg, no significant changes in any production parameter were noted.

Squires and Naber (1993b) studied the changes produced in the riboflavin content of eggs when breeding hens were supplemented with 1.55, 2.20, 4.4, and 8.8 mg/kg for 27 weeks. In the first week of treatment, significant differences were observed between the 2 lower levels of supplementation and the 2 higher ones. In another study, Naber and Squires (1993a) found that when multiplying the requirements by 1 or 2, the transfer efficiency of riboflavin from the diet to the egg was 45%. In contrast, transfer efficiency decreased markedly when the required level was given 4 times. This reduction in egg riboflavin content related to deficient levels of supplementation became even more important as the hens got older.

In the study by Squires and Naber (1993b), blood spots were lower in the eggs of hens that had received supplements of 4.4 and 8.8 mg/kg than those with lower doses. However, these levels of supplementation reduced shell thickness for several weeks. This deterioration in shell quality is probably linked more to the increase in egg production and weight than to the riboflavin level per se. Riboflavin deficiency reduces the ability of the hens to deal with heat stress. Onwudike and Adegbola (1984) have documented that riboflavin requirements by layers increases with heat stress. It would also be advisable to increase the dosage of riboflavin in the ration in cases of immunological stress (vaccinations, infections) because of its involvement in antibody synthesis. These studies indicate that 2.5 mg/kg riboflavin in layer rations may be inadequate.

It has been seen that supplementation with 4.4 and 8.8 mg/kg may benefit certain production parameters and egg quality. This review found no references to studies using supplementation levels between 2.2 and 4.4 mg/kg. However, Leiber *et al.* (2021) evaluated riboflavin supplementation in layer diets for organic production during Swiss winter conditions. A basal diet contained 4.5 mg/kg; the other diets were supplemented with 1.5 and 3.0 mg/kg for 6 and 7.5 mg riboflavin/kg feed. Based on these results, adding 3 mg/kg riboflavin to the winter diet appeared to be sufficient for the health and performance of laying hens. Supplementation with only 1.5 mg/kg resulted in some metabolic signs of deficiency.

Vitamin B_6 (pyridoxine)

Details about current vitamin B_6 recommendations for layers, provided by institutional sources and genetic companies, can be found in Tables 7.1 to 7.3.

The minimum established requirements are 2.5 ppm (NRC, 1994) based on old studies carried out in the 1960s. Vitamin B_6 being present in many feedstuffs often receives scant attention by nutritionists, but the availability of pyridoxine in common feed materials is only 50% on average of the total.

Vitamin B_6 is a cofactor for many enzymes, most of which catalyze reactions involving amino acids. It also takes part in fatty acid and carbohydrate metabolism and energy production. Requirements are higher when there is an increase in the protein content of the diet and for feeds formulated to contain high energy levels derived from fat. A level of normally adequate pyridoxine could become marginal in the presence of illness or heat stress.

Abend *et al.* (1975) observed no significant changes in the carcass or the egg's chemical composition or in the pattern of deposition of amino acids in the pectoral muscle on adding gradual increments of vitamin B_6 to the ration. When the ration was deficient in pyridoxine, the body's protein levels fell. There was a reduction in the glycine-serine quotient.

Weiser *et al.* (1991) indicated, in a study of layers aged 71 and 90 weeks, that a level of 6 mg/kg pyridoxine, mostly provided in the basal diet, is sufficient to prevent bone deformities. The results of Kucuk *et al.* (2008) suggested that pyridoxine (8 mg/kg) along with zinc (30 mg/kg) supplements improved performance and egg quality, especially eggshell weight, in laying hens.

Khan (2019) evaluated pyridoxine supplementation at 40 mg/kg in layer diets with 5% flaxseed cake and 2% flaxseed crushed. Hens fed diets supplemented with pyridoxine had better incorporation of omega-3 fatty acids into the egg and reduced liver toxicity.

Pyridoxine does not cause toxicity problems even when given in very large amounts. A study carried out on layers between 78 and 82 weeks of age, before molt, in which the ration was supplemented with 100 mg/kg pyridoxine, found no changes in egg production or shell formation

(Hupfauer, 1993). This may indicate that an excess of pyridoxine in environmental conditions without much stress brings no additional benefits in production.

Flaxseed cake is a feed ingredient used to increase the content of PUFA in eggs in later diets. However, it contains the antinutritional factor linatine, N-(D-2-carboxy-1-pyrrolidinyl)-L-glutamine, which has antagonistic activity toward pyridoxine. Despite the benefits of improving PUFA content, flaxseed cake is associated with reducing hen performance and liver damage.

Vitamin B_{12} (cyanocobalamin)

Details about current vitamin B_{12} recommendations for layers, provided by institutional sources and genetic companies, can be found in Tables 7.1 to 7.3.

Cobalamin contains cobalt in its structure and is the only vitamin with a trace element in its composition. Unlike the other B group vitamins, cobalamin does not have to be utilized immediately after absorption. It can be accumulated, mainly in the liver and, to a lesser degree, in the kidney, muscles, bone, and skin. The capacity of the hen to deposit reserves of vitamin B_{12} has not been sufficiently studied. Denton *et al.* (1954) noted that deposits were significantly depleted after 2 unsupplemented weeks, but Scott *et al.* (1982) proposed that it takes around 12 weeks to exhaust body reserves completely.

Birds obtain a certain quantity of vitamin B_{12} from bacterial synthesis in the intestine. However, it is still necessary to provide vitamin B_{12} in the diet of layers, albeit in small amounts, particularly if the main diet is of vegetable origin and coprophagy is not possible or relevant, like in birds housed in cages. Levels suggested by the NRC in 1994 are 0.004 mg/kg and are based on studies from the 1950s.

Since vitamin B_{12} is related to choline (via methionine), reducing the intake of methionine and choline will increase the requirement for cyanocobalamin. It is generally believed that vitamin B_{12} deficiency does not affect commercial egg production, but the early reference was made to a drop in egg weight caused by vitamin B_{12} deficiency (Skinner *et al.*, 1951). In a study on breeders, Squires and Naber (1992) observed that the best egg production, egg weight, shell thickness, hen weight, and optimum hatchability were obtained when the diet contained 8 μg/kg vitamin B_{12} of which 7.5 μg/kg were supplemented. Slight improvements were obtained with levels greater than 8 μg/kg, but the differences were not statistically significant. It may be that the nature of the study, carried out over a long period (27 weeks), allowed the detection of differences that had not been observed in shorter-term studies.

Dzhambulatov *et al.* (1996) and Akhmedkhanova and Alisheikhov (1997) estimated that in hot conditions, 36 μg/kg is an adequate level to optimize egg production based on different variables (egg production, egg weight, and FCR). These authors suggested that vitamin B_{12} levels above minimum established requirements are necessary for optimum feeding of breeders.

El-Husseiny *et al.* (2008a) evaluated the interactive effect of methionine (0.40, 0.45, and 0.50%), FA (6, 9, and 12 mg/kg) and vitamin B_{12} (0.01 and 0.02 mg/kg) in Bovans White laying hens between 28 and 43 weeks of age. The highest levels of these 3 nutrients supplemented gave the best productivity, eggshell percentage, hemoglobin concentration, and economic efficiency.

As for egg quality, studies by Squires and Naber (1992) and Naber and Squires (1993a) noted that the concentration of vitamin B_{12} in yolk responds rapidly to dietary levels, so the vitamin B_{12} content of the egg could be used as an indicator of the vitamin B_{12} level in the hen and as a standard of egg quality. This observation confirms the old results of Denton *et al.* (1954), which suggest that vitamin B_{12} deposits in the body do not sustain the vitamin B_{12} content of the egg over a long period. The same authors noted that the minimum concentration of vitamin B_{12} in the egg for maximum hatchability and egg weight is between 1–3 and 2–6 µg/100 g yolk, respectively. Whitehead (1995a) puts vitamin B_{12} requirements for layers at 8 µg/kg, based on the study by Squires and Naber (1992).

Niacin (vitamin B_3)

Details about current niacin recommendations for layers, provided by institutional sources and genetic companies, can be found in Tables 7.1 to 7.3.

Niacin is present in 2 forms, nicotinic acid and nicotinamide, and nicotinic acid must be converted to nicotinamide to undertake vitamin activity. Many foods of layers' diets, both of vegetable and animal origin, contain high quantities of niacin. However, a large part of this niacin is bound and unavailable for absorption. Therefore, laying hens diets must be supplemented with niacin (Leclercq *et al.*, 1987).

Another source is the conversion of tryptophan to niacin in the body, a process that is very inefficient. Sashidhar *et al.* (1988) suggested that mycotoxins in the diet could limit the conversion of tryptophan to niacin. Minimum requirements indicated by the NRC in 1994 are 10 mg/kg, based on studies by Ringrose *et al.* (1965). Several studies have evaluated both production parameters and the metabolism and the cholesterol content in the bird as affected by niacin intake.

Jensen *et al.* (1976) observed no changes in egg production, weight, food consumption, or body weight when supplementing layer diets with 44 mg/kg niacin. Similar results were obtained by Ouart *et al.* (1987), evaluating niacin levels from 0 to 22 mg/kg in diets containing 21.02 mg/kg (corn-based diet) or 46.11 mg/kg (wheat-based diet).

Leeson *et al.* (1991) conducted a study with several strains of laying hens to determine the niacin requirements of highly productive birds in terms of production characteristics. The control diet contained 22 mg/kg niacin, and niacin treatment ranged from a supplement level of 44 to 1,022 mg/kg. A slight increase in production was observed when supplementing with 44 mg/kg compared to the control group. This increase became significant when supplementing with 66 mg/kg or more. Shell quality (measured as the degree of shell deformity) improved in those hens treated with 44 or 132 mg/kg. There were no egg weight, feed consumption, or bird weight changes.

Similar results were obtained by Dikicioglu *et al.* (2000) feeding rations containing niacin levels varying between 250 and 1,500 mg/kg and observed significant improvements in shell quality and feed conversion efficiency. Body weight was influenced negatively. In 2019, Baghban-Kanani *et al.* evaluated the effect of different levels of sunflower meal and niacin on performance, biochemical parameters, antioxidant status, and egg yolk cholesterol of laying hens. The dietary addition of 225 and 275 mg/kg niacin improved egg production and eggshell strength (Figures 7.13 and 7.14). In addition, feeding laying hens with diets containing 15% sunflower meal and 275 mg/kg niacin decreased plasma and egg yolk cholesterol levels.

Kucukersan's (2000) results agreed with the conclusions on production parameters. He found that with 100 mg/kg niacin supplements, bird weight, egg production, and feed conversion efficiency increased. Still, his results differ on shell quality since shell thickness, and weight was reduced with this same supplementation level. There were no differences between the controls and birds receiving 50 mg/kg niacin.

In other animal species and humans, a relationship had been observed between niacin and fat and cholesterol metabolism. In humans, it is thought that niacin treatment helps reduce

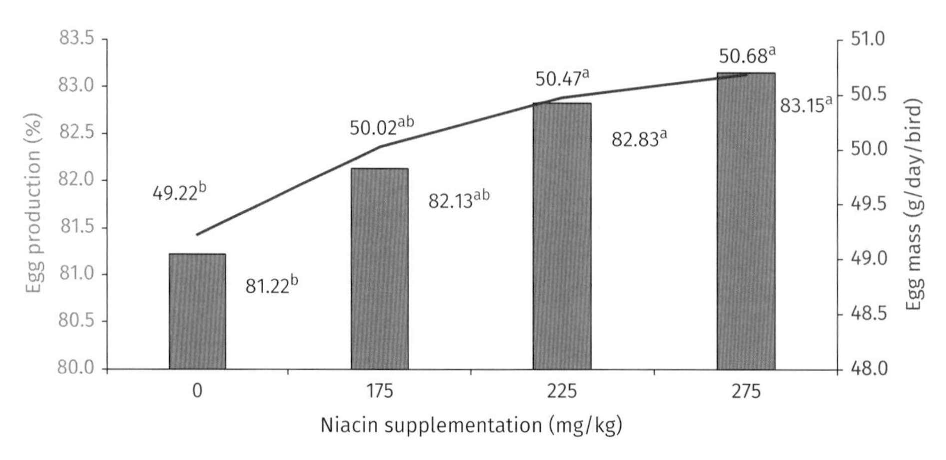

Figure 7.13 Effect of Niacin supplementation on performance in laying hens, values with no common superscripts differ significantly, $P < 0.05$ (adapted from Baghban-Kanani *et al.*, 2019)

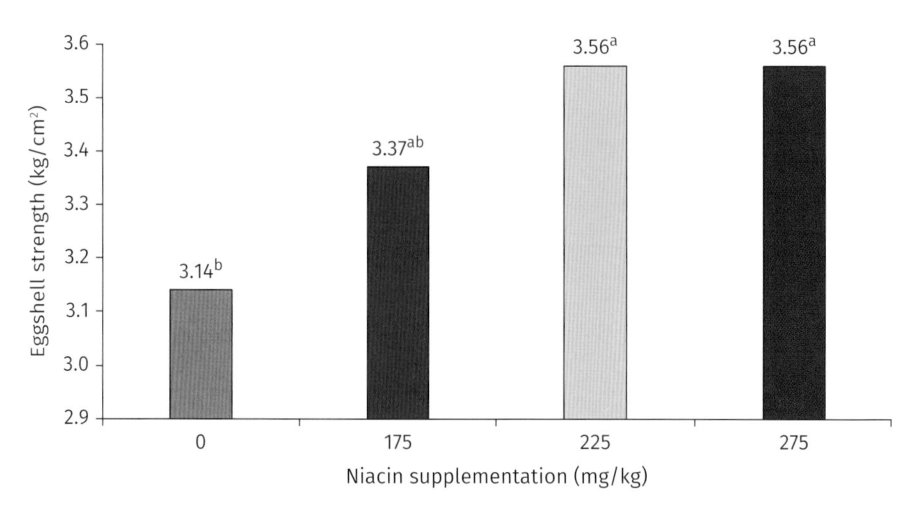

Figure 7.14 Effect of Niacin supplementation on egg quality in laying hens, values with no common superscripts differ significantly, $P < 0.05$ (adapted from Baghban-Kanani, *et al.*, 2019)

blood cholesterol levels. Alderman *et al.* (1989) suggested that supplementation with 2 g/day effectively reduced total cholesterol in blood serum and improved humans' high-density cholesterol-lipoprotein quotient. Witzum (1989) also described reductions of 25–35% in human cholesterol levels when treating with high levels of niacin.

Leeson *et al.* (1991) did not observe effects on the cholesterol content of eggs during the 28 days of the experiment. They did not observe effects on the incidence of fatty liver evaluated according to fat accumulation in the liver. This latter point agrees with the results previously obtained by Jensen *et al.* (1976) that adding 44 mg/kg niacin to the ration failed to alter liver weight or lipid content significantly. Concerning the cholesterol content of the egg, similar results were obtained by Kucukersan (2000) by supplementing 50 and 100 mg/kg niacin.

On the other hand, Dikicioglu *et al.* (2000) described that adding levels of niacin from 250 to 1,500 mg/kg to the ration increased blood cholesterol levels, while the cholesterol content in yolk was significantly reduced. It has been suggested that this vitamin controls hysteria or nervousness in birds at a dosage of 200 mg/kg. At this level mortality rate was reduced when birds were housed at high densities, and the conversion ratio improved. North (1984) agreed that large doses of niacin help alleviate hysteria problems in caged birds. However, Ouart *et al.* (1987) observed no differences between groups that received different levels of supplementation, from 0 to 22 ppm, over diets containing 21.02 or 46.11 mg/kg niacin.

In a review published in 1992, Jackson indicated that genetic companies suggested niacin levels of 18–38 mg/kg, and economic benefits could be achieved by using higher dosages than those recommended by the NRC (1994). Based on the studies referred to here, 22 mg/kg niacin is a marginal level if the aim is to maximize egg yield. A 66 mg/kg is sufficient for a good egg production rate. Feed conversion efficiency probably improves with a ration supplemented with 100 mg/kg, and with 132–250 mg/kg, positive effects on shell quality would be obtained. In a review published by Whitehead (2001), the practical level of supplementation for layers is 50 mg/kg niacin.

Pantothenic acid (vitamin B_5)

Details about current pantothenic acid recommendations for layers, provided by institutional sources and genetic companies, can be found in Tables 7.1 to 7.3.

As a constituent of coenzyme A and the carrier protein for acyl groups (ACP), pantothenic acid plays a fundamental role in fatty acid metabolism. Requirements for this vitamin in laying hens stand at 2 mg/kg (NRC, 1994), with a great variation between individuals of the same breed or strain.

Pantothenic acid requirements depend on interactions with other vitamins like vitamin C, biotin, and vitamin B_{12}, and the fat content of the ration. Low levels of vitamin B_{12} and high levels of fat increase pantothenic acid requirements, while the presence of vitamin C could reduce requirements.

Initially, a deficiency in this vitamin might not affect egg production but might reduce hatchability and embryo survival. Beer *et al.* (1963), feeding White leghorn pullets with purified diets, concluded that these hens require a minimum of 1.9 mg/kg to optimize egg production, at least 4 mg/kg to maximize hatchability, and 8 mg/kg to ensure the viability of the chicks. Bootwalla and Harms (1991), in their study on minimum pantothenic acid requirements of Single Comb White leghorn chicks, concluded that a minimum of 4.8 mg/kg in the diet is necessary to optimize sexual maturity and future performance.

In 2011, Zang *et al.* evaluated the effects of different dietary vitamin combinations on the egg quality and vitamin concentrations in the eggs of commercial laying hens. They found that the hens receiving OVN™ vitamins (11.3 mg pantothenic acid) produced eggs containing higher levels of most vitamins, with the least impact seen for dirty and cracked eggs.

Insufficient information is available to conclude the pantothenic acid requirements of layers. The requirement has not been re-evaluated for 40 years, and due to its relationship with energy metabolism, it should be adjusted according to the energy content of the diet.

Biotin (vitamin B_7)

Details about current biotin recommendations for layers, provided by institutional sources and genetic companies, can be found in Tables 7.1 to 7.3.

Biotin is involved in the metabolism of carboxylation reactions, gluconeogenesis, and protein synthesis. For these reasons, it is considered essential for life, growth, maintenance of epidermal tissue, and reproduction. Carboxylation reactions are important in fatty acid synthesis, so biotin is necessary for synthesizing long-chain fatty acids and essential fatty acid metabolism.

The level of biotin recommended by the NRC in 1994 is 0.1 mg/kg. Marginal levels of biotin may lead to the appearance of fatty liver or kidney syndrome, especially when there is a low level of fat in the diet and lipogenesis is necessary. This scenario may be aggravated by stress since this drains glycogen reserves.

Jensen *et al.* (1976) conducted a study to determine the effects of niacin, biotin, or both on the accumulation of lipids in the liver. They used a diet of maize and soy for 12 weeks, supplemented with 44 mg/kg niacin and 110 µg/kg biotin, and saw no changes in the liver weight or lipid content. There were no significant differences in production parameters or body weight. It seems that biotin may prevent fatty liver syndrome, but once signs have appeared, it does not seem to have beneficial effects on the accumulation of lipids in the liver.

In a study by Whitehead *et al.* (1976b), supplements of thiamine, riboflavin, nicotinic acid, pyridoxine, pantothenic acid, biotin, FA, vitamin B_{12}, ascorbic acid, choline, and inositol were given separately or in combination to layers. Of all of these, only biotin proved effective in preventing the occurrence of fatty liver or kidney syndrome. The supplementation levels required to avoid this condition were greater than those needed to maximize the live weight of the animal, being between 0.05 and 0.15 mg/kg, depending on the diet.

Recently, Huang *et al.* (2020) evaluated a biotin supplementation of 300 µg/kg feed in high-energy low protein diets fed to 43-week-old Hy-Line Brown layers for 60 days. These high-energy, low protein diets decreased gene expression of important lipoproteins carriers of lipids. The liver gene expression was measured for apolipoprotein A I (apoA I), involved in the formation of high-density lipoprotein (HDL), and Apolipoprotein B100 (apoB100), a specific ligand for the low-density lipoprotein (LDL) receptor involved in the synthesis and secretion of VLDL. Biotin increased mRNA levels of apoA I and apoB100, indicating that this level of 300 µg/kg feed could effectively alleviate the pathological changes induced by this diet that caused fatty liver hemorrhagic syndrome and improve egg production rate.

Highly productive layers may benefit from biotin supplementation to maximize their productive capacity. On the other hand, young hens are less efficient than the older ones in transferring biotin to the yolk, so they need higher supplementation to optimize hatchability (World Poultry-Elsevier, 2001). However, other studies have found a positive relationship between diet biotin levels and yolk levels (Buenrostro and Kratzer, 1984; Whitehead, 1984). Several researchers have observed the benefits of supplementing biotin in local Egyptian layer breeds. Abdel-Mageed and Shabaan (2012), using 52-week-old Fayoumi hens, watched that biotin addition to layers diets at levels of 325.5 µg/kg diet gave the best improvement in egg production, egg number, egg mass, and FCR as well as the highest increase in egg shape index, yolk index, and Haugh unit.

Okasha *et al.* (2019) and El-Garhy *et al.* (2019) recently evaluated 100, 150, and 200 µg/kg supplementation using a local Egyptian breed, Benha line, fed corn-soybean diets. Compared to the other levels, biotin supplementation at a 150 µg/kg level improved feed conversion, early sexual maturity, egg production, egg mass, and plasma calcium. It also increased the relative weight of eggshell and albumin, yolk index, and Haugh unit. The authors concluded that 150 µg/kg had the highest economic efficiency, followed by hens fed diets with 100 µg/kg biotin. Manson *et al.* (2019) also reported positive results on the same breed with 150 µg/kg.

The positive results of biotin can be explained by the role of biotin in growing ovarian follicles (Taniguchi and Watanabe, 2007). Free biotin is abundant in the yolk, and the serum and liver biotin concentrations in layers are about 10 times and 3 times higher than those in mice. This indicates the importance of biotin for laying hens.

Folic acid (vitamin B_9)

Details about current FA recommendations for layers, provided by institutional sources and genetic companies, can be found in Tables 7.1 to 7.3.

The term folacin describes a series of compounds derived from FA. Many active biological forms of folates make the amount present in feedstuffs difficult to evaluate. Principal food sources of folacin include leafy green vegetables and offal such as liver or kidneys. Folate metabolism is entirely related to the metabolism of many other single-carbon atom donors, including S-adenosylmethionine, serine, vitamin B_{12}, and choline. These nutrients interact so that their respective requirements may be changed. The nutritional importance of these interactions is greater for birds since they have a high rate of uric acid synthesis. This metabolic pathway uses single-carbon atoms from excreted nitrogen. Furthermore, the requirements for methionine and cysteine are very high. Methionine is usually the first limiting amino acid, making other sources of methyl groups necessary.

Inadequate levels of other methyl group donors (serine, vitamin B_{12}, choline, etc.) therefore increase requirements, in the same way, that high levels of protein in the diet increase requirements to above the recommended levels due to the need to synthesize high quantities of uric acid for the excretion of nitrogen. Any circumstance affecting microorganisms' intestinal synthesis of folates will also affect requirements.

Dietary requirements for folates set by NRC (1994) are 0.25 mg/kg, despite ARC in 1984 previously indicated a minimum of 0.3 mg/kg. Sherwood *et al.* (1993) fed layers with a purified diet deficient in folates (0.07 mg/kg), harming egg production. By increasing the supplementation of folates, folate deposition in yolk and plasma reached saturation point. With 0.72 mg/kg folates in the diet, the eggs contained less than half the maximum possible folate content in the yolk.

The study by Keshavarz (2003b) used combinations of reduced supplies of methionine, choline, FA, and vitamin B_{12} and obtained smaller eggs but improved shell quality in the final phases of the laying period. Abas *et al.* (2008) evaluated FA supplementation in 5 and 10 mg/kg diets with and without ascorbic acid (200 mg/kg diet). Results indicated that FA caused a reduction in egg production with an increment in egg weight and eggshell thickness that was more pronounced in the vitamin C supplemented diets.

El-Husseiny *et al.* (2008a) also showed that supplementation up to 12 mg/kg diet with FA significantly increased egg weight. Nofal *et al.* (2018) evaluated the effect of dietary FA (0, 10, and 20 mg/kg feed) supplementation on diets of low energy levels (2,800 and 2,600 kcal/kg diet) and methionine (0.40 to 0.30%) of developed laying hens in the summer season on performance, physiological status, and immune response. In that study, the authors concluded that feeding hens on a diet with a metabolizable energy level of 2,800 kcal/kg with a level of 0.40% DL-methionine supplemented with FA at 20 mg/kg which can improve daily egg mass, shell thickness (Figure 7.15), and hatchability of fertile eggs in Silver Montazah laying hens. FA increased egg numbers, plasma total protein, globulin, and egg folate. Increasing dietary FA improved daily feed intake and decreased plasma triglycerides.

Concerning the deposition of FA in the eggs, studies by Hebert *et al.* (2005) and House *et al.* (2002) focused on the enrichment of folate in the egg. They used levels between 0 and 128 mg folic acid/kg feed and showed how the content in the egg responds to levels above 0.25 mg/kg

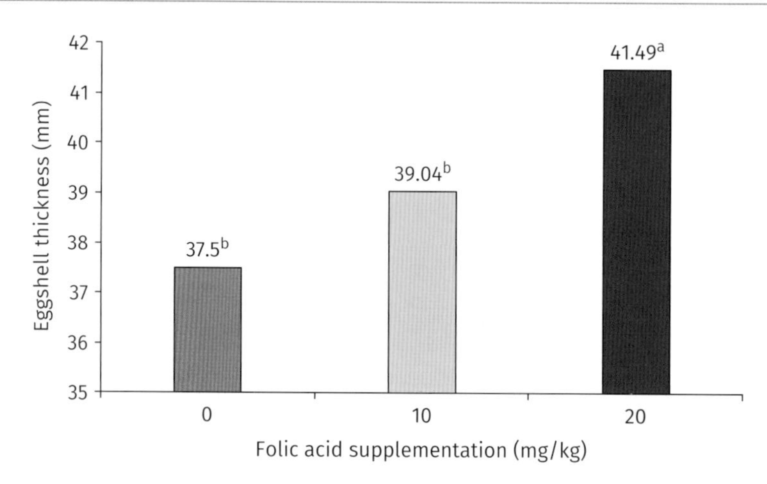

Figure 7.15 Means of egg quality measurements as affected by dietary levels of metabolizable energy, methionine, and added FA in Silver Montazah laying hens, values with no common superscripts differ significantly, $P < 0.05$ (adapted from Nofal *et al.*, 2018)

up to deposit saturation. They observed no changes in production parameters, but suggested strains differ in their folate requirements and that a re-evaluation of the recommendations is important for highly productive birds.

Other authors found similar results confirming that hens can convert high doses of FA added to the feed into natural folates in their eggs (Bunchasak and Kachana, 2009; Hoey *et al.*, 2009; Krishnan-Rajalekshmy, 2010). Dickson *et al.* (2010) determined that it is possible to enhance the folate content as 5-methyltetrahydrofolate of egg yolks two- to three-fold by feeding hens FA at 4 mg/kg feed. These researchers also observed that sensitivity and responsiveness to increasing dietary FA concentration in egg folate content were similar for Hy-Line W36, W98, and CV20 hens throughout the production cycle. Tactacan *et al.* (2012) found that the egg and plasma folate concentrations of birds fed 10 or 100 mg/kg FA supplemented diets significantly increased compared with those fed the control diet. Sun *et al.* (2021) observed that total folate in yolks could range from 147 to 760 μg/100 g when hens' diet was supplemented from 0 to 10 mg/kg feed. These authors identified 4 folate vitamers in egg yolks: 5-methyltetrahydrofolate accounted for 91–98% of total folates, whereas FA, 5-formyltetrahydrofolate, and 10-formylfolic acid together accounted for 2–9%. Folate-enriched eggs could offer consumers a practical means of increasing folate intake and potentially protecting against disease without the safety concerns relating to folic acid–fortified foods (Ward, 2017).

Since FA is essential, dietary supplementation would probably bring similar benefits to breeding hens and layers. It would appear prudent to increase dietary recommendations to 2–3 times the minimum established requirements. Liu and Feng (1992) suggested reviewing the minimum requirements established by the NRC in 1984 (0.25 mg/kg) since they observed that levels of 1.5 ppm FA increased productive yield in old hens.

Vitamin C

Details about current vitamin C recommendations for layers, provided by institutional sources and genetic companies, can be found in Tables 7.1 to 7.3.

Vitamin C is involved in different metabolic reactions, which means it has important repercussions on the well-being and production of animals. It is engaged in calcitriol biosynthesis, regulating calcium homeostasis in the body, collagen, and aldosterone. Aldosterone regulates and maintains the electrolytic balance of tissues. It has a preventive rather than reparative function.

Modern layer lines and intensive production lead to an increased demand for vitamin C, especially if there are other stressful situations. Various results support higher levels in the birds' diets, particularly in specific handling and environmental conditions, which may cause stressful situations.

Studies examining the influence of supplementation with vitamin C on production parameters have given conflicting results. Some authors (Bell and Marion, 1990; Cheng *et al.*, 1990; Peebles *et al.*, 1992) did not observe differences in egg production with feed supplementation levels from 0 to 400 mg/kg vitamin C, nor even with levels of 1,000 mg/kg in feed or water (Keshavarz, 1996; Puthpongsiriporn *et al.*, 2001).

However, other studies did find an improvement in production after supplementation with vitamin C. In a survey carried out by Zapata and Gernat (1995), an increase in production of approximately 5% was observed on supplying 250 or 500 mg/kg vitamin C in feed compared to the unsupplemented control group. Where there was heat stress, the increase in egg production in supplemented hens was 20% higher than the unsupplemented hens, and this result appeared more quickly the greater the dosage. This is corroborated by other studies (Sahota and Gillani, 1995; Sushil *et al.*, 1998a,b; Seven, 2008) and in a review carried out by Kolb and Seehawer (2001). The authors concluded that supplementing 100–300 mg/kg vitamin C at high ambient temperatures improved production. Njoku and Nwazota (1989) found that adding ascorbic acid at elevated temperatures improved egg production and the feed conversion index, and 400 mg/kg proved the most effective supplementation.

Keshavarz (1996) observed no effect on shell quality or bone calcium content when supplementing with 0, 250, 500, or 1,000 ppm vitamin C hens exposed to temperatures within the thermoneutral range.

In 2021, Reyes *et al.* found that dietary supplementation of vitamin C improves the productive performance of laying hens raised under normal temperature conditions with little effect on egg quality and tibia characteristics. The quadratic improvements in production (Figures 7.16 and 7.17) suggest that dietary supplementation of 250 mg/kg vitamin C is recommended for laying hens raised under normal temperature conditions.

A positive effect has been observed of supplementing hens subjected to low temperatures (6°C). The addition of 250 mg/kg vitamin C and 250 mg/kg vitamin E, particularly as a combination, improved the performance of cold-stressed laying hens, offering a potential protective management practice in preventing cold stress-related losses in performance of laying hens. The present study's results also indicated that vitamin C and E's effects are additive (Kucuk *et al.*, 2003b).

Sahin and Sahin (2002) showed that a combined supplementation with chromium (400 μg/kg) and vitamin C (250 mg/kg) might be a strategy for improving production in laying hens subjected to low temperatures (6.2°C). They demonstrated better mineral retention and reduced the excretion of nitrogen, calcium, zinc, iron, and chromium.

Some studies indicate that vitamin C prevents increases in body temperature, and it is suggested that, in heat stressed birds, it might increase heat loss in animals and their capacity to tolerating high temperatures. Several studies (Pardue *et al.*, 1984, 1985; Abd-Ellah, 1995; Andrews *et al.*, 1987; Cheng *et al.*, 1988; Bell and Marion, 1990; Cheng *et al.*, 1990; Dzhambulatov *et al.*, 1996; Torki *et al.*, 2013) have confirmed that supplementing ascorbic acid during periods of heat stress, during molt or in old birds results in a significant reduction in mortality.

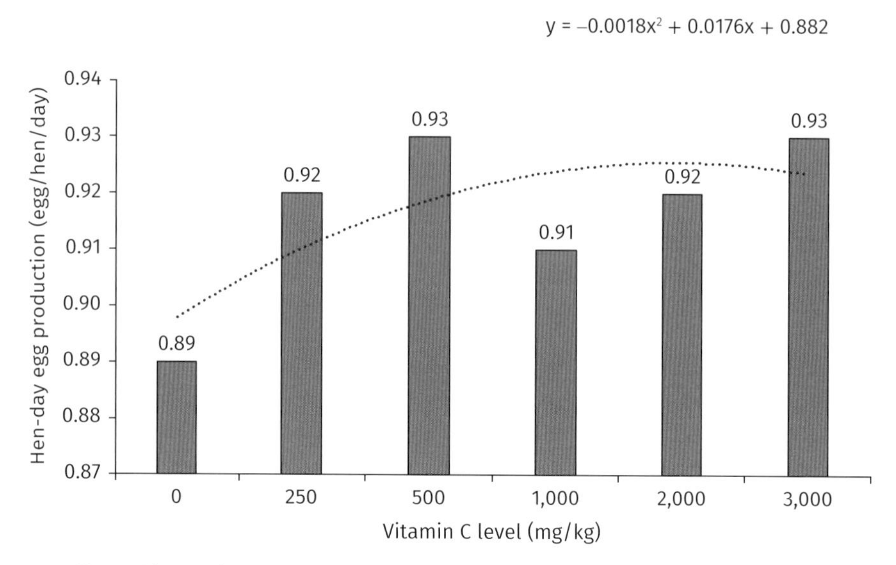

Figure 7.16 Effects of increasing supplementation of vitamin C in diets on egg production of laying hens from 46 to 51 weeks of age (adapted from Reyes et al. 2021)

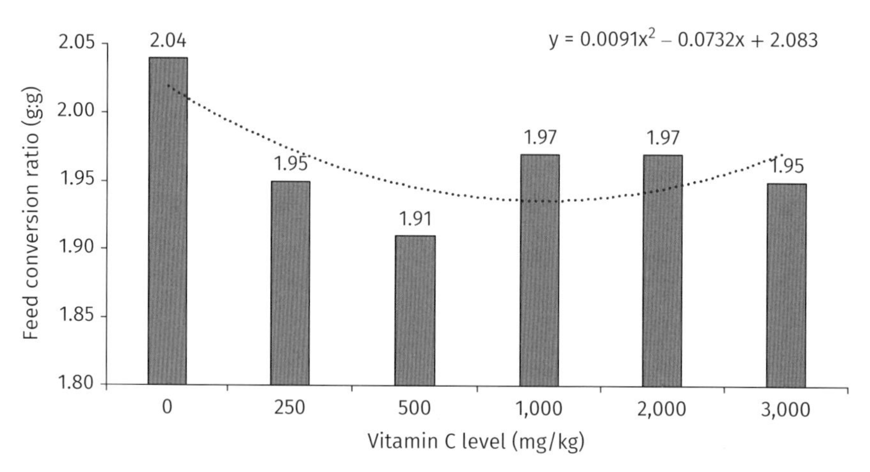

Figure 7.17 Effects of increasing supplementation of vitamin C in diets on feed conversion ratio of laying hens from 46 to 51 weeks of age (adapted from Reyes et al. 2021)

In an evaluation of the effects of betaine (1,000 mg/kg), vitamin C (200 mg/kg ascorbic acid), and vitamin E (150 mg/kg α-tocopherol acetate) and their possible combinations in feed for laying hens under chronic heat stress, Attia *et al.* (2016) observed that vitamin C had the best results in production. Egg production of vitamin C and betaine-supplemented hens was the highest among heat-stressed birds, and feed conversion was similar to the non-heat-stressed group.

Abd-Ellah (1995) studied layers during summer months and observed that hens receiving feed supplemented with 250 or 500 mg/kg laid eggs significantly heavier than those receiving unsupplemented feed or feed supplemented at a level below 125 ppm.

For bone growth, supplementation with ascorbic acid (250–300 mg/kg) during the development of layer pullets did not affect the formation and structure of the bones at 15 weeks of age (Fleming *et al.*, 1998) nor alter the volume of the medullary or trabecular bone at the end of laying (Rennie *et al.*, (1997). But ascorbic acid biosynthesis is reduced in layers over 40–45 weeks of age. This is reflected in the low rate of calcitriol biosynthesis, which may affect eggshell properties. Torki *et al.* (2014) evaluated the supplementation of chromium picolinate (0, 200, and 400 µg/kg) and 2 levels (0 and 250 mg/kg) of vitamin C in 66- to 74-week-old Lohmann LSL-lite hens under heat stress. Chromium or vitamin C provided separately produced eggs with higher shell mass and thickness and higher calcium and phosphorus than the control. It indicated that vitamin C could improve eggshell and mineral metabolism.

Ascorbic acid has a protective effect on macrophages during phagocytosis, improving cellular immune response. This vitamin is also necessary to regulate corticosterone production during environmental or immunological stress (Sahin and Önderci, 2002). In a review by Kolb and Seehawer (2001), supplementing 300 mg/kg vitamin C in the feed or 5,000 mg/kg vitamin C in water 5 days before and after vaccination contributed to the stimulation of antibody formation, and supplementing 500 mg/kg vitamin C in feed increased immune response capacity in cases of infection or coccidiosis. Vitamin C has an antistress effect when adding 1.000 mg/kg to water administered 24 hours before transportation.

Layers that suffered high temperatures improved their egg weight and immune response thanks to supplementation with ascorbic acid (Lin *et al.*, 2003; Asli *et al.*, 2007). A greater response has also been observed in lymphocyte proliferation due to immune challenges to combining vitamin C with 65 mg/kg vitamin E (Puthpongsiriporn *et al.*, 2001).

Combination with trace minerals also potentiates the effects of vitamin C. Skřivan *et al.* (2013) evaluated the supplementation of selenium (0.3 mg/kg) and vitamin C (200 mg/kg) in 20-week-old Isa Brown hens under thermoneutral conditions observing improved egg production and increased vitamin E in the yolk. However, the combination of vitamin C and sodium selenite decreased egg production. Mirfendereski and Jahanian (2015) investigated the combination of vitamin C (500 mg/kg) with chromium-methionine (0, 500, and 1,000 ppb) in Hy-Line W-36 hens, 26-week-old and subjected to high stocking density. They observed that vitamin C improved egg production, feed conversion and reduced corticosterone. The combination with chromium improved more the immunological responses post-vaccination.

Rajabi and Torki (2021) investigated the effects of dietary supplemental vitamin C (240 mg/kg), and zinc sulfate (40 mg/kg) on performance, egg quality, and blood parameters of Lohmann LSL lite hens (65-week-old) reared under cold stress (13–15°C). This combination improved egg weight, mass, and FCR, while vitamin C improved Haugh units and shell thickness.

Concerning egg weight, studies carried out by Balnave *et al.* (1991), Cheng *et al.* (1990), Keshavarz (1996), Khalafalla and Bessei (1997), and Puthpongsiriporn *et al.* (2001) revealed no significant differences as a result of supplementing with ascorbic acid. On the other hand, Bell and Marion (1990) reported that supplementing with 400 mg/kg feed slightly increased egg weight compared to the eggs of the unsupplemented hens.

Orban *et al.* (1993) devised a study examining 76- and 96-week-old layers that received a diet supplemented with 0, 1,000, 2,000, or 3,000 mg/kg for 4 weeks. Egg weight increased between 1 and 5% in the birds receiving 2,000 or 3,000 mg/kg vitamin C. These authors linked egg weight and density improvement with the influence of vitamin C on intestinal absorption of calcium and bone reabsorption, increasing the blood concentration of calcium, thereby improving the bone mass of the bird and shell quality. Zapata and Gernat (1995) also observed greater egg density when supplementing with ascorbic acid: they measured an improvement in shell quality when increasing with 250–500 mg/kg vitamin C in feed. This was corroborated by other studies (Kassim and Norziha, 1995; Oruwari *et al.*, 1995; Lin *et al.*, 1997; Ahmed *et al.*, 2008). This improvement appears to be linked to an increase in shell thickness.

Some studies have looked at the capacity of ascorbic acid to mitigate the effects of ingesting toxic elements, such as vanadium (Toussant and Latshaw, 1994). Balnave *et al.* (1991) carried out a study in which saline water was combined with supplementation of ascorbic acid (from 0.25 to 1 g/l) and concluded that vitamin C helps to reduce the damaging effect of saline water on shell quality and that in these situations vitamin C is better as a preventive measure than as a remedial treatment (Balnave and Zhang, 1992). Odabaşi *et al.* (2006) showed that supplementation with 100 mg/kg vitamin C effectively prevents and reverses pigment loss caused by an excess of vanadium in hens' diet laying brown eggs.

In conclusion, laying hens under stress conditions, specifically heat stress, responds positively to ascorbic acid supplementation. Concentrations of vitamin C between 250 and 500 mg/kg improve survival, feed consumption, production, and egg quality. Doses of ascorbic acid between 1 and 2 g/kg feed or liter of drinking water effectively counteract the adverse effects of consuming water with high salt concentrations on shell quality.

Choline

Details about current choline recommendations for layers, provided by institutional sources and genetic companies, can be found in Tables 7.1 to 7.3.

Although it is an essential nutrient, choline should not be classed as a vitamin since it is a structural component of fat and nervous tissue. This is why it is required in large amounts, generally more than other vitamins. Choline is also very important in laying hens to form the phospholipid lecithin or phosphatidylcholine, the egg yolk component.

Choline is widely distributed among feedstuffs of both vegetable and animal origin and is often found in combined form as a component of phospholipids. Soybean meal, fish meal, egg yolk, offal, vegetables, milk products, and wholegrain cereals are all rich sources of choline. Levels shown in the NRC (1994) tables of the natural content of choline in raw foods must be used with caution as the bioavailability varies widely, giving rise to over-estimation of choline levels contained in the feedstuffs (Workel *et al.*, 1998).

The NRC (1994) indicates a minimum requirement for layers of 1,050 mg/kg choline. Its commercial form is choline chloride. Birds can synthesize choline in the liver from methionine, an amino acid. The ability of layers to synthesize choline is insufficient to meet requirements in intensive production conditions, even in diets with adequate levels of methionine. Both choline and methionine may become limiting in diets with poor protein and marginal levels of sulfur amino acids.

Studies have been carried out to look at the effect of choline in the diet of layers. The results have varied widely. In most cases, the purpose was to observe the response to supplementing diets with different levels of protein or sulfur amino acids to determine the influence of choline levels on egg production.

Pourreza and Smith (1988) suggested that choline supplementation is more or less efficient depending on the dietary methionine content. That is to say, diets with low levels of sulfur amino acids increase the requirements for choline (Workel *et al.*, 1998).

Parsons and Leeper (1984) evaluated the addition of choline and methionine to layer feed containing differing levels of raw protein. They concluded that with crude protein levels of 13–15%, hens respond to supplementation of both nutrients, increasing egg production, feed conversion efficiency, and egg weight, with a greater response to supplementation with methionine than with choline. However, with diets containing a crude protein level of 16%, the response to supplementation is not significant.

Likewise, Harms *et al.* (1990b) and Miles *et al.* (1986) observed that response to supplementation with respective levels of 660 or 440 mg/kg choline was evident only when there was a sulfur amino acid deficiency. In these studies, the egg's weight correlated more to the methionine than the choline level in the ration.

Tsiagbe *et al.* (1982) found that layers fed a diet based on maize-soy and meat meal had to be supplemented with choline to maximize production and egg weight. In the absence of supplementary methionine, choline requirements appear to be greater than 1,000 but not more than 1,500 mg/kg. Sljivovacki *et al.* (1988) tried different combinations of choline and methionine. When they combined 1,100 mg/kg choline and 200 mg/kg methionine, egg production and feed intake increased, whereas no changes were observed in feed conversion.

Schexnailder and Griffith (1973) found improvements in egg production and weight by supplementing 5 μg vitamin B_{12} and 850 mg choline to a diet containing a low or adequate protein level and proper methionine. Furthermore, this increase in production by supplementing choline was in addition to the increase obtained by giving vitamin B_{12} and methionine, indicating that choline cannot be substituted. These authors also observed greater feed intake in layers supplemented with choline, attributing this to increased production.

Vogt and Harnisch (1991) observed no benefits when supplementing choline levels between 386 and 1,222 mg/kg. These authors concluded that choline content in the basal diet (325–386 mg/kg) is sufficient to meet requirements.

Nesheim *et al.* (1971) found no response in production parameters when supplementing practical layer diets with choline. Only when the diet had been purified to contain very low levels of choline did they improve production, gain in body weight, and reduce liver fat content following supplementation. Furthermore, the same author stated that, based on the choline content of the egg, layers appear to be capable of synthesizing a considerable quantity of choline for egg production when they are fed diets free of choline.

Couch and Grossie (1970), in a study aimed at establishing whether the addition of choline, with or without inositol, could influence production parameters, observed that supplementing the basal diet with 660 and 1,320 mg/kg choline chloride did not affect egg production but did improve egg weight and feed conversion efficiency.

Ruiz *et al.* (1983) concluded that layers of 50 weeks of age require very little choline supplementation when fed a maize-soy diet with adequate methionine levels. Another important parameter when evaluating the addition of choline to the diet of layers is its effect on reducing excess fat deposited in the liver. This is due to the role of choline in fat metabolism, both in the utilization and transport of fat, thereby preventing the abnormal accumulation of fat in the liver. Fatty infiltration of the liver is cited as a clinical sign of choline deficiency, caused by the inability of hepatocytes to export triglycerides and phospholipids, secondary to limited plasma lipoprotein biosynthesis. The phosphatidylcholine is an integral part of these lipoproteins' structure and the microsomal membranes that join them (Mookerjea, 1969). Phosphatidylcholine may be synthesized from pre-existing choline molecules via cytidine diphosphocholine (CDP) (Zeisel, 1981) or via transmethylase, allowing *de novo* synthesis of choline (Blusztajn *et al.*, 1979). March (1981) confirmed a significant reduction in the fat content of the liver when supplementing with 1,000 mg/kg choline. However, March did not guarantee that this was directly linked with the prevention of fatty liver since he did not indicate how much fat in the liver was considered pathological. He did not see differences in the mortality rate between supplemented and unsupplemented hens, nor did he observe changes in production parameters.

The reduction in the fat content of the liver has been confirmed by various authors, such as Mendonca *et al.* (1989), who conducted a study with laying hens of 63–64 days of age, giving them supplements with choline at 500, 1,000, 1,500 or 2,000 mg/kg. After 4 periods of 28 days, it was observed that with supplements of 1,500 and 2,000 mg/kg choline, fat deposition in the liver was reduced significantly. There was a negative correlation between the level of choline in the diet and the total blood concentration of lipids. Similar results were obtained by Schexnailder and Griffith (1973). They also confirmed that choline supplementation might be particularly interesting in heat-stress conditions since fat deposition in the liver increased significantly at higher temperatures.

A study by Armanious *et al.* (1973) touches on the usefulness of choline to combat tannic acid toxicity arising from using sorghum grain, which has a high tannin content, in the diets of laying hens. By adding choline, the authors observed a reduction in tannic acid's toxic effects, such as a reduction in body weight, egg weight, egg production, feed intake, and pimpling of the yolk. This beneficial effect of choline and methionine confirms the hypothesis that tannic acid and tannins increase the requirements for methyl group donors.

Since choline is generally not expensive, it is recommended to be added routinely to the vitamin-mineral premix to ensure that methionine is available for protein synthesis. When formulating metabolic requirements of methyl groups in terms of minimum cost, it is better to meet them by supplementation with choline (118 mg/hen/day) than methionine (Workel *et al.*, 1998).

Zhai *et al.* (2013) evaluated the long-term effects of choline on productive performance and egg quality of Hy-Line Brown-egg caged laying hens from 19 weeks to 68 weeks. Six choline levels were evaluated (0, 425, 850, 1,700, 3,400, and 6,800 mg/kg) in corn-soybean meal diets. Albumen height and Haugh units increased linearly as choline increased from 59 to 68 weeks of age. Diets supplemented with choline at 425 or 850 mg/kg improved yolk color from 19 to 58 weeks.

Tsiagbe *et al.* (1988) studied the effect of supplementing with choline and methionine on the composition of phospholipids in the yolk. They used a basal diet containing 976 mg/kg betaine (equimolar to 1,000 mg/kg choline) and 250 mg/kg methionine, supplemented with 500 or 1,000 mg/kg choline, methionine, or both combined. The content of phospholipids and phosphatidylcholine in the yolk increased significantly when supplementing with choline, while the phosphatidylethanolamine content diminished during the peak of production (at 36 weeks of age). Furthermore, they observed greater egg and yolk weight when the hen had been supplemented with 1,000 mg/kg choline than with the control birds. The results demonstrated that the increase in egg weight seen when supplementing the ration with choline might be linked to changes in the yolk composition of phospholipids. However, Vogt and Harnisch (1991) observed no increase in yolk phosphatidylcholine content when supplementing the diet with choline. Krishnan-Rajalekshmy (2010) supplemented choline (0, 500, and 1,000 mg/kg) and FA (0, 2, and 4 mg/kg), and vitamin B_{12} (0.01 and 0.02 mg/kg) in 2 factorial experiments. All 3 vitamins help increase phosphatidylcholine content by 20 to 25% compared to no supplementation.

Phosphatidylcholine or lecithin constitutes the majority of phospholipids in the egg yolk. A 60 g egg contains 1.9 g of phospholipids, of which 73% is phosphatidylcholine. Egg consumers can benefit from higher yolk phosphatidylcholine because it inhibits intestinal cholesterol absorption, improves memory, and reduces risks of neural defects, cardiovascular disease, and breast cancer.

Recently, Dong *et al.* (2019) evaluated 6 different dosages of choline in a corn-soybean meal diet in layers (0, 425, 850, 1,700, 3,400, and 6,800 mg/kg). Choline supplementation positively impacted the different parameters at dosage depending on the endpoint. The differences

($P < 0.001$) were caused by choline treatments in yolk phosphatidylcholine (at 850 mg/kg or more choline), serum VLDL, and liver triglyceride (at 1,700 and 3,400 mg/kg choline), at weeks 58 and 68 of age, and yolk total lipids were elevated ($P < 0.05$) by supplemental choline at 3,400 mg/kg whereas liver total lipids were reduced ($P < 0.05$) by 1,700 and 3,400 mg/kg choline addition. Hens fed diets supplemented choline had higher ($P = 0.005$) liver GSH-Px activity (with 3,400 mg/kg choline) and greater ($P = 0.014$) T-AOC (with 1,700 mg/kg choline) than those fed diets with 0 and 425 mg/kg choline additions. The authors concluded in that study that dietary choline supplementation elevated yolk total lipid and phosphatidylcholine and serum VLDL, reduced liver total lipid and triglyceride, and enhanced hepatic glutathione peroxidase (GSH-Px) activity and total antioxidant capacity (T-AOC) (Figure 7.18) in laying hens.

Janist *et al.* (2019) supplemented hen diets with choline, FA, and vitamin B_{12} to observe the impact on egg production, egg quality, and yolk phospholipids. The authors concluded that adding choline at 1,500 mg/kg diet maximizes yolk phosphatidylcholine concentration. The results indicated that supplementation with FA, vitamin B_{12}, or both did not affect yolk phosphatidylcholine or yolk phosphatidylethanolamine concentration, production performance, and egg quality. No other effects of choline were observed on production performance or egg quality.

Choline supplementation can also help increase docosahexaenoic acid (22:6 n-3 DHA) in egg yolks of hens fed diets with high-DHA content, which is becoming popular in design-egg production enriched eggs. Wang *et al.* (2017) concluded that choline chloride (1,000 mg/kg) for more than 14 days enhanced egg yolk omega-3 PUFA, particularly DHA, when 28-week-old Hy-Line W-36 hens were fed diets with 2% *shizochytrium* powder.

Yonke and Cherian (2019) evaluated the addition of 1,000 and 2,000 mg/kg choline chloride into corn-soybean meal diets with 1% microalgae product (DHA Gold S17-B, DSM Nutritional Products) in 24-week-old white leghorn hens for 16 weeks. The product provided 0.93 to 1.05% DHA (22:6 omega-3), doubled the total omega-3 from 1.01 to 1.97–2.03%, and changed the omega-6: omega-3 ratio from 27.29 to 13.43–15.20. Higher content of PUFAs reduce the antioxidant stability of the animals and eggs, causing a risk for long-term application. Choline at

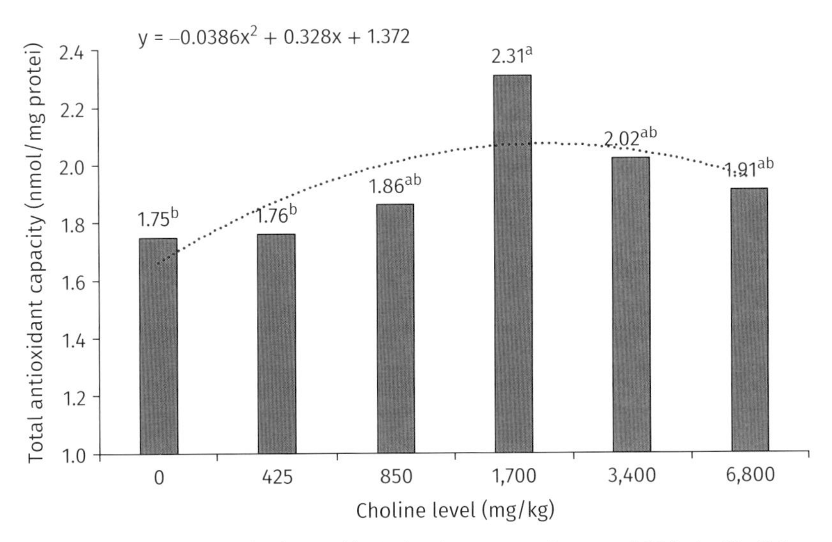

Figure 7.18 Total antioxidant capacity (T-AOC) in laying hens at weeks 58 and 68 fed with diets supplemented with different levels of choline chloride, values with no common superscripts differ significantly, $P < 0.05$ (source: Dong *et al.*, 2019)

1.000 mg/kg increased hen day egg production and Haugh unit, reduced FCR and liver lipid peroxidation caused by the algae product, and increased γ-tocopherol in eggs. Choline, at both levels, increased gamma and α-tocopherol liver content. In conclusion, choline chloride can improve egg production, feed conversion, and egg quality and protect the hen from liver oxidative stress.

More recently, Moghadam *et al.* (2021) used choline chloride (1,500 mg/kg) or methionine (50% more than the requirement) to improve the production of hens fed diets with 15% flaxseed and enhance the egg phosphatidylcholine, omega-3 PUFA and lipid stability. This flaxseed inclusion increased sixfold the omega-3 PUFA. Both supplements improved egg production and egg mass. Choline improved egg weight, egg α-tocopherol content, reduced lipid oxidation products, and maximized phosphatidylcholine. Neither choline nor methionine affected total lipid, phosphatidylethanolamine, and DHA, but both increased docosapentaenoic acid (22:5 omega-3). Choline can improve egg production, weight, and vitamin E, phosphatidylcholine, and oxidative stability of hens fed diets containing flaxseed or other ingredients with high levels of PUFA.

Commercial recommendations for choline content in layer feed are between 1,200 and 1,400 mg/kg. Supplementation with choline chloride will depend on the quantity provided in the feed ingredients and the objectives to enrich eggs. Levels between 1,200 and 1,500 mg/kg could be necessary for hens producing enriched eggs.

NUTRITIONAL COMPOSITION OF EGGS

There is a great variation in data published on egg nutrient composition (Table 7.7). These differences are partly due to the analytical methods and factors such as hen genetics, bird age, management practices, and hens' diet. The variation is especially evident in feed ingredients of a lipid nature and specifically in the dietary level of fat-soluble vitamins. It has been demonstrated that there is a direct relationship between the level of vitamins in the feed and deposition in the egg for certain vitamins.

Table 7.7 Nutritional composition of whole eggs in the US and countries of the European Union (adapted from Seuss-Baum and Nau, 2011)

Composition per 100 g of edible portion	Spain 2008[1]	USD 2009[2]	France 2008[3]	Germany 2009[4]	Italy 1997[5]	UK 2002[6]
Water (g)	76.9	75.84	75.6	74.09	77.1	75.2
Energy (kcal)	141	143	142	154	128	147
Proteins (g)	12.7	12.57	12.6	12.9	12.4	12.6
Carbohydrates (g)	0.68	0.78	0.8	0.7	–*	–
Lipids (g)	9.7	9.94	9.86	11.2	8.7	10.9
SFA (g)	2.8	3.10	2.64	3.33	3.17	3.1
MUFA (g)	3.6	3.81	3.66	4.46	2.58	4.7
PUFA (g)	1.6	1.36	1.65	1.51	1.26	1.2
Cholesterol (mg)	410	423	378	396	371	–
Vitamin A (Retinol eq.; µg)	227	140	179	278	225	190
Carotenoids (β-carotene eq.; µg)	10		–	–	–	–

Table 7.7 (continued)

Composition per 100 g of edible portion	Spain 2008[1]	USD 2009[2]	France 2008[3]	Germany 2009[4]	Italy 1997[5]	UK 2002[6]
Vitamin D (μg)	1.8	1.2	1.62	2.9	1.79	1.7
Vitamin E (α-tocopherol eq.; mg)	1.9	1.51	1.42	2	1.11	1.1
Vitamin K (μg)	8.9	0.3	–	48	–	–
Thiamine B_1 (mg)	0.11	0.07	0.08	0.1	0.09	0.1
Riboflavin B_2 (mg)	0.37	0.48	0.46	0.3	0.3	–
Vitamin B_6 (mg)	0.12	0.14	0.13	0.12	0.12	0.12
Folate Eq. (μg)	51.2	47	45	65	50	50.4
Vitamin B_{12} (μg)	2.1	1.29	1.36	2	2.5	2.5
Niacin (mg)	3.3(a)	0.07	0.08	3.10(a)	0.1	3.80
Pantothenic acid (mg)	1.8	1.44	1.58	1.6	1.77	1.8
Biotin (μg)	20	–	–	25	20	19.4
Vitamin C (mg)	0	0	0	0	0	0
Calcium (mg)	56.2	53	72.4	56	48	56
Phosphorus (mg)	216	191	181	216	210	200
Iron (mg)	2.2	1.83	1.7	2.1	1.5	1.9
Iodine (μg)	12.7	–	38.3	10	53	52.3
Zinc (mg)	2	1.11	1.01	1.35	1.2	1.4
Magnesium (mg)	12.1	12	11.1	12	13	12
Sodium (mg)	144	140	125	144	137	140
Potassium (mg)	147	134	104	147	133	130
Copper (mg)	0.014	0.10	0.06	0.14	0.06	0.1
Selenium (μg)	10	31.7	13	–	5.8	11.6
Fluoride (μg)	0.11	1.1	–	0.11	–	–

Notes: SFA: saturated fatty acids; MUFA: monounsaturated fatty acids; PUFA: polyunsaturated fatty acids. *Some databases or tables do not include all nutrients, or values are not indicated. (a) Niacin equivalents (niacin + tryptophan).

Sources: (1) Aparicio *et al.* (2008) (2) USDA (2009) (3) Composition nutritionnelle des aliments (2008) (4) BLS (2009) (5) Tabelle di composizione degli alimenti – Istituto Nazionale della Nutrizione, Edra, Milan (1997) (6) McCance and Widdowson (2002).

FORTIFICATION OF EGGS WITH VITAMINS

The use of vitamins in animal feeds has moved from being exclusively to avoid deficiency symptoms to playing an important role in improving the quality of food. Using high dosages of some vitamins fortifies eggs with these vitamins. This fortification allows diversification of the egg market and enables the production of products with added nutritional and commercial value.

In Table 7.8 we included a summary of the concentrations of vitamins in the egg or egg yolk that have been observed in some published studies. Values were standardized per gram of egg or gram of yolk, and, later, the value for either an 18 g yolk or 60 g egg was calculated to establish how many eggs would supply the daily reference requirement. It can be observed that, according to several studies, 1 to 3 enriched eggs per day could provide 100% of the human daily vitamin A, D, K, B_{12}, pantothenic, and biotin requirements. More detailed information on the topic can be found in the studies by Naber (1993), Squires and Naber (1993a,b), Leeson and Caston (2003), Leeson (2007), Sirri and Barroeta (2007), Schiavone and Barroeta (2011), and Ward (2017) examining the efficiency of vitamin transfer to the egg.

The linear relationship between vitamin D_3 supplementation (0 to 25.000 IU/kg diet) for hens with vitamin D_3 in their egg yolks is presented in Figure 7.19. The relationship between vitamin D_3 (2,500, 5,000, and 10,000 IU/kg) in conjunction with $25OHD_3$ (34.5 and 69 µg/kg feed) is shown in Figure 7.20. These are linear relationships, and $25OHD_3$ enhances the ability of vitamin D to accumulate in the egg yolk.

Vitamin E has a lower transfer rate from feed to diet (0 to 625 mg/kg), as is illustrated in Figure 7.21. Selenium sources do not seem to affect tocopherol in the yolk, but sodium selenite affects retinol in the yolk (Skřivan *et al.*, 2010). Folate transfer from feed to diet is linear from 0 to 15 mg/kg and very efficient from 0 to 5 mg/kg (Figure 7.22).

Other factors, such as hen health status, heat stress, and housing systems, may affect vitamin deposition in the egg. Ogunwole *et al.* (2020) concluded that housing systems impact thiamine, FA, and vitamin D_3 transfer to the eggs. The eggs of hens housed in open-sided deep litter had more vitamin D_3 and FA deposition than the eggs of hens housed in cages, but more thiamine was observed in the latter.

The enrichment of eggs with most vitamins and lutein, omega-3 fatty acids, and selenium does not negatively impact table eggs' physical-chemical, functional properties, and sensory qualities (e.g., appearance, texture, and flavor profile) (Yao *et al.*, 2013; Kralik *et al.*, 2018). In fact, most of the studies indicate that the oxidative stability of eggs is improved and their shelf life extended by higher supplementation (Botsoglou *et al.*, 2005). The presence of Vitamin E

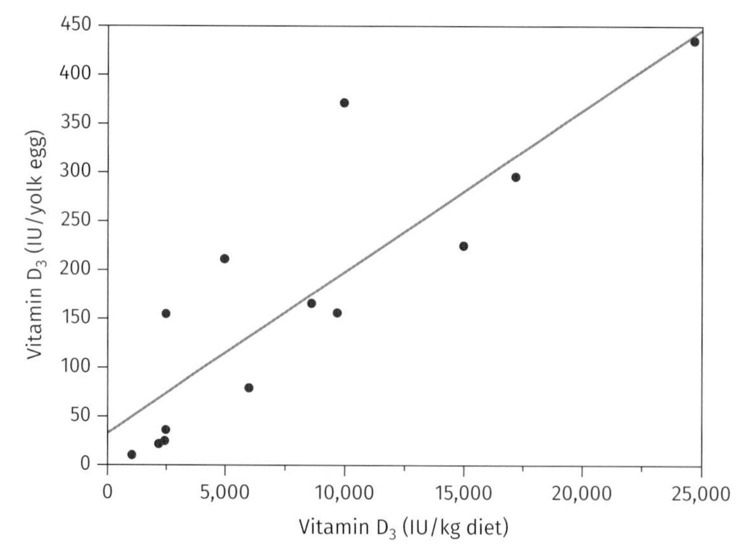

Figure 7.19 Vitamin D_3 content of eggs from hens fed various dietary levels of vitamin D_3. The line represents this linear effect: vitamin D_3 (IU/yolk egg) = 32.150184 + 0.0164989 × vitamin D_3 (IU/kg diet) (R^2 = 0.73) (adapted from Mattila *et al.*, 1999; Mattila *et al.*, 2004; Yao *et al.*, 2013; Browning and Cowieson, 2014)

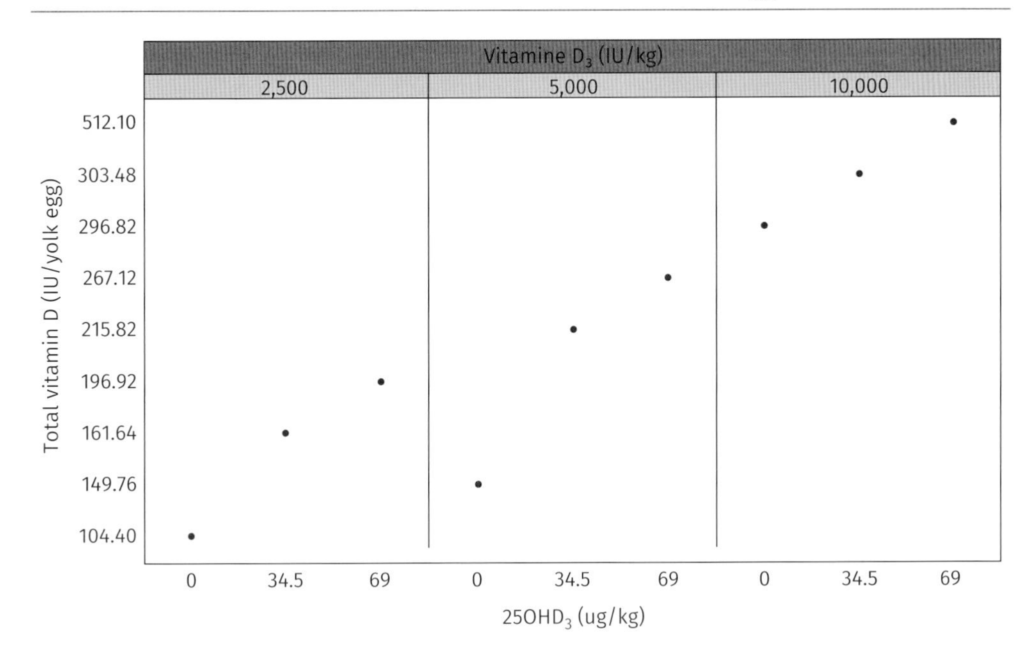

Figure 7.20 Analyzed content of vitamin D_3 and 25-hydroxycholecalciferol ($25OHD_3$) in egg yolks and their combined vitamin D activity after 9 weeks of feeding the dietary treatments to Isa brown laying hens (adapted from Browning and Cowieson, 2014)

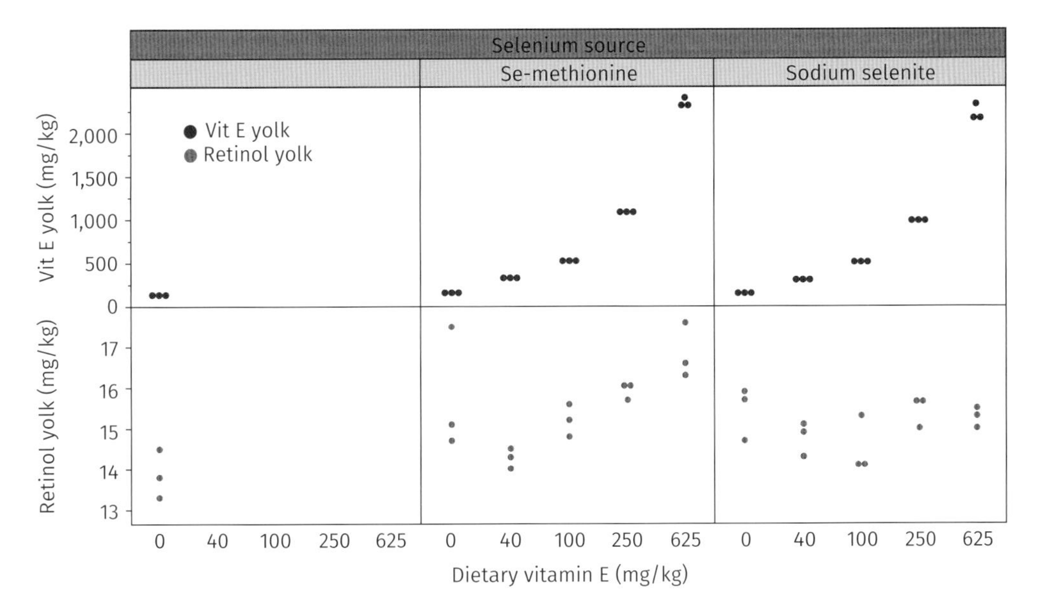

Figure 7.21 Concentration of vitamin E and retinol in egg yolk from hens fed vitamin E from 3 to 11 weeks with different sources of selenium (adapted from Skřivan *et al.*, 2010)

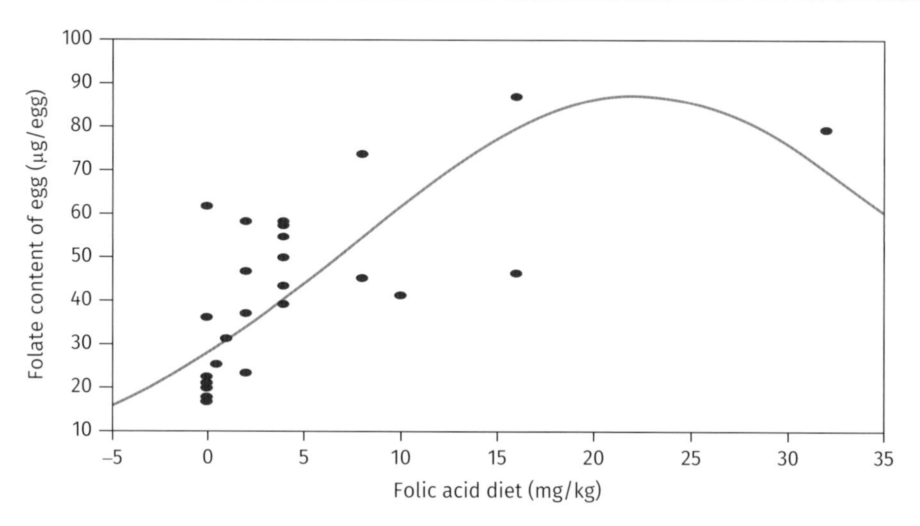

Figure 7.22 Folate content of eggs from hens fed various levels of dietary FA (adapted from House *et al.*, 2002; Bunchasak and Kachana, 2009; Hoey *et al.*, 2009; Dickson *et al.*, 2010; Hebert *et al.*, 2011)

(200 mg/kg), choline (1,000–1,500 mg/kg), and pyridoxine (40 mg/kg) can also improve the absorption of PUFAs in enriched eggs, their stability, and minimize the negative effects that feeding diets higher in PUFAs may have on the hen (Jiang *et al.*, 2013; Wang *et al.*, 2017; Khan, 2019; Yonke and Cherian, 2019; Moghadam *et al.*, 2021).

Table 7.8 Fortification of eggs with vitamins relative to the human daily reference intake

	IU or u g/g yolk		IU or mg/g egg		18 g yolk		60 g egg		Daily requirements		No. of eggs required		Reference
	Min	Max	Min	Max	Min	Max	Min	Max	Male	Female	Male	Female	
Vitamin A (IU)	10,300	24,000	–	–	185	432	–	–	900	700	3	2	Squires and Naber (1993a)
	13,300	283,700	–	–	239	5.107	–	–			1	1	Surai *et al.* (1998a)
	23,800	35,900	–	–	428	646	–	–			2	2	Mendonça *et al.* (2002)
	24,600	37,700	–	–	443	679	–	–			2	2	Mori *et al.* (2003)
	–	–	–	–	–	–	197	250			4	3	Lima and Souza (2018)
Vitamin D (µg)	0.053	0.298	–	–	0.95	5.36	–	–	15	15	3	3	Mattila *et al.* (2003)
	0.042	0.302	–	–	0.76	5.44	–	–			3	3	Mattila *et al.* (2003)
	0.050	0.312	–	–	0.90	5.62	–	–			3	3	Mattila *et al.* (2004)
	0.050	0.133	–	–	0.90	2.39	–	–			7	7	Mattila *et al.* (2004)
	0.058	0.269	–	–	1.04	4.84	–	–			4	4	Browning and Cowieson (2014)
	0.029	8,704	–	–	0.52	156.67	–	–			1	1	Yao *et al.* (2013)
	–	0.200	–	–	–	3.60	–	–			5	5	Barnkob *et al.* (2020)
Vitamin E (IU)	–	–	0.023	0.252	–	–	1,374	15,144	600	600	4	4	Galobart *et al.* (2001a)
	0.122	0.373	–	–	2.19	6.72	–	–			9	9	Scheideler *et al.* (2010)
	0.128	2,325	–	–	2.30	41.85	–	–			1.5	1.5	Skrivan *et al.* (2010)
Vitamin K (µg)	1.04	19.08	–	–	18.72	343.44	–	–	120	90	1	1	Suzuki and Okamoto (1997) (K_1)
	0.67	1.92	–	–	12.06	34.56	–	–			4	3	Suzuki and Okamoto (1997) (K_2)
	1.15	2.4	–	–	20.7	43.2	–	–			3	3	Suzuki and Okamoto (1997) (K_2)
	–	–	0.111	0.530	–	–	6.66	31.8			4	3	Park *et al.* (2005)
	–	–	0.46	0.510	–	–	27.6	30.6			4	3	O'Sullivan *et al.* (2020)
Niacin (mg)	–	–	0.010	0.012	–	–	0.047	0.077	16	14	21	18	Leeson and Caston (2003)
	–	–	0.010	0.018	–	–	0.599	1,103			15	13	Zang *et al.* (2011)

Table 7.8 (continued)

	IU or u g/g yolk		IU or mg/g egg		18 g yolk		60 g egg		Daily requirements		No. of eggs required		Reference
	Min	Max	Min	Max	Min	Max	Min	Max	Male	Female	Male	Female	
Pantothenic acid (mg)	–	–	0.013	0.020	–	–	0.80	1.20	5	5	5	5	Leeson and Caston (2003)
	–	–	0.041	0.099	–	–	2.44	5.91			1	1	Zang *et al.* (2011)
Pyridoxine (mg)	–	–	0.0005	0.0006	–	–	0.027	0.033	1.3	1.3	40	40	Leeson and Caston (2003)
Riboflavin (mg)	0.0049	0.0065	–	–	0.087	0.116	–	–	1.3	1.1	12	10	Tuite and Austic (1974)
	0.0044	0.0054	–	–	0.079	0.098	–	–			14	12	Tuite and Austic (1974)
	0.0051	0.0080	–	–	0.092	0.144	–	–			10	8	Squires and Naber (1993)
Thiamine (mg)	–	–	0.0008	0.0011	–	–	0.049	0.067	1.2	1.1	18	17	Leeson and Caston (2003)
	–	–	0.0017	0.0024	–	–	0.102	0.144			9	8	Zang *et al.* (2011)
Vitamin B_{12} (µg)	0.005	0.048	–	–	0.090	0.864	–	–	2.4	2.4	3	3	Squires and Naber (1993)
	–	–	0.015	0.057	–	–	0.9	3.4			1	1	Leeson and Caston (2003)
	–	–	0.005	0.041	–	–	0.29	2.48			1	1	Zang *et al.* (2011)
Folate (µg)	–	–	–	–	–	–	17.5	41.0	400	400	10	10	House *et al.* (2002)
	–	–	–	–	–	–	16.7	46.2			9	9	House *et al.* (2002)
	3.4	5.4	–	–	61.2	97.2	–	–			5	5	Bunchasak and Kachana (2009)
	–	–	0.6	1.3	–	–	36.0	79.1			6	6	Hoey *et al.* (2009)
	–	–	–	–	–	–	17.7	49.6			9	9	Dickson *et al.* (2010)
	–	–	–	–	–	–	20.8	57.2			7	7	Dickson *et al.* (2010)
	–	–	–	–	–	–	19.7	39.0			11	11	Hebert *et al.* (2011)
	1.5	7.6	–	–	26.5	136.8	–	–			3	3	Sun *et al.* (2021)
Biotin (µg)	–	–	–	–	–	–	17.0	18.0	30	30	2	2	Leeson and Caston (2003)
	–	–	0.525	1,115	–	–	31.5	66.9			1	1	Zang *et al.* (2011)

Bibliography

Abas, I., Kahraman, R., Eseceli, H. and Toker, N. (2008) The effect of high levels of folic acid on performance and egg quality of laying hens fed on diets with and without ascorbic acid from 28–36 weeks of age. J. Anim. Vet. Adv. 7(4):389–395. https://medwelljournals.com/abstract/?doi=javaa.2008.389.395.

Abawi, F.G., Sullivan, T.W. and Scheideler, S.E. (1985) Interaction of dietary fat with levels of vitamins A and E in broiler chicks. Poult. Sci. 64(6):1192–1198. https://doi.org/10.3382/ps.0641192.

Abawi, F.G. and Sullivan, T.W. (1989) Interactions of vitamins A, D_3, E and K in the diet of broiler chicks. Poult. Sci. 68(11):1490–1498. https://doi.org/10.3382/ps.0681490.

Abbaspour, B., Sharifi, S.D., Ghazanfari, S., Mohammadi-Sangcheshmeh, A. and Honarbakhsh, S. (2020) Effect of dietary supplementation of whole flaxseed on sperm traits and sperm fatty acid profile in aged broiler breeder roosters. Reprod. Domest. Anim. 55(5):594–603. https://doi.org/10.1111/rda.13658.

Abd El-Azeem, N.A., Abdo, M.S., Madkour, M. and El-Wardany, I. (2014) Physiological and histological responses of broiler chicks to *in ovo* injection with folic acid or l-carnitine during embryogenesis. Glob. Vet. 13(4):544–551. https://doi.org/10.5829/idosi.gv.2014.13.04.85231.

Abd El-Hack, M.E., Mahrose, K., Askar, A.A., Alagawany, M., Arif, M., Saeed, M., Abbasi, F., Soomro, R.N., Siyal, F.A. and Chaudhry, M.T. (2017) Single and combined impacts of vitamin A and selenium in diet on productive performance, egg quality, and some blood parameters of laying hens during hot season. Biol. Trace Elem. Res. 177(1):169–179. https://doi.org/10.1007/s12011-016-0862-5.

Abd El-Hack, M.E., Alagawany, M., Mahrose, K.M., Arif, M., Saeed, M., Arain, M.A., Soomro, R.N., Siyal, F.A., Fazlani, S.A. and Fowler, J. (2019) Productive performance, egg quality, hematological parameters and serum chemistry of laying hens fed diets supplemented with certain fat-soluble vitamins, individually or combined, during summer season. Anim. Nutr. 5(1):49–55. https://doi.org/10.1016/j.aninu.2018.04.008.

Abd-Ellah, A.M. (1995) Effect of ascorbic acid supplementation on performance of laying hens during hot summer months. Assiut. Vet. Med. J. 34(1):83–95. https://doi.org/10.21608/avmj.1995.184294.

Abd El-Wahab, A., Radko, D. and Kamphues, J. (2013) High dietary levels of biotin and zinc to improve health of foot pads in broilers exposed experimentally to litter with critical moisture content. Poult. Sci. 92(7):1774–1782. https://doi.org/10.3382/ps.2013-03054.

Abdel-Halim, A.A., Mohamed, F.R., El-Menawey, M.A.R. and Gharib, H.B. (2020) Impact of *in ovo* injection of folic acid and glucose on hatchability, and post-hatching performance of broiler chicken. World Vet. J. 10(4):481–491. https://doi.org/10.54203/scil.2020.wvj58.

Abdel-Mageed, M. and Shabaan, S.A.M. (2012) Effect of supplemental biotin on the performance of aged Fayoumi hens and progeny performance. Egypt. Poult. Sci. J. 32(4):895–908.

Abdukalykova, S.T. and Ruiz-Feria, C.A. (2006) Arginine and vitamin E improve the cellular and humoral immune response of broiler chickens. Int. J. Poult. Sci. 5(2):121–127. https://doi.org/10.3923/ijps.2006.121.127.

Abdukalykova, S.T., Zhao, X. and Ruiz-Feria, C.A. (2008) Arginine and vitamin E modulate the subpopulations of T lymphocytes in broiler chickens. Poult. Sci. 87(1):50–55. https://doi.org/10.3382/ps.2007-00315.

Abdulrahim, S.M., Patel, M.B. and McGinnis, J. (1979) Effects of vitamin D_3 and D_3 metabolites on production parameters and hatchability of eggs. Poult. Sci. 58(4):858–863. https://doi.org/10.3382/ps.0580858.

Abed, M.K., Razuki, W.M. and Al-Naif, H.H.N. (2018) Effects of omitting vitamin-trace mineral premixes from finisher ration on performance, carcass parameters and blood characteristics of broilers fed corn- or wheat-based diets. J. Vet. Sci. Anim. Husb. 6(2):1–7. ISSN: 2348–9790. https://doi.org/10.15744/2348-9790.6.205.

Abend, R., Jeroch, H. and Hennig, A. (1975) Studies on the influence of various vitamin B_6 uptake in the hen on the nutrient content of liver, pectoral muscle, total body and egg. Arch. Tierernahr. 25(8):565–573. https://doi.org/10.1080/17450397509423222.

Abidin, Z. and Khatoon, A. (2013) Heat stress in poultry and the beneficial effects of ascorbic acid (vitamin C) supplementation during periods of heat stress. Worlds Poult. Sci. J. 69(1):135–152. https://doi.org/10.1017/S0043933913000123.

Abrams, J.T. (1978) Nutrient deficiencies in animals: vitamin D. In Rechcigl, M. Jr. (ed.) "Handbook series in nutrition and food". CRC Press, West Palm Beach, FL.

Aburto, A. and Britton, W.M. (1998a) Effects of different levels of vitamins A and E on the utilization of cholecalciferol by broiler chickens. Poult. Sci. 77(4):570–577. https://doi.org/10.1093/ps/77.4.570.

Aburto, A. and Britton, W.M. (1998b) Effects and interactions of dietary levels of vitamins A and E and cholecalciferol in broiler chickens. Poult. Sci. 77(5):666–673. https://doi.org/10.1093/ps/77.5.666.

Aburto, A., Edwards, H.M. and Britton, W.M. (1998) The influence of vitamin A on the utilization and amelioration of toxicity of cholecalciferol, 25-hydroxycholecalciferol, and 1,25 dihydroxy cholecalciferol in young broiler chickens. Poult. Sci. 77(4):585–593. https://doi.org/10.1093/ps/77.4.585.

Adams, C.R. (1973) Effect of environmental conditions on the stability of vitamins in feeds. In "Effect of processing on the nutritional value of feeds". National Academy of Sciences, National Research Council, USA.

Adams, C.R., Eoff, H.J. and Zimmerman, C.R. (1975) Protecting feeds from vitamin E and A deficits in light weight moldy and blighted corn. Feedstuffs 47(36):24.

Adams, C.R. (1978) Vitamin product forms for animal feeds. In "Vitamin nutrition update-seminar". Hoffman-La Roche Inc. RCD, Nutley, NJ.

Adebowale, T.O., Liu, H., Oso, A.O., Oke, O.E., Hussain, T., Bamgbose, A.M., Yao, K. and Yulong, Y. (2019) Effect of dietary niacin supplementation on performance, total tract nutrient retention, carcass yield and meat lipid profile of growing turkeys. Anim. Prod. Sci. 59(6):1098–1107. https://doi.org/10.1071/AN17806.

Adewole, D.I., MacIsaac, J. and Yang, C. (2021) Effect of dietary energy density and folic acid supplementation on white striping occurrence and growth performance of broiler chickens. Can. J. Anim. Sci. 101(4):788–792. https://doi.org/10.1139/cjas-2020-0175.

Afsarmaneh, M., Pourreza, J. and Samie, A.H. (2004) Influences of citric and ascorbic acids as mineral chelators, and vitamin D_3 on efficacy of microbial phytase in broilers fed wheat-based diets. Proc. 22nd World's Poult. Congr. Istanbul, Turkey.

Afsarmaneh, M. and Pourreza, J. (2005) Effects of calcium, citric acid, ascorbic acid, vitamin D, on the efficacy of microbial phytase in broilers starters fed wheat-based diets I. Performance, bone mineralization and ileal digestibility. Int. J. Poult. Sci. 4(6):418–424. https://doi.org/10.3923/ijps.2005.418.424.

Aguilera-Quintana, I., Munn, B.J. and Krautmann, B.A. (1989) The influence of ascorbic acid on broiler preslaughter levels and heterophil/lymphocyte ratios. Poult. Sci. 68(1):166.

Ahmadian, A., Bouyeh, M. and Seidavi, A.R. (2021) A review of the effects of niacin on broiler productivity. Poult. Sci. 77(3):589–604. https://doi.org/10.1080/00439339.2021.1959275.

Ahmadu, S., Mohammed, A.A., Buhari, H. and Auwal, A. (2016) An overview of vitamin C as an antistress in poultry. Malays. J. Vet. Res. 7(2):9–22.

Ahmed, F., Jones, D.B. and Jackson, A.A. (1990) The interaction of vitamin A deficiency and rotavirus infection in the mouse. Br. J. Nutr. 63(2):363–373. https://doi.org/10.1079/BJN19900122.

Ahmed, W., Ahmad, S., Ahsan-ul-Haq, and Kamran, Z. (2008) Response of laying hens to vitamin C supplementation through drinking water under sub-tropical conditions. Avian Biol. Res. 1(2):59–63. https://doi.org/10.3184/175815508X360461.

Ahn, D.U., Wolfe, F.H. and Sim, J.S. (1995) Dietary α-linolenic acid and mixed tocopherols and packaging influences on lipid stability in broiler chicken breast and leg muscle. J. Food Sci. 60(5):1013–1018. https://doi.org/10.1111/j.1365-2621.1995.tb06282.x.

Ahn, D.U., Sell, J.L., Jeffery, M., Jo, C., Chen, X., Wu, C. and Lee, J.I. (1997) Dietary vitamin E affects lipid oxidation and total volatiles of irradiated raw turkey meat. J. Food Sci. 62(5):954–958. https://doi.org/10.1111/j.1365-2621.1997.tb15014.X.

Ahn, D.U., Sell, J.L., Jo, C., Chen, X., Wu, C. and Lee, J.I. (1998) Effects of dietary vitamin E supplementation on lipid oxidation and volatiles content of irradiated, cooked turkey meat patties with different packaging. Poult. Sci. 77(6):912–920. https://doi.org/10.1093/ps/77.6.912.

Ajafar, M., Zaghari, M., Zhandi, M. and Lotfi, L. (2018) Effect of high dietary levels of α-tocopherol acetate on immune response of light and heavy weight male broiler breeders. Comp. Clin. Pathol. 27(5):1281–1288. https://doi.org/10.1007/s00580-018-2736-z.

Ajuyah, A.O., Ahn, D.U., Hardin, R.T. and Sim, J.S. (1993) Dietary antioxidants and storage affect chemical characteristics of omega-3 fatty acid enriched broiler chicken meats. J. Food Sci. 58(1):43–46. https://doi.org/10.1111/j.1365-2621.1993.tb03206.x.

Akhmedkhanova, R.R. and Alisheikhov, A.M. (1997) Use of vitamins C and B_{12} under laying hens heat stress. 11th Eur. Symp. Poult. Nutr. Faaborg, Denmark.

Akinyemi, F. and Adewole, D. (2021) Environmental stress in chickens and the potential effectiveness of dietary vitamin supplementation. Front. Anim. Sci. 2. https://doi.org/10.3389/fanim.2021.775311.

Alcocer, H.M., Xu, X., Gravely, M.E. and Gonzalez, J.M. (2021) *In ovo* feeding of commercial broiler eggs: an accurate and reproducible method to affect muscle development and growth. J. Vis. Exp. 175(175). https://doi.org/10.3791/63006.

Alderman, J.D., Pasternak, R.C., Sacks, F.M., Smith, H.S., Monrad, E.S. and Grossman, W. (1989) Effect of a modified, well-tolerated niacin regimen on serum total cholesterol, high density lipoprotein cholesterol and the cholesterol to high density lipoprotein ratio. Am. J. Cardiol. 64(12):725–729. https://doi.org/10.1016/0002-9149(89)90754-6.

Alisheilkhov, A.M., Akhmedkhanova, R.R. and Jamboulatov, M.M. (2000) The problem of inter-reaction of vitamins C and B_{12} and fermentation preparations in broiler feeding Proc. 12th World's Poult. Congr. Istanbul, Turkey.

Aljamal, A.A., Masa'deh, M.K. and Scheideler, S.E. (2008) Vitamin E and selenium supplementation in laying hens. Poult. Sci. 87 (Suppl. 1):50.

Alkubaisy, S.A., Majid, A.A., Abdulateef, S.M., Al-Bazy, F.A., Attallah, O.K., Abdualmajeed, O.M., Mohammed, T.T., Abdulateef, F.M. and Mahmud, K.I. (2021) Effects of *in ovo* injection of biotin on chick's embryonic development and physiological traits. IOP Conf. Ser. Earth Environ. Sci. 761(1):12–11. https://doi.org/10.1088/1755-1315/761/1/012111.

Allen, P.C. (1988) Physiological basis for carotenoid malabsorption during coccidiosis. In Proc. 1988 Maryland Nutr. Conf. Feed Manuf., College Park, MD.

Allen, P.C., Danforth, H.D., Morris, V.C. and Levander, O.A. (1996) Association of lowered plasma carotenoids with protection against cecal coccidiosis by diets high in n-3 fatty acids. Poult. Sci. 75(8):966–972. https://doi.org/10.3382/ps.0750966.

Allen, P.C. (1997) Production of free radical species during *Eimeria maxima* infections in chickens. Poult. Sci. 76(6):814–821. https://doi.org/10.1093/ps/76.6.814.

Allen, P.C. and Fetterer, R.H. (2002) Interaction of dietary vitamin E with *Eimeria maxima* infections in chickens. Poult. Sci. 81(1):41–48. https://doi.org/10.1093/ps/81.1.41.

Almquist, H.J. (1978) Effect of nutrient deficiencies in animals: vitamin K. In Rechcigl Jr., M. (ed.) "CRC Handbook series in nutrition and foods, section E: nutrition disorders". CRC Press, Boca Raton, FL.

Amakye-Anim, J., Lin, T.L., Hester, P.Y., Thiagarajan, D., Watkins, B.A. and Wu, C.C. (2000) Ascorbic acid supplementation improved antibody response to infectious bursal disease vaccination in chickens. Poult. Sci. 79(5):680–688. https://doi.org/10.1093/ps/79.5.680.

Ameenudin, S., Sunde, M.L. and Cook, M.E. (1985) Essentiality of vitamin D_3 and its metabolites in poultry nutrition: a review. World's. Poult. Sci. 41(1):52–63. https://doi.org/10.1079/WPS19850005.

Amer, S.A., Mohamed, W.A.M., Gharib, H.S.A., Al-Gabri, N.A., Gouda, A., Elabbasy, M.T., Abd El-Rahman, G.I.A. and Omar, A.E. (2021) Changes in the growth, ileal digestibility, intestinal histology, behaviour, fatty acid composition of the breast muscles, and blood biochemical parameters of broiler chickens by dietary inclusion of safflower oil and vitamin C. BMC Vet. Res. 17(1):68. https://doi.org/10.1186/s12917-021-02773-5.

Amevor, F.K., Cui, Z., Du, X., Ning, Z., Shu, G., Jin, N., Deng, X., Tian, Y., Zhang, Z., Kang, X., Xu, D., You, G., Zhang, Y., Li, D., Wang, Y., Zhu, Q. and Zhao, X. (2021) Combination of quercetin and vitamin E supplementation promotes yolk precursor synthesis and follicle development in aging breeder hens via liver-blood-ovary signal axis. Animals (Basel) 11(7):1915. https://doi.org/10.3390/ani11071915.

An, B.K., Tanaka, K. and Ohtani, S. (1995) Effects of dietary vitamin B_6 levels on lipid concentration and fatty acid composition in growing chicks. Asian. Australas. J. Anim. Sci. 8(6):627–633. https://doi.org/10.5713/ajas.1995.627.

An, S.Y., Guo, Y.M., Ma, S.D., Yuan, J.M. and Liu, G.Z. (2010) Effects of different oil sources and vitamin E in breeder diet on egg quality, hatchability, and development of the neonatal offspring. Asian. Australas. J. Anim. Sci. 23(2):234–239. https://doi.org/10.5713/ajas.2010.90140.

Anderson, R. and Lukey, P.T. (1987) A biological role for ascorbate in the selective neutralization of extracellular phagocyte-derived oxidants. Ann. N. Y. Acad. Sci. 498:229–247. https://doi.org/10.1111/j.1749-6632.1987.tb23764.x.

Andi, M.A., Shivazad, M., Pourbakhsh, S.A. Afshar, M, Rokni, H., Shiri, N.E. Mohammadi, A. and Salahi, Z. (2006) Effects of vitamin E in broiler breeder diet on hatchability, egg quality and breeder and day-old chick immunity. Pak. J. Biol. Sci. 9(5):789–794. https://doi.org/10.3923/pjbs.2006.789.794.

Andreasen, C.B. and Frank, D.E. (1999) The effects of ascorbic acid on in vitro heterophil function. Avian Dis. 43(4):656–663. https://doi.org/10.2307/1592734.

Andrews, D.K., Berry, W.D. and Brake, J. (1987) Effect of lighting program and nutrition on reproductive performance of molted single comb White leghorn hens. Poult. Sci. 66(8):1298–1305. https://doi.org/10.3382/ps.0661298.

Ang, C.Y.W., Jung, H.C., Benoff, F.H. and Charles, O.W. (1984) Effect of feeding three levels of riboflavin, niacin and vitamin B_6 to male chickens on the nutrient composition of broiler breast meat. J. Food Sci. 49(2):590–592. https://doi.org/10.1111/j.1365-2621.1984.tb12475.x.

Angel, R., Dhandu, A.S., Applegate, T.J. and Christman, M. (2001a) Phosphorus sparing effect of phytase, 25-hydroxycholecalciferol, and citric acid when fed to broiler chicks. Poult. Sci. 80(1):133–134.

Angel, R., Dhandu, A.S., Applegate, T.J. and Christman, M. (2001b) Non-phytate phosphorus sparing effect of phytase and citric acid when fed to poults. Poult. Sci. 8(1):134 (abstract).

Angel, R., Saylor, W.W., Dhandu, A.S., Powers, P. and Applegate, T.J. (2005) Effects of dietary phosphorus, phytase, and 25-hydroxycholecalciferol on performance of broiler chickens growing in floor pens. Poult. Sci. 84(7):1031–1044. https://doi.org/10.1093/ps/84.7.1031.

Angel, R., Saylor, W.W., Mitchell, A.D., Powers, W. and Applegate, T.J. (2006) Effects of dietary phosphorus, phytase, and 25-hydroxycholecalciferol on broiler chicken bone mineralization, litter phosphorus, and processing yields. Poult. Sci. 85(7):1200–1211. https://doi.org/10.1093/ps/85.7.1200.

Angela, S.G., Flachowsky, G. and Schubert, R. (1999) Effects of high vitamin E dosage on the concentration of various lipid soluble substances in the organism of laying hens. 7th Symp. Jena-Thuringen. (pp. 403–406).

Anonymous (1977) Vitamin A and retinolo-binding protein in fetal growth and development of the rat. Nutr. Rev. 35(11):305–309. https://doi.org/10.1111/j.1753-4887.1977.tb06506.x.

Aparicio, A., Barroeta, A.C., López-Sobaler, A.M. and Ortega, R.M. (2008) Etiquetado nutricional. In "Guía de etiquetado del huevo". Instituto de Estudios del Huevo.

Applegate, T.J. and Sell, J.L. (1996) Effect of dietary linoleic to linolenic acid ratio and vitamin E supplementation on vitamin E status of poults. Poult. Sci. 75(7):881–890. https://doi.org/10.3382/ps.0750881.

Applegate, T.J., Angel, R. and Classen, H.L. (2003) Effect of dietary calcium, 25-hydroxycholecalciferol, or bird strain on small intestinal phytase activity in broiler chickens. Poult. Sci. 82(7):1140–1148. https://doi.org/10.1093/ps/82.7.1140.

Applegate, T.J. and Angel, R. (2014) Nutrient requirements of poultry publication: history and need for an update. J. Appl. Poult. Res. 23(3):567–575. https://doi.org/10.3382/japr.2014-00980.

Araújo, I.C.S., Café, M.B., Noleto, R.A., Martins, J.M.S., Ulhoa, C.J., Guareshi, G.C., Reis, M.M. and Leandro, N.S.M. (2019a) Effect of vitamin E *in ovo* feeding to broiler embryos on hatchability, chick quality, oxidative state, and performance. Poult. Sci. 98(9):3652–3661. https://doi.org/10.3382/ps/pey439.

Araújo, L.F., Araujo, C.S.S., Pereira, R.J.G., Bittencourt, L.C., Silva, C.C., Cisneros, F., Hermes, R.G., Sartore, Y.G.A. and Dias, M.T. (2019b) The dietary supplementation of canthaxanthin in combination with $25OHD_3$ results in reproductive, performance, and progeny quality gains in broiler breeders. Poult. Sci. 98(11):5801–5808. https://doi.org/10.3382/ps/pez377.

Arijeniwa, A., Ikhimioya, I., Bamidele, O.K. and Ogunmodede, B.K. (1996) Riboflavin requirement of breeding hens in a humid tropical environment. J. Appl. Anim. Res. 10(2):163–166. https://doi.org/10.1080/09712119.1996.9706144.

Armanious, M.W., Britton, W.M. and Fuller, H.L. (1973) Effect of methionine and choline and tannic acid and tannin toxicity in the laying hen. Poult. Sci. 52(6):2160–2168. https://doi.org/10.3382/ps.0522160.

Arscott, G.H. and Kuhns, R.V. (1969) Packed sperm volume versus optical density as a measure of semen concentration. Poult. Sci. 48(3):1126–1127. https://doi.org/10.3382/ps.0481126.

Arscott, G.H. and Parker, J.E. (1967) Effectiveness of vitamin E in reversing sterility of male chickens fed a diet high in linoleic acid. J. Nutr. 91(2):219–222. https://doi.org/10.1093/jn/91.2.219.

Aseltine, M. (1990) Practical applications of vitamin nutrition in dairy cattle. In Proc. Missouri 1990 National Feed Ingred. Assoc. Nutr. Inst. Development in Vitamin Nutrition and Health Application. Kansas City. National Feed Ingredients Association (NFIA), Des Moines, Iowa.

Asensio, X., Abdelli, N., Piedrafita, J., Soler, M.D. and Barroeta, A.C. (2020) Effect of fibrous diet and vitamin C inclusion on uniformity, carcass traits, skeletal strength, and behavior of broiler breeder pullets. Poult. Sci. 99(5):2633–2644. https://doi.org/10.1016/j.psj.2020.01.015.

Asghar, A., Lin, C.F., Gray, J.I., Buckley, D.J., Booren, A.M. and Flegal, C.J. (1990) Effects of dietary oils and α-tocopherol supplementation on membrane lipid oxidation in broiler meat. J. Food Sci. 55(1):46–50. https://doi.org/10.1111/j.1365-2621.1990.tb06013.x.

Asl, R.S., Shariatmadari, F., Sharafi, M., Karimi Torshizi, M.A. and Shahverdi, A. (2018) Dietary fish oil supplemented with vitamin E improves quality indicators of rooster cold-stored semen through reducing lipid peroxidation. Cryobiology 84:15–19. https://doi.org/10.1016/j.cryobiol.2018.08.008.

Aslam, S.M., Garlich, J.D. and Qureshi, M.A. (1998) Vitamin D deficiency alters the immune responses of broiler chicks. Poult. Sci. 77(6):842–849. https://doi.org/10.1093/ps/77.6.842.

Asli, M.M., Shariatmad, F., Hosseini, S.A. and Lotfollahi, H. (2007) Effect of probiotics, yeast, vitamin E and vitamin C supplements on performance and immune response of laying hen during high environmental temperature. Int. J. Poult. Sci. 6(12):895–900. https://doi.org/10.3923/ijps.2007.895.900.

Asmar, J.A., Daghir, N.J. and Azar, H.A. (1968) Effects of pyridoxine deficiency on the lymphatic organs and certain blood components of the neonatal chicken. J. Nutr. 95(2):153–159. https://doi.org/10.1093/jn/95.2.153.

Asson-Batres, M.A., Smith, W.B. and Clark, G. (2009) Retinoic acid is present in the postnatal rat olfactory organ and persists in vitamin A–depleted neural tissue. J. Nutr. 139(6):1067–1072. https://doi.org/10.3945/jn.108.096040.

Atef, S.H. (2018) Vitamin D assays in clinical laboratory: past, present and future challenges. J. Steroid Biochem. Mol. Biol. 175:136–137. https://doi.org/10.1016/j.jsbmb.2017.02.011.

Atencio, A., Edwards, H.M. and Pesti, G.M. (2005a) Effect of the level of cholecalciferol supplementation of broiler breeder hen diets on the performance and bone abnormalities of the progeny fed diets containing various levels of calcium or 25-hydroxycholecalciferol. Poult. Sci. 84(10):1593–1603. https://doi.org/10.1093/ps/84.10.1593.

Atencio, A., Edwards, H.M. and Pesti, G.M. (2005b) Effects of vitamin D_3 dietary supplementation of broiler breeder hens on the performance and bone abnormalities of the progeny. Poult. Sci. 84(7):1058–1068. https://doi.org/10.1093/ps/84.7.1058.

Atencio, A., Pesti, G.M. and Edwards, H.M. (2005c) Twenty-five hydroxycholecalciferol as a cholecalciferol substitute in broiler breeder hen diets and its effect on the performance and general health of the progeny. Poult. Sci. 84(8):1277–1285. https://doi.org/10.1093/ps/84.8.1277.

Atencio, A., Edwards, H.M., Pesti, G.M. and Ware, G.O. (2006) The vitamin D_3 requirement of broiler breeders. Poult. Sci. 85(4):674–692. https://doi.org/10.1093/ps/85.4.674.

Atia, F.A., Waibel, P.E., Hermes, I. and Carlson, C.W. (1994) Effect of dietary cholecalciferol and 1,25-dihydroxycholecalcif-erol on turkey poults in the absence and presence of ascorbic acid. Poult. Sci. 73(1):91.

Atkinson, R.L., Ferguson, T.M., Quisenberry, J.H. and Couch, J.R. (1955) Vitamin E and reproduction in turkeys. J. Nutr. 55(3):387–397. https://doi.org/10.1093/jn/55.3.387.

Attia, Y.A., Abd El-Hamid, A.E.E., Abedalla, A.A., Berika, M.A., Al-Harthi, M.A., Kucuk, O., Sahin, K. and Abou-Shehema, B.M. (2016) Laying performance, digestibility and plasma hormones in laying hens exposed to chronic heat stress as affected by betaine, vitamin C, and/or vitamin E supplementation. SpringerPlus 5(1):1–12. https://doi.org/10.1186/s40064-016-3304-0.

Attia, Y.A., Al-Harthi, M.A., El-Shafey, A.S., Rehab, Y.A. and Kim, W.K. (2017) Enhancing tolerance of broiler chickens to heat stress by supplementation with vitamin E, vitamin C and/or probiotics. Ann. Anim. Sci. 17(4):1155–1169. https://doi.org/10.1515/aoas-2017-0012.

Attia, Y.A., Abou-Shehema, B.M. and Abdellah, A.A. (2020a) Effect of ascorbic acid and/or alpha-tocopherol fortification on semen quality, metabolic profile, antioxidants status and DNA of roosters exposed to heat stress. J. Anim. Plant Sci. 30(2):325–335. https://doi.org/10.36899/JAPS.2020.2.0051.

Attia, Y.A., Al-Harthi, M.A. and Abo El-Maaty, H.M.A. (2020b) Calcium and cholecalciferol levels in late-phase laying hens: effects on productive traits, egg quality, blood biochemistry, and immune responses. Front. Vet. Sci. 7:389. https://doi.org/10.3389/fvets.2020.00389.

Augustine, P.C. and Ruff, M.D. (1983) Changes in carotenoid and vitamin A levels in young turkeys infected with *Eimeria meleagrimitis* or *E. adenoeides*. Avian Dis. 27(4):963–971. https://doi.org/10.2307/1590197.

Augustine, P.C., McNaughton, J.L., Virtanen, E. and Rosi, L. (1997) Effect of betaine on the growth performance of chicks inoculated with mixed cultures of avian Eimeria species and on invasion and development of *Eimeria tenella* and *Eimeria Acervulina in vitro* and *in vivo*. Poult. Sci. 76(6):802–809. https://doi.org/10.1093/ps/76.6.802.

Austic, R.E. and Scott, M.L. (2000) Nutritional diseases. In "Diseases of poultry" 10th edition Calnek, B.W. (ed.). Iowa State University Press. (pp. 48–64).

Aviagen (2020) Feeding guidelines for Nicholas and B.U.T. Heavy lines. https://www.aviagenturkeys.com/en-gb/documents.

Aviagen (2021) Parent stock nutrituin specifications. https://en.aviagen.com/brands/ross/.

Aviagen (2022) Ross broiler nutrition specifications. https://en.aviagen.com/brands/ross/.

Axelrod, A.E. (1971) Immune processes in vitamin deficiency states. Am. J. Clin. Nutr. 24(2):265–271. https://doi.org/10.1093/ajcn/24.2.265.

Aye, P.P., Morishita, T.Y., Saif, Y.M. and Jonas, M. (2000) The effect of hypovitaminosis A on the pathogenesis of *Pasteurella multocida* in turkeys. Avian Dis. 44(4):818–826.

Babior, B.M. (1984) The respiratory burst of phagocytes. J. Clin. Invest. 73(3):599–601. https://doi.org/10.1172/JCI111249.

Babu, S. and Srikantia, S.G. (1976) Availability of folates from some foods. Am. J. Clin. Nutr. 29(4):376–379. https://doi.org/10.1093/ajcn/29.4.376.

Bachmann, H., Autzen, S., Frey, U., Wehr, U., Rambeck, W., McCormack, H. and Whitehead, C.C. (2013) The efficacy of a standardized product from dried leaves of *Solanum glaucophyllum* as source of 1,25-dihydroxycholecalciferol for poultry. Br. Poult. Sci. 54(5):642–652. https://doi.org/10.1080/00071668.2013.825692.

Bäckermann, S., Poel, C. and Ternes, W. (2008) Thiamin phosphates in egg yolk granules and plasma of regular and embryonated eggs of hens and in five- and seven-day-old embryos. Poult. Sci. 87(1):108–115. https://doi.org/10.3382/ps.2007-00158.

Badwey, J.A. and Karnovsky, M.L. (1980) Active oxygen species and the functions of phagocytic leukocytes. Annu. Rev. Biochem. 49:695–726. https://doi.org/10.1146/annurev.bi.49.070180.003403.

Baghban-Kanani, P., Janmohammadi, H. and Ostadrahimi, A.R. (2019) Effect of different levels of sunflower meal and niacin on performance, biochemical parameters, antioxidant status, and egg yolk cholesterol of laying hens. Iran. J. Appl. Anim. Sci. 9(4):737–746.

Baghbanzadeh, A. and Decuypère, E. (2008) Ascites syndrome in broilers: physiological and nutritional perspectives. Avian Pathol. 37(2):117–126. https://doi.org/10.1080/03079450801902062.

Bailey, L.B. and Gregory, J.F. (2006) Folate. In "Present knowledge in nutrition" Bowman, B. and Russell, R. (ed.). International Life Sciences Institute. (pp. 278–301).

Bailey, L.B., Da-Silva, V., West, A.A. and Caudill, M.A. (2013) Folate. In "Handbook of vitamins" 5th edition Zempleni, J., Suttie, J., Gregory, J. and Stover P.J. (ed.). CRC Press, Taylor & Francis Group, LLC ISBN 9781466515567. (pp. 421–446).

Bain, M.M., Nys, Y. and Dunn, I.C. (2016) Increasing persistency in lay and stabilizing egg quality in longer laying cycles. What are the challenges? Br. Poult. Sci. 57(3):330–338. https://doi.org/10.1080/00071668.2016.1161727.

Bain, S.D., Newbrey, J.W. and Watkins, B.A. (1988) Biotin deficiency may alter tibiotarsal bone growth and modeling in broiler chicks. Poult. Sci. 67(4):590–595. https://doi.org/10.3382/ps.0670590.
Bains, B. (1997) Important role for vitamins during stress. World's. Poult. Sci. 13(2):30–35.
Bains, B. (1999) "A guide to the application of vitamins in commercial poultry feed". Rath Design Communications, Australia.
Bains, B. (2001) Impaired health reduces impact of vitamins. World's Poult. Vitam. Special:(9–11).
Bains, B.S. (1994) Broilers suffer from dyschondroplasia and femoral necrosis. World's. Poult. Sci. 10(10): 109–111.
Bains, B.S. (2001) Vitamin nutrition for hatchability and chick livability. World's Poult. Vitam. Specail:(7–8).
Bains, B., Brake, J.T. and Pardue, S.L. (1996) Reducing leg weakness in commercial broilers. World's. Poult. Sci. 14(1):24–27.
Bains, B.S., Brake, J.T. and Pardue, S.L. (1998) Reducing leg weakness in commercial broilers. World's. Poult. Sci. 14(1):24–27.
Baker, D.H., Allen, N.K. and Kleiss, A.J. (1973) Efficiency of tryptophan as a niacin precursor in young chicks. J. Anim. Sci. 36(2):299–302. https://doi.org/10.2527/jas1973.362299x.
Baker, D.H., Biehl, R.R. and Emmert, J.L. (1998) Vitamin D_3 requirement of young chicks receiving diets varying in calcium and available phosphorus. Br. Poult. Sci. 39(3):413–417. https://doi.org/10.1080/00071669888980.
Baker, S.S. and Cohen, H.J. (1983) Altered oxidative metabolism in selenium-deficient rat granulocytes. J. Immunol. 130(6):2856–2860. PMID:6304192.
Balaghi, M. and Wagner, C. (1992) Methyl group metabolism in the pancreas of folate-deficient rats. J. Nutr. 122(7):1391–1396. https://doi.org/10.1093/jn/122.7.1391.
Balaghi, M., Horne, D.W., Woodward, S.C. and Wagner, C. (1993) Pancreatic one-carbon metabolism in early folate deficiency in rats. Am. J. Clin. Nutr. 58(2):198–203. https://doi.org/10.1093/ajcn/58.2.198.
Baldi, G., Soglia, F. and Petracci, M. (2021) Spaghetti meat abnormality in broilers: current understanding and future research directions. Front. Physiol. 12:684497. https://doi.org/10.3389/fphys.2021.684497.
Balios, J. and Poupulis, C. (1992) Effect of biotin on the fatty acid composition of abdominal fat, liver fat and blood serum fat of broilers fed high fat diets Proc. 19th World's Pult. Congr., Amsterdam, The Netherlands.
Ballard, R. and Edwards, H.M. (1988) Effects of Dietary zeolite and vitamin A on tibial dyschondroplasia in chickens. Poult. Sci. 67(1):113–119. https://doi.org/10.3382/ps.0670113.
Balloun, S.L. and Phillips, R.E. (1957) Interaction effects of vitamin B_{12} and pantothenic acid in breeder hen diets on hatchability, chick growth and livability. Poult. Sci. 36(5):929–934. https://doi.org/10.3382/ps.0360929.
Balnave, D. (2004) Challenges of accurately defining the nutrient requirements of heat- stressed poultry. Poult. Sci. 83(1):5–14. https://doi.org/10.1093/ps/83.1.5.
Balnave, D. and Brake, J. (2005) Nutrition and management of heat-stressed pullets and laying hens. Worlds Poult. Sci. J. 61(3):399–406. https://doi.org/10.1079/WPS200565.
Balnave, D. and Zhang, D. (1992) Responses in eggshell quality from dietary ascorbic acid supplementation of hens receiving saline drinking water. Aust. J. Agric. Res. 43(6):1259–1264. https://doi.org/10.1071/AR9921259.
Balnave, D., Berry, M.N. and Cumming, R.B. (1977) Clinical signs of fatty liver and kidney syndrome in broilers and their alleviation by the short-term use of biotin or animal tallow. Br. Poult. Sci. 18(6):749–753. https://doi.org/10.1080/00071667708416430.
Balnave, D., Zhang, D. and Moreng, R.E. (1991) Use of ascorbic acid to prevent the decline in eggshell quality observed with saline drinking water. Poult. Sci. 70(4):848–852. https://doi.org/10.3382/ps.0700848.
Bar, A., Sharvit, M., Noff, D., Edelstein, S. and Hurwitz, S. (1980) Absorption and excretion of cholecalciferol and of 25-hydroxycholecalciferol and metabolites in birds. J. Nutr. 110(10):1930–1934. https://doi.org/10.1093/jn/110.10.1930.
Bar, A., Rosenberg, J., Perlman, R. and Hurwitz, S. (1987) Field rickets in turkeys: relationship to vitamin D. Poult. Sci. 66(1):68–72. https://doi.org/10.3382/ps.0660068.
Bar, A., Vax, E. and Striem, S. (1999) Relationships among age, eggshell thickness and vitamin D metabolism and its expression in the laying hen. Comp. Biochem. Physiol. A Mol. Integr. Physiol. 123(2):147–154. https://doi.org/10.1016/S1095-6433(99)00039-2.

Bar, A., Razaphkovsky, V., Vax, E. and Plavnik, I. (2003) Performance and bone development in broiler chickens given 25-hydroxycholecalciferol. Br. Poult. Sci. 44(2):224–233. https://doi.org/10.1080/0007166031000087029.

Barash, P.G. (1978) Nutrient toxicities of vitamin K. In "CRC handbook series in nutrition and food" Rechcigl, M. Jr. (ed.). CRC Press.

Barnkob, L.L., Argyraki, A. and Jakobsen, J. (2020) Naturally enhanced eggs as a source of vitamin D: a review. Trends Food Sci. Technol. 102:62–70. https://doi.org/10.1016/j.tifs.2020.05.018.

Barroeta, A.C. and King, A.J. (1991) Effects of carotenoids on lipid oxidation in stored poultry muscle. Poult. Sci. 70 (suppl. 1).

Barroeta, A.C. (2007) Nutritive value of poultry meat: relationship between vitamin E and PUFA. Poult. Sci. 63(2):277–284. https://doi.org/10.1017/S0043933907001468.

Barth, C.A., Frigg, M. and Hagemeister, H. (1986) Biotin absorption from the hindgut of the pig. J. Anim. Physiol. Anim. Nutr. 55(1–5):128–134. https://doi.org/10.1111/j.1439-0396.1986.tb00711.x.

Bartov, I. (1997) Moderate excess of dietary vitamin E does not exacerbate cholecalciferol deficiency in young broiler chicks. Br. Poult. Sci. 38(4):442–444. https://doi.org/10.1080/00071669708418018.

Bartov, I. and Frigg, M. (1992) Effect of high concentrations of dietary vitamin E during various age periods on performance, plasma vitamin E and meat stability of broiler chicks at 7 weeks of age. Br. Poult. Sci. 33(2):393–402. https://doi.org/10.1080/00071669208417477.

Bartov, I. and Kanner, J. (1996) Effect of high levels of dietary iron, iron injection, and dietary vitamin E on the oxidative stability of turkey meat during storage. Poult. Sci. 75(8):1039–1046. https://doi.org/10.3382/ps.0751039.

Bartov, I., Weisman, Y. and Wax, E. (1991) Effects of high concentrations of dietary vitamin E and ethoxyquin on the performance of laying hens. Br. Poult. Sci. 32(3):525–534. https://doi.org/10.1080/00071669108417377.

Bartov, I., Sklan, D. and Friedman, A. (1997) Effect of vitamin A on the oxidative stability of broiler meat during storage: lack of interactions with vitamin E. Br. Poult. Sci. 38(3):255–257. https://doi.org/10.1080/00071669708417982.

Basmacioğlu, H., Toku ğlu, Ö. and Ergül, M. (2004) Effect of dietary natural antioxidants on lipid oxidation in stored broiler meat enriched with N-3 PUFAs. Proc. 12th World's Poultr. Congr., Istanbul, Turkey.

Bates, C.J. (2006) Thiamine. In "Present knowledge in nutrition" 9th edition Bowman, B.A. and Russell, R.M. (ed.). International Life Sciences Institute. (pp. 242–249).

Batifoulier, F., Mercier, Y., Gatellier, P. and Renerre, M. (2002) Influence of vitamin E on lipid and protein oxidation induced by H_2O_2-activated MetMb in microsomal membranes from turkey muscle. Meat Sci. 61(4):389–395. https://doi.org/10.1016/S0309-1740(01)00209-1.

Bauernfeind, J.C. (1974) Pyridoxine-A use appraisal in animal feeds. Feedstuffs 46(45):30.

Baugh, C.M. and Krumdieck, C.L. (1971) Naturally occurring folates. Ann. N. Y. Acad. Sci. 186:7–28. PMID:4943577.

Bayyari, G.R., Huff, W.E., Rath, N.C., Balog, J.M., Newberry, L.A., Villines, J.D., Skeeles, J.K., Anthony, N.B. and Nestor, K.E. (1997) Effect of the genetic selection of turkeys for increased body weight and egg production on immune and physiological responses. Poult. Sci. 76(2):289–296. https://doi.org/10.1093/ps/76.2.289.

Bealish, A., Assaf, I., Mousa, S., Hamed, S., Soliman, M., Bahakaim, A. and Elden, A.A. (2019) Effect of dietary supplementation and injecting hatching eggs with pyridoxine on some hatchability and incubation characters and some physiological traits of chicks. J. Product. Dev. 24(1):135–151. https://doi.org/10.21608/jpd.2019.41326.

Bearse, G.E., McClary, C.F. and Saxena, H.C. (1960) Blood spots and vitamin A. Poult. Sci. 39(4):860–865. https://doi.org/10.3382/ps.0390860.

Bechtel, H.E. (1964) Folic acid in poultry and animal nutrition. Feedstuffs. Minneap. 36(14):18–20.

Becker, E.M., Christensen, J., Frederiksen, C.S. and Haugaard, V.K. (2003) Front-face fluorescence spectroscopy and chemometrics in analysis of yogurt: rapid analysis of riboflavin. J. Dairy Sci. 86(8):2508–2515. https://doi.org/10.3168/jds.S0022-0302(03)73845-4.

Beer, A.E., Scott, M.L. and Nesheim, M.C. (1963) The effects of graded levels of pantothenic acid on the breeding performance of white leghorn pullets. Br. Poult. Sci. 4(3):243–253. https://doi.org/10.1080/00071666308415501.

Beheshti Moghadam, M.H., Aziza, A.E. and Cherian, G. (2021) Choline and methionine supplementation in layer hens fed flaxseed: effects on hen production performance, egg fatty acid composition, tocopherol content, and oxidative stability. Poult. Sci. 100(9):101299. https://doi.org/10.1016/j.psj.2021.101299.

Beirne, M.J. and Jensen, L.S. (1981) Influence of high levels of pyridoxine on twisted legs in broilers. Poult. Sci. 60(5):1026–1029. https://doi.org/10.3382/ps.0601026.

Bell, D.E. and Marion, J.E. (1990) Vitamin C in laying hen diets. Poult. Sci. 69(11):1900–1904. https://doi.org/10.3382/ps.0691900.

Bello, A., Nascimento, M., Pelici, N., Womack, S.K., Zhai, W., Gerard, P.D. and Peebles, E.D. (2015) Effects of the *in ovo* injection of 25-hydroxycholecalciferol on the yolk and serum characteristics of male and female broiler embryos. Poult. Sci. 94(4):734–739. https://doi.org/10.3382/ps/pev017.

Bender, D.A. (1992) "Nutritional biochemistry of the vitamins". Cambridge University Press. https://doi.org/10.1017/CBO9780511615191.

Bendich, A. (1987) Role of antioxidant vitamins on immune function. In Proc. Roche Technical Symp.: "The and immune response." RCD 7442. Hoffmann–La Roche Inc.

Bermudez, A.J., Swayne, D.E., Squires, M.W. and Radin, M.J. (1993) Effects of vitamin A deficiency on the reproductive system of mature white leghorn hens. Avian Dis. 37(2):274–283. https://doi.org/10.2307/1591649.

Bernadette, P.M., Diane, F.B., Virginia, A.S. and Allison, A.Y. (2020) "Present knowledge in nutrition: basic nutrition and metabolism" 11th edition. Academic Press, New York. https://doi.org/10.1016/C2018-0-02422-6.

Berri, C., Praud, C., Raud, E., Godet, M. and Duclos, M.J. (2013) Effect of dietary 25-hydroxycholecalciferol on muscle tissue and primary cell culture properties in broiler chicken. WPSA Egg Meat Symposia, Bergamo. Worlds Poult. Sci. J. 69(1).

Bettendorff, L. (2013) Vitamin B_1. In "Handbook of vitamins" 5th edition Zempleni, J., Suttie, J., Gregory, J. and Stover P.J. (ed.). CRC Press, Taylor & Francis Group. (pp. 267–324).

Bhandari, S.D. and Gregory, J.F. (1992) Folic acid, 5-methyl-tetrahydrofolate and 5-formyl-tetrahydrofolate exhibit equivalent intestinal absorption, metabolism and *in vivo* kinetics in rats. J. Nutr. 122(9): 1847–1854. https://doi.org/10.1093/jn/122.9.1847.

Bhanja, S.K., Mandal, A.B., Agarwal, S.K. and Majumdar, S. (2006) Modulation of post hatch growth and immunocompetence development through *in ovo* injection of vitamin E and linoleic acid Proc. 12th Eur. Poult. Nutr., Verona, Italy.

Bhanja, S.K., Mandal, A., Bagarwal, S.K., Majumdar, S. and Bhattacharyya, A. (2007) Effect of in ovo injection of vitamins on the chick weight and post-hatch growth performance in broiler chickens Proc. 16th Eur. Symp. Poult. Nutr. Strasbourg, France.

Bhanja, S.K., Mandal, A.B., Majumdar, S., Mehra, M. and Goel, A. (2012) Effect of in ovo injection of vitamins on the chick weight and post-hatch growth performance in broiler chickens. Indian J. Poult. Sci. 47(3):306–310.

Bhavanishankar, T.N., Shantha, T. and Ramesh, H.P. (1986) Counteraction of the toxicity of aflatoxin B_1 by thymine and folic acid in experimental animals. Nutr. Rep. Int. 33(4):603–612.

Biagi, E., Mengucci, C., Barone, M., Picone, G., Lucchi, C., P., Litta, G., Candela, M., Manfreda, G., Brigidi, P., Capozzi, F. and De Cesare, A. (2021) Effects of vitamin B_2 supplementation in broilers microbiota and metabolome. Microorganisms 8(8):1134–1145. https://doi.org/10.3390/microorganisms8081134.

Bieber-Wlaschny, M. (1988) Vitamin E in swine nutrition. In "Update of vitamins and nutrition management in swine production technical conference" RCD 7776/988. Hoffmann–La Roche Inc., Nutley, NJ, USA.

Biehl, R.R., Baker, D.H. and DeLuca, H.F. (1995) 1alpha-hydroxylated cholecalciferol compounds act additively with microbial phytase to improve phosphorus, zinc and manganese utilization in chicks fed soy-based diets. J. Nutr. 125(9):2407–2416. https://doi.org/10.1093/jn/125.9.2407.

Biehl, R.R. and Baker, D.H. (1997) Utilization of phytate and non-phytate phosphorus in chicks as affected by source and amount of vitamin D. J. Anim. Sci. 75(11):2986–2993. https://doi.org/10.2527/1997.75112986x.

Bilgili, S.F., Alley, M.A., Hess, J.B. and Moran, E.T. (2005) Influence of strain-cross, sex, and feeding programs on broiler chicken paw (feet) yield and quality. Proc. 17th Eur. Symp. Ther. Qual. Poult. Meat, Doorwerth, The Netherlands. (pp. 342–349).

Binkley, N.C. and Suttie, J.W. (1995) Vitamin K nutrition and osteoporosis. J. Nutr. 125(7):1812–1821. https://doi.org/10.1093/jn/125.7.1812.

Bird, N. and Boren, B. (1999) Vitamin E and immunity in commercial broiler production. World's. Poult. Sci. 15(7):20–21.

Birdsall, J.J. (1975) "Technology of fortification of foods". Proc. Natl. Acad. Sci. USA. https://doi.org/10.17226/20201.

Biswas, A., Mohan, J., Sastry, K.V. and Tyagi, J.S. (2007) Effect of dietary vitamin E on the cloacal gland, foam and semen characteristics of male Japanese quail. Theriogenology 67(2):259–263. https://doi.org/10.1016/j.theriogenology.2006.07.010.

Biswas, A., Mohan, J. and Sastry, K.V. (2009) Effect of higher dietary vitamin E concentrations on physical and biochemical characteristics of semen in Kadaknath cockerels. Br. Poult. Sci. 50(6):733–738. https://doi.org/10.1080/00071660903264369.

Blair, M.E. (1993) Niacin (vitamin B_3) in poultry nutrition. Zootec. Int. 16:70.

Blalock, T.L. and Thaxton, J.P. (1984) Hematology of chicks experiencing marginal vitamin B_6 deficiency. Poult. Sci. 63(6):1243–1249. https://doi.org/10.3382/ps.0631243.

Blalock, T.L., Thaxton, J.P. and Garlich, J.D. (1984) Humoral immunity in chicks experiencing marginal vitamin B_6 deficiency. J. Nutr. 114(2):312–322. https://doi.org/10.1093/jn/114.2.312.

Blaxter, K.L. (1962) The significance of selenium and vitamin E in nutrition. Muscular dystrophy in farm animals: its cause and prevention. Proc. Nutr. Soc. 21(2):211–216. https://doi.org/10.1079/PNS19620034.

Blesbois, E., Grasseau, I. and Blum, J.C. (1993) Effects of vitamin E on fowl semen storage at 4 degrees C. Theriogenology 39(3):771–779. https://doi.org/10.1016/0093-691x(93)90260-c.

Blesbois, E., Lessire, M., Grasseau, I., Hallouis, J.M. and Hermier, D. (1997) Effect of dietary fat on the fatty acid composition and fertilizing ability of fowl semen. Biol. Reprod. 56(5):1216–1220. https://doi.org/10.1095/biolreprod56.5.1216.

Blomhoff, R., Green, M.H., Green, J.B., Berg, T. and Norum, K.R. (1991) Vitamin A metabolism: new perspectives on absorption, transport, and storage. Physiol. Rev. 71(4):951–990. https://doi.org/10.1152/physrev.1991.71.4.951.

BLS (Bundeslebensmittelschlüssel – Federal foodstuffs database (Germany)) (2009) www.blsdb.de.

Blum, J.C., Touraille, C., Salichon, Y. and Ricard, F.H. (1990) Influence des apports elevés de vitamin E sur les performances de croissance du "broiler" et la conservation des carcasses refrigereés. 8th Eur. Poult. Nutr. Barcelona, Spain. (pp. 228–231).

Blusztajn, J.K., Zeisel, S.H. and Wurtman, R.J. (1979) Synthesis of lecithin (phosphatidylcholine) from phosphatidylethanolamine in bovine brain. Brain Res. 179(2):319–327. https://doi.org/10.1016/0006-8993(79)90447-5.

Boa-Amponsem, K., Price, S.E., Geraert, P.A., Picard, M. and Siegel, P.B. (2001) Antibody responses of hens fed vitamin E and passively acquired antibodies of their chicks. Avian Dis. 45(1):122–127.

Boa-Amponsem, K., Picard, M., Blair, M.E., Meldrum, B. and Siegel, P.B. (2006) Memory antibody responses of broiler and leghorn chickens as influenced by dietary vitamin E and route of sheep red blood cell administration. Poult. Sci. 85(2):173–177. https://doi.org/10.1093/ps/85.2.173.

Bodle, B.C., Alvarado, C., Shirley, R.B., Mercier, Y. and Lee, J.T. (2018) Evaluation of different dietary alterations in their ability to mitigate the incidence and severity of woody breast and white striping in commercial male broilers. Poult. Sci. 97(9):3298–3310. https://doi.org/10.3382/ps/pey166.

Bollengier-Lee, S., Mitchell, M.A., Utomo, D.B., Williams, P.E.V. and Whitehead, C.C. (1998) Influence of high dietary vitamin E supplementation on egg production and plasma characteristics in hens subjected to heat stress. Br. Poult. Sci. 39(1):106–112. https://doi.org/10.1080/00071669889466.

Bollengier-Lee, S., Williams, P.E.V. and Whitehead, C.C. (1999) Optimal dietary concentration of vitamin E for alleviating the effect of heat stress on egg production in laying hens. Br. Poult. Sci. 40(1):102–107. https://doi.org/10.1080/00071669987917.

Bond, P.L., Meinecke, C.F., Miller, M.A. and Stephenson, E.L. (1985) Choline-methionine interrelationships in broiler diets when measuring at different growth stages. Poult. Sci. 64(1):6–28.

Bonilla, C.E.V., Rosa, A.P., Londero, A., Giacomini, C.B.S., Orso, C., Fernandes, M.O., Paixão, S.J. and Bonamigo, D.V. (2017) Effect of broiler breeders fed with corn or sorghum diet and canthaxanthin supplementation on production and reproductive performance. Poult. Sci. 96(6):1725–1734. https://doi.org/10.3382/ps/pew442.

Bonjour, J.P. (1991) Biotin. In "Handbook of vitamins" 2nd edition Machlin, L.J. (ed.). Marcel Dekker Inc., New York.

Booth, S.L. (1997) Skeletal functions of vitamin K-dependent proteins: not just for clotting anymore. Nutr. Res. Rev. 55(7):282–284. https://doi.org/10.1111/j.1753-4887.1997.tb01619.x.

Bootwalla, S.M. and Harms, R.H. (1990) Reassessment of riboflavin requirement for single comb White leghorn pullets from 0 to 6 weeks of age fed on maize-soyabean meal diets and its subsequent effect on sexual maturity and egg production. Br. Poult. Sci. 31(4):779–784. https://doi.org/10.1080/00071669008417308.

Bootwalla, S.M. and Harms, R.H. (1991) Reassessment of pantothenic acid requirement for single comb white leghorn pullets for 0 to 6 weeks of age and its subsequent effect on sexual maturity. Poult. Sci. 70(1):80–84. https://doi.org/10.3382/ps.0700080.

Boren, B. and Bond, P. (1996) Vitamin E and immunocompetence. Broiler Ind., November:26–33.

Boren, J.C., Engle, D.M., Palmer, M.W., Masters, R.E. and Criner, T. (1999) Land use change effects on breeding bird community composition. J. Range Manag. 52(5):420–430. https://doi.org/10.2307/4003767.

Bortolotti, G.R., Negro, J.J., Surai, P.F. and Prieto, P. (2003) Carotenoids in eggs and plasma of red-legged partridges: effects of diet and reproductive output. Physiol. Biochem. Zool. 76(3):367–374. https://doi.org/10.1086/375432.

Botsoglou, N.A., Florou-Paneri, P., Christaki, E., Fletouris, D.J. and Spais, A.B. (2002) Effect of dietary oregano essential oil on performance of chickens and on iron- induced lipid oxidation of breast, thigh and abdominal fat tissues. Br. Poult. Sci. 43(2):223–230. https://doi.org/10.1080/00071660120121436.

Botsoglou, N., Florou-Paneri, P., Botsoglou, E., Dotas, V., Giannenas, I., Koidis, A. and Mitrakos, P. (2005) The effect of feeding rosemary, oregano, saffron and alpha- tocopheryl acetate on hen performance and oxidative stability of eggs. S. Afr. J. Anim. Sci. 35:143–151. https://doi.org/10.2141/jpsa.43.143.

Bottje, W.G., Enkvetchakul, B., Moore, R. and McNew, R. (1995) Effect of α-tocopherol on antioxidants, lipid peroxidation, and the incidence of pulmonary hypertension syndrome (ascites) in broilers. Poult. Sci. 74(8):1356–1369. https://doi.org/10.3382/ps.0741356.

Bottje, W.G. and Wideman, R.F. (1995) Potential role of free radicals in the pathogenesis of pulmonary hypertension syndrome. Poult. Biol. Rev. 6:221–231.

Bottje, W.G., Erf, G.F., Bersi, T.K., Wang, S., Barnes, D. and Beers, K.W. (1997) Effect of dietary DL- α-tocopherol on tissue α- and γ-tocopherol and pulmonary hypertension syndrome (ascitis) in broilers. Poult. Sci. 76(11):1506–1512. https://doi.org/10.1093/ps/76.11.1506.

Bottje, W.G., Wang, S., Beers, K.W. and Cawthon, D. (1998) Lung lining fluid antioxidants in male broilers: age-related changes under thermoneutral and cold temperature conditions. Poult. Sci. 77(12):1905–1912. https://doi.org/10.1093/ps/77.12.1905.

Bou, R., Guardiola, F., Grau, A., Grimpa, S., Manich, A., Barroeta, A. and Codony, R. (2001) Influence of dietary fat source, α-tocopherol, and ascorbic acid supplementation on sensory quality of dark chicken meat. Poult. Sci. 80(6):800–807. https://doi.org/10.1093/ps/80.6.800.

Bou, R., Guardiola, F., Tres, A., Barroeta, A.C. and Codony, R. (2004) Effect of dietary fish oil, alpha-tocopheryl acetate, and zinc supplementation on the composition and consumer acceptability of chicken meat. Poult. Sci. 83(2):282–292. https://doi.org/10.1093/ps/83.2.282.

Bou, R., Grimpa, S., Guardiola, F., Barroeta, A.C. and Codony, R. (2006) Effect of various fat sources. Poult. Sci. 85(8):1472–1481. https://doi.org/10.1093/ps/85.8.1472.

Bozkurt, M., Yalçin, S., Koçer, B., Tüzün, A.E., Akşit, H., Özkan, S., Uygun, M., Ege, G., Güven, G. and Yildiz, O. (2017) Effects of enhancing vitamin D status by 25-hydroxycholecalciferol supplementation, alone or in combination with calcium and phosphorus, on sternum mineralisation and breast meat quality in broilers. Br. Poult. Sci. 58(4):452–461. https://doi.org/10.1080/00071668.2017.1327703.

Brandon, S., Morrissey, P.A., Buckley, D.J. and Frigg, M. (1993) Influence of dietary α-tocopheryl acetate on the oxidative stability of chicken tissues. 11th Eur. Symp. Qual. Poult. Meat. (pp. 397–403).

Brass, E.P. (1993) Hydroxycobalamin [c-lactam] increases total coenzyme A content in primary culture hepatocytes by accelerating coenzyme A biosynthesis secondary to acyl-CoA accumulation. J. Nutr. 123(11):1801–1807. https://doi.org/10.1093/jn/123.11.1801.

Braun, F. (1986) The effect of bile on intestinal absorption of calcium and vitamin D. Wien. Klin. Wochenschr. 98(166):23.

Bräunlich, K. (1974) "Vitamin B_6". 1451. F Hoffmann-La Roche and Co, Ltd.

Bräunlich, K. and Zintzen, H. (1976) "Vitamin B_1". 1593. F Hoffmann-La Roche and Co, Ltd.

Brenes, A., Viveros, A., Goñi, I., Centeno, C., Sáyago-Ayerdy, S.G., Arija, I. and Saura-Calixto, F. (2008) Effect of grape pomace concentrate and vitamin E on digestibility of polyphenols and antioxidant activity in chickens. Poult. Sci. 87(2):307–316. https://doi.org/10.3382/ps.2007-00297.

Brent, B.E. (1985) Is supplementation necessary? Feed Manag. 36(12):8.

Bréque, C., Surai, P. and Brillard, J.P. (2003) Roles of antioxidants on prolonged storage of avian spermatozoa *in vivo* and *in vitro*. Mol. Reprod. Dev. 66(3):314–323. https://doi.org/10.1002/mrd.10347.

Brewer, L.E. and Edwards, H.M. (1972) Studies on the biotin requirement of broiler breeders. Poult. Sci. 51(2):619–624. https://doi.org/10.3382/ps.0510619.

Briggs, G.M. (1946) Nicotinic acid deficiency in turkey poults and the occurrence of perosis. J. Nutr. 31(1): 79–84. https://doi.org/10.1093/jn/31.1.79.

Briggs, G.M., Mill, R.C., Elvehjem, C.A. and Hart, E.B. (1942) Nicotinic acid in chick nutrition. Exp. Biol. Med. 51(1):59-61. https://doi.org/10.3181/00379727-51-13826.

Briggs, G.M., Hill, E.G. and Canfield, T.H. (1953) The need for choline, folic acid and nicotinic acid by goslings fed purified diets. Sci. J. S. Minn. Agric. Exp. Stn. 32(4):678–680. https://doi.org/10.3382/ps.0320678.

Britton, W.M. (1994) Effects of dietary vitamin A at marginal levels of cholecalciferol. Poult. Sci. 73(1):52.

Bronner, F. and Stein, W.D. (1995) Calcium homeostasis an old problem revisited. J. Nutr. 125(7) Supplement:1987S-1995S. https://doi.org/10.1093/jn/125.suppl_7.1987S.

Brown, E.S. (1964) Isolation and assay of dipalmityl lecithin in lung extracts. Am. J. Physiol. 207:402–406. https://doi.org/10.1152/ajplegacy.1964.207.2.402.

Brown, G.M. (1962) The biosynthesis of folic acid. II. Inhibition by sulfonamides. J. Biol. Chem. 237(2): 536–540. https://doi.org/10.1016/S0021-9258(18)93957-8.

Browning, L.C. and Cowieson, A.J. (2014) Effect of vitamin D_3 and strontium on performance, nutrient retention, and bone mineral composition in broiler chickens. Anim. Prod. Sci. 54(7):942–949. https://doi.org/10.1071/AN13091.

Brownlee, N.R., Huttner, J.J., Panganamala, R.V. and Cornwell, D.G. (1977) Role of vitamin E and glutathione-induced oxidant stress: methemoglobin, lipid peroxidation and hemolysis. J. Lipid Res. 18(5):635–644. https://doi.org/10.1016/S0022-2275(20)41605-0.

Broz, J. and Ward, N.E. (2007) The role of vitamins and feed enzymes in combating metabolic challenges and disorders. J. Appl. Poult. Res. 16(1):150–159. https://doi.org/10.1093/japr/16.1.150.

Brufau, J., Llauradó, L.L., Pérez-Vendrell, A. and Esteve-García, E. (1995) Effect of biotin supplementation on broiler diets based on wheat or corn. Poult. Sci. 74(1):398.

Bryden, W.L. (1991) Tissue depletion of biotin in chickens and the development of deficiency lesions and the fatty liver and kidney syndrome. Avian Pathol. 20(2):259–269. https://doi.org/10.1080/03079459108418762.

Buda, S. (2000) Effects of biotin on the skin of turkey foot pads. World Poult. 16(12):47–48.

Buenrostro, J.L. and Kratzer, F.H. (1984) Use of plasma and egg yolk biotin of white leghorn hens to assess biotin availability from feedstuffs. Poult. Sci. 63(8):1563–1570. https://doi.org/10.3382/ps.0631563.

Bunchasak, C. and Kachana, S. (2009) Dietary folate and vitamin B_{12} supplementation and consequent vitamin deposition in chicken eggs. Trop. Anim. Health Prod. 41(7):1583–1589. https://doi.org/10.1007/s11250-009-9350-7.

Burgos, S., Bohorquez, D.V. and Burgos, S.A. (2006) Vitamin deficiency-induced neurological disease in poultry. Int. J. Poult. Sci. 5(9):804–807. https://doi.org/10.3923/ijps.2006.804.807.

Burkholder, W.J. and Swecker, W.S. (1990) Seminars in Vet. Med. Surg. (Small Animal) 5(3):154–166 PMID: 2236979.

Buzała, M., Janicki, B. and Czarnecki, R. (2015) Consequences of different growth rates in broiler breeder and layer hens on embryogenesis, metabolism and metabolic rate: a review. Poult. Sci. 94(4):728–733. https://doi.org/10.3382/ps/pev015.

Calderón-Ospina, C.A. and Nava-Mesa, M.O. (2020) B vitamins in the nervous system: current knowledge of the biochemical modes of action and synergies of thiamine, pyridoxine, and cobalamin. CNS Neurosci. Ther. 26(1):5–13. https://doi.org/10.1111/cns.13207.

Calini, F. and Sirri, F. (2007) Breeder nutrition and offspring performance. Rev. Bras. Cienc. Avic. 9(2):77–83. https://doi.org/10.1590/S1516-635X2007000200001.

Camporeale, G. and Zempleni, J. (2006) Biotin. In "Present knowledge in nutrition" 9th edition Bowman, B.A. and Russell, R.M. (ed.). International Life Sciences Institute. (pp. 250–259).

Cantatore, F.P., Loperfido, M.C., Magli, D.M., Mancini, L. and Carrozzo, M. (1991) The importance of vitamin C for hydroxylation of vitamin D_3 to 1,25$(OH)_2D_3$ in man. Clin. Rheumatol. 10(2):162–167. https://doi.org/10.1007/BF02207657.

Cantor, A. and Bacon, W.L. (1978) Performance of caged broilers fed vitamin D_3 and 25-hydroxyvitamin D_3. Poult. Sci. 57:1123–1124.

Cantorna, M.T. (2006) Vitamin D and its role in immunology: multiple sclerosis, and inflammatory bowel disease. Prog. Biophys. Mol. Biol. 92(1):60–64. https://doi.org/10.1016/j.pbiomolbio.2006.02.020.

Carmel, R. (1994) *In vitro* studies of gastric juice in patients with food-cobalamin malabsorption. Dig. Dis. Sci. 39(12):2516–2522. https://doi.org/10.1007/BF02087684.

Carpenter, K.J. (1981) "Pellagra". Hutchinson Ross, Stroudsburg, PA.

Carpenter, K.J., Schelstraete, M., Vilicich, V.C. and Wall, J.S. (1988) Immature corn as a source of niacin for rats. J. Nutr. 118(2):165–169. https://doi.org/10.1093/jn/118.2.165.

Carreras, I., Castellari, M., García Regueiro, J.A., Guerrero, L., Esteve-Garcia, E. and Sárraga, C. (2004) Influence of enrofloxacin administration and α-tocopheryl acetate supplemented diets on oxidative stability of broiler tissues. Poult. Sci. 83(5):796–802. https://doi.org/10.1093/ps/83.5.796.

Carson, D.A., Seto, S. and Wasson, D.B. (1987) Pyridine nucleotide cycling and poly(ADP-ribose) synthesis in resting human lymphocytes. J. Immunol. 138(6):1904–1907.

Carter, E.G. and Carpenter, K.J. (1982) The available niacin values of foods for rats and their relation to analytical values. J. Nutr. 112(11):2091–2103.

Carter, S.D., Cromwell, G.L., Combs, T.R., Colombo, G. and Fanti, P. (1996) The determination of serum concentrations of osteocalcin in growing pigs and its relationship to end-measures of bone mineralization. J. Anim. Sci. 74:2719–2729. https://doi.org/10.2527/1996.74112719x.

Cashman, K.D. (2018) Vitamin D requirements for the future-lessons learned and charting a path forward. Nutrients 10(5):533–545. https://doi.org/10.3390/nu10050533.

Cashman, K.D. and O'Connor, E. (2008) Does high vitamin K_1 intake protect against bone loss in later life? Nutr. Rev. 66(9):532–538. https://doi.org/10.1111/j.1753-4887.2008.00086.x.

Castaing, J., Larroudé, P., Pcyhorgue, A., Hamelin, C. and Manroufi, C. (2003) Incidence de deux niveaux d'apports en vitamines sur les performances du poulet de chair. V Journées Rech. Avicoles.

Castaing, J., Larroudé, P., Hamelin, C. and Ball, A. (2007) Effect de deux niveaux d'apports en vitamines sur les performances zootechniques de poulets type labels. Journées Rech. Avicoles VII: (288–292).

Castaldo, D.J., Jones, J.E. and Maurice, D.V. (1990) Growth and carcass composition of female turkeys implanted with anabolic agents and fed high-protein and low-protein diets. Arch. Tierernahr. 40(8): 703–712. https://doi.org/10.1080/17450399009428419.

Catani, M.V., Savini, I., Rossi, A., Melino, G. and Avigliano, L. (2005) Biological role of vitamin C in keratinocytes. Nutr. Rev. 63(3):81–90. https://doi.org/10.1111/j.1753-4887.2005.tb00125.x.

Çelik, L., Öztürkcan, O., Inal, T.C., Canacankatan, N. and Kayrin, L. (2003) Effects of l-carnitine and niacin supplied by drinking water on fattening performance, carcass quality and plasma l-carnitine concentration of broiler chicks. Arch. Tierernahr. 57(2):127–136. https://doi.org/10.1080/0003942031000107325.

Celik, L., Tekeli, A., Kutlu, H.R. and Gorgulu, M. (2006) Effects of dietary vitamin B_6 and L-carnitine on growth performance and carcass characteristics of broilers reared under high temperature regime Proc. 12th Eur. Poult. Nutr. Verona, Italy.

Cerolini, S., Pizzi, F., Gliozzi, T., Maldjian, A., Zaniboni, L. and Parodi, L. (2003) Lipid manipulation of chicken semen by dietary means and its relation to fertility: a review. Poult. Sci. 59(1):65–75. https://doi.org/10.1079/WPS20030003.

Cerolini, S., Surai, P.F., Speake, B.K. and Sparks, N.H. (2005) Dietary fish and evening primrose oil with vitamin E effects on semen variables in cockerels. Br. Poult. Sci. 46(2):214–222. https://doi.org/10.1080/00071660500065839.

Cerolini, S., Zaniboni, L., Maldjian, A. and Gliozzi, T. (2006) Effect of docosahexaenoic acid and alpha-tocopherol enrichment in chicken sperm on semen quality, sperm lipid composition and susceptibility to peroxidation. Theriogenology 66(4):877–886. https://doi.org/10.1016/j.theriogenology.2006.02.022.

Cerrate, S. and Corzo, A. (2018) Lysine and energy trends in feeding modern commercial broilers. Int. J. Poult. Sci. 18(1):28–38. https://doi.org/10.3923/ijps.2019.28.38.

Chan, A.C. (1993) Partners in defense, vitamin E, and vitamin C. Can. J. Physiol. Pharmacol. 71(9):725–731. https://doi.org/10.1139/y93-109.

Chan, A.C., Tran, K., Raynor, T., Ganz, P.R. and Chow, C.K. (1991) Regeneration of vitamin E in human platelets. J. Biol. Chem. 266(26):17290–17295. https://doi.org/10.1016/S0021-9258(19)47372-9.

Chan, M.M. (1991) Choline and carnitine. In "Handbook of vitamins" 2nd edition Machlin, L.J. (ed.). Marcel Dekker. (pp. 537–556).

Chang, A., Halley, J. and Silva, M. (2016) Can feeding the broiler breeder improve chick quality and offspring performance? Anim. Prod. Sci. 56(8):1254–1262. https://doi.org/10.1071/AN15381.

Chang, W.P., Marsh, J.A., Dietert, R.R. and Combs, G.F. (1990) The effect of dietary vitamin E and selenium deficiencies on chicken lymphocyte surface marker expression and proliferation. Poult. Sci. 69(1):32.

Charles, O.W., Roland, D.A. and Edwards, H.M. (1972) Thiamine deficiency identification and treatment in commercial turkey and coturnix quail. Poult. Sci. 51(2):419–423. https://doi.org/10.3382/ps.0510419.

Chee, K.W. and Chang, M.I. (1995) Biotin deficiency and plasma fatty acids patterns in broilers. Poult. Sci. 74(1):398.

Chen, B., Shen, T. and Austic, R.E. (1996) Efficiency of tryptophan-niacin conversion in chickens and ducks. Nutr. Res. 16(1):91–104. https://doi.org/10.1016/0271-5317(95)02063-2.

Chen, C., Turner, B., Applegate, T.J., Litta, G. and Kim, W.K. (2020a) Role of long-term supplementation of 25-hydroxyvitamin D_3 on laying hen bone 3-dimensional structural development. Poult. Sci. 99(11): 5771–5782. https://doi.org/10.1016/j.psj.2020.06.080.

Chen, C., Turner, B., Applegate, T.J., Litta, G. and Kim, W.K. (2020b) Role of long-term supplementation of 25-hydroxyvitamin D_3 on egg production and egg quality of laying hen. Poult. Sci. 99(12):6899–6906. https://doi.org/10.1016/j.psj.2020.09.020.

Chen, C., White, D.L., Marshall, B. and Kim, W.K. (2021) Role of 25-hydroxyvitamin D_3 and 1,25-dihydroxyvitamin D_3 in chicken embryo osteogenesis, adipogenesis, myogenesis, and vitamin D_3 metabolism. Front. Physiol. 12:637629. https://doi.org/10.3389/fphys.2021.637629.

Chen, F., Noll, S.L. and Waibel, P.E. (1994) Dietary biotin and turkey breeder performance. Poult. Sci. 73(5):682–686. https://doi.org/10.3382/ps.0730682.

Chen, F., Jiang, Z., Jiang, S., Li, L., Lin, X., Gou, Z. and Fan, Q. (2016) Dietary vitamin A supplementation improved reproductive performance by regulating ovarian expression of hormone receptors, caspase-3 and Fas in broiler breeders. Poult. Sci. 95(1):30–40. https://doi.org/10.3382/ps/pev305.

Chen, J. (1990) "Technical service internal reports". BASF Corp.

Chen, J.Y., Latshaw, J.D., Lee, H.O. and Min, D.B. (1998) α-tocopherol content and oxidative stability of egg yolk as related to dietary α-tocopherol. J. Food Sci. 63(5):919–922. https://doi.org/10.1111/j.1365-2621.1998.tb179 27.x.

Chen, W. and Chen, G. (2014) The roles of vitamin A in the regulation of carbohydrate, lipid, and protein metabolism. J. Clin. Med. 3(2):453–479. https://doi.org/10.3390/jcm3020453.

Chen, W., Fouada, A. M., Ruana, D., Wanga, S., Xia, W. G. and Zhenga, C. T. (2018) Effects of dietary thiamine supplementation on performance, egg quality, and antioxidant-related enzymes in Chinese egg-laying ducks. The J. Anim. Plant Sci. 28(6).

Chen, Y.F., Huang, C.F., Liu, L., Lai, C.H. and Wang, F.L. (2019) Concentration of vitamins in the 13 feed ingredients commonly used in pig diets Anim. Feed Sci. Techn. 247:1–8 https://doi.org/10.1016/j.anifeed sci.2018.10.011.

Cheng, T., Coon, C. and Hamre, M. (1988) Effect of vitamin C and environmental stress on layer performance. Poult. Sci. 67:67.

Cheng, T.K., Coon, C.N. and Hamre, M.L. (1990) Effect of environmental stress on the ascorbic acid requirement of laying hens. Poult. Sci. 69(5):774–780. https://doi.org/10.3382/ps.0690774.

Chennaiah, S., Qadri, S.S.Y.H., Rao, S.V.R., Shyamsunder, G. and Raghuramulu, N. (2004) Cestrum diurnum leaf as a source of 1,25(OH)$_2$ vitamin D$_3$ improves eggshell thickness. J. Steroid Biochem. Mol. Biol. 89–90(1–5):589–594. https://doi.org/10.1016/j.jsbmb.2004.03.101.

Cherian, G., Wolfe, F.W. and Sim, J.S. (1996a) Dietary oils with added tocopherols: effects on egg or tissue tocopherols, fatty acids, and oxidative stability. Poult. Sci. 75(3):423–431. https://doi.org/10.3382/ps.0750423.

Cherian, G., Wolfe, F.H. and Sim, J.S. (1996b) Feeding dietary oils with tocopherols: effects on internal qualities of eggs during storage. J. Food Sci. 61(1):15–18. https://doi.org/10.1111/j.1365-2621.1996.tb14716.x.

Cherian, G. and Sim, J.S. (1997) Egg yolk polyunsaturated fatty acids and vitamin E content alters the tocopherol status of hatched chicks. Poult. Sci. 76(12):1753–1759. https://doi.org/10.1093/ps/76.12.1753.

Cherian, G. and Sim, J.S. (2003) Maternal and post hatch dietary polyunsaturated fatty acids alter tissue tocopherol status of chicks. Poult. Sci. 82(4):681–686. https://doi.org/10.1093/ps/82.4.681.

Chew, B.P. (1995) Antioxidant vitamins affect food animal immunity and health. J. Nutr. 125(6) Supplement:1804S–1808S.

Chew, B.P. (1996) Importance of antioxidant vitamins in immunity and health in animals. Anim. Feed Sci. Technol. 59(1–3):103–114. https://doi.org/10.1016/0377-8401(95)00891-8.

Chew, B.P. and Park, J.S. (2004) Carotenoid action on the immune response. J. Nutr. 134(1):257S-261S. https://doi.org/10.1093/jn/134.1.257S.

Chien, C.T., Chang, W.T., Chen, H.W., Wang, T.D., Liou, S.Y., Chen, T.J., Chang, Y.L., Lee, Y.T. and Hsu, S.M. (2004) Ascorbate supplement reduces oxidative stress in dyslipidemic patients undergoing apheresis. Arterioscler. Thromb. Vasc. Biol. 24(6):1111–1117. https://doi.org/10.1161/01.ATV.0000127620.12310.89.

Choi, Y., Lee, S., Kim, S., Lee, J., Ha, J., Oh, H., Lee, Y., Kim, Y. and Yoon, Y. (2020) Vitamin E (α-tocopherol) consumption influences gut microbiota composition. Int. J. Food Sci. Nutr. 71(2):221–225. https://doi.org/10.1080/09637486.2019.1639637.

Chou, P.C., Chen, Y.H., Chung, T.K., Walzem, R.L., Lai, L.S. and Chen, S.E. (2020) Supplemental 25-hydroxycholecalciferol alleviates inflammation and cardiac fibrosis in hens. Int. J. Mol. Sci. 21(21):8379. https://doi.org/10.3390/ijms21218379.

Chow, C.K. (1979) Nutritional influence on cellular antioxidant defense systems. Am. J. Clin. Nutr. 32(5): 1066–1081. https://doi.org/10.1093/ajcn/32.5.1066.

Christensen, K. (1983) Pools of cellular nutrients. In "Dynamic biochemistry of animal production" Riis, P.M. (ed.). Elsevier, Amsterdam.

Christensen, S. (1973) The biological fate of riboflavin in mammals. A survey of literature and own investigations. Acta Pharmacol. Toxicol. (Copenh) 32(2):3–72. https://doi.org/10.1111/j.1600-0773.1973.tb03313.x.

Christmas, R.B. and Harms, R.H. (1988) The choline requirement of the four- to twelve-week-old turkey poult as affected by dietary methionine. Poult. Sci. 67(1):9.

Christmas, R.B. and Harms, R.H. (1989) Further evaluation on the methionine effect on the supplemental choline needs of the four- to twelve-week-old male turkey poult. Poult. Sci. 68(1):30 (abstract).

Christmas, R.B., Harms, R.H. and Sloan, D.R. (1995) The absence of vitamins and trace minerals and broiler performance. J. Appl. Poult. Res. 4(4):407–410. https://doi.org/10.1093/japr/4.4.407.

Chung, M.K., Choi, J.H., Chung, Y.K. and Chee, K.M. (2005) Effects of dietary vitamins C and E on eggshell quality of broiler breeder hens exposed to heat stress. Asian. Australas. J. Anim. Sci. 18(4):545–551. https://doi.org/10.5713/ajas.2005.545.

Chung, T.K. (2006) Vitamins and poultry products quality. Int. Poult. Prod. 14(5):11–15.

Chung, T.K. and Baker, D.H. (1990) Riboflavin requirement of chicks fed purified amino acid and conventional corn-soybean meal diets. Poult. Sci. 69(8):1357–1363. https://doi.org/10.3382/ps.0691357.

Chung, T.K. and Boren, B. (1999) Vitamin E use in commercial flocks examined. Feedstuffs 71(37):11–14.

Cier, D., Rimsky, Y., Rand, N., Polishuk, O., Gur, N., Ben-Shoshan, A., Frish, Y. and Ben-Moshe, A. (1992) The effects of supplementing ascorbic acid on broilers performance under summer conditions Proc. 19th World's Poult. Congr., Amsterdam, The Netherlands (pp. 586–589).

Clagett, C.O. (1971) Genetic control of the riboflavin carrier protein. Fed. Proc. 30(1):127–129. PMID:5539866.

Clagett-Dame, M. and Knutson, D. (2011) Vitamin A in reproduction and development. Nutrients 3(4):385–428. https://doi.org/10.3390/nu3040385.

Clark, N.B., Lee, S.K. and Murphy, M.J. (1990) Vitamin D action on calcium regulation and osmoregulation in embryonic chicks. In "Endocrinology of birds" Wada, M., Ishii, S. and Scanes, C.G. (ed.). Springer Verlag, Berlin. (pp. 159–170).

Clark, S., Hansen, G., Mclean, P., Bond, P., Wakeman, W., Meadows, R. and Buda, S. (2002) Pododermatitis in turkeys. Avian Dis. 46(4):1038–1044. https://doi.org/10.1637/0005-2086(2002)046[1038:PIT]2.0.CO;2.

Clifford, A.J., Jones, A.D. and Bills, N.D. (1990) Bioavailability of folates in selected foods incorporated into amino acid-based diets fed to rats. J. Nutr. 120(12):1640–1647. https://doi.org/10.1093/jn/120.12.1640.

Cobb-Vantress (2020) Cobb breeder management supplement. https://www.cobb-vantress.com/resource/product-supplements.

Cobb-Vantress (2022) Cobb 500 Nutrition and management guide. https://www.cobb-vantress.com/resource/product-supplements.

Coelho, M.B. (1991) Vitamin stability in premixes and feeds: a practical approach. BASF Tech. Symp. (p. 56).

Coelho, M.B. (1996a) Stability of vitamins affected by feed processing. Feedstuffs 69(32):9.

Coelho, M.B. (1996b) Optimum vitamin supplementation needed for turkey performance and profitability. Feedstuffs 68(19):13.

Coelho, M.B. (2000) "Update on commercial poultry, swine and dairy vitamin supplement. https://www.feedinfo.com/home/global-news/update-on-commercial-poultry-swine-and-dairy-vitamin-supplementation/52417.

Coelho, M.B. and McNaughton, J.L. (1995) Effect of composite vitamin supplementation on broilers. J. Appl. Poult. Res. 4(3):219–229. https://doi.org/10.1093/japr/4.3.219.

Coelho, M.B., McKnight, W. and Cousins, B. (2001) Impact of a targeted B-vitamin regimen on rate and efficiency of fast-growing broilers from 0 to 49 days Proc. Poultry Science Association Symp., Indianapolis, IN.

Coetzee, G.J.M. and Hoffman, L.C. (2001) Effect of dietary vitamin E on the performance of broilers and quality of broiler meat during refrigerated storage. S. Afr. J. Anim. Sci. 31(3):161–176. https://doi.org/10.4314/sajas.v31i3.3799.

Cogburn, L.A., Smarsh, D.N., Wang, X., Trakooljul, N., Carré, W. and White, H.B. (2018) Transcriptional profiling of liver in riboflavin-deficient chicken embryos explains impaired lipid utilization, energy depletion, massive hemorrhaging and delayed feathering. BMC Genomics 19(1):177. https://doi.org/10.1186/s12864-018-4568-2.

Cohen, N., Scott, C.G., Neukon, C., Lopresti, R.L., Weber, G. and Saucy, G. (1981) Total synthesis of all 8 stereoisomers of α-tocopheryl acetate. Analysis of their diastereomeric and enantiomeric purity by gas chromatography. Helv. Chim. Acta 64:1158–1173. https://doi.org/10.1002/HLCA.19810640422.

Colet, S., Garcia, R.G., Almeida Paz, I.C.L., Caldara, F.R., Borille, R., Royer, A.F.B., Nääs, I.A. and Sgavioli, S. (2015) Bone characteristics of broilers supplemented with vitamin D. Rev. Bras. Cienc. Avic. 17(3):325–332. https://doi.org/10.1590/1516-635x1703325-332.

Colnago, G.L., Jensen, L.S. and Long, P.L. (1984) Effect of selenium and vitamin E on the development of immunity to coccidiosis in chickens. Poult. Sci. 63(6):1136–1143. https://doi.org/10.3382/ps.0631136.

Combs, G.F. (1976) Differential effects of high dietary levels of vitamin A on the vitamin e-selenium nutrition of young and adult chickens. J. Nutr. 106(7):967–975. https://doi.org/10.1093/jn/106.7.967.

Combs Jr., G.F. and Combs, S.B. (1986) "The role of selenium in nutrition". Academic Press, New York. https://doi.org/10.1016/B978-0-12-183495-1.X5001-5.

Combs Jr., G.F. and McClung, J.P. (2022) "The vitamins. Fundamental aspects in nutrition and health" 6th edition. Elsevier, Amsterdam.

Commission on Biochemical Nomenclature of Tocopherols and Related Compounds, Recommendations (IUPAC-IUB) (1973) (1974) Eur J Biochem. 46(2):217-219219.

Composition nutritionnelle des aliments – Table CIQUAL (2008) http://www.afssa.fr/TableCIQUAL/.

Cook, M.E. (1988) Factors enhancing the incidence of skeletal deformities Proc. Md. Nutr. Conf. (pp. 24–29).

Cook, M.E. (1990) Vitamin-mycotoxin interactions Proc. Natl. Feed Ingred. Assoc. Nutr. Inst. Development in Vitamin Nutrition and Health Applications.

Cook, M.E. (1992) "Performance of turkeys fed thiamine, riboflavin and vitamin E in excess of NRC requirements". BASF Technical Seminar, Fresno, CA, USA.

Cook, M.E. (2000) Skeletal deformities and their causes: introduction. Poult. Sci. 79(7):982–984. https://doi.org/10.1093/ps/79.7.982.

Cook, M.E., Springer, W.T. and Hebert, J.A. (1984a) Enhanced incidence of leg abnormalities in reovirus WVU 2937-infected chickens fed various dietary levels of selected vitamins. Avian Dis. 28(3):548–561. https://doi.org/10.2307/1590224.

Cook, M.E., Springer, W.R., Kerr, K.M. and Herbert, J.A. (1984b) Severity of tenosynovitis reovirus-infected chickens fed various dietary levels of choline, folic acid, manganese, biotin or niacin. Avian Dis. 28(3):562–573. https://doi.org/10.2307/1590225.

Cooke, B.C. and Raine, H.D. (1987) The application of nutritional principles by the commercial nutritionist. In "Nutrient requirements of poultry and nutritional research" Fisher, C. and Boorman, K.N. (ed.). Butterworths, E.D. (pp. 191–200).

Cooper, J.R., Roth, R.H. and Kini, M.M. (1963) Biochemical and physiological function of thiamine in nervous tissue. Nature 199:609–610. https://doi.org/10.1038/199609a0.

Cope, F.O., Stuart, M. and Stake, P.E. (1979) Reducing the incidence and severity of curled toes and perosis-like leg abnormalities in cage-reared broilers by high dietary levels of pyridoxine or choline. Poult. Sci. 58:1046.

Cort, W.M., Vicente, T.S., Waysek, E.H. and Williams, B.D. (1983) Vitamin E content of feedstuffs determined by high-performance liquid chromatographic fluorescence. J. Agric. Food Chem. 31(6):1330–1333. https://doi.org/10.1021/jf00120a045.

Cortinas, L., Galobart, J., Barroeta, A.C., Castillo, M.S. and Jensen, S.K. (2001) Influencia del nivel de insaturación dietética sobre el depósito y efecto antioxidante del α-tocopherol en muslo de pollo (crudo, cocido y cocido-refrigerado). 38th Symp. Cient. Avic. (pp. 141–148).

Cortinas, L., Villaverde, C., Baucells, M.D., Guardiola, F. and Barroeta, A.C. (2003) Interaction between dietary unsaturation and α-tocopherol levels: vitamin E content in thigh meat. 16th Eur. Symp. Qual. Poult. Meat. Saint-Brieuc, France.

Cortinas, L., Barroeta, A., Galobart, J. and Jensen, S.K. (2004) Distribution of α-tocopherol stereoisomers in liver and thigh of chickens. Br. J. Nutr. 92(2):295–301. https://doi.org/10.1079/BJN20041188.

Cortinas, L., Barroeta, A.C., Villaverde, C., Galobart, J., Guardiola, F. and Baucells, M.D. (2005) Influence of the dietary polyunsaturation level on chicken meat quality: lipid oxidation. Poult. Sci. 84(1):48–55. https://doi.org/10.1093/ps/84.1.48.

Cortinas, L., Baucells, M.D., Villaverde, C., Guardiola, F., Jensen, S.K. and Barroeta, A.C. (2006) Influence of dietary polyunsaturation level on α-tocopherol content in chicken meat. Arch. Geflügelk 70(3): 98–105.

Coşkun, B., Inal, F., Celik, I., Erganiş, O., Tiftik, A.M., Kurtoglu, F., Kuyucuoglu, Y. and Ok, U. (1998) Effects of dietary levels of vitamin A on the egg yield and immune responses of laying hens. Poult. Sci. 77(4):542–546. https://doi.org/10.1093/ps/77.4.542.

Couch, J.R. and Grossie, B. (1970) Choline and inositol in laying hen nutrition. Poult. Sci. 49(6):1731–1733. https://doi.org/10.3382/ps.0491731.

Cravens, W.W., McGibbon, W.H. and Sebesta, E.E. (1944) Effect of biotin deficiency on embryonic development in the domestic fowl. Anat. Rec. 90(1):55–64. https://doi.org/10.1002/ar.1090900109.

Crawford, J.S., Griffith, M., Teekell, R.A. and Watts, A.B. (1969) Choline requirement and synthesis in laying hens. Poult. Sci. 48(2):620–626. https://doi.org/10.3382/ps.0480620.

Creech, B.G., Feldman, G.L., Ferguson, T.M., Reid, B.L. and Couch, J.R. (1957) Exudative diathesis and vitamin E deficiency in turkey poults. J. Nutr. 62(1):83–95. https://doi.org/10.1093/jn/62.1.83.

Creek, R.D. and Vasaitis, V. (1963) The effect of excess dietary protein on the need for folic acid by the chick. Poult. Sci. 42(5):1136–1141. https://doi.org/10.3382/ps.0421136.

Crevieu-Gabriel, I. and Naciri, M. (2001) Effect de l'alimentation sur les coccidiosis chez le poulet. INRA Prod. Anim. 14(4):231–246. https://doi.org/10.20870/productions-animales.2001.14.4.3746.

Cruickshank, J.J. and Sim, J.S. (1987) Effects of excess vitamin D_3 and cage density on the incidence of leg abnormalities in broiler chickens. Avian Dis. 31(2):332–338. https://doi.org/10.2307/1590881.

Csallany, A.S., Menken, B.Z. and Waibel, P.E. (1988) Hepatic tocopherol concentration in turkeys as influenced by dietary vitamin and fat. Poult. Sci. 67(12):1814–1816. https://doi.org/10.3382/ps.0671814.

Cunha, T.J. (1982a) Niacin in animal feeding and nutrition. In "Vitamins: the life essentials". National Feed Ingredients Association.

Cunha, T.J. (1982b) Niacin's role in animal feeds should be re-evaluated. Feedstuffs 54(25):20.

Cunha, T.J. (1985) Nutrition and disease interaction. Feedstuffs 57(41):37.

Cunha, T.J. (1987) Variables in animal nutrition keep shifting the requirements. Feedstuffs 59(42):1.

Curça, D., Andonie, V., Andronie, I.C. and Pop, A. (2006) The influence of feed supplementation with ascorbic acid and sodium ascorbate on broilers, under thermal stress. Proc. 12th Eur. Poult. Nutr., Verona, Italy.

Daghir, N.J. (1995) Broiler feeding and management in hot climates. In Poultry production in hot climates. CA B International. Google Books. (pp. 185–218).

Daghir, N.J. (1996) Nutrition and climatic stress. Proc. 20th World's Poult. Congress Delhi, India. (pp. 141–150).

Daghir, N.J. and Haddad, K.S. (1981) Vitamin B_6 in the etiology of gizzard erosion in growing chickens. Poult. Sci. 60(5):988–992. https://doi.org/10.3382/ps.0600988.

Daghir, N.J. and Shah, M.A. (1973) Effect of dietary protein level on vitamin B_6 requirement of chicks. Poult. Sci. 52(4):1247–1252. https://doi.org/10.3382/ps.0521247.

Dagnelie, P.C., Van Staveren, W.A. and Van den Berg, H. (1991) Vitamin B_{12} from algae appears not to be bioavailable. Am. J. Clin. Nutr. 53(3):695–697. https://doi.org/10.1093/ajcn/53.3.695.

Dakshinamurti, S. and Dakshinamurti, K. (2013) Vitamin B_6. In "Handbook of vitamins" 5th edition Zempleni, J., Suttie, J., Gregory, J. and Stover P.J. (ed.). CRC Press, Taylor & Francis Group. (pp. 351–396).

Dal Bosco, A., Mugnai, C., Rosati, A., Paoletti, A., Caporali, S. and Castellini, C. (2014) Effect of range enrichment on performance behavior, and forage intake of free-range chickens. J. Appl. Poult. Res. 23(2): 137–145. https://doi.org/10.3382/JAPR.2013-00814.

Dal Bosco, A., Mugnai, C., Mattioli, S., Rosati, A., Ruggeri, S., Ranucci, D. and Castellini, C. (2016) Transfer of bioactive compounds from pasture to meat in organic free-range chickens. Poult. Sci. 95(10):2464–2471. https://doi.org/10.3382/ps/pev383.

Dale, N.M. and Villacres, A. (1986) Dietary factors affecting the incidence of ascites in broilers. Proc. Georgia Nutr. Conference.

Dalloul, R.A., Lillehoj, H.S. and Doerr, J.A. (2000) Effect of vitamin A deficiency on local and systemic immune responses of broiler chickens. Poult. Sci. 79(1):98–99.

Dalloul, R.A., Lillehoj, H.S., Shellem, T.A. and Doerr, J.A. (2002) Effect of vitamin A deficiency on host intestinal immune response to *Eimeria Acervulina* in broiler chickens. Poult. Sci. 81(10):1509–1515. https://doi.org/10.1093/ps/81.10.1509.

Dalloul, R.A. and Lillehoj, H.S. (2005) Recent advances in immunomodulation and vaccination against coccidiosis. Avian Dis. 49(1):8. https://doi.org/10.1637/7306-11150R.

Damaziak, K., Michalczuk, M., Zdanowska-Sąsiadek, Ż, Niemiec, J. and Gozdowski, D. (2015) Variation in growth performance and carcass yield of pure and reciprocal crossbred turkeys. Ann. Anim. Sci. 15(1): 51–66. https://doi.org/10.2478/aoas-2014-0058.

Damjanov, I., Neilsen, S.W., Van der Heide, L. and Eaton, H.D. (1980) Testicular changes of acute vitamin A deficiency of cockerels. Am. J. Vet. Res. 41(4):586–590. PMID: 7406277.

Danikowski, S., Sallmann, H.P., Halle, I. and Flachowsky, G. (2002) Influence of high levels of vitamin E on semen parameters of cocks. J. Anim. Physiol. Anim. Nutr. (Berl) 86(11–12):376–382. https://doi.org/10.1046/j.1439-0396.2002.00396.x.

Darby, W.J., McNutt, K.W. and Todhunter, E.N. (1975) Niacin. Nutr. Rev. 33(10):289–297. https://doi.org/10.1111/j.1753-4887.1975.tb05075.x.

Daryabari, H., Akhlaghi, A., Zamiri, M.J., Mianji, G.R., Pirsaraei, Z.A., Deldar, H. and Eghbalian, A.N. (2014) Reproductive performance and oviductal expression of avidin and avidin-related protein-2 in young and old broiler breeder hens orally exposed to supplementary biotin. Poult. Sci. 93(9):2289–2295. https://doi.org/10.3382/ps.2013-03862.

Das, R., Mishra, P. and Jha, R. (2021) *In ovo* feeding as a tool for improving performance and gut health of poultry: a review. Front. Vet. Sci. 8:754246. https://doi.org/10.3389/fvets.2021.754246.

Dash, S.K. and Mitchell, D.J. (1976) Storage, processing reduce vitamin A. Anim. Nutr. Health 31(7):16.

Davelaar, F.G. and Van Den Bos, J. (1992) Ascorbic acid and infectious bronchitis infections in broilers. Avian Pathol. 21(4):581–589. https://doi.org/10.1080/03079459208418879.

David, V., Dai, B., Martin, A., Huang, J., Han, X. and Quarles, L.D. (2013) Calcium regulates FGF-23 expression in bone. Endocrinology 154(12):4469–4482. https://doi.org/10.1210/en.2013-1627.

Davis, C.Y. and Sell, J.L. (1989) Immunoglobulin concentrations in serum and tissues of vitamin A-deficient broiler chicks after Newcastle disease virus vaccination. Poult. Sci. 68(1):136–144. https://doi.org/10.3382/ps.0680136.

Dawson, E., Ferguson, T.M., Deyoe, C.W. and Couch, J. (1962) Pantothenic acid deficient turkey embryos. Poult. Sci. 41:1639.

De Boer-van den Berg, M.A., Verstijnen, C.P. and Vermeer, C. (1986) Vitamin K-dependent carboxylase in skin. J. Invest. Dermatol. 87(3):377–380. https://doi.org/10.1111/1523-1747.ep12524848.

De la Huerga, J. and Popper, H. (1952) Factors influencing choline absorption in the intestinal tract. J. Clin. Invest. 31(6):598–603. https://doi.org/10.1172/JCI102646.

De Lima, M.B., Da Silva, E.P., Pereira, R., Romano, G.G., De Freitas, L.W., Dias, C.T.S. and Menten, J.F.M. (2018) Estimate of choline nutritional requirements for chicks from 1 to 21 days of age. J. Anim. Physiol. Anim. Nutr. (Berl) 102(3):780–788. https://doi.org/10.1111/jpn.12881.

De Winne, A. and Dirinck, P. (1996) Studies on vitamin E and meat quality. 2. Effect of feeding high vitamin E levels on chicken meat quality. J. Agric. Food Chem. 44(7):1691–1696. https://doi.org/10.1021/jf9506848.

Decuypere, E., Vega, C., Bartha, T., Buyse, J., Zoons, J. and Albers, G.A. (1994) Increased sensitivity to triiodothyronine (T3) of broiler lines with a high susceptibility for ascites. Br. Poult. Sci. 35(2):287–297. https://doi.org/10.1080/00071669408417693.

Degkwitz, E. (1987) Some effects of vitamin C may be indirect, since it affects the blood levels of cortisol and thyroid hormones. Ann. NY Acad. Sci. 498(1):470–472. https://doi.org/10.1111/j.1749-6632.1987.tb23786.x.

DeLuca, H.F. (2008) Evolution of our understanding of vitamin D. Nutr. Rev. 66(10) Supplement 2:S73-S87. https://doi.org/10.1111/j.1753-4887.2008.00105.x.

DeLuca, H.F. (2014) History of the discovery of vitamin D and its active metabolites. BoneKEy Rep. 3:479. https://doi.org/10.1038/bonekey.2013.213.

DeLuca, H.F. and Zierold, C. (1998) Mechanisms and functions of vitamin D. Nutr. Rev. 56(2 Pt 2):S4–10; discussion S 54. https://doi.org/10.1111/j.1753-4887.1998.tb01686.x.

DeLuca, H.F., Uyeda, J.A., Mericq, V., Mancilla, E.E., Yanovski, J.A., Barnes, K.M., Zile, M.H. and Baron, J. (2000) Retinoic acid is a potent regulator of growth plate chondrogenesis. Endocrinology 141(1):346–353. https://doi.org/10.1210/endo.141.1.7283.

Denisova, N.A. and Booth, S.L. (2005) Vitamin K and sphingolipid metabolism: evidence to date. Nutr. Rev. 63(4):111–121. https://doi.org/10.1111/j.1753-4887.2005.tb00129.x.

Denton, C.A., Kellog, W.L., Sizemore, J.R. and Lillie, R.J. (1954) Effect of injecting and feeding vitamin B_{12} to hens on content of the vitamin in the egg and blood. J. Nutr. 54(4):571–577. https://doi.org/10.1093/jn/54.4.571.

Derilo, Y.L. and Balnave, D. (1980) The choline and sulphur amino acid requirements of broiler chickens fed on semi-purified diets. Br. Poult. Sci. 21(6):479–487. https://doi.org/10.1080/00071668008416700.

Desoky, A.A. (2018) Growth performance and immune response of broiler chickens reared under high stocking density and vitamin E supplementation. Egypt. Poult. Sci. J. 38(2):607–620.

Deyhim, F. and Teeter, R.G. (1993) Dietary vitamin and/or trace mineral premix effects on performance, humoral mediated immunity, and carcass composition of broilers during thermoneutral and high ambient temperature distress. J. Appl. Poult. Res. 2(4):347–355. https://doi.org/10.1093/japr/2.4.347.

Deyhim, F. and Teeter, R.G. (1996) Vitamin withdrawal effects on performance, carcass composition, and tissue vitamin concentration of broilers exposed to various stress types. Poult. Sci. 75(1):113. https://doi.org/10.3382/ps.0750201.

Deyhim, F., Wiernusz, C.J., Belay, T., Teeter, R.G., Coelho, M.B. and Halley, J.T. (1990) Riboflavin and pantothenic acid requirement of broilers through eight weeks post hatching. Poult. Sci. 69(1):195–201. PMID: 19921444882.

Deyhim, F., Wiernusz, C.J., Belay, T., Teeter, R.G., Coelho, M.B. and Halley, J.T. (1991) A re-evaluation of the male broilers riboflavin and pantothenic acid dietary requirement in thermoneutral and heat distress environment. Poult. Sci. 70(1):157.

Deyhim, F., Belay, T. and Teeter, R.G. (1992) An elevation of dietary pantothenic acid needs of broilers through eight weeks posthatching. Nutr. Res. 12(12):1549–1554. https://doi.org/10.1016/S0271-5317(05)80195-2.

Deyhim, F., d'Offay, J.M. and Teeter, R.G. (1994) The effects of heat distress environment and vitamin or trace mineral supplementation on growth and cell mediated immunity in broiler chickens. Nutr. Res. 14(4):587–592. https://doi.org/10.1016/S0271-5317(05)80222-2.

Deyhim, F., Stoecker, B.S., Adeleye, B.G. and Teeter, R.G. (1995) The effects of heat distress environment, vitamin, and trace mineral supplementation on performance, blood constituents, and tissue mineral concentration in broiler chickens. Nutr. Res. 15(4):521–526. https://doi.org/10.1016/0271-5317(95)00019-4.

Deyhim, F., Stoecker, B.J. and Teeter, R.G. (1996) Vitamin and trace mineral withdrawal effects on broiler breast tissue riboflavin and thiamin content. Poult. Sci. 75(2):201–202. https://doi.org/10.3382/ps.0750201.

Dhur, A., Galan, P. and Hercberg, S. (1991) Folate status and the immune system. Prog. Food Nutr. Sci. 15(1–2):43–60. PMID: 1887065.

Diaz, V.E.S.M. (2018). Effects of 1-α-hydroxycholecalciferol and other vitamin D analogs on live performance, bone development, meat yield and quality, and mineral digestibility on broilers.

Díazí-Cruz, A., Avila, G.E., Guinzberg, P.R. and Iña, E.P. (2001) Effects of vitamins E and C and lipoic acid on productive performance and oxidative stress in broiler chicks. 13th Eur. Symp. Poult. Nutr., Blankenberge, Belgium. (p. 335).

Dickson, T.M., Tactacan, G.B., Hebert, K., Guenter, W. and House, J.D. (2010) Optimization of folate deposition in eggs through dietary supplementation of folic acid over the entire production cycle of Hy-line W36, Hy-line W98, and CV20 laying hens. J. Appl. Poult. Res. 19(1):80–91. https://doi.org/10.3382/japr.2009-00099.

Dikicioglu, T., Yigit, A.A. and Ozdemir, E. (2000) The effects of niacin on egg production and egg quality. Lalahan Hayvancilik Araştırma Enstitüsü Derg. 40(2):65–74.

Dilger, R.N., Garrow, T.A. and Baker, D.H. (2007) Betaine can partially spare choline in chicks but only when added to diets containing a minimal level of choline. J. Nutr. 137(10):2224–2228. https://doi.org/10.1093/jn/137.10.2224.

Dimanov, D.J., Petkov, G.S., Georgiev, S.G. and Mitev, J.E. (1994) Influence of selenium and ascorbic acid on the activity of plasma glutathione peroxidase and peroxidase resistance of erythrocyte lipids in chickens. Proc. 9th Eur. Poult. Nutrerence, Glasgow, UK. (pp. 183–185).

Dinev, I. (2012a) Clinical and morphological investigations on the incidence of forms of rickets and their association with other pathological states in broiler chickens. Res. Vet. Sci. 92(2):273–277. https://doi.org/10.1016/j.rvsc.2011.02.011.

Dinev, I. (2012b) Leg weakness pathology in broiler chickens. J. Poult. Sci. 49(2):63–67. https://doi.org/10.2141/jpsa.011109.

Doan, B.H. (2000) Effects of different levels of dietary calcium and supplemental vitamin C on growth, survivability, leg abnormalities, total ash in the tibia, serum calcium and phosphorus in 0–4 week old chicks under tropical conditions. Livest. Res. Rural Dev. 12(1). http://www.lrrd.org/lrrd12/1/doa121.htm.

Dobson, D.C. (1970) Biotin requirement of turkey poults. Poult. Sci. 49(2):546–553. https://doi.org/10.3382/ps.0490546.

Doerr, J.A. (1987) Influence of aflatoxin on broiler nutrition: where do we go from here? Proc. of the Arkansas Nutrition Conference, North Little Rock, Arkansas. (p. 48).

Dolgorukova, A.M., Titov, V.Y., Fisinin, V.I. and Zotov, A.A. (2020) Prenatal nutrition of poultry and its postnatal effects (review). Agric. Biol. 55(6):1061–1072. https://doi.org/10.15389/agrobiology.2020.6.1061eng.

Donaldson, W.E. (1986) Interaction of lead toxicity and riboflavin status in chicks (*Gallus domesticus*). Comp. Biochem. Physiol. C Comp. Pharmacol. Toxicol. 85(1):1–3. https://doi.org/10.1016/0742-8413(86)90042-3.

Donaldson, W.E., Wineland, M.J. and Christensen, V.I. (1996) The effect of flock age and egg storage on fatty acid composition of yolk membranes from two broiler crosses. Poult. Sci. 75(1):5.

Dong, X.F., Zhai, Q.H. and Tong, J.M. (2019) Dietary choline supplementation regulated lipid profiles of egg yolk, blood, and liver and improved hepatic redox status in laying hens. Poult. Sci. 98(8):3304–3312. https://doi.org/10.3382/ps/pez139.

Donnez, J., Dolmans, M.M., Pellicer, A., Diaz-Garcia, C., Ernst, E., Macklon, K.T. and Andersen, C.Y. (2015) Fertility preservation for age-related fertility decline. Lancet 385(9967): 506–507. https://doi.org/10.1016/S0140-6736(15)60198-2.

Dos Santos, E.O., Freitas, E.R., Nepomuceno, R.C., Watanabe, P.H., Souza, D.H., Fernandes, D.R., Freita, C.A., Nascimiento, G.A.J., Costa-Aguiar, G. and de Melo, M.C.A. (2021) Organic zinc and manganese and 25-hydroxycholecalciferol improves eggshell thickness in late-phase laying hens. Trop. Anim. Health Prod. 53(6):1–9. https://doi.org/10.1007/s11250-021-02959-x.

Dove, C.R. and Ewan, R.C. (1991) Effect of trace minerals on the stability of vitamin E in swine grower diets. J. Anim. Sci. 69(5):1994–2000. https://doi.org/10.2527/1991.6951994x.

Downs, K.M., Hess, J.B ,Macklin, K.S. and Norton, P.A.(1999) The effectiveness of dietary vitamin E and organic zinc complexes for reducing the incidence of cellulitis. J. Appl. Poult. Res. 78(3):319–323. https://doi.org/10.1093/japr/9.3.319.

Downs, K.M., Norton, P.A., Macklin, K.S. and Hess, J.B. (2000) The influence of supplemental vitamin E and zinc-amino acid complex on avian cellulitis. Poult. Sci. 23(1):108.

Driver, J.P., Pesti, G.M., Bakalli, R.I. and Edwards, H.M. (2005) Phytase and 1-α-hydroxycholecalciferol supplementation of broiler chickens during the starting and growing/finishing phases. Poult. Sci. 84(10):1616–1628. https://doi.org/10.1093/ps/84.10.1616.

Driver, J.P., Atencio, A., Pesti, G.M., Edwards, H.M. and Bakalli, R.I. (2006) The effect of maternal dietary vitamin D_3 supplementation on performance and tibial dyschondroplasia of broiler chicks. Poult. Sci. 85(1):39–47. https://doi.org/10.1093/ps/85.1.39.

DSM Nutritional Products (2022) OVN Optimum Vitamin Nutrition® guidelines. https://www.dsm.com/anh/products-and-services/tools/ovn.html.

Dudley-Cash, W.A. (1994) Supplemental vitamin use in poultry feeds varies considerably. Feedstuffs 66(6):12.

Du, M. and Ahn, D.U. (2002) Effect of antioxidants on the quality of irradiated sausages prepared with turkey thigh meat. Poult. Sci. 81(8):1251–1256. https://doi.org/10.1093/ps/81.8.1251.

DuCoa, L.P. (1994) Choline functions and requirements. DuCoa L.P., Higland, IL.

Dunn, N. (1996) The vital vitamin boost for broilers under stress. World Poult. Sci. 12(6):45–47.

Dunnington, E.A. and Siegel, P.B. (1996) Long-term divergent selection for eight-week body weight in white Plymouth Rock chickens. Poult. Sci. 75(10):1168–1179. https://doi.org/10.3382/ps.0751168.

Dutta-Roy, A.K., Gordon, M.J., Campbell, F.M., Duthie, G.G. and James, W.P.T. (1994) Vitamin E requirements, transport, and metabolism: role of α-tocopherol-binding proteins. J. Nutr. Biochem. 5(12):562–570. https://doi.org/10.1016/0955-2863(94)90010-8.

Dzhambulatov, M.M., Viktorov, P.I., Alisheikhov, A.M. and Akhemedkhanova, R.R. (1996) Setting norms for vitamins C and B_{12} in feeds for laying hens and broiler chickens subjected to heat stress. Russ. Agric. Sci. 10:14–16.

Ebeid, T.A. (2012) Vitamin E and organic selenium enhances the antioxidative status and quality of chicken semen under high ambient temperature. Br. Poult. Sci. 53(5):708–714. https://doi.org/10.1080/00071668.2012.722192.

Eder, K., Skufca, P. and Brandsch, C. (2002) Thermally oxidized dietary fats increase plasma thyroxine concentrations in rats irrespective of the vitamin E and selenium supply. J. Nutr. 132(6):1275–1281. https://doi.org/10.1093/jn/132.6.1275.

Edrise, B.M., Khair El-Din, A.W. and Soliman, R. (1986) The immunopotentiating effect of ascorbic acid against Newcastle disease in chickens. Vet. Med. 34:251–264.

Edwards, H.M. (1989a) Effect of vitamin C, environmental temperature, chlortetracycline and vitamin D_3 on the development of tibial dyschondroplasia in chickens. Poult. Sci. 68(11):1527–1534. https://doi.org/10.3382/ps.0681527.

Edwards, H.M. (1989b) The effect of dietary cholecalciferol, 25-hydroxycholecalciferol and 1,25-dihydroxycholecalciferol on the development of tibial dyschondroplasia in broiler chickens in the absence and presence of disulfiram. J. Nutr. 119(4):647–652. https://doi.org/10.1093/jn/119.4.647.

Edwards, H.M. (1990) Efficacy of several vitamin D compounds in the prevention of tibial dyschondroplasia in broiler chickens. J. Nutr. 120(9):1054–1061. https://doi.org/10.1093/jn/120.9.1054.

Edwards, H.M. (1992) Nutritional factors and leg disorders. In Bone biology and skeletal disorders in poultry. 10 Whitehead, C.C. (ed.). Carfax Pub., Oxfordshire, UK. (pp. 167–193).

Edwards, H.M. (1993) Dietary 1,25-dihydroxycholecalciferol supplementation increases natural phytate phosphorus utilization in chickens. J. Nutr. 123(3):567–577. https://doi.org/10.1093/jn/123.3.567.

Edwards, H.M. (1995a) Factors influencing leg disorders in broilers. Proc. Maryland Nutrition Conference. Feed Ind. Council:(21–19).

Edwards, H.M. (1995b) Efficacy of several vitamin D compounds in increasing phytate phosphorus utilization in chickens. Poult. Sci. 74(1):107.

Edwards, H.M. (1999) Responses to vitamin D_3 metabolites tend to vary. Feedstuffs 5:14–15.

Edwards, H.M. (2000) Nutrition and skeletal problems in poultry. Poult. Sci. 79(7):1018–1023. https://doi.org/10.1093/ps/79.7.1018.

Edwards, H.M. (2002) Studies on the efficacy of cholecalciferol and derivatives for stimulating phytate utilization in broilers. Poult. Sci. 81(7):1026–1031. https://doi.org/10.1093/ps/81.7.1026.

Edwards, H.M., Elliot, M.A. and Sooncharernying, S. (1992a) Effect of dietary calcium on tibial dyschondroplasia. Interaction with light, cholecalciferol, 1,25-dihydroxycholecalciferol, protein, and synthetic zeolite Poult. Sci. 71(12):2041–2055. https://doi.org/10.3382/ps.0712041.

Edwards, H.M., Elliot, M.A. and Sooncharernying, S. (1992b) Quantitative substitution of 1,25-dihydroxycholecalciferol and 1-hydroxycholecalciferol for cholecalciferol in broiler diets. 19th World´s Poultr. Congress, Amsterdam. (pp. 567–571).

Edwards, H.M., Elliot, M.A., Sooncharernying, S. and Britton, W.M. (1994) Quantitative requirement for cholecalciferol in the absence of ultraviolet light. Poult. Sci. 73(2):288–294. https://doi.org/10.3382/ps.0730288.

Edwards, H.M., Shirley, R.B., Escoe, W.B. and Pesti, G.M. (2002) Quantitative evaluation of 1-α-hydroxycholecalciferol as a cholecalciferol substitute for broilers. Poult. Sci. 81(5):664–669. https://doi.org/10.1093/ps/81.5.664.

Edwards, H.M., Shirley, R.B., Atencio, A. and Pesti, G.M. (2004) Effect of dietary Ca levels on the efficacy of 1-α-hydroxycholecalciferol in the diets of young broilers. Proc. 22nd World's Poult. Congress, Paris, France.

Eggersdorfer, M., Laudert, D., Létinois, U., McClymont, T., Medlock, J., Netscher, T. and Bonrath, W. (2012) One hundred years of vitamins a success story of the natural sciences. Angew. Chem. Int. Ed. Engl. 51(52):12960–12990. https://doi.org/10.1002/anie.201205886.

Eichner, G., Vieira, S.L., Torres, C.A., Coneglian, J.L.B., Freitas, D.M. and Oyarzabal, O.A. (2007) Litter moisture and footpad dermatitis as affected by diets formulated on an all-vegetable basis or having the inclusion of poultry by-product. J. Appl. Poult. Res. 16(3):344–350. https://doi.org/10.1093/japr/16.3.344.

Eid, Y., Ebeid, T. and Younis, H. (2006) Vitamin E supplementation reduces dexamethasone- induced oxidative stress in chicken semen. Br. Poult. Sci. 47(3):350–356. https://doi.org/10.1080/00071660600753912.

Ekanayake, A. and Nelson, P.E. (1990) Effect of thermal processing on lima bean vitamin B_6 availability. J. Food Sci. 55(1):154–157. https://doi.org/10.1111/j.1365-2621.1990.tb06040.x.

Ekstrand, C., Algers, B. and Svedberg, J. (1997) Rearing conditions and foot-pad dermatitis in Swedish broiler chickens. Prev. Vet. Med. 31(3–4):167–174. https://doi.org/10.1016/S0167-5877(96)01145-2.

Ekunseitan, D.A., Yusuf, A.O., Ekunseitan, O.F., Alao, S.O. and Allinson, A.Z. (2021) Dietary supplementation of vitamin E and selenium on performance and oxidative stability of meat of broiler chickens in a hot climate. Agric. Trop. Subtrop. 54(1):24–31. https://doi.org/10.2478/ats-2021-0003.

Elad, O., Uribe-Diaz, S., Losada-Medina, D., Yitbarek, A., Sharif, S. and Rodriguez-Lecompte, J.C. (2020) Epigenetic effect of folic acid (FA) on the gene proximal promoter area and mRNA expression of chicken B cell as antigen presenting cells. Br. Poult. Sci. 61(6):725–733. https://doi.org/10.1080/00071668.2020.1799332.

Elaroussi, M.A., Uhland-Smith, A., Hellwig, W. and DeLuca, H.F. (1994) The role of vitamin D in chorioallantoic membrane calcium transport. Biochim. Biophys. Acta 1192(1):1–6. https://doi.org/10.1016/0005-2736(94)90135-x.

El-Garhy, O.H., El-Gendi, G.M. and Okasha, H.M. (2019) Effect of housing system and dietary biotin supplementation on productive performance, some blood constituents and economic efficiency of Benha line chicken. Egypt. Poult. Sci. J. 39(1):219–234. https://doi.org/10.21608/epsj.2019.29132.

El-Husseiny, O.M., Abo-El-Ella, M.A., Abd-Elsamee, M.O., Magda, M. and Abd-Elfattah, M.M. (2007) Response of broilers performance to dietary betaine and folic acid at different methionine levels. Int. J. Poult. Sci. 6(7):515–523. https://doi.org/10.3923/ijps.2007.515.523.

El-Husseiny, O.M., Soliman, A.Z., Omara, I.I. and El – Sheri, H.M.R. (2008a) Evaluation of dietary methionine, folic acid and cyanocobalamin (B_{12}) and their interactions in laying hen performance. Int. J. Poult. Sci. 7(5):461–469. https://doi.org/10.3923/ijps.2008.461.469.

El-Husseiny, O.M., Abd-Elsame, M.O., Omara, I.I. and Fouad, A.M. (2008b) Effect of dietary zinc and niacin on laying hens performance and egg quality. Int. J. Poult. Sci. 7(8):757–764. https://doi.org/10.3923/ijps.2008.757.764.

El-Hussein, O.M., Soliman, A.Z.M. and Elsherif, H.M.R. (2018) Influence of dietary methionine, folic acid and cyanocobalamin and their interactions on the performance of broiler breeder. Int. J. Poult. Sci. 17(4):189–196. https://doi.org/10.3923/ijps.2018.189.196.

Elliot, M.A. and Edwards, H.M. (1994) Effect of genetic strain, calcium, and feed withdrawal on growth, tibial dyschondroplasia, plasma 1,25-dihydroxycholecalciferol, and plasma 25-hydroxycholecalciferol in sixteen-day-old chickens. Poult. Sci. 73(4):509–519. https://doi.org/10.3382/ps.0730509.

Elliot, M.A. and Edwards, H.M. (1997) Effect of 1,25-dihydroxycholecalciferol, cholecalciferol, and fluorescent lights on the development of tibial dyschondroplasia and rickets in broiler chickens. Poult. Sci. 76(4):570–580. https://doi.org/10.1093/ps/76.4.570.

Elliot, M.A., Roberson, K.D., Rowland, G.N. and Edwards, H.M. (1995) Effects of dietary calcium and 1,25-dihydroxycholecalciferol on the development of tibial dyschondroplasia in broilers during the starter and grower periods. Poult. Sci. 74(9):1495–1505. https://doi.org/10.3382/ps.0741495.

Elmadfa, I., Majchrzak, D., Rust, P. and Genser, D. (2001) The thiamine status of adult humans depends on carbohydrate intake. Int. J. Vitam. Nutr. Res. 71(4):217–221. https://doi.org/10.1024/0300-9831.71.4.217.

El-Senousey, H.K., Chen, B., Wang, J.Y., Atta, A.M., Mohamed, F.R. and Nie, Q.H. (2018) *In ovo* injection of ascorbic acid modulates antioxidant defense system and immune gene expression in newly hatched local Chinese yellow broiler chicks. Poult. Sci. 97(2):425–429. https://doi.org/10.3382/ps/pex310.

Elvehjem, C. A., Madden, R.J., Strong, F.M. and Wolley, D.W. (2002) The isolation and identification of the anti-black tongue factor. 1937, in J. Biol. Chem, 277(34)e22.

Emmert, J.L. and Baker, D.H. (1997) A chick bioassay approach for determining the bioavailable choline concentration in normal and overheated soybean meal, canola meal and peanut meal. J. Nutr. 127(5):745–752. https://doi.org/10.1093/jn/127.5.745.

Emmert, J.L., Garrow, T.A. and Baker, D.H. (1996) Development of an experimental diet for determining bioavailable choline concentration and its application in studies with soybean lecithin. J. Anim. Sci. 74(11):2738–2744. https://doi.org/10.2527/1996.74112738x.

Engelmann, D., Flachowsky, G., Halle, I. and Sallmann, H.P. (2001) Effects of feeding high dosages of vitamin E to laying hens on thyroid hormone concentrations of hatching chicks. J. Exp. Zool. 290(1):41–48. https://doi.org/10.1002/jez.1034.

Engberg, R.M., Lauridsen, C., Jensen, S.K. and Jakobsen, K. (1996) Inclusion of oxidized vegetable oil in broiler diets. Its influence on nutrient balance and on the antioxidative status of broilers. Poult. Sci. 75(8):1003–1011. https://doi.org/10.3382/ps.0751003.

Engstrom, G.W. and Littledike E.T. (1986) Vitamin D metabolism in the pig. In "Swine in biomedical research," Vol. 2 Tumbleson, M.E. (ed.). Plenum Press, New York.

Engstrom, G.W., Goff, J.P., Horst, R.L. and Reinhardt, T.A. (1987) Regulation of calf renal 25-hydroxyvitamin D- hydroxylase activities by calcium-regulating hormones. J. Dairy Sci. 70(11):2266–2271. https://doi.org/10.3168/jds.S0022-0302(87)80286-2.

Engström, A., Skerving, S., Lidfeldt, J., Burgaz, A., Lundh, T., Samsioe, G., Vahter, M. and Akesson, A. (2009) Cadmium-induced bone effect is not mediated via low serum 1,25-dihydroxy vitamin D. Environ. Res. 109(2):188–192. https://doi.org/10.1016/j.envres.2008.10.008.

Enkvetchakul, B., Bottje, W., Anthony, N., Moore, R. and Huff, W. (1993) Compromised antioxidant status associated with ascites in broilers. Poult. Sci. 72(12):2272–2280. https://doi.org/10.3382/ps.0722272.

Ensminger, A.H., Ensminger, M.E., Konlande, J.E. and Robson, J.R.K. (1983) In Ensminger, A.H. (ed.). 'Foods and Nutrition Encyclopedia', Ensminger pub., Colorado, USA.

Erf, G.F., Bottje, W.G., Bersi, T.K., Headrick, M.D. and Fritts, C.A. (1998) Effects of dietary vitamin E on the immune system in broilers: altered proportions of CD4 T cells in the thymus and spleen. Poult. Sci. 77(4):529–537. https://doi.org/10.1093/ps/77.4.529.

Erf, G.F., Noll, S., Bersi, T.K., Wang, X., Kalbfleisch, J., Bottje, W.G. and Erf, G.F. (2000) Effects of dietary vitamin E supplementation in young male turkey poults. II. Tissue levels of vitamin E, proportions and concentrations of immune cells. Poult. Sci. 79(1):47–48 (abstract).

Erhan, M.K. and Bölükbaşi, S.C. (2011) Effects of feeding diets supplemented with vitamin E and vitamin C on performance, egg quality and stereological and structural analysis of the liver of laying hens exposed to heat stress. Ital. J. Anim. Sci. 10(4):e58. https://doi.org/10.4081/2032.

Eslick, N.L., Ahn, D. and Sell, J. (1997) Effect of vitamin E and irradiation on tocopherol content and lipid oxidation of turkey breast and thigh meat. Poult. Sci. 75 (Suppl. 1):352.

Esmail, S.H.M. (2002) Nutrition is a major player in disease prevention. World Poult. 18(6):16–17.

Esmon, C.T., Sadowski, J.A. and Suttie, J.W. (1975) A new carboxylation reaction. The vitamin K-dependent incorporation of $H\text{-}_{14}\text{-}CO_3\text{-}$ into prothrombin. J. Biol. Chem. 250(12):4744–4748. https://doi.org/10.1016/S0021-9258(19)41365-3.

Esteban-Pretel, G., Marín, M.P., Renau-Piqueras, J., Barber, T. and Timoneda, J. (2010) Vitamin A deficiency alters rat lung alveolar basement membrane: reversibility by retinoic acid. J. Nutr. Biochem. 21(3): 227–236. https://doi.org/10.1016/j.jnutbio.2008.12.007.

Evans, W.C. (1975) Thiaminases and their effects on animals. Vitam. Horm. 33:467–504. https://doi.org/10.1016/S0083-6729(08)60970-X.

Eyles, D., Anderson, C., Ko, P., Jones, A., Thomas, A., Burne, T., Mortensen, P.B., Nørgaard-Pedersen, B., Hougaard, D.M. and McGrath, J. (2009) A sensitive LC/MS/MS assay of 25OH vitamin D_3 and 25OH vitamin D_2 in dried blood spots. Clin. Chim. Acta 403(1–2):145–151. https://doi.org/10.1016/j.cca.2009.02.005.

Falleiros, F.T., Oliveira Cesco, M.A., Temponi Lebre, D. and Luvizotto, J.M. (2019) 25-Hydroxycholecalciferol blood levels by dried blood spot (DBS) technology evaluation for broilers. Proc. Poult. Sci. Ass. Meeting, Montreal, Canada.

Fan, S., Han, Y. and Li, R. (1998) Effect of adding anti-oxidative micronutrients to the diets on the performance of layers exposed to high ambient temperature. Chin. J. Vet. Sci. 18(6):606–610.

Fan, X., Liu, S., Liu, G., Zhao, J., Jiao, H., Wang, X., Song, Z. and Lin, H. (2015) Vitamin A deficiency impairs mucin expression and suppresses the mucosal immune function of the respiratory tract in chicks. PLoS One 10(9):e0139131. https://doi.org/10.1371/journal.pone.0139131.

Fares, W.A., Ahmed, R.M.M. and El-Deken, M.R. (2018) Effect of vitamin K_3 on chicken production performance and bone quality 1. Late phase of egg production Egypt. Poult. Sci. 38(II):637–656. https://doi.org/10.21608/epsj.2018.22902.

Faria, D.E., Junqueira, O.M., Souza, P.A., Mazalli, M.R. and Salvador, D. (1999) Influence of different levels of vitamins D and C and age of laying hens on performance and egg quality. 1-summer. Rev. Bras. Cien. Avic. 1(3):193–201.

Farina, G., Kessler, AdM., Ebling, P.D., Marx, F.R., César, R. and Ribeiro, A.M.L. (2017) Performance of broilers fed different dietary choline sources and levels. Ciênc. anim. bras. 18:1–14. https://doi.org/10.1590/1089-6891v18e-37633.

Farqhuarson, C., Berny, E.B., Barbara-Mawer, E., Seawright, E. and Whitehead, C.C. (1998) Ascorbic acid-induced chondrocyte differentiation: the role of the extracellular matrix and 1,25 dihydroxycholecalciferols. Eur. J. Cell Biol. 76(2):110–118. https://doi.org/10.1016/S0171-9335(98)80023-X.

Farr, A.J., Salman, H.K., Krautmann, B.A., Gonzales, L. and Mcdonald, A. (1988) Effect of high level of vitamin C dosage 32 hours prior to slaughter on processing parameters of broiler chickens. Poult. Sci. 67(1):85.

Fatemi, S.A., Alqhtani, A.H., Elliott, K.E.C., Bello, A., Levy, A.W. and Peebles, E.D. (2021a) Improvement in the performance and inflammatory reaction of ross 708 broilers in response to the *in ovo* injection of 25-hydroxyvitamin D_3. Poult. Sci. 100(1):138–146. https://doi.org/10.1016/j.psj.2020.10.010.

Fatemi, S.A., Alqhtani, A., Elliott, K.E.C., Bello, A., Zhang, H. and Peebles, E.D. (2021b) Effects of the in ovo injection of vitamin D_3 and 25-hydroxyvitamin D_3 in Ross 708 broilers subsequently fed commercial or calcium and phosphorus-restricted diets. I. Performance, carcass characteristics and incidence of woody breast myopathy1,2,3. Poult. Sci. 100(8):101220. https://doi.org/10.1016/j.psj.2021.101220.

Fatemi, S.A., Elliott, K.E.C., Bello, A. and Peebles, E.D. (2021c) Effects of the in ovo injection of vitamin D_3 and 25-hydroxyvitamin D_3 in ross 708 broilers subsequently challenged with coccidiosis. I. Performance, meat yield and intestinal lesion incidence. Poult. Sci. 100(10):101382. https://doi.org/10.1016/j.psj.2021.101382.

FEDNA (Federacion Española para el Desarrollo Nutricion Animal) (2018) Necesidades nutricionales en avicultura: normas para la formulacion de piensos http://www.fundacionfedna.org/node/75.

FEFANA (EU association of specialty feed ingredients and their mixtures) (2015) Vitamins in animal nutrition https://fefana.org/app/uploads/2022/06/2015-04-15_booklet_vitamins.pdf.

Feingold, I.B. and Colby, H.D. (1992) Sex differences in adrenal and hepatic α-tocopherol concentrations in rats. Pharmacology 44(2):113–116. https://doi.org/10.1159/000138880.

Fell, H.B. and Thomas, L. (1960) Comparison of the effects of papain and vitamin A on cartilage. II. The effects on organ cultures of embryonic skeletal tissue. J. Exp. Med. 111(5):719–744. https://doi.org/10.1084/jem.111.5.719.

Fellenberg, M.A. and Speisky, H. (2006) Antioxidants: their effects on broiler oxidative stress and its meat oxidative stability. World Poult. Sci. J. 62(1):53–70. https://doi.org/10.1079/WPS200584.

Feng, Y.L., Xie, M., Tang, J., Huang, W., Zhang, Q. and Hou, S.S. (2019) Effects of vitamin A on growth performance and tissue retinol of starter white Pekin ducks. Poult. Sci. 98(5):2189–2192. https://doi.org/10.3382/ps/pey571.

Fenstermacher, D.K. and Rose, R.C. (1986) Absorption of pantothenic acid in rat and chick intestine. Am. J. Physiol. 250(2 Pt 1):G155-G160. https://doi.org/10.1152/ajpgi.1986.250.2.G155.

Ferguson, R.M. and Couch, J.R. (1954) Further gross observations on the B_{12} deficient chick embryo. J. Nutr. 54(3):361–370. https://doi.org/10.1093/jn/54.3.361.

Ferguson, T.M., Whiteside, C.H., Creger, C.R., Jones, M.L., Atkinson, R.L. and Couch, J.R. (1961) B-vitamin deficiency in the mature turkey hen. Poult. Sci. 40(5):1151–1159. https://doi.org/10.3382/ps.0401151.

Ferket, P.R. and Allen, E. (1994) How nutrition and management influence PSE in poultry meat. Broiler Ind. 57(9).

Ferket, P.R. and Qureshi, M.A. (1992) Performance and immunity of heat-stressed broilers fed vitamin- and electrolyte-supplemented drinking water. Poult. Sci. 71(1):88–97. https://doi.org/10.3382/ps.0710088.

Ferket, P.R. and Qureshi, M.A. (1999) The turkey immune system and nutritional immunomodulators. Proc. 12th Eur. Symp. Poult. Nutr., Veldhoven, The Netherlands. (pp. 17–29).

Ferket, P.R., Garlich, J.D. and Thomas, L.N. (1993) Dietary choline and labile methyl donor requirement of turkey poults. Poult. Sci. 72(1):13.

Ferland, G. (2006) Vitamin K. In "Present knowledge in nutrition" 9th edition Bowman, B.A. and Russell, R.M. (ed.). International Life Sciences Institute. (pp. 220–230).

Fernandes, J.I.M., Murakami, A.E., Scapinello, C., Moreira, I. and Varela, E.V. (2009) Effect of vitamin K on bone integrity and eggshell quality of white hen at the final phase of the laying cycle R. R. Bras. Zootec. 38(3):488–492. https://doi.org/10.1590/S1516-35982009000300013.

Fernandes, J.I.M., Prokoski, K., Oliveira, B.C., Oro, C.S., Oro, P.J. and Fernandes, N.L.M. (2016) Evaluation of incubation yield, vaccine response, and performance of broilers submitted to *in ovo* vaccination at different embryonic ages. Rev. Bras. Cienc. Avic. 18(spe2):55–63. https://doi.org/10.1590/1806-9061-2015-0216.

Fichter, S.A. and Mitchell, G.E. (1997) Sheep blood response to orally supplemented vitamin K dissolved in coconut oil. J. Anim. Sci. 72(1):266 (abstr.).

Finkelstein, J.D., Martin, J.J., Harris, B.J. and Kyle, W.E. (1982) Regulation of the betaine content of rat liver. Arch. Biochem. Biophys. 218(1):169–173. https://doi.org/10.1016/0003-9861(82)90332-0.

Fisher, C. and Willemsen, M.H.A. (1999) Nutrition of broiler breeders. In "Recent advances in animal nutrition" Garnsworthy, P.C. and Wiseman, J. (ed.). Nottingham University Press, Nottingham. (pp. 165–168).

Fisher, C. and Kemp, C. (2000) Impact of breeder nutrition on broiler performance. Int. Hatchery Pract. 15:13–15.

Fisher, H.H. (1974) Niacin requirements. Proc. Roche Symposium. (pp. 11–29).

Flachowsky, G., Engelman, D., Sünder, A., Halle, I. and Sallmann, H.P. (2002) Eggs and poultry meat as tocopherol sources in dependence on tocopherol supplementation of poultry diets. Food Res. Int. 35(2–3):239–243. https://doi.org/10.1016/S0963-9969(01)00191-0.

Fleming, R.H., McCormack, H.A. and Whitehead, C.C. (1998) Bone structure and strength at different ages in laying hens and effects of dietary particulate limestone, vitamin K and ascorbic acid. Br. Poult. Sci. 39(3):434–440. https://doi.org/10.1080/00071669889024.

Fleming, R.H., McCormack, H.A., McTeir, L. and Whitehead, C.C. (2003) Effects of dietary particulate limestone, vitamin K3 and fluoride and photostimulation on skeletal morphology and osteoporosis in laying hens. Br. Poult. Sci. 44(5):683–689. https://doi.org/10.1080/00071660310001643688.

Fletcher, D.L. and Cason, J.A. (1991) Influence of ascorbic acid on broiler shrink and processing yields. Poult. Sci. 70(10):2191–2196. https://doi.org/10.3382/ps.0702191.

Flores-Garcia, W. (1992) Einfluß verschiedener B-vitamine, speziell des riboflavins, auf reproduktionsmerkmale bei legehennen. Agricultural dissertation.

Flores-Garcia, W. and Scholtyssek, S. (1992) Effects of levels of riboflavin in the diet on the reproductivity of layer-breeding stocks. Proc. World's 19th World's Poult. Congress, Amsterdam the Netherlands. (pp. 622–623).

Florou-Paneri, P., Dotas, D., Mitsopoulos, I., Dotas, V., Botsoglou, E., Nikolakakis, I. and Botsoglou, N. (2006) Effect of feeding rosemary and alpha-tocopheryl acetate on hen performance and egg quality. J. Poult. Sci. 43(2):143–149. https://doi.org/10.2141/jpsa.43.143.

Folegatti, E., Sirri, F., Meluzzi, A. and Toscani, T.T. (2006) Prevalence of foot pad lesions and carcass injuries as indicators of broiler welfare conditions in Italy. Proc. 12th Eur. Poultry Conf.

Fox, H.M. (1991) Pantothenic acid. In "Handbook of vitamins" 2nd edition Machlin, L.J. (ed.). Marcel Dekker, New York. (pp. 429–451).

Franceschi, R.T. (1992) The role of ascorbic acid in mesenchymal differentiation. Nutr. Rev. 50(3):65–70. https://doi.org/10.1111/j.1753-4887.1992.tb01271.x.

Franchini, A., Bertuzzi, S. and Meluzzi, A. (1986) The influence of high doses of vitamin E on immune response of chicks to inactivated oil adjuvant vaccine. Clin. Vet. 109:117–127.

Franchini, A. and Bertuzzi, S. (1991) Micronutrients and immune functions. 8th Eur. Symp. on Poult. Nutr., Venezia, Italy. (pp. 63–80).

Franchini, A., Canti, M., Manfreda, G., Bertuzzi, S., Asdrubali, G. and Franciosi, C. (1991) Vitamin E as adjuvant in emulsified vaccine for chicks. Poult. Sci. 70(8):1709–1715. https://doi.org/10.3382/ps.0701709.

Franchini, A., Bertuzzi, S., Tosarelli, C., Ianelli, S., Nanni-Costa, A. and Stefoni, S. (1994) Chronobiological influence of vitamin C on chicken immune functions. Archiv. Geflugelk 58:165–170.

Franchini, A., Bertuzzi, S., Tosarelli, C. and Manfreda, G. (1995) Vitamin E in viral inactivated vaccines. Poult. Sci. 74(4):666–671. https://doi.org/10.3382/ps.0740666.

Franchini, A., Bergonzoni, M.L., Melotti, D. and Minelli, G. (2001) The effects of dietary supplementation with high doses of vitamin E and C on the quality traits of chicken semen. Arch. Geflügelk 65(2):76–81.

Franchini, A., Sirri, F., Tallarico, N., Minelli, G., Iaffaldano, N. and Meluzzi, A. (2002) Oxidative stability and sensory and functional properties of eggs from laying hens fed supranutritional doses of vitamins E and C. Poult. Sci. 81(11):1744–1750. https://doi.org/10.1093/ps/81.11.1744.

Frank, J., Weiser, H. and Biesalski, H.K. (1997) Interaction of vitamins E and K: effect of high dietary vitamin E on phylloquinone activity in chicks. Int. J. Vitam. Nutr. Res. 67(4):242–247. PMID: 9285253.

Fraser, D.R. (2021) Vitamin D toxicity related to its physiological and unphysiological supply. Trends Endocrinol. Metab. 32(11):929–940. https://doi.org/10.1016/j.tem.2021.08.006.

Fraser, D.R. and Emtage, J.S. (1976) Vitamin-D in avian egg its molecular identity and mechanism of incorporation into yolk. Biochem. J. 160(3):671–682. https://doi.org/10.1042/bj1600671.

Frei, B., England, L. and Ames, B.N. (1989) Ascorbate is an outstanding antioxidant in human blood plasma. Proc. Natl. Acad. Sci. U. S. A. 86(16):6377–6381. https://doi.org/10.1073/pnas.86.16.6377.

Freiser, H. and Jiang, Q. (2009) Optimization of the enzymatic hydrolysis and analysis of plasma conjugated gamma-CEHC and sulfated long-chain carboxychromanols, metabolites of vitamin E. Anal. Biochem. 388(2):260–265. https://doi.org/10.1016/j.ab.2009.02.027.

Friedman, A. and Sklan, D. (1989) Antigen-specific immune response impairment in the chick as influenced by dietary vitamin A. J. Nutr. 119(5):790–795. https://doi.org/10.1093/jn/119.5.790.

Friedman, A. and Sklan, D. (1997) Effects of retinoids on immune response impairment in birds. Word Poult. Sci. 53(2):185–195. https://doi.org/10.1079/WPS19970016.

Friedman, A., Meidovsky, A., Leitner, G. and Sklan, D. (1991) Decreased resistance and immune response to *E. coli* infection in chickens with low and high intakes of vitamin A. J. Nutr. 121(3):395–400. https://doi.org/10.1093/jn/121.3.395.

Friedman, A., Bartov, I. and Sklan, D. (1998) Humoral immune response impairment following excess vitamin E nutrition in the chick and turkey. Poult. Sci. 77(7):956–962. https://doi.org/10.1093/ps/77.7.956.

Friedrichsen, J.V., Arscott, G.H. and Willis, D.L. (1980) Improvement in fertility of white leghorn males by vitamin E following a prolonged deficiency. Nutr. Rep. Int. 22:41.

Friesecke, H. (1980). Vitamin B_{12}. 1728. F Hoffmann-La Roche, and Co., Ltd, Basel.

Frigg, M. (1976) Bio-availability of biotin in cereals. Poult. Sci. 55(6):2310–2318. https://doi.org/10.3382/ps.0552310.

Frigg, M. (1984) Available biotin content of various feed ingredients. Poult. Sci. 63(4):750–753. https://doi.org/10.3382/ps.0630750.

Frigg, M. (1987) Biotin in poultry and swine rations and its significance for optimum performance. Proc. Maryland Nutr. Conf. (pp. 101–108).

Frigg, M. and Volker, L. (1994) Biotin inclusion helps optimize animal performance. Feedstuffs 66(1):12–13.

Frigg, M., Whitehead, C.C. and Weber, S. (1992) Absence of effects of dietary alpha- tocopherol on egg yolk pigmentation. Br. Poult. Sci. 33(2):347–353. https://doi.org/10.1080/00071669208417473.

Fritts, C.A. and Waldroup, P.W. (2003) Effect of source and level of vitamin D on live performance and bone development in growing broilers. J. Appl. Poult. Res. 12(1):45–52. https://doi.org/10.1093/japr/12.1.45.

Fritts, C.A. and Waldroup, P.W. (2005) Comparison of cholecalciferol and 25-hydroxycholecalciferol in broiler diets designed to minimize phosphorus excretion. J. Appl. Poult. Res. 14(1):156–166. https://doi.org/10.1093/japr/14.1.156.

Fritts, C.A., Erf, G.F., Bersi, T.K. and Waldroup, P.W. (2004) Effect of source and level of vitamin D on immune function in growing broilers. J. Appl. Poult. Res. 13(2):263–273. https://doi.org/10.1093/japr/13.2.263.

Fritz, J.C., Mislivec, P.B., Pla, G.W., Harrison, B.N., Weeks, C.E. and Dantzman, J.G. (1973) Toxicogenicity of moldy feed for young chicks. Poult. Sci. 52(4):1523–1530. https://doi.org/10.3382/ps.0521523.

Frost, T.J., Roland, D.A.S. and Untawale, G.G. (1990) Influence of vitamin D_3, 1alpha-hydroxyvitamin D_3, and 1,25-dihydroxyvitamin D_3 on eggshell quality, tibia strength, and various production parameters in commercial laying hens. Poult. Sci. 69(11):2008–2016. https://doi.org/10.3382/ps.0692008.

Frost, T.J., Roland, D.A.S. and Marple, D.N. (1991 The Effects of Various Dietary Phosphorus Levels on the Circadian Patterns of Plasma 1,25-Dihydroxycholecalciferol, Total Calcium, Ionized Calcium, and Phosphorus in Laying Hens Poult. Sci. 70(7):1564–1570. https://doi.org/10.3382/ps.0701564.

Frye, T.M. (1978). Vitamin compatibility in custom premixes. In Proceedings of the Roche Vitamin Update Meeting, Arkansas Nutrition Conference. RCD 5483/1078., Hoffman La Roche, Nutley, NJ. (pp. 70–79).

Frye, T.M. (1994) The performance of vitamins in multicomponent premixes. Proc. Roche Technical Symposium.

Fuhrmann, H. and Sallmann, H.P. (1995) α-tocopherol and phospholipase A_2 in liver and brain of chicks post hatching: the influence of dietary fat and vitamin E. Ann. Nutr. Metab. 39(5):302–309. https://doi.org/10.1159/000177877.

Fuller, H.L. and Kifer, P.E. (1959) The vitamin B_6 requirement of chicks. Poult. Sci. 38(2):255–260. https://doi.org/10.3382/ps.0380255.

Fuller, H.L., Field, R.C., Roncalli-Amici, R., Dunahoo, W.S. and Edwards, H.M. (1961) Vitamin B_6 requirement of breeder hens. Poult. Sci. 40(1):249–253. https://doi.org/10.3382/ps.0400249.

Funada, U., Wada, M., Kawata, T., Mori, K., Tamai, H., Isshiki, T., Onoda, J., Tanaka, N., Tadokoro, T. and Maekawa, A. (2001) Vitamin B_{12} deficiency affects immunoglobulin production and cytokine levels in mice. Int. J. Vitam. Nutr. Res. 71(1):60–65. https://doi.org/10.1024/0300-9831.71.1.60.

Funk, C. and Dubin, H.E. (1922). "The vitamins". Williams & Wilkins, Co., Baltimore, MD.

Gaál, T., Mézes, M., Noble, R.C., Dixon, J. and Speake, B.K. (1995) Development of antioxidant capacity in tissues of the chick embryo. Comp. Biochem. Physiol. Part B: Biochem Mol. Biol. 112(4):711–716 https://doi.org/10.1016/0305-0491(95)00125-5.

Gadient, M. (1986) Effect of pelleting on nutritional quality of feed. In Proc. Maryland Nutr. Conf. Feed Manuf., College Park, MD.

Gallop, P.M., Lian, J.B. and Hauschka, P.V. (1980) Carboxylated calcium-binding proteins and vitamin K. N. Engl. J. Med. 302(26):1460–1466. https://doi.org/10.1056/NEJM198006263022608.

Galobart, J., Barroeta, A.C., Baucells, M.D., Cortinas, L. and Guardiola, F. (2001a) α-tocopherol transfer efficiency and lipid oxidation in fresh and spray-dried eggs enriched with omega3-polyunsaturated fatty acids. Poult. Sci. 80(10):1496–1505. https://doi.org/10.1093/ps/80.10.1496.

Galobart, J., Barroeta, A.C., Baucells, M.D. and Guardiola, F. (2001b) Lipid oxidation in fresh and spray-dried eggs enriched with $omega_3$ and $omega_6$ polyunsaturated fatty acids during storage as affected by dietary vitamin E and canthaxanthin supplementation. Poult. Sci. 80(3):327–337. https://doi.org/10.1093/ps/80.3.327.

Galobart, J., Barroeta, A.C., Baucells, M.D., Codony, R. and Ternes, W. (2001c) Effect on dietary supplementation with rosemary extract and α-tocopheryl acetate on lipid oxidation in eggs enriched with omega3 fatty acids. Poult. Sci. 80(4):460–467. https://doi.org/10.1093/ps/80.4.460.

Galvin, K., Morrissey, P.A., Buckley, D.J. and Rigg, M. (1993) Influence of oil quality and α-tocopheryl acetate supplementation on α-tocopherol and lipid oxidation in chicken tissues. 11th Eur. Symp. Qual. Poult. Meat. Tours, France. (pp. 423–429).

Galvin, K., Morrissey, P.A. and Buckley, D.J. (1997) Influence of dietary vitamin E and oxidized sunflower oil on the storage stability of cooked chicken muscle. Br. Poult. Sci. 38(5):499–504. https://doi.org/10.1080/00071669708418028.

Galvin, K., Morrissey, P.A. and Buckley, D.J. (1998) Cholesterol oxides in processed chicken muscle as influenced by dietary α -tocopherol supplementation. Meat Sci. 48(1–2):1–9. https://doi.org/10.1016/S0309-1740(97)00069-7.

Gan, L., Zhao, Y., Mahmood, T. and Guo, Y. (2020) Effects of dietary vitamins supplementation level on the production performance and intestinal microbiota of aged laying hens. Poult. Sci. 99(7):3594–3605. https://doi.org/10.1016/j.psj.2020.04.007.

Gannon, B., Herrmann, R., Sinha, A., Ghezzi-Kopel, K., Rogers, L., Nieves Garcia-Casal, M.N., Peña-Rosas, J.P. and Mehta, S. (2020) The accuracy of dried blood spots compared to plasma or serum retinol for the diagnosis of vitamin A deficiency: a DTA systematic review and meta-analysis. Curr. Dev. Nutr. 4(Supplement_2):106. https://doi.org/10.1093/cdn/nzaa041_010.

Gao, J., Lin, H., Wang, X.J., Song, Z.G. and Jiao, H.C. (2010) Vitamin E supplementation alleviates the oxidative stress induced by dexamethasone treatment and improves meat quality in broiler chickens. Poult. Sci. 89(2):318–327. https://doi.org/10.3382/ps.2009-00216.

Gao, S., Heng, N., Liu, F., Guo, Y., Chen, Y., Wang, L., Ni, H., Sheng, X., Wang, X., Xing, K., Xiao, L. and Qi, X. (2021) Natural astaxanthin enhanced antioxidant capacity and improved semen quality through the MAPK/Nrf2 pathway in aging layer breeder roosters. J. Anim. Sci. Biotechnol. 12(1):112. https://doi.org/10.1186/s40104-021-00633-8.

Garcia, A.F., Murakami, Q.M., Amaral, A.E., Duarte, C.R., Ospina Rojas, I.C., Picoli, K.P. and Puzotti, M.M. (2013) Use of vitamin D_3 and its metabolites in broiler chicken feed on performance, bone parameters and meat quality. Asian. Aust. J. Anim. Sci. 26(3):408–415. https://doi.org/10.5713/ajas.2012.12455.

García, M.N., Pesti, G.M. and Bakalli, R.J. (1999) The effects of three methyl sources (methionine, betaine and choline) on the performance of growing chicks. Poult. Sci. J. 78(1):137.

Garcia Regueiro, J.A., Diaz, I. and Hortós, M. (1998) Volatile compounds of meat from broilers fed with different dietary oils and antioxidants. Proc. 44th Int. Congr. Meat Sci.

Gardner, H.W. (1989) Oxygen radical chemistry of polyunsaturated fatty acids. Free Radic. Biol. Med. 7(1):65–86. https://doi.org/10.1016/0891-5849(89)90102-0.

Garlich, J.D., Qureshi, M.A., Ferket, P.R. and Aslam, S.M. (1992) Immune system modulation by dietary calcium. Proc. 19th World's Poult. Congr., Amsterdam, The Netherlands. (pp. 618–619).

Garrow, T.A. (2007) Choline. In "Handbook of vitamins" 4th edition Zempleni, J., Rucker, R.B., McCormick, D.B. and Suttie, J.W. (ed.). CRC Press, Boca Raton, FL. (pp. 459–487).

Gasperi, V., Sibilano, M., Savini, I. and Catani, M.V. (2019) Niacin in the central nervous system: an update of biological aspects and clinical applications. Int. J. Mol. Sci. 20(4):974. https://doi.org/10.3390/ijms20040974.

Gatellier, P., Mercier, Y., Remignon, H. and Renerre, M. (1998) Effects of dietary fat and vitamin E content on lipid and protein oxidation in turkey meat homogenates after a chemical induction. Proc. 44th Int. Congr. Meat Sci. (pp. 636–637).

Gatellier, P., Lessire, M., Hermier, D., Maaroufi, C. and Renerre, M. (2003) Influence of nitrite and vitamin E percentage on myoglobin and lipid oxidation in packaged cooked cured hams. Br. Poult. Sci. Spr. meeting of the WPSA French branch 44(5):786–787. https://doi.org/10.1080/00071660410001666772.

Geng, Y., Ma, Q., Wang, Z. and Guo, Y. (2018) Dietary vitamin D_3 supplementation protects laying hens against lipopolysaccharide-induced immunological stress. Nutr. Metab. (Lond) 15(1):58. https://doi.org/10.1186/s12986-018-0293-8.

Genot, C., Meynier, A., Viau, M., Métro, B. and Gandemer, G. (1998) Dietary fat and vitamin E supplementation affect lipid oxidation in cooked turkey meat. Proc. 48th Int. Congr. Meat Sci. (pp. 632–633).

Gershoff, S.N., Legg, M.A., O'Connor, F.J. and Hegsted, D.M. (1957) The effect of vitamin D-deficient diets containing various Ca : P ratios on cats. J. Nutr. 63(1):79–93. https://doi.org/10.1093/jn/63.1.79.

Gershoff, S.N. (1993) Vitamin C (ascorbic acid): new roles, new requirements? Nutr. Rev. 51(11):313–326. https://doi.org/10.1111/j.1753-4887.1993.tb03757.x.

Ghane, F., Qotbi, A.A.A., Slozhenkina, M., Mosolov, A.A., Gorlov, I., Seidavi, A., Colonna, M.A., Laudadio, V. and Tufarelli, V. (2021) Effects of *in ovo* feeding of vitamin E or vitamin C on egg hatchability, performance, carcass traits and immunity in broiler chickens. Anim. Biotechnol.:1–6. https://doi.org/10.1080/10495398.2021.1950744.

Gheisari, A.A., Samie, A., Pourreza, J., Khoddami, A. and Gheisari, M.M. (2004) Effect of dietary fat, α-tocopherol, and ascorbic acid supplementation on the performance and meat oxidative stability of heat stressed broiler chicks. Proc. 12th World's Poult. Congr., Istanbul, Turkey.

Gheisari, A.A., Taheri, R., Rahmani, H.R., Toghyani, M., Bahadoran, R. and Khoddami, A. (2006) Effects of dietary vitamin E and green tea powder on performance of broiler chicks and meat lipid peroxidation during different storage times. Proc. 12th Eur. Poult. Nutr., Verona, Italy.

Gholami, J., Qotbi, A.A.A., Seidavi, A., Meluzzi, A., Tavaniello, S. and Maiorano, G. (2015) Effects of *in ovo* administration of betaine and choline on hatchability results, growth and carcass characteristics and immune response of broiler chickens. Ital. J. Anim. Sci. 14(2):3694. https://doi.org/10.4081/ijas.2015.3694.

Ghosh, H.P., Sarkar, P.K. and Guha, B.C. (1963) Distribution of the bound form of nicotinic acid in natural materials. J. Nutr. 79(4):451–453. https://doi.org/10.1093/jn/79.4.451.

Gibson, G.E. and Zhang, H. (2002) Interactions of oxidative stress with thiamine homeostasis promote neurodegeneration. Neurochem. Int. 40(6):493–504. https://doi.org/10.1016/S0197-0186(01)00120-6.

Gill, C. (2002) Vitamin D_3 metabolite versus MAS in broilers. Feed Int.:16–17.

Godoy-Parejo, C., Deng, C., Zhang, Y., Liu, W. and Chen, G. (2020) Roles of vitamins in stem cells. Cell. Mol. Life Sci. 77(9):1771–1791. https://doi.org/10.1007/s00018-019-03352-6.

Goeger, M.P. and Arscott, G.H. (1984) Effect of pantothenic acid on reproductive performance of adult white leghorn cockerels. Nutr. Rep. Int. 30:1193.

Goff, J.P., Reinhardt, T.A. and Horst, R.L. (1991) Enzymes and factors controlling vitamin D metabolism and action in normal and milk fever cows. J. Dairy Sci. 74(11):4022–4032. https://doi.org/10.3168/jds.S0022-0302(91)78597-4.

Golub, M.S. and Gershwin, M.E. (1985) Stress-induced immunomodulation: what is it, if it is? In "Animal stress" Moberg, G.P. (ed.). Springer, New York. https://doi.org/10.1007/978-1-4614-7544-6_11.

Golzar Adabi, S.H., Cooper, R.G., Kamali, M.A. and Hajbabaei, A. (2011) The influence of inclusions of vitamin E and corn oil on semen traits of Japanese quail (Coturnix coturnix japonica). Anim. Reprod. Sci. 123(1–2):119–125. https://doi.org/10.1016/j.anireprosci.2010.11.006.

Goñi, I., Brenes, A., Centeno, C., Viveros, A., Saura-Calixto, F., Rebolé, A., Arija, I. and Estevez, R. (2007) Effect of dietary grape pomace and vitamin E on growth performance, nutrient digestibility, and susceptibility to meat lipid oxidation in chickens. Poult. Sci. 86(3):508–516. https://doi.org/10.1093/ps/86.3.508.

Gonnerman, W.A., Toverud, S.U., Ramp, W.K. and Mechanic, G.L. (1976) Effects of dietary vitamin D and calcium on lysyl oxidase activity in chick bone metaphysis. Proc. Soc. Exp. Biol. Med. 151(3):453–456. https://doi.org/10.3181/00379727-151-39233.

Gonzales, E., Cruz, C.P.D., Leandro, N.S.M., Stringhini, J.H. and Brito, A.B.D. (2013) *In ovo* supplementation of 25 (OH) D_3 to broiler embryos. Rev. Bras. Cienc Avic 15(3):199–202. https://doi.org/10.1590/S1516-635X2013000300005.

Gonzales, E., Oliveira, A.S. and Cruz, C.P. (2003) *In ovo* supplementation of 25(OH)D_3 to broiler embryos. In Eur. Symp. on Poult. Nutri., Lillehammer, Norway. (pp. 72–74).

Gonzales, M. (1987). Nutricion y alimentacion del ganado Ed. Mundi Prensa. Madrid.

Goodson-Williams, R., Roland, D.A. and McGuire, J.A. (1986) Effects of feeding graded levels of vitamin D_3 on eggshell pimpling in aged hens. Poult. Sci. 65(8):1556–1560. https://doi.org/10.3382/ps.0651556.

Goodwin, T.W. (1984) "The biochemistry of carotenoids. Vol II. Animals". Chapman Hall. (pp. 1–21).

Gore, A.B. and Qureshi, M.A. (1997) Enhancement of humoral and cellular immunity by vitamin E after embryonic exposure. Poult. Sci. 76(7):984–991. https://doi.org/10.1093/ps/76.7.984.

Gouda, A., Amer, S.A., Gabr, S. and Tolba, S.A. (2020) Effect of dietary supplemental ascorbic acid and folic acid on the growth performance, redox status, and immune status of broiler chickens under heat stress. Trop. Anim. Health Prod. 52(6):2987–2996. https://doi.org/10.1007/s11250-020-02316-4.

Gouda, A., Tolba, S.A. and M El-Moniary, M.M. (2021) Impact of *in ovo* injection of certain vitamins to improve the physiological conditions of hatching chicks. Pak. J. Biol. Sci. 24(2):268–273. https://doi.org/10.3923/pjbs.2021.268.273.

Gous, R.M. and Morris, T.R. (2005) Nutritional interventions in alleviating the effects of high temperatures in broiler production. Worlds Poult. Sci. J. 61(3):463–475. https://doi.org/10.1079/WPS200568.

Grashorn, M.A. and Völker, L. (1993) Effects of an application of vitamin C before transportation on carcass yield of broiler chickens. Proc. 11th Eur. Symp. Ther. Qual. Poult. Meat, Tours, France. (pp. 191–195).

Grashorn, M.A. and Steinhilber, S. (1999) Effect of dietary fat with different relations between omega6 and omega3 fatty acids on egg quality. Proc. 8th Eur. Symp. Ther. Qual. of eggs and egg Prod., Bologna, Italy. (pp. 95–100).

Grashorn, M.A. and Steinberg, W. (2002) Deposition rates of canthaxanthin in egg yolks. Arch. Geflügelk 66:258–262.

Grau, A., Guardiola, F., Bou, R. and Codony, R. (2000) Influencia de la dosis y el tiempo de suplementación del pienso con acetato de α-tocoferol en la calidad de la carne de pollo. Aliment. nutr. salud 7(4):91–98.

Grau, A., Codony, R.L., Grimpa, S., Baucells, M.D. and Guardiola, F. (2001a) Cholesterol oxidation in frozen dark chicken meat: influence of dietary fat source, and α-tocopherol and ascorbic acid supplementation. Meat Sci. 57(2):197–208. https://doi.org/10.1016/S0309-1740(00)00094-2.

Grau, A., Guardiola, F., Grimpa, S., Barroeta, A.C. and Codony, R. (2001b) Oxidative stability of dark chicken meat through frozen storage: influence of dietary fat and α-tocopherol and ascorbic acid supplementation. Poult. Sci. 80(11):1630–1642. https://doi.org/10.1093/ps/80.11.1630.

Green, R. and Miller, J.W. (2013) Vitamin B_{12}. In Handbook of vitamins 5th edition Zempleni, J., Suttie, J., Gregory, J. and Stover P. J.(ed.). CRC Press, Taylor & Francis Group, LLC ISBN 9781466515567. (pp. 447–490).

Gregory, J.F. (1989) Chemical and nutritional aspects of folate research: analytical procedures, methods of folate synthesis, stability and bioavailability of dietary folates. Adv. Food Nutr. Res. 33:1–101. https://doi.org/10.1016/S1043-4526(08)60126-6.

Gregory, J.F. (2001) Case study: folate bioavailability. J. Nutr. 131(4) suppl.:1376S-1382S. https://doi.org/10.1093/jn/131.4.1376S.

Gregory, J.F., Trumbo, P.R., Bailey, L.B., Toth, J.P., Baumgartner, T.G. and Cerda, J.J. (1991a) Bioavailability of pyridoxine-5′-beta-D-glucoside determined in humans by stable-isotopic methods. J. Nutr. 121(2):177–186. https://doi.org/10.1093/jn/121.2.177.

Gregory, J.F., Bhandari, S.D., Bailey, L.B., Toth, J.P., Baumgartner, T.G. and Cerda, J.J. (1991b) Relative bioavailability of deuterium-labeled monoglutamyl and hexaglutamyl folates in human subjects. Am. J. Clin. Nutr. 53(3):736–740. https://doi.org/10.1093/ajcn/53.3.736.

Gries, C.L. and Scott, M.L. (1972) The pathology of thiamine, riboflavin, pantothenic acid and niacin deficiencies in the chick. J. Nutr. 102(10):1269–1285. https://doi.org/10.1093/jn/102.10.1269.

Griminger, P. (1966) Influence of maternal vitamin D intake on growth and bone ash of offspring. Poult. Sci. 45(4):849–851. https://doi.org/10.3382/ps.0450849.

Griminger, P. (1984) Vitamin K in animal nutrition: deficiency can be fatal. Part 1. Feedstuffs 56(38):24–25.

Griminger, P. and Donis, O. (1960) Potency of vitamin K_1 and two analogues in counteracting the effects of dicumarol and sulfaquinoxaline on the chick. J. Nutr. 70(3):361–368. https://doi.org/10.1093/jn/70.3.361.

Griminger, P. and Brubacher, G. (1966) The transfer of vitamin K_1 and menadione from the hen to the egg. Poult. Sci. 45(3):512–519. https://doi.org/10.3382/ps.0450512.

Grobas, S., Méndez, J., Lopez, B.C., De, B.C. and Mateos, G.G. (2002) Effect of vitamin E and A supplementation on egg yolk α-tocopherol concentration. Poult. Sci. 81(3):376–381. https://doi.org/10.1093/ps/81.3.376.

Gross, W.B. (1988) Effect of environmental stress on the responses of ascorbic-acid-treated chicks to Escherichia coli challenge infection. Avian Dis. 32(3):432–436. https://doi.org/10.2307/1590908.

Gross, W.B. (1992) Effects of ascorbic acid on stress and disease in chickens. Avian Dis. 36(3):688–692. https://doi.org/10.2307/1591766.

Gross, W.B., Jones, D. and Cherry, J. (1988) Effect of ascorbic acid on the disease caused by *Escherichia coli* challenge infection. Avian Dis. 32(3):407–409. https://doi.org/10.2307/1590904.

Groziak, S.M. and Kirksey, A. (1987) Effects of maternal dietary restriction in vitamin B_6 on neocortex development in rats: B_6 vitamer concentrations, volume and cell estimates. J. Nutr. 117(6):1045–1052. https://doi.org/10.1093/jn/117.6.1045.

Groziak, S.M. and Kirksey, A. (1990) Effects of maternal dietary restriction in vitamin B6 on neocortex development in rats: neuron differentiation and synaptogenesis. J. Nutr. 120(5):485–492. https://doi.org/10.1093/jn/120.5.485.

Gualtieri, M., Poli, B.M. and Rapaccini, S. (1993) Fatty acid composition of broiler meat as influenced by diet supplementation with fish oil. Proc. 11th Eur. Symp Ther. Qual. Poultr. Meat, Tours, France. (pp. 136–143).

Guetchom, B., Venne, D., Chénier, S. and Chorfi, Y. (2012) Effect of extra dietary vitamin E on preventing nutritional myopathy in broiler chickens. J. Appl. Poult. Res. 21(3):548–555. https://doi.org/10.3382/japr.2011-00440.

Guggenheim, K.Y. (1995). Basic issues of the history of nutrition. Magnes Press, Hebrew University.

Guo, S., Xv, J., Li, Y., Bi, Y., Hou, Y. and Ding, B. (2020) Interactive effects of dietary vitamin K_3 and Bacillus subtilis PB_6 on the growth performance and tibia quality of broiler chickens with sex separate rearing. Animal:1–9. https://doi.org/10.1017/S1751731120000178.

Guo, S., Niu, J., Xv, J., Fang, B., Zhang, Z., Zhao, D., Wang, L. and Ding, B. (2021) Interactive effects of vitamins A and K3 on laying performance, egg quality, tibia attributes and antioxidative status of aged Roman Pink laying hens Animal 15(6)100242. https://doi.org/10.1016/j.animal.2021.100242.

Guo, X., Yan, S., Shi, B. and Feng, Y. (2010) Effect of excessive vitamin A on alkaline phosphatase activity and concentrations of calcium-binding protein and bone gla-protein in culture medium and CaBP mRNA expression in osteoblasts of broiler chickens. Asian. Australas. J. Anim. Sci. 24(2):239–245. https://doi.org/10.5713/ajas.2011.10059.

Guo, Y., Tang, Q., Yuan, J. and Jiang, Z. (2001) Effects of supplementation with vitamin E on the performance and the tissue peroxidation of broiler chicks and the stability of thigh meat against oxidative deterioration. Anim. Feed Sci. Technol. 89(3–4):165–173. https://doi.org/10.1016/S0377-8401(00)00228-5.

Guo, Y., Zhang, G., Yuan, J. and Nie, W. (2003) Effects of source and level of magnesium and vitamin E on prevention of hepatic peroxidation and oxidative deterioration of broiler meat. Anim. Feed Sci. Technol. 107(1–4):143–150. https://doi.org/10.1016/S0377-8401(03)00116-0.

Gursu, M.F., Onderci, M., Gulcu, F. and Sahin, K. (2004) Effects of vitamin C and folic acid supplementation on serum paraoxonase activity and metabolites induced by heat stress *in vivo*. Nutr. Res. 24(2):157–164. https://doi.org/10.1016/j.nutres.2003.11.008.

Ha, J., Daniel, S., Broyles, S.S. and Kim, K.H. (1994) Critical phosphorylation sites for acetyl-CoA carboxylase activity. J. Biol. Chem. 269(35):22162–22168. https://doi.org/10.1016/S0021-9258(17)31770-2.

Hadden, J.W. (1987) Neuroendocrine modulation of the thymus-dependent immune system. Agonists and mechanisms. Ann. N. Y. Acad. Sci. 496(1):39–48. https://doi.org/10.1111/j.1749-6632.1987.tb35744.x.

Halevy, O., Arazi, Y., Melamed, D., Friedman, A. and Sklan, D. (1994) Retinoic acid receptor-gene expression is modulated by dietary vitamin A and by retinoic acid in chicken T lymphocytes. J. Nutr. 124(11):2139–2146. https://doi.org/10.1093/jn/124.11.2139.

Halle, I., Henning, M. and Kohler, P. (2011) Influence of vitamin B_{12} and cobalt on growth of broiler chickens and Pekin ducks. Landbauforsch Volkenrode 61(4):299–306.

Hamidi, M.S., Gajic-Veljanoski, O. and Cheung, A.M. (2013) Vitamin K and bone health. J. Clin. Densitom. 16(4):409–413. https://doi.org/10.1016/j.jocd.2013.08.017.

Han, J.C., Chen, G.H., Wang, J.G., Zhang, J.L., Qu, H.X., Zhang, C.M., Yan, Y.F. and Cheng, Y.H. (2016) Evaluation of relative bioavailability of 25-hydroxycholecalciferol to cholecalciferol for broiler chickens. Asian-Australas. J. Anim. Sci. 29(8):1145–1151. https://doi.org/10.5713/ajas.15.0553.

Han, J.C., Yang, X.D., Zhang, T., Li, H., Li, W.L., Zhang, Z.Y. and Yao, J.H. (2009) Effects of 1α-hydroxycholecalciferol on growth performance, parameters of tibia and plasma, meat quality, and type IIb sodium phosphate cotransporter gene expression of one- to twenty-one-day-old broilers. Poult. Sci. 88(2):323–329. https://doi.org/10.3382/ps.2008-00252.

Hankes, L.V. (1984) Nicotinic acid and nicotinamide. In "Handbook of vitamins" Machlin, L.J. (ed.). Marcel Dekker Inc.

Hannah, S.S. and Norman, A.W. (1994) 1 alpha,25$(OH)_2$ vitamin D_3-regulated expression of the eukaryotic genome. Nutr. Rev. 52(11):376–382. https://doi.org/10.1111/j.1753-4887.1994.tb01368.x.

Haq, A.U. and Bailey, C.A. (1996) Time course evaluation of carotenoid and retinol concentrations in post hatch chick tissue. Poult. Sci. 75(10):1258–1260. https://doi.org/10.3382/ps.0751258.

Haq, A.U., Bailey, C.A. and Chinnah, A. (1996) Effect of beta-carotene, canthaxanthin, lutein and vitamin E on neonatal immunity of chicks when supplemented in the broiler breeder diets. Poult. Sci. 75(9):1092–1097. https://doi.org/10.3382/ps.0751092.

Harms, R.H. and Simpson, C.F. (1975) Biotin deficiency as a possible cause of swelling and ulceration of foot pads. Poult. Sci. 54(5):1711–1713. https://doi.org/10.3382/ps.0541711.

Harms, R.H. and Miles, R.D. (1984) Effects of supplemental methionine and potassium sulfate on the choline requirement of the turkey poult. Poult. Sci. 63(7):1464–1466. https://doi.org/10.3382/ps.0631464.

Harms, R.H. and Bootwalla, S.M. (1992) Do turkey starter diets need pantothenic acid supplementation? J. Appl. Poult. Res. 1(1):19–21. https://doi.org/10.1093/japr/1.1.19.

Harms, R.H. and Nelson, D.S. (1992) Research note: A lack of response to pantothenic acid supplementation to a corn and soybean meal broiler diet. Poult. Sci. 71(11):1952–1954. https://doi.org/10.3382/ps.0711952.

Harms, R.H., Damron, B.L. and Simpson, C.F. (1977) Effect of wet litter and supplemental biotin and/or whey on the production of foot pad dermatitis in broilers. Poult. Sci. 56(1):291–296. https://doi.org/10.3382/ps.0560291.

Harms, R.H., Voitle, R.A., Janky, D.M. and Wilson, H.R. (1979) Influence of biotin supplementation on performance of broiler breeder hens and foot pad dermatitis in the progeny. Nutr. Rep. Int. 19(5):603–606.

Harms, R.H., Ruiz, N., Buresh, R.E. and Wilson, H.R. (1988a) Research note: Effect of niacin supplementation of corn-soybean meal diet on performance of turkey breeder hens. Poult. Sci. 67(2):336–338. https://doi.org/10.3382/ps.0670336.

Harms, R.H., Wilson, H.R. and Miles, R.D. (1988b) Influence of 1,25-dihydroxyvitamin D_3 on the performance of commercial laying hens. Poult. Sci. 67(8):1233–1235. https://doi.org/10.3382/ps.0671233.

Harms, R.H., Bootwalla, S.M., Woodward, S.A., Wilson, H.R. and Untawale, G.A. (1990a) Some observations on the influence of vitamin D metabolites when added to the diet of commercial laying hens. Poult. Sci. 69(3):426–432. https://doi.org/10.3382/ps.0690426.

Harms, R.H., Ruiz, N. and Miles, R.D. (1990b) Conditions necessary for a response by the commercial laying hen to supplemental choline and sulfate. Poult. Sci. 69(7):1226–1229. https://doi.org/10.3382/ps.0691226.

Harris, H.F. (1919). Pellagra. Macmillan Co., New York, NY.

Harrison, H.E. and Harrison, H.C. (1963) Sodium, potassium, and intestinal transport of glucose, l-tyrosine, phosphate, and calcium. Am. J. Physiol. 205(1):107–111. https://doi.org/10.1152/ajplegacy.1963.205.1.107.

Hart, L.E. and DeLuca, H.F. (1985) Effect of vitamin D_3 metabolites on calcium and phosphorus metabolism in chick embryos. Am. J. Physiol. 248(3 Pt 1):E281-E285. https://doi.org/10.1152/ajpendo.1985.248.3.E281.

Hartcher, K.M. and Lum, H.K. (2020) Genetic selection of broilers and welfare consequences: a review. Worlds Poult. Sci. J. 76(1):154–167. https://doi.org/10.1080/00439339.2019.1680025.

Haslam, S.M., Knowles, T.G., Brown, S.N., Wilkins, L.J., Kestin, S.C., Warriss, P.D. and Nicol, C.J. (2007) Factors affecting the prevalence of foot pad dermatitis, hock burn and breast burn in broiler chicken. Br. Poult. Sci. 48(3):264–275. https://doi.org/10.1080/00071660701371341.

Hassan, R.A., Attia, Y.A. and El-Ganzory, E.H. (2005) Growth, carcass quality and serum constituents of slow growing chicks as affected by betaine addition to diets containing different levels of choline. Int. J. Poult. Sci. 4(11):840–850. https://doi.org/10.3923/ijps.2005.840.850.

Hassan, S., Hakkarainen, J., Jönsson, L. and Työppönen, J. (1990) Histopathological and biochemical changes associated with selenium and vitamin E deficiency in chicks. Zentralbl. Veterinarmed. A 37(9):708–720. https://doi.org/10.1111/j.1439-0442.1990.tb00964.x.

Hatfield, D.L. and Gladyshev, V.N. (2002) How selenium has altered our understanding of the genetic code. Mol. Cell. Biol. 22(11):3565–3576. https://doi.org/10.1128/MCB.22.11.3565-3576.2002.

Hatta, H., Hamada, N., Nishii, M., Hayakawa, T. and Hernández, J.M. (2009) Effects of enriched multi-vitamin and canthaxanthin combination on performance of laying hens and egg quality. 17th Eur. Symp. Poult. Nutr. Edinb., Scotland.

Havenstein, G.B., Ferket, P.R., Scheideler, S. and Larson, B.T. (1994) Carcass composition and yield of 1957 vs 1991 broilers when fed "typical" 1957 and 1991 broiler diets. Poult. Sci. 73(12):1785–1804. https://doi.org/10.3382/ps.0731795.

Havenstein, G.B., Ferket, P.R. and Qureshi, M.A. (2003) Growth, livability, and feed conversion of 1957 versus 2001 broilers when fed representative 1957 and 2001 broiler diets. Poult. Sci. 82(10):1500–1508. https://doi.org/10.1093/ps/82.10.1500.

Hayashi, K., Yoshizaki, R., Ohtsuka, A., Torada, T. and Tuduki, T. (2004) Effects of ascorbic acid on performance and antibody production in broilers vaccinated against infectious bursal disease under a hot environment. Proc. 22nd World's Poult. Congr. Istanbul, Turkey.

Hayat, Z., Cherian, G., Pasha, T.N., Khattak, F.M. and Jabbar, M.A. (2010) Oxidative stability and lipid components of eggs from flax-fed hens: effect of dietary antioxidants and storage. Poult. Sci. 89(6):1285–1292. https://doi.org/10.3382/ps.2009-00256.

Heaney, R.P. and Holick, M.F. (2011) Why the IOM recommendations for vitamin D are deficient. J. Bone Miner. Res. 26(3):455–457. https://doi.org/10.1002/jbmr.328.

Hebert, K., House, J.D. and Guenter, W. (2005) Effect of dietary folic acid supplementation on egg folate content and the performance and folate status of two strains of laying hens. Poult. Sci. 84(10):1533–1538. https://doi.org/10.1093/ps/84.10.1533.

Hebert, K., Tactacan, G.B., Dickson, T.M., Guenter, W. and House, J.D. (2011) The effect of cereal type and exogenous enzyme use on total folate content of eggs from laying hens consuming diets supplemented with folic acid. J. Appl. Poult. Res. 20(3):303–312. https://doi.org/10.3382/japr.2010-00243.

Heffels-Redmann, U., Redmann, Th., Lange, K., Schröder-Gravendyck, S.E. and Sallmenn, H.P. (2000) Influence of vitamin E on immune reactions of turkeys. Arch. Geflügelk 65(2):68–75.

Heffels-Redmann, U., Redmann, T.H. and Weber, G. (2001) Vitamin E supplementation in turkeys influences immune reactions and performance. World Poultry special issue on vitamins.

Heffels-Redmann, U., Redmann, T. and Weber, G. (2003) Vitamin E supplementation influences immune reactions and performance. World Poult. 19(Special):18–19.

Heidari, M., Mohebalian, H. and Hassanabadi, A. (2021) The effects of *in ovo* injection of nanocurcumin and vitamin E on immune responses and growth performance of broiler chickens under heat stress. J. Anim. Vet. Adv. 20(5):124–133.

Hekal, A.M. (2018) Effect of in-ovo injection of pyridoxine on hatchability and physiological response of hatched turkey poults. Egypt. Poult. Sci. J. 38(4):1127–1140. https://doi.org/10.21608/epsj.2018.22910.

Henderson, L.M. (1984) Vitamin B_6. In "Nutrition reviews, present knowledge in nutrition" 5th edition Olson, R.E., Broquist, H.P., Chichester, O., Darby, W.J., Kolbye, A.C. and Stalvey, R.M. (ed.) The Nutrition Foundation, Inc.

Henderson, L.M. and Gross, C.J. (1979) Metabolism of niacin and niacinamide in perfused rat intestine. J. Nutr. 109(4):654–662. https://doi.org/10.1093/jn/109.4.654.

Henderson, S.N., Vicente, J.L., Pixley, C.M., Hargis, B.M. and Tellez, G. (2008) Effect of an early nutritional supplement on broiler performance. Int. J. Poult. Sci. 7(3):211–214. https://doi.org/10.3923/ijps.2008.211.214.

Hendrix Genetics (2016) Vitamin and trace mineral supplementation for turkeys. https://www.hybridturkeys.com/en/resources/commercial-management/feed-and-water/.

Hendrix Genetics (2022) Nutrition guide. https://layinghens.hendrix-genetics.com/en/technical-support/nutrition/.

Herendy, V., Suto, Z., Horn, P. and Szalay, I. (2004) Effect of the housing system on the meat production of turkey. Acta Agric. Slov. suppl. 1:209–2013.

Hernández, J.M., Blanch, A. and Bird, N. (2001) Why consumers need carotenoids in poultry. Int. Poult. Prod. 9:15–16.

Hernández, J.M., Pérez-Vendrell, A.M. and Brufau, J. (2002) Effect of vitamin level in broiler diets on the production parameters and meat deposition. 11th Eur. Symp. Poult. Nutr. Faaborg, Denmark. (pp. 6–10).

Herrick, J.B. (1972) The influence of vitamin A on disease states. Vet.Med. 67:906.

Hesabi, H. (2007) Effect of vitamin E on performance and immune response of broiler chicks. Proc. 16th Eur. Symp. Poult. Nutr. Strasbourg, France. (p. 321).

Heuser, G.F. and Norris, L.C. (1929) The effectiveness of midsummer sunshine and irradiation from a quartz mercury vapor arc in preventing rickets in chickens. Poult. Sci. 8:89–98.

Higgins, F.M., Kerry, J.P., Buckley, D.J. and Morrissey, P.A. (1998a) Assessment of α-tocopheryl acetate supplementation, addition of salt and packaging on the oxidative stability of raw turkey meat. Br. Poult. Sci. 39(5):596–600. https://doi.org/10.1080/00071669888458.

Higgins, F.M., Kerry, J.P., Buckley, D.J. and Morrissey, P.A. (1998b) Effect of dietary α-tocopheryl acetate supplementation on α-tocopherol distribution in raw turkey muscles and its effect on the storage stability of cooked turkey meat. Meat Sci. 50(3):373–383. https://doi.org/10.1016/s0309-1740(98)00045-x.

Higgins, F.M., Kerry, J.P., Buckley, D.J. and Morrissey, P.A. (1999) Effects of dietary α-tocopheryl acetate supplementation and salt addition on the oxidative stability (TBARS) and warmed-over flavor (WOF) of cooked turkey meat. Br. Poult. Sci. 40(1):59–64. https://doi.org/10.1080/00071669987845.

Hill, C.H. and Garren, H.W. (1958) Plasma ascorbic acid levels of chicks with fowl typhoid. Poult. Sci. 37(1):236–237. https://doi.org/10.3382/ps.0370236.

Hill, C.H. and Baker, V.C. (1961) Dietary protein levels as they affect blood citric acid levels of chicks subjected to certain stresses. Poult. Sci. 40(3):762–765. https://doi.org/10.3382/ps.0400762.

Hill, F.W., Scott, M.L., Norris, L.C. and Hetjser, G.F. (1961) Reinvestigation of the vitamin A requirement of laying and breeding hens and their progeny. Poult. Sci. 40(5):1245–1254. https://doi.org/10.3382/ps.0401245.

Hirsch, A. (1982) Vitamin D history, manufacture, analysis and metabolism: an overview. In "Vitamins the life essentials", National Feed Ingredients Association (NIFA) (Pub), Des Moines, IA.

Hocking, P.M. (2007) Optimum feed composition of broiler breeder diets to maximize progeny performance. Proc. 16th Eur. Symp. Poult. Nutr. (pp. 101–108).

Hocking, P.M. (2014) Unexpected consequences of genetic selection in broilers and turkeys: problems and solutions. Br. Poult. Sci. 55(1):1–12. https://doi.org/10.1080/00071668.2014.877692.

Hocking, P.M., Wilson, S., Dick, L., Dunn, L.N., Robertson, G.W. and Nixey, C. (2002) Role of dietary calcium and available phosphorus in the aetiology of tibial dyschondroplasia in growing turkeys. Br. Poult. Sci. 43(3):432–441. https://doi.org/10.1080/00071660120103729.

Hocking, P.M., Stevenson, E. and Beard, P.M. (2013) Supplementary biotin decreases tibial bone weight, density and strength in riboflavin-deficient starter diets for turkey poults. Br. Poult. Sci. 54(6):801–809. https://doi.org/10.1080/00071668.2013.860213.

Hodges, R.E., Ohlson, M.A. and Bean, W.B. (1958) Pantothenic acid deficiency in man. J. Clin. Invest. 37(11):1642–1657. https://doi.org/10.1172/JCI103756.

Hoekstra, W.G. (1975) Biochemical function of selenium and its relation to vitamin E. Fed. Proc. 34(11): 2083–2089. PMID:1100437.

Hoey, L., McNulty, H., McCann, E.M.E., McCracken, K.J., Scott, J.M., Marc, B.B., Molloy, A.M., Graham, C. and Pentieva, K. (2009) Laying hens can convert high doses of folic acid added to the feed into natural folates in eggs providing a novel source of food folate. Br. J. Nutr. 101(2):206–212. https://doi.org/10.1017/S0007114508995647.

Hoffmann-La Roche (1967) Vitamin A, the keystone of animal nutrition. Hoffmann–La Roche Inc., Nutley, NJ.

Hoffmann-La Roche (1969) Riboflavin. No. 1170. Hoffmann–La Roche Inc., Nutley, NJ.

Hoffmann–La Roche (1972) Vitamin E. No. 1206. Hoffmann–La Roche Inc., Nutley, NJ.

Hoffmann-La Roche (1979) Rationale for Roche recommended vitamin fortification poult. rations. RCD 5692/979. Hoffmann–La Roche Inc., Nutley, NJ.

Hoffmann–La Roche (1984) Roche technical Bulletin-Vitamin B_{12}. RCD 6723. Hoffmann–La Roche Inc., Nutley, NJ.

Hofmann, P., Siegert, W., Ahmadi, H., Krieg, J., Novotny, M., Naranjo, V.D. and Rodehutscord, M. (2020) Interactive effects of glycine equivalent, cysteine, and choline on growth performance, nitrogen excretion characteristics, and plasma metabolites of broiler chickens using neural networks optimized with genetic algorithms. Animals (Basel) 10(8):1392. https://doi.org/10.3390/ani10081392.

Hogan, J.S., Smith, K.L., Weiss, W.P., Todhunter, D.A. and Schockey, W.L. (1990) Relationships among vitamin E, selenium and bovine blood neutrophils. J. Dairy Sci. 73(9):2372–2378. https://doi.org/10.3168/jds.S0022-0302(90)78920-5.

Hogan, J.S., Weiss, W.P., Todhunter, D.A., Smith, K.L. and Schoenberger, P.S. (1992) Bovine neutrophil responses to parenteral vitamin E. J. Dairy Sci. 75(2):399–405. https://doi.org/10.3168/jds.S0022-0302(92)77775-3.

Hogan, J.S., Weiss, W.P., Smith, K.L., Sordillo, L.M. and Williams, S.N. (1996) Alpha-tocopherol concentration in milk and plasma during clinical. J. Dairy Sci. 79(1):71–75. https://doi.org/10.3168/jds.S0022-0302(96)76335-X.

Holick, M.F. (2007) Vitamin D deficiency. N. Engl. J. Med. 357(3):266–281. https://doi.org/10.1056/NEJMra070553.

Hollander, D. (1973) Vitamin K_1 absorption by everted intestinal sacs of the rat. Am. J. Physiol. 225(2): 360–364. https://doi.org/10.1152/ajplegacy.1973.225.2.360.

Höller, U., Bakker, S.J., Düsterloh, L., Frei, A., Körrle, B., Konz, J., Lietz, T., McCann, G. and Michels, A. (2018) Micronutrient status assessment in humans: current methods of analysis and future trends. TrAC Trends in Analytical Chemistry 102:110-122. https://doi.org/10.1016/j.trac.2018.02.001.

Hooda, S., Tyagi, P.K., Mohan, J., Mandal, A.B., Elangovan, A.V. and Pramod, K.T. (2007) Effects of supplemental vitamin E in diet of Japanese quail on male reproduction, fertility and hatchability. Br. Poult. Sci. 48(1):104–110. https://doi.org/10.1080/00071660601157378.

Hooper, C.L., Lightsey, S.F., Toler, J.E. and Maurice, D.U. (1989) Effect of age, sex and food deprivation on the biosynthesis of ascorbic acid in meat-type chickens. Poult. Sci. 68(1):116.

Hornig, B., Glatthar, B. and Mosw, U. (1984) General aspects of ascorbic acid and metabolism. In Proc. workshop Ascorbic Acid in Domest. Anim. The Royal Danish Agriculture Society Wegger, I., Tagwerker, F.J. and Moustgaard, J. (ed.). Copenhagen, Denmark.

Horsted, K., Hermansen, J.E. and Ranvig, H. (2007) Crop content in nutrient-restricted versus non-restricted organic laying hens with access to different forage vegetations. Br. Poult. Sci. 48(2):177–184. https://doi.org/10.1080/00071660701227501.

Horváth, M. and Babinszky, L. (2018) Impact of selected antioxidant vitamins (vitamin A, E and C) and micro minerals (Zn, Se) on the antioxidant status and performance under high environmental temperature in poultry. A review. Acta Agric. Scand. A 68(3):152–160. https://doi.org/10.1080/09064702.2019.1611913.

Hossain, S.M., Barreto, S.L., Bertechini, A.G., Ríos, A.M. and Silva, C.G. (1998) Influence of dietary vitamin E level on egg production of broiler breeders and on the growth and immune response of progeny in comparison with the progeny from eggs injected with vitamin E. Anim. Feed Sci. Technol. 73(3–4):307–317. https://doi.org/10.1016/S0377-8401(98)00149-7.

House, J.D., Braun, K., Ballance, D.M., O'Connor, C.P. and Guenter, W. (2002) The enrichment of eggs with folic acid through supplementation of the laying hen diet. Poult. Sci. 81(9):1332–1337. https://doi.org/10.1093/ps/81.9.1332.

Howell, J.C. and Thompson, J.N. (1967) Lesions associated with the development of ataxia in vitamin A-deficient chicks. Br. J. Nutr. 21(3):741–750. https://doi.org/10.1079/BJN19670075.

Hsieh, H.F., Chiang, S.H. and Lu, M.Y. (2002) Effect of dietary monounsaturated/saturated fatty acid ratio on fatty acid composition and oxidative stability of tissues in broilers. Anim. Feed Sci. Technol. 95(3–4):189–204. https://doi.org/10.1016/S0377-8401(01)00292-9.

Hsu, J.C., Tanaka, K. and Ohtani, H.S. (1988) Effects of dietary choline deficiency, and the supplementation of methionine and/or vitamin B_{12} to the choline-free diet on the growth and contents of various lipid fractions in the liver and serum of ducklings. J. Poult. Sci. 25(1):34–40. https://doi.org/10.2141/jpsa.25.34.

Huang, H.Y. and Appel, L.J. (2003) Supplementation of diets with α-tocopherol reduces serum concentrations of γ-and δ-tocopherol in humans. J. Nutr. 133(10):3137–3140. https://doi.org/10.1093/jn/133.10.3137.

Huang, J., Li, G., Cao, H., Yang, F., Xing, C., Zhuang, Y., Zhang, C., Liu, P., Cao, H. and Hu, G. (2020) The improving effects of biotin on hepatic histopathology and related apolipoprotein mRNA expression

in laying hens with fatty liver hemorrhagic syndrome. Can. J. Anim. Sci. 100(3):494–501. https://doi.org/10.1139/cjas-2019-0147.
Huang, S., Kong, A., Cao, Q., Tong, Z. and Wang, X. (2019) The role of blood vessels in broiler chickens with tibial dyschondroplasia. Poult. Sci. 98(12):6527–6532. https://doi.org/10.3382/ps/pez497.
Huang, X.X. and Miller, E.L. (1994) Stability of meat from broilers fed vitamin E in conjunction with lipids from fish oil and fish meal. Proc. 9th Eur. Poult. Nutr., Glasgow, UK. (pp. 217–218).
Hubbard Breeders Nutrition Guide (2019) https://www.hubbardbreeders.com/documentation/.
Huff, G.R., Huff, W.E., Balog, J.M. and Rath, N.C. (2000) The effect of vitamin D_3 on resistance to stress-related infection in an experimental model of turkey osteomyelitis complex. Poult. Sci. 79(5):672–679. https://doi.org/10.1093/ps/79.5.672.
Huff, G.R., Huff, W.E., Balog, J.M., Rath, N.C., Xie, H. and Horst, R.L. (2002) Effect of dietary supplementation with vitamin D metabolites in an experimental model of turkey osteomyelitis complex. Poult. Sci. 81(7):958–965. https://doi.org/10.1093/ps/81.7.958.
Hughes, B.O. and Wood-Gush, D.G.M. (1971) Investigations into specific appetites for sodium and thiamine in domestic fowls. Physiol. Behav. 6(4):331–339. https://doi.org/10.1016/0031-9384(71)90164-8.
Hulan, H.W., Proudfoot, F.G. and Mcrae, K.B. (1980) Effect of vitamins on the incidence of mortality and acute death syndrome ('flip-over') in broiler chickens. Poult. Sci. 59(4):927–931. https://doi.org/10.3382/ps.0590927.
Hupfauer, M. (1993). Effect of vitamins C and B_6 and various vitamin D_2 and D_3 metabolites on laying performance and eggshell quality in old layers. Ludwig Maximilian Universität, München. (p. 117).
Hussein, A.S. (1995) Effects of dietary energy and vitamin C on growth performance of broiler chicks raised in hot climates. Poult. Sci. 74(1):151. https://doi.org/10.9755/ejfa.v8i1.5247.
Hustmyer, F.G., Beitz, D.C., Goff, J.P., Nonnecke, B.J., Horst, R.L. and Reinhardt, T.A. (1994) Effects of in vivo administration of 1,25-dihydroxyvitamin D_3 on in vitro proliferation of bovine lymphocytes. J. Dairy Sci. 77(11):3324–3330. https://doi.org/10.3168/jds.S0022-0302(94)77273-8.
Hutton, K.C., Vaughn, M.A., Litta, G., Turner, B.J. and Starkey, J.D. (2014) Effect of vitamin D status improvement with 25-hydroxycholecalciferol on skeletal muscle growth characteristics and satellite cell activity in broiler chickens. J. Anim. Sci. 92(8):3291–3299. https://doi.org/10.2527/jas.2013-7193.
Huyghebaert, A. (1991) Stability of vitamin K in a mineral premix. World Poult. 7:71.
Huyghebaert, G., Lippens, M., Lescoat, P. and Nys, Y. (2005) The interaction between the macrominerals calcium and phosphorus, vitamin D and phytase in broilers. Proc. 15th Eur. Symp. Poult. Nutr. Balatonfured, Hungary. (pp. 151–165).
Hy-Line (2021) Management guide. https://www.hyline.co.uk/services/management-guides/.
Ibrahim, M. (1998) Riboflavin deficiency in chicken World Poultry, 20-21.
Ibrahim, W., Lee, U.S., Yeh, C.C., Szabo, J., Bruckner, G. and Chow, C.K. (1997) Oxidative stress and antioxidant status in mouse liver: effects of dietary lipid, vitamin E and iron. J. Nutr. 127(7):1401–1406. https://doi.org/10.1093/jn/127.7.1401.
Igwe, I.R., Okonkwo, C.J., Uzoukwu, U.G. and Onyenegecha, C.O. (2015) The effect of choline chloride on the performance of broiler chickens. Annu. Res. Rev. Biol. 8(3):1–8. https://doi.org/10.9734/ARRB/2015/19372.
Ikeda, S., Takasu, M., Matsuda, T., Kakinuma, A. and Horio, F. (1997) Ascorbic acid deficiency decreases the renal level of kidney fatty acid-binding protein by lowering the $alpha_{2u}$-globulin gene expression in liver in scurvy-prone ods rats. J. Nutr. 127(11):2173–2178. https://doi.org/10.1093/jn/127.11.2173.
Inal, F., Coşkun, B., Gülşen, N. and Kurtoğlu, V. (2001) The effects of withdrawal of vitamin and trace mineral supplements from layer diets on egg yield and trace mineral composition. Br. Poult. Sci. 42(1):77–80. https://doi.org/10.1080/713655024.
Ingram, R.T., Park, Y.K., Clarke, B.L. and Fitzpatrick, L.A. (1994) Age- and gender-related changes in the distribution of osteocalcin in the extracellular matrix of normal male and female bone. Possible involvement of osteocalcin in bone remodeling. J. Clin. Invest. 93(3):989–997. https://doi.org/10.1172/JCI117106.
Institut Scientifique de Recherche Agronomique (INRA) (1985). Alimentatión de animales monogástriques. Mundi-prensa, Madrid.
Ipek, A. and Dikmen, B.Y. (2014) The effects of vitamin E and vitamin C on sexual maturity body weight and hatching characteristics of Japanese quails (*Coturnix coturnix japonica*) reared under heat stress. Anim. Sci. Pap. 32:261–268.

Iqbal, M., Cawthon, D., Wideman, R.F. and Bottje, W.G. (2001) Lung mitochondrial dysfunction in pulmonary hypertension syndrome. II. Oxidative stress and inability to improve function with repeated additions of adenosine diphosphate. Poult. Sci. 80(5):656–665. https://doi.org/10.1093/ps/80.5.656.

Iqbal, M., Cawthon, D., Beers, K., Wideman, R.F. and Bottje, W.G. (2002) Antioxidant enzyme activities and mitochondrial fatty acids in pulmonary hypertension syndrome (PHS) in broilers. Poult. Sci. 81(2):252–260. https://doi.org/10.1093/ps/81.2.252.

Ishii M, Yamauchi T, Matsumoto K, Watanabe, G., Taya, K., and Chatani, F. (2012) Maternal age and reproductive function in female Sprague-Dawley rats. J. Toxicol. Sci. 37(3):631–638. https://doi.org/10.2131/jts.37.631.

Iskakova, M., Karbyshev, M., Piskunov, A. and Rochette-Egly, C.R. (2015 Dec) Nuclear and extranuclear effects of vitamin A. Can. J. Physiol. Pharmacol. 93(12):1065–1075. https://doi.org/10.1139/cjpp-2014-0522.

Jackson, D.W., Law, G.R. and Nockels, C.F. (1978) Maternal vitamin E alters passively acquired immunity of chicks. Poult. Sci. 57(1):70–73. https://doi.org/10.3382/ps.0570070.

Jackson, M. (1992) "Feeding layers: nutritional considerations" Multi-state Poult. Meeting.

Jacob, R.A., Wu, M.M., Henning, S.M. and Swendseid, M.E. (1994) Homocysteine increases as folate decreases in plasma of healthy men during short-term dietary folate and methyl group restriction. J. Nutr. 124(7):1072–1080. https://doi.org/10.1093/jn/124.7.1072.

Jacob, R.A. (1995) The integrated antioxidant system. Nutr. Res. 15(5):755–766. https://doi.org/10.1016/0271-5317(95)00041-G.

Jacob, R.A. (2006) Niacin. In Present knowledge in nutrition 9th edition Bowman, B.A. and Russell, R.M. (ed.). International Life Sciences Institute. (pp. 261–268).

Jager, N. (1977). New York State College of Veterinary Medicine Cornell University Annual Report 1975–76.

Jain, G. and Pandey, R. (2018) Effect of vitamin C on growth performance of caged broilers. Adv. Biol. Res. 9(2):178–181.

Jakobsen, K., Engberg, R.M., Andersen, J.O., Jensen, S.K., Lauridsen, C., Sørensen, P., Henckel, P., Bertelsen, G., Skibsted, L.H. and Jensen, C. (1995) Supplementation of broiler diets with all- rac- α-tocopheryl acetate or a mixture of RRR-α-γ- tocopheryl acetate. Effect on the vitamin status of broilers in vivo and at slaughter. Poult. Sci. 74(12):1984–1994. https://doi.org/10.3382/ps.0741984.

Janist, N., Srichana, P., Asawakarn, T. and Kijparkorn, S. (2019) Effect of supplementing the laying hen diets with choline, folic acid, and vitamin B12 on production performance, egg quality, and yolk phospholipid. Livest. Sci. 223:24–31. https://doi.org/10.1016/j.livsci.2019.02.019.

Janssens, G., Cheetham, V., Fitt, T. and Taylor, A. (1999) Effect of dietary vitamin E on consumer acceptance of fresh poultry meat. Quality, Bologna, Italy. 14th Eur. Symp. Poult. Meat. (pp. 173–179).

Javed, M.T., Ellahi, M., Abbas, N., Yasmin, R. and Mazhar, M. (2010) Effects of dietary chromium chloride, nicotinic acid and copper sulphate on meat of broilers. Br. Poult. Sci. 51(3):354–360. https://doi.org/10.1080/00071668.2010.496773.

Jegede, A.V., Ogunsola, I.A., Fafiolu, A.O., Oluwatosin, O.O., Lawal, R.F., Odejayi, O.A. and Adeniran, A.C. (2018) Growth performance, nutrient digestibility and hematological indices of broiler chickens fed diets supplemented with riboflavin and pyridoxine. Nig. J. Anim. Prod. 45(1):259–267. https://doi.org/10.51791/njap.v45i1.364.

Jena, B.P., Panda, N., Patra, R.C., Mishra, P.K., Behura, N.C. and Panigrahi, B. (2013) Supplementation of vitamin E and C reduces oxidative stress in broiler breeder hens during summer. Food Nutr. Sci. 04(8):33–37. https://doi.org/10.4236/fns.2013.48A004.

Jensen, C., Engberg, R., Jakobsen, K., Skibsted, L.H. and Bertelsen, G. (1997) Influence of the oxidative quality of dietary oil on broiler meat storage stability. Meat Sci. 47(3–4):211–222. https://doi.org/10.1016/S0309-1740(97)00052-1.

Jensen, C., Lauridsen, C. and Bertelsen, G. (1998) Dietary vitamin E: quality and storage stability of pork and poultry. Trends Food Sci. Technol. 9(2):62–72. https://doi.org/10.1016/S0924-2244(98)00004-1.

Jensen, L.S. (1965) Vitamin A requirement of breeding Turkeys. Poult. Sci. 44(6):1609–1610. https://doi.org/10.3382/ps.0441609.

Jensen, L.S. (1968) Vitamin E and essential fatty acids in avian reproduction. Fed. Proc. 27(3):914–919.

Jensen, L.S. (1986) Interaction of nutrition with stress and disease. Proc. GA Nutr. Conf. (pp. 27–37).

Jensen, L.S. and McGinnis, J. (1957a) Improvement in hatchability of turkey eggs by injection with water soluble vitamin E. Poult. Sci. 36(1):212–213. https://doi.org/10.3382/ps.0360212.

Jensen, L.S. and McGinnis, J. (1957b) Studies on the vitamin E requirement of turkeys for reproduction. Poult. Sci. 36(6):1344–1350. https://doi.org/10.3382/ps.0361344.

Jensen, L.S., Chang, C.H. and Maurice, D.V. (1976) Effect of biotin and niacin on lipid content of livers in the laying hen. Poult. Sci. 55(5):1771–1773. https://doi.org/10.3382/ps.0551771.

Jensen, L.S., Fletcher, D.L., Lilburn, M.S. and Akiba, Y. (1981) Relationship of level of dietary vitamin A supplementation to broiler performance. Poult. Sci. 59(1):1603.

Jensen, L.S., Fletcher, D.L., Lilburn, M.S. and Akiba, Y. (1983) Growth depression in broiler chicks fed high vitamin A levels. Nutr. Rep. Int. 28:171–179.

Jensen, S.K. and Edberg, R.M. (1999) Bioavailability of various α-tocopherol esters in relation to age and feed formulation and vitamin A activity of β-carotene in broilers. Proc. 12th Eur. Symp. Poult. Nutr., Veldhoven, The Netherlands. (pp. 132–133).

Jensen, S.K., Nørgaard, J.V. and Lauridsen, C. (2006) Bioavailability of α-tocopherol stereoisomers in rats depends on dietary doses of all-rac- or RRR-α-tocopheryl acetate. Br. J. Nutr. 95(3):477–487. https://doi.org/10.1079/BJN20051667.

Jian, L., Shuisheng, H. and Hunchun, H. (1996) Studies of the biotin deficiency and its requirement for broiler chicks. Proc. 20th World's Poult. Congr., Delhi, India. (p. 179).

Jiang, R.R., Zhao, G.P., Chen, J.L., Zheng, M.Q., Zhao, J.P., Li, P., Hu, J. and Wen, J. (2011) Effect of dietary supplemental nicotinic acid on growth performance, carcass characteristics and meat quality in three genotypes of chicken. J. Anim. Physiol. Anim. Nutr. (Berl) 95(2):137–145. https://doi.org/10.1111/j.1439-0396.2010.01031.x.

Jiang, S., Jiang, Z., Yang, K., Chen, F., Zheng, C. and Wang, L. (2015) Dietary vitamin D_3 requirement of Chinese yellow-feathered broilers. Poult. Sci. 94(9):2210–2220. https://doi.org/10.3382/ps/pev163.

Jiang, W., Zhang, L. and Shan, A. (2013) The effect of vitamin E on laying performance and egg quality in laying hens fed corn dried distillers grains with solubles. Poult. Sci. 92(11):2956–2964. https://doi.org/10.3382/ps.2013-03228.

Jiang, X., Yan, J. and Caudill, M.A. (2013) Choline. In "Handbook of vitamins" 5th edition, Zempleni, J., Suttie, J., Gregory, J. and Stover P. J.(ed.). CRC Press, Taylor & Francis Group. (pp. 491–514).

Jiang, Y.H., McGeachin, R.B. and Bailey, C.A. (1994) Alpha-tocopherol, beta-carotene and retinol enrichment of chicken eggs. Poult. Sci. 73(7):1137–1143. https://doi.org/10.3382/ps.0731137.

Jiang, W., Zhang, L. and Shan, A. (2013) The effect of vitamin E on laying performance and egg quality in laying hens fed corn dried distillers grains with solubles. Poult. Sci. 92(11):2956–2964. https://doi.org/10.3382/ps.2013-03228.

Jin, S. and Sell, J.L. (2001) Dietary vitamin K_1 requirement and comparison of biopotency of different vitamin K sources for young turkeys. Poult. Sci. 80(5):615–620. https://doi.org/10.1093/ps/80.5.615.

Johnson, M.A. and Kimlin, M.G. (2006) Vitamin D, aging, and the 2005 dietary guidelines for Americans. Nutr. Rev. 64(9):410–421. https://doi.org/10.1111/j.1753-4887.2006.tb00226.x.

Johnson, N.E., Harland, B.F., Ross, E., Gautz, L. and Dunn, M.A. (1992) Effects of dietary aluminium and niacin on chick tibiae. Poult. Sci. 71(7):1188–1195. https://doi.org/10.3382/ps.0711188.

Johnson, N.E., Qiu, X.L., Gautz, L.D. and Ross, E. (1995) Changes in dimensions and mechanical properties of bone in chicks fed high levels of niacin. Food Chem. Toxicol. 33(4):265–271. https://doi.org/10.1016/0278-6915(94)00143-C.

Johnston, C.S. (2006) Vitamin C. In "Present knowledge in nutrition" 9th edition Bowman, B.A. and Russell, R.M. (ed.). International Life Sciences Institute, Washington, DC. (pp. 233–241).

Johnston, C.S., Steinberg, F.M. and Rucker, R.B. (2013) Ascorbic acid. In "Handbook of vitamins" 5th edition Zempleni, J., Suttie, J., Gregory, J. and Stover P. J. (ed.). CRC Press, Taylor & Francis Group. (pp. 515–550).

Johnston, L. and Laverty, G. (2007) Vitamin C transport and SVCT1 transporter expression in chick renal proximal tubule cells in culture. Comp. Biochem. Physiol. A Mol. Integr. Physiol. 146(3):327–334. https://doi.org/10.1016/j.cbpa.2006.11.025.

Jolly, D.W., Craig, C. and Nelson, T.E. (1977) Estrogen and prothrombin synthesis: effect of estrogen on absorption of vitamin K1. Am. J. Physiol. 232(1):H12-H17. https://doi.org/10.1152/ajpheart.1977.232.1.H12.

Jones, R.B. (1996) Fear and adaptability in poultry: insights, implications, and imperatives. World's. Poult. Sci. 52(2):131–174. https://doi.org/10.1079/WPS19960013.

Jones, R.B. and Satterlee, D.G. (1997) Vitamin C and fear in poultry: an overview. Poult. Sci. 76(1):104. https://doi.org/10.1093/ps/76.3.469.

Kadhim, A.H., Al-Jebory, H.H., Ali, M.A. and Al-Khafaji, F.R. (2021) Effect of early feeding (*in ovo*) with nano-selenium and vitamin E on body weight and glycogen level in broiler chickens exposed to fasting condition. In IOP Conf. Ser. Earth Environ. Sci. 910(1):012009. https://doi.org/10.1088/1755-1315/910/1/012009.

Kaempf-Rotzoll, D.E., Traber, M.G. and Arai, H. (2003) Vitamin E and transfer proteins. Curr. Opin. Lipidol. 14(3):249–254. https://doi.org/10.1097/00041433-200306000-00004.

Kafri, I. and Cherry, J.A. (1984) Supplemental ascorbic acid and heat stress in broiler chicks. Poult. Sci. J. 63(1):125.

Kafri, I., Rosebrough, R.W., McMurtry, J.P. and Steele, N.C. (1988) Corticosterone implants and supplemental ascorbic acid effects on lipid metabolism in broiler chicks. Poult. Sci. 67(9):1356–1359. https://doi.org/10.3382/ps.0671356.

Kakhki, R., Heuthorst, T., Wornath-Vanhumbeck, A., Neijat, M. and Kiarie, E. (2019) Medullary bone attributes in aged Lohmann LSL-lite layers fed different levels of calcium and top-dressed 25-hydroxyvitamin D_3. Can. J. Anim. Sci. 99(1):138–149. https://doi.org/10.1139/cjas-2018-0062.

Kalantar, M., Hosseini, S.M., Hosseini, M.R., Kalantar, M.H., Farmanullah, F. and Yang, L.G. (2019) Effects of *in ovo* injection of coenzyme Q10 on hatchability, subsequent performance, and immunity of broiler chickens. BioMed Res. Int. 2019:7167525. https://doi.org/10.1155/2019/7167525.

Kalbfleisch, J., Erf, G.F., Brannon, J. and Noll, S. (2000) Effects of dietary vitamin E supplementation in young male poults. Growth performance and lymphoid organ characteristics. Poult. Sci. 79(1):116.

Kallner, A., Hartmann, D. and Hornig, D. (1977) On the absorption of ascorbic acid in man. Int. J. Vitam. Nutr. Res. 47(4):383–388. PMID:591210.

Kan, P., Mitchell, M.A. and Carlisle, A.J. (1993) Effect of vitamin E on thyroid hormone production in heat stressed broiler chickens. Proc. 4th Eur. Symp. Poultry Welfare, Edinburgh, Scotland, UK. (pp. 295–297).

Kaneko, K., Kiyose, C., Ueda, T., Ichikawa, H. and Igarashi, O. (2000) Studies of the metabolism of a-tocopherol stereoisomers in rats using [5-methyl-14C]SRR- and RRR-a-tocopherol. J. Lipid Res. 41(3):357–367. https://doi.org/10.1016/S0022-2275(20)34474-6.

Kang, D.K., Kim, S.I., Cho, C.H., Yim, Y.H. and Kim, H.S. (2003) Use of lycopene, an antioxidant carotenoid, in laying hens for egg pigmentation. Asian Aust. J. Anim. Sci. 16(12):1799–1803. https://doi.org/10.5713/ajas.2003.1799.

Kao, C. and Robinson, R.J. (1972) *Aspergillus flavus* deterioration of grain: its effect on amino acids and vitamins in whole wheat. J. Food Sci. 37(2):261–263. https://doi.org/10.1111/j.1365-2621.1972.tb05831.x.

Käppeli, S., Fröhlich, E., Gebhardt-Henrich, S.G., Pfulg, A., Schäublin, H., Zweifel, R., Wiedmer, H. and Stoffel, M.H. (2011) Effects of dietary supplementation with synthetic vitamin D_3 and 25-hydroxycholecalciferol on blood calcium and phosphate levels and performance in laying hens. Archiv. Geflügelkunde 75:179–184.

Karadas, F., Pappas, A.C., Surai, P.F. and Speake, B.K. (2005) Embryonic development within carotenoid-enriched eggs influences the post-hatch carotenoid status of the chicken. Comp. Biochem. Physiol. B Biochem. Mol. Biol. 141(2):244–251. https://doi.org/10.1016/j.cbpc.2005.04.001.

Kasim, A.B. and Edwards, H.M. (2000) Evaluation of cholecalciferol sources using broiler chick bioassays. Poult. Sci. 79(11):1617–1622. https://doi.org/10.1093/ps/79.11.1617.

Kasner, P., Chambon, P. and Leid, M. (1994) Role of nuclear retinoic acid receptors in the regulation of gene expression. In Vitamin A in health and disease Blomhoff, R. (ed.). CRC Press. (p. 189).

Kassim, H. and Norziha, I. (1995) Effects of ascorbic acid (vitamin C) supplementation in layer and broiler diets in the tropics. Asian. Australas. J. Anim. Sci. 8(6):607–610. https://doi.org/10.5713/ajas.1995.607.

Kaya, S., Umucalilar, H., Haliloglu, S. and Ipek, H. (2001) Dietary vitamin A and zinc on egg yield and some blood parameters of laying hens. Proc. 14th Symp. Egg and Egg Prod. Qual., Leipzig, Germany.

Kazemi-Fard, M., Kermanshahi, H., Rezaei, M. and Golian, M. (2013) Effect of different levels of fennel extract and vitamin D_3 on performance, hatchability and immunity in post molted broiler breeders. Iran. J. Appl. Anim. Sci. 3(4):729–741.

Ke, Z.J. and Gibson, G.E. (2004) Selective response of various brain cell types during neurodegeneration induced by mild impairment of oxidative metabolism. Neurochem. Int. 45(2–3):361–369. https://doi.org/10.1016/j.neuint.2003.09.008.

Kechik, I.T. and Sykes, A.H. (1979) The effect of intestinal coccidiosis (*Eimeria acervulina*) on blood and tissue ascorbic acid concentrations. Br. J. Nutr. 42(1):97–103. https://doi.org/10.1079/bjn19790093.

Kelley, K. and Easter, R. (1987) Nutritional factors can influence immune response of swine. Feedstuffs 59(22):14.

Kennedy, D.G., Rice, D.A., Bruce, D.W., Goodall, E.A. and McIlroy, S.G. (1992) Economic effects of increased vitamin E supplementation of broiler diets on commercial broiler production. Br. Poult. Sci. 33(5):1015–1023. https://doi.org/10.1080/00071669208417544.

Kesavan, V. and Noronha, J.M. (1983) Folate malabsorption in aged rats related to low levels of pancreatic folyl conjugase. Am. J. Clin. Nutr. 37(2):262–267. https://doi.org/10.1093/ajcn/37.2.262.

Keshavarz, K. (1996) The effect of different levels of vitamin C and cholecalciferol with adequate or marginal levels of dietary calcium on performance and eggshell quality of laying hens. Poult. Sci. 75(10):1227–1235. https://doi.org/10.3382/ps.0751227.

Keshavarz, K. (2003a) A comparison between cholecalciferol and 25-OH-cholecalciferol on performance and eggshell quality of hens fed different levels of calcium and phosphorus. Poult. Sci. 82(9):1415–1422. https://doi.org/10.1093/ps/82.9.1415.

Keshavarz, K. (2003b) Effects of reducing dietary protein, methionine, choline, folic acid, and vitamin B12 during the late stages of the egg production cycle on performance and eggshell quality. Poult. Sci. 82(9):1407–1414. https://doi.org/10.1093/ps/82.9.1407.

Keshavarz, K. and Nakajima, S. (1993) Re-evaluation of calcium and phosphorous requirements of laying hens for optimum performance and eggshell quality. Poult. Sci. 72(1):144–153. https://doi.org/10.3382/ps.0720144.

Kettunen, H., Peuranen, S., Remus, J.C., Tiihonen, K. and Virtanen, E. (1999) The bioefficacy of dietary betaine and choline in broiler chicks. Poult. Sci. 78(1):140.

Khajali, F., Khoshoei, E.A. and Moghaddam, A.K. (2006) Effect of vitamin and trace mineral withdrawal from finisher diets on growth performance and immunocompetence of broiler chickens. Br. Poult. Sci. 47(2):159–162. https://doi.org/10.1080/00071660600610732.

Khakpour Irani, F., Daneshyar, M. and Najafi, R. (2015) Growth and antioxidant status of broilers fed supplemental lysine and pyridoxine under high ambient temperature. Vet. Res. Forum 6(2):161–165 PMID: 26261713.

Khalafalla, M.K. and Bessei, W. (1997) Effect of ascorbic acid supplementation on eggshell quality of laying hens receiving saline drinking water. Arch. Geflügelk 61(4):172–175.

Khalifa, O.A., Al Wakeel, R.A., Hemeda, S.A., Abdel-Daim, M.M., Albadrani, G.M., El Askary, A., Fadl, S.E. and Elgendey, F. (2021) The impact of vitamin E and/or selenium dietary supplementation on growth parameters and expression levels of the growth-related genes in broilers. BMC Vet. Res. 17(1):251. https://doi.org/10.1186/s12917-021-02963-1.

Khaligh, F., Hassanabadi, A., Nassiri-Moghaddam, H., Golian, A. and Kalidari, G.A. (2018) Effects of *in ovo* injection of chrysin, quercetin and ascorbic acid on hatchability, somatic attributes, hepatic oxidative status and early post-hatch performance of broiler chicks. J. Anim. Physiol. Anim. Nutr. (Berl) 102(1):e413-e420. https://doi.org/10.1111/jpn.12760.

Khan, R.U., Naz, S., Nikousefat, Z., Selvaggi, M., Laudadio, V. and Tufarelli, V. (2012a) Effect of ascorbic acid in heat-stressed poultry. Worlds Poult. Sci. J. 68(3):477–490. https://doi.org/10.1017/S004393391200058X.

Khan, R.U., Rahman, Z.U., Nikousefat, Z., Javdani, M., Laudadio, V. and Tufarelli, V. (2012b) Vitamin E: pharmaceutical role in poultry male fecundity. Poult. Sci. 68(1):63–70. https://doi.org/10.1017/S0043933912000074.

Khan, R.U., Rahman, Z.U., Nikousefat, Z., Javdani, M., Tufarelli, V., Dario, C., Selvaggi, M. and Laudadio, V. (2012c) Immunomodulating effects of vitamin E in broilers. World's Poult. Sci. 68(1):31–40. https://doi.org/10.1017/S0043933912000049.

Khan, R.U., Rahman, Z.U., Javed, I. and Muhammad, F. (2013) Effect of vitamins, probiotics and protein level on semen traits and seminal plasma biochemical parameters of post-moult male broiler breeders. Br. Poult. Sci. 54(1):120–129. https://doi.org/10.1080/00071668.2012.753511.

Khan, S.A. (2019) Inclusion of pyridoxine to flaxseed cake in poultry feed improves productivity of omega-3 enriched eggs. Bioinformation 15(5):333–341. https://doi.org/10.6026/97320630015333.

Khan, S.H., Shahid, R., Mian, A.A., Sardar, R. and Anjum, M.A. (2010) Effect of the level of cholecalciferol supplementation of broiler diets on the performance and tibial dyschondroplasia. J. Anim. Physiol. Anim. Nutr. (Berl) 94(5):584–593. https://doi.org/10.1111/j.1439-0396.2009.00943.x.

Khan, W.A., Khan, M.Z., Khan, A. and Hussain, I. (2010) Pathological effects of aflatoxin and their amelioration by vitamin E in white leghorn layers. Pak. Vet. J. 30(3):155–162.

Khan, W.A., Khan, M.Z., Khan, A., Ul Hassan, Z. and Saleemi, M.K. (2014) Potential for amelioration of aflatoxin b1-induced immunotoxic effects in progeny of white leghorn breeder hens co-exposed to vitamin E. J. Immunotoxicol. 11(2):116–125. https://doi.org/10.3109/1547691X.2013.804134.

Khattak, F.M., Scaife, J.R. and Acamovic, T. (1996) Influence of whole mustard seed and supplemental vitamin E on lipid oxidation in broiler meat. Br. Poult. Sci. 37:S58-S59.

Khoramabadi, V., Akbari, M.R., Khajali, F., Noorani, H. and Rahmatnejad, E. (2014) Influence of xylanase and vitamin A in wheat-based diet on performance, nutrients digestibility, small intestinal morphology and digesta viscosity in broiler chickens. Acta Scient. Acta Sci. Anim. Sci. 36(4):379. https://doi.org/10.4025/actascianimsci.v36i4.23910.

Kidd, M.T. (2003) A treatise on chicken dam nutrition that impacts on progeny. World's Poult. Sci. 59(4): 475–494. https://doi.org/10.1079/WPS20030030.

Kidd, M.T. (2004) Nutritional modulation of immune function in broilers. Poult. Sci. 83(4):650–657. https://doi.org/10.1093/ps/83.4.650.

Kim, Y.I., Miller, J.W., Da Costa, K.A., Nadeau, M., Smith, D., Selhub, J., Zeisel, S.H. and Mason, J.B. (1994) Severe folate deficiency causes secondary depletion of choline and phosphocholine in rat liver. J. Nutr. 124(11):2197–2203. https://doi.org/10.1093/jn/124.11.2197.

King, A.J., Uijttenboogaart, T.G. and De Vries, A.W. (1993) A comparative study: α-tocopherol, beta-carotene and ascorbic acid as antioxidants in stored poultry muscle. Proc. 11th Eur. Symp. Qual. Poult. Meat. (pp. 435–441).

King, A.J., Uijttenboogaart, T.G. and De Vries, A.W. (1995) α-tocopherol, β-carotene and ascorbic acid as antioxidants in stored poultry muscle. J. Food Sci. 60(5):1009–1012. https://doi.org/10.1111/j.1365-2621.1995.tb06281.x.

Kirichenko, A. (1991) Proportion of group B vitamins in diets for table hens. Ptitsevodstvo 5:13–14.

Kirkland, J.B. (2013) Niacin. In "Handbook of vitamins" 5th edition Zempleni, J., Suttie, J., Gregory, J. and Stover P J. (ed.). Taylor & Francis Group. (pp. 149–190).

Kirunda, D.F., Scheideler, S.E. and McKee, S.R. (2001) The efficacy of vitamin E (DL-alpha-tocopheryl acetate) supplementation in hen diets to alleviate egg quality deterioration associated with temperature exposure. Poult. Sci. 80(9):1378–1383. https://doi.org/10.1093/ps/80.9.1378.

Kiyose, C., Muramatsu, R., Ueda, T. and Igarashi, O. (1995) Change in the distribution of a-tocopherol stereoisomers in rats after intravenous administration. Biosci. Biotechnol. Biochem. 59(5):791–795. https://doi.org/10.1271/bbb.59.791.

Kjaer, J.B., Su, G., Nielsen, B.L. and Sørensen, P. (2006) Foot pad dermatitis and hock burn in broiler chickens and degree of inheritance. Poult. Sci. 85(8):1342–1348. https://doi.org/10.1093/ps/85.8.1342.

Klasing, K.C. (1998) "Comparative avian nutrition". CAB International.

Klasing, K.C. (2007) Nutrition and the immune system. Br. Poult. Sci. 48(5):525–537. https://doi.org/10.1080/00071660701671336.

Klein, D.L., Novilla, M. N. and Watkins, K. L. (1994) Nutritional encephalomalacia in turkeys: diagnosis and growth performance Avian Diseases 38:653–659. https://doi.org/10.2307/1592094.

Klein-Hessling, H. (2006) Chondrodystrophy in turkeys and broilers. World Poult. 22(9):35–36.

Kliewer, S.A., Umesono, K., Mangelsdorf, D.J. and Evans, R.M. (1992) Retinoid X receptor interacts with nuclear receptors in retinoic acid, thyroid hormone and vitamin D_3 signaling. Nature 355(6359):446–449. https://doi.org/10.1038/355446a0.

Kodentsova, V.M., Yakusina, L.M., Vrzhesinskaya, O.A., Beketova, N.A. and Sprichev, V.B. (1993) Effect of riboflavin status on pyridoxine metabolism. Vopr. pitan. 5:32.

Kodicek, E., Ashby, D.R., Muller, M. and Carpenter, K.J. (1974) The conversion of bound nicotinic acid to free nicotinamide on roasting sweet corn. Proc. Nutr. Soc. 33(3):105A-106A. PMID:4282141.

Kolb, E. (1984) Metabolism of ascorbic acid in livestock under pathological conditions. In "Ascorbic acid in domestic animals" Wegger, I., Tagwerker, F.J. and Moustgaard, J. (ed.). Workshop. Danish, R. Agr. Society, Copenhagen:(162–175).

Kolb, E. and Seehawer, J. (2001) Significance and application of ascorbic acid in poultry. Archiv. Geflügelk 65(3):106–113.

Kominato T. (1971) Speed of vitamin B_{12} turnover and its relation to the intestine in the rat. Vitamins. 44:76–83.

Konieczka, P., Rozbicka-Wieczorek, A.J., Czauderna, M. and Smulikowska, S. (2017) Beneficial effects of enrichment of chicken meat with n-3 polyunsaturated fatty acids, vitamin E and selenium on health parameters: a study on male rats. Animal 11(8):1412–1420. https://doi.org/10.1017/S1751731116002652.

Konjufca, V.K., Bottje, W.G., Bersi, T.K. and Erf, G.F. (2004) Influence of dietary vitamin E on phagocytic functions of macrophages in broilers. Poult. Sci. 83(9):1530–1534. https://doi.org/10.1093/ps/83.9.1530.

Koreleski, J. and Świątkiewicz, S. (2005) Performance and tibia bones quality in broilers fed diet supplemented with particular limestone and 25-hydroxycholecalciferol. Proc. 15th Eur. Symp. Poult. Nutr., Balatonfured, Hungary. (pp. 215–218).

Koreleski, J. and Świątkiewicz, S. (2006) Fatty acids and T-BARS in frozen stored breast meat of chickens fed diets with rapeseed oil supplemented with fish oil and vitamin E. Proc. 12th Eur. Poult. Nutr., Verona, Italy.

Kostadinović, L., Teodosin, S., Lević, J., Čolović, R., Banjac, V., Vukmirović, Đ. and Sredanović, S. (2014) Effect of pelleting and expanding processes on vitamin A stability in animal feeds. Process. Energy Agric. 18(1):44–46.

Koutsos, E. (2003) Carotenoids in avian immunity. Proc. Calif. Anim. Nutr. Conf. (p. 179).

Koutsos, E.A., Clifford, A.J., Calvert, C.C. and Klasing, K.C. (2003) Maternal carotenoid status modifies the incorporation of dietary carotenoids into immune tissues of growing chickens (*Gallus gallus domesticus*). J. Nutr. 133(4):1132–1138. https://doi.org/10.1093/jn/133.4.1132.

Koutsos, E.A., García López, J.C. and Klasing, K.C. (2006) Carotenoids from *in ovo* or dietary sources blunt systemic indices of the inflammatory response in growing chicks (*Gallus gallus domesticus*). J. Nutr. 136(4):1027–1031. https://doi.org/10.1093/jn/136.4.1027.

Koutsos, E.A., Tell, L.A., Woods, L.W. and Klasing, K.C. (2003) Adult cockatiels (*Nymphicus hollandicus*) at maintenance are more sensitive to diets containing excess vitamin A than to vitamin A-deficient diets. J. Nutr. 133(6):1898–1902. https://doi.org/10.1093/jn/133.6.1898.

Kovar, S.J., Ingram, D.R., Hagedorn, T.K., Klemperer, M.D., Barnes, D.G. and Laurent, S.M. (1990) Broiler performance as influenced by dietary sodium zeolite-A and ascorbic acid. Poult. Sci. 69(1):75.

Kralik, Z., Kralik, G., Grčević, M., Kralik, I. and Gantner, V. (2018) Physical-chemical characteristics of designer and conventional eggs. Rev. Bras. Cienc Avic 20(1):119–126. https://doi.org/10.1590/1806-9061-2017-0631.

Kranen, R.W., Lambooij, E., Veerkamp, C.H., Van Kuppevelt, T.H. and Veerkamp, J.H. (2000) Hemorrhages in muscles of broiler chickens. World's. Poult. Sci. 56(2):93–126. https://doi.org/10.1079/WPS20000009.

Krautmann, B.A. (1989) Practical application of ascorbic acid in combating stress. in "The role of vitamin C in poultry stress management". Roche Tech, Symp., Atlanta, GA, USA. (pp. 48–67).

Krautmann, B.A., Gwyther, M.J., Lentz, E.L. and Peterson, L.A. (1991) Effect of ascorbic acid on carcass yield in broiler chickens. Poult. Sci. 70(1):67–73.

Krinke, G.J. and Fitzgerald, R.E. (1988) The pattern of pyridoxine-induced lesion: difference between the high and the low toxic level. Toxicology 49(1):171–178. https://doi.org/10.1016/0300-483X(88)90190-4.

Krishnan, S., Bhuyan, U.N., Talwar, G.P. and Ramalingaswami, R. (1974) Effect of vitamin A and protein calorie undernutrition on immune responses. Immunol. 27(3):383–392.

Krishnan-Rajalekshmy, P. (2010). Effects of dietary choline, folic acid and vitamin B_{12} on laying hen performance, egg components and egg phospholipid composition. University of Nebraska, Lincoln.

Kristiansen, F. (1973) Conditions in poultry associated with deficiencies of vitamin E in Norway. Acta Agric. Scand. 19:51–57.

Kríz, H. and Holman, J. (1969) Histology of onset of skin changes in hypervitaminosis A in chickens. Int. Z. Vitaminforsch. 39(1):3–12. PMID:5784665.

Krumdieck, C.L. (1990) Folic acid. In "Present knowledge in nutrition" 6th edition Brown, M.L. (ed.) Int. Life Sci. Institute/Nutrition Foundation. (pp. 179–188).

Kubota, M., Abe, E., Shinki, T. and Suda, T. (1981) Vitamin D metabolism and its possible role in the developing chick embryo. Biochem. J. 194(1):103–109. https://doi.org/10.1042/bj1940103.

Kucuk, O., Sahin, N. and Sahin, K. (2003a) Supplemental zinc and vitamin A can alleviate negative effects of heat stress in broiler chickens. Biol. Trace Elem. Res. 94(3):225–235. https://doi.org/10.1385/BTER:94:3:225.

Kucuk, O., Sahin, N., Sahin, K., Gursu, M.F., Gulcu, F., Ozcelik, M. and Issi, M. (2003b) Egg production, egg quality, and lipid peroxidation status in laying hens maintained at a low ambient temperature (6 degrees C) and fed a vitamin C and vitamin E supplemented diet. Vet. Med. 48(1):33–40. https://doi.org/10.17221/5747-VETMED.

Kucuk, O., Kahraman, A., Kurt, I., Yildiz, N. and Onmaz, A.C. (2008) A combination of zinc and pyridoxine supplementation to the diet of laying hens improves performance and egg quality. Biol. Trace Elem. Res. 126(1–3):165–175. https://doi.org/10.1007/s12011-008-8190-z.

Kucukersan, S. (2000) The effect of niacin added to the laying hen rations on egg production and egg quality with some blood metabolites. Ank. Univ. Vet. Fak. Derg. 47(2):201–212.

Kurnick, A.A., Hanold, F.J. and Stangeland, V.A. (1972) Problems in the use of feed ingredient vitamin values in formulating feeds. Proc. 1972 Georgia Nutr. Conf. Feed Ind.

Kurkure, N.V., Kalorey, D.R. and Bhandarkar, A.G. (2004) The effect of vitamin E and selenium on reversal of ochratoxicosis in broilers: growth, hematological and immunological study. Proc. 12th World's Poultr. Congr., Istanbul, Turkey.

Kutlu, H.R. (2001) Influence of wet-feeding and supplementation with ascorbic acid on performance and carcass composition of broiler chicks exposed to high ambient temperature. Archiv Geflügelk 61(2):172–175. https://doi.org/10.1080/17450390109381972.

Kutlu, H.R. and Forbes, J.M. (1994) Responses of broiler chicks to dietary ascorbic acid and corticosterone. Br. Poult. Sci. 35(1):184–185. https://doi.org/10.1080/00071669408417682.

Kutlu, H.R. and Forbes, J.M. (1994) Self-selection for ascorbic acid by broiler chicks in response to changing environmental temperature. Livest. Prod. Sci. 36(5):820.

Kuttappan, V.A., Goodgame, S.D., Bradley, C.D., Mauromoustakos, A., Hargis, B.M., Waldroup, P.W. and Owens, C.M. (2012b) Effect of different levels of dietary vitamin E (DL-α-tocopherol acetate) on the occurrence of various degrees of white striping on broiler breast fillets. Poult. Sci. 91(12):3230–3235. https://doi.org/10.3382/ps.2012-02397.

Ladmakhi, M.H., Buys, N., Dewil, E., Rahimi, G. and Decuypere, E. (1997) The prophylactic effect of vitamin C supplementation on broiler ascites incidence and plasma thyroid hormone concentration. Avian Pathol. 26(1):33–44. https://doi.org/10.1080/03079459708419191.

Lakritz, L. and Thayer, D.W. (1994) Effect of gamma radiation on total tocopherols in fresh chicken breast muscle. Meat Sci. 37(3):439–448. https://doi.org/10.1016/0309-1740(94)90059-0.

Lakritz, L., Fox, J.B., Hampson, J., Richardson, R., Kohout, K. and Thayer, D.W. (1995) Effect of gamma radiation on levels of α-tocopherol in red meats and turkey. Meat Sci. 41(3): 261–271. https://doi.org/10.1016/0309-1740(94)00003-P.

Lakshmi, A.V., Prasad, R.K. and Bamji, M.S. (1990) Effect of riboflavin deficiency on collagen content of cornea and bone. J. Clin. Biochem. Nutr. 9(2):115–118. https://doi.org/10.3164/jcbn.9.115.

Lakshmi, R., Lakshmi, A.V. and Bamji, M.S. (1989) Skin wound healing in riboflavin deficiency. Biochem. Med. Metab. Biol. 42(3):185–191. https://doi.org/10.1016/0885-4505(89)90054-6.

Lal, H., Pandey, R. and Aggarwal, S.K. (1999) Vitamin D: non-skeletal actions and effects on growth. Nutr. Res. 19(11):1683–1718. https://doi.org/10.1016/S0271-5317(99)00124-4.

Lambertz, C., Leopold, J., Damme, K., Vogt-Kaute, W., Ammer, S. and Leiber, F. (2020) Effects of a riboflavin source suitable for use in organic broiler diets on performance traits and health indicators. Animal 14(4):716–724. https://doi.org/10.1017/S175173111900243X.

Landauer, W. (1967) The hatchability of chicken eggs was influenced by environment and heredity. Storrs Agricultural Experimental Station Monograph 1 (revised). Storrs Agricultural Experiment Station (SAES).

Larbier, M. and Leclercq, B. (1992) Nutrition et alimentation des volailles. Institut National de la Recherche Agronomique (INRA). (pp. 139–170).

Larbier, M. and Leclercq, B. (1994) "Nutrition and feeding of poultry". Nottingham University Press.

Larroudé, P., Castaing, J., Hamelin, C. and Ball, A. (2005) Effet d'une supplementation en Hy-D® pour deux niveaux d'apports en vitamins sur les performances, le development osseux et les troubles locomoteurs des dindons. 6th Journées de la Recherche Avicole. Paris, France. (pp. 244–248).

Latshaw, J.D. (1991) Nutrition-mechanisms of immunosuppression. Vet. Immunol. Immunopathol. 30(1): 111–120. https://doi.org/10.1016/0165-2427(91)90012-2.

Latshaw, J.D. and Jensen, L.S. (1972) Choline deficiency and synthesis of choline from precursors in mature Japanese quail. J. Nutr. 102(6):749–755. https://doi.org/10.1093/jn/102.6.749.

Latymer, E.A. and Coates, M.E. (1981) The effects of high dietary supplements of copper sulphate on pantothenic acid metabolism in the chick. Br. J. Nutr. 45(2):431–439. https://doi.org/10.1079/BJN19810118.

Lauridsen, C., Buckley, D.J. and Morrissey, P.A. (1997) Influence of dietary fat and vitamin E supplementation on α-tocopherol levels and fatty acid profiles in chicken muscle membranal fractions and on susceptibility to lipid peroxidation. Meat Sci. 46(1):9–22. https://doi.org/10.1016/s0309-1740(97)00010-7.

Lauzon, D.A., Johnston, S.L., Southern, L.L. and Xu, Z. (2008) The effect of carrier for vitamin E on liver concentrations of vitamin E and vitamin E excretion in broilers. Poult. Sci. 87(5):934–939. https://doi.org/10.3382/ps.2007-00241.

Lavelle, P.A., Lloyd, Q.P., Gay, C.V. and Leach, R.M. (1994) Vitamin K deficiency does not functionally impair skeletal metabolism of laying hens and their progeny. J. Nutr. 124(3):371–377. https://doi.org/10.1093/jn/124.3.371.

Leach, R.M. and Burdette, J.H. (1985) The influence of ascorbic acid on the occurrence of tibial dyschondroplasia in young broiler chickens. Poult. Sci. 64(6):1188–1191. https://doi.org/10.3382/ps.0641188.

Leach, R.M. and Monsonego-Ornan, E. (2007) Tibial dyschondroplasia 40 years later. Poult. Sci. 86(10):2053–2058. https://doi.org/10.1093/ps/86.10.2053.

Lechowski, J. and Nagórna-Stasiak, B. (1993) The effect of biotin supplementation on ascorbic acid metabolism in chickens. Arch. vet. pol. 33(1–2):19–27. PMID:8055051.

Leclercq, B., Blum, J.C., Sauveur, B. and Stevens, P. (1987) Nutrition of laying hens. In Feeding of non-ruminant livestock Wiseman, J. (ed.). Butterworths. (pp. 78–85).

Ledwaba, M.F. and Roberson, K.D. (2003) Effectiveness of twenty-five hydroxycholecalciferols in the prevention of tibial dyschondroplasia in Ross cockerels depends on calcium level. Poult. Sci. 82(11):1769–1777. https://doi.org/10.1093/ps/82.11.1769.

Lee, D.J.W. (1982) Growth, erythrocyte glutathione reductase and liver flavine as indicators of riboflavin status in turkey poults. Br. Poult. Sci. 23(3):263–272. https://doi.org/10.1080/00071688208447956.

Lee, C.M. and White, H.B. (1996) Riboflavin-binding protein induces early death of chicken embryos. J. Nutr. 126(2):523–528. https://doi.org/10.1093/jn/126.2.523.

Lee, L.C., Carlson, R.W., Judge, D.L. and Ogawa, M. (1973) The absorption cross sections of N_2, O_2, CO, NO, CO_2, N_2O, CH_4, C_2H_4, C_2H_6 and C_4H_{10} from 180 to 700A. J. Quant. Spectrosc. Radiati Transf. 13(10):1023–1031. https://doi.org/10.1016/0022-4073(73)90075-7.

Leeson, S. (2007) Vitamin requirements: is there basis for re-evaluating dietary specifications? Worlds Poult. Sci. J. 63(2):255–266. https://doi.org/10.1017/S0043933907001444.

Leeson, S. (2008) Dietary allowances for poultry. Feedstuffs 7 :53–61.

Leeson, S. and Caston, L.J. (2003) Vitamin enrichment of eggs. J. Appl. Poult. Res. 12(1):24–26. https://doi.org/10.1093/japr/12.1.24.

Leeson, S. and Marcotte, M. (1993) Irradiation of poultry feed. II. Effect on nutrient composition. Worlds Poult. Sci. J. 49(1):19–33. https://doi.org/10.1079/WPS19930003.

Leeson, S. and Summers, J.D. (1978) Effect of vitamin deficiencies on hatchability. Poult. Sci. 5:1152–1152.

Leeson, S. and Summers, J.D. (2008) Commercial poult. Nutr. 3rd edn. Nottingham University Press (digital edition) https://www.agropustaka.id/wp-content/uploads/2020/04/agropustaka.id_buku_Commercial-Poultry-Nutrition-3rd-Edition-by-S.-Leeson-J.-D.-Summers.pdf.

Leeson, S., Reinhart, B.S. and Summers, J.D. (1979a) Response of white leghorn and Rhode-Ssland red breeder hens to dietary deficiencies of synthetic vitamins. 1. Egg production, hatchability and chick growth. Can. J. Anim. Sci. 59(3):561–567. https://doi.org/10.4141/cjas79-070.

Leeson, S., Reinhart, B.S. and Summers, J.D. (1979b) Response of white leghorn and Rhode Island Red breeder hens to dietary deficiencies of synthetic vitamins. 2. Embryo mortality and abnormalities. Can. J. Anim. Sci. 59(3):569–575. https://doi.org/10.4141/cjas79-071.

Leeson, S., Caston, L.J. and Summers, J.D. (1991) Response of laying hens to supplemental niacin. Poult. Sci. 70(5):1231–1235. https://doi.org/10.3382/ps.0701231.

Leeson, S., Díaz, G. and Summers, J.D. (1995) Poultry metabolic disorders and mycotoxins. Ed. Guelph by University Books. (pp. 351).

Lehninger, A.L. (1982) Principles of biochemistry. Worth Publishers, New York.

Leiber, F., Holinger, M., Amsler, Z., Maeschli, A., Maurer, V., Früh, B., Lambertz, C. and Ayrle, H. (2022) Riboflavin for laying hens fed organic winter diets: effects of different supplementation rates on health, performance and egg quality. Biol. Agric. Hortic. 38(1):1–16. https://doi.org/10.1080/01448765.2021.1955005.

Lemire, J.M. (1992) Immunomodulatory role of 1,25 dihydroxy. J. Cell. Biochem. 49(1):26–31. https://doi.org/10.1002/jcb.240490106.

Leonard, S.W., Terasawa, Y., Farese, R.V. and Traber, M.G. (2002) Incorporation of deuterated RRR- or all-rac-a-tocopherol in plasma and tissues of a-tocopherol transfer protein-null mice. Am. J. Clin. Nutr. 75(3):555–560. https://doi.org/10.1093/ajcn/75.3.555.

Leshchinsky, T.V. and Klasing, K.C. (2001) Relationship between the level of dietary vitamin E and the immune response of broiler chickens. Poult. Sci. 80(11):1590–1599. https://doi.org/10.1093/ps/80.11.1590.

Leshchinsky, T.V. and Klasing, K.C. (2003) Profile of chicken cytokines induced by lipopolysaccharide is modulated by dietary α-tocopheryl acetate. Poult. Sci. 82(8):1266–1273. https://doi.org/10.1093/ps/82.8.1266.

Leskovec, J., Levart, A., Perić, L., Đukić Stojčić, M.Đ., Tomović, V., Pirman, T., Salobir, J. and Rezar, V. (2019) Antioxidative effects of supplementing linseed oil-enriched diets with α-tocopherol, ascorbic acid, selenium, or their combination on carcass and meat quality in broilers. Poult. Sci. 98(12):6733–6741. https://doi.org/10.3382/ps/pez389.

Lessard, M., Hutchings, D. and Cave, N.A. (1997) Cell-mediated and humoral immune responses in broiler chickens maintained on diets containing different levels of vitamin A. Poult. Sci. 76(10):1368–1378. https://doi.org/10.1093/ps/76.10.1368.

Lewis, E.D., Meydani, S.N. and Wu, D. (2019) Regulatory role of vitamin E in the immune system and inflammation. IUBMB Life 71(4):487–494. https://doi.org/10.1002/iub.1976.

Lewis, L.L., Stark, C.R., Fahrenholz, A.C., Bergstrom, J.R. and Jones, C.K. (2015) Evaluation of conditioning time and temperature on gelatinized starch and vitamin retention in a pelleted swine diet. J. Anim. Sci. 93(2):615–619. https://doi.org/10.2527/jas.2014-8074.

Leyva-Jimenez, H., Khan, M., Gardner, K., Abdaljaleel, R.A., Al-Jumaa, Y., Alsadwi, A.M. and Bailey, C.A. (2019) Developing a novel oral vitamin D_3 intake bioassay to re-evaluate the vitamin D_3 requirement for modern broiler chickens. Poult. Sci. 98(9):3770–3776. https://doi.org/10.3382/ps/pez074.

Li, D., Zhang, K., Bai, S., Wang, J., Zeng, Q., Peng, H., Su, Z., Xuan, Y., Qi, S. and Ding, X. (2021) Effect of 25-hydroxycholecalciferol with different vitamin D_3 levels in the hens diet in the rearing period on growth performance, bone quality, egg production, and eggshell quality. Agriculture 11(8):698. https://doi.org/10.3390/agriculture11080698.

Li, J., Hou, S.S. and Huang, J.C. (1994) Studies of the biotin deficiency and requirement of broiler chicks. Acta vet. zootech. sin. 25:295.

Li, J., Bi, D., Pan, S., Zhang, Y. and Zhou, D. (2008) Effects of high dietary vitamin A supplementation on tibial dyschondroplasia, skin pigmentation and growth performance in avian broilers. Res. Vet. Sci. 84(3):409–412. https://doi.org/10.1016/j.rvsc.2007.11.008.

Li, S.X., Cherian, G. and Sim, J.S. (1996) Cholesterol oxidation in egg yolk powder during storage and heating as affected by dietary oils and tocopherol. J. Food Sci. 61(4):721–725. https://doi.org/10.1111/j.1365-2621.1996.tb12189.x.

Li, W., Maeda, N. and Beck, M.A. (2006) Vitamin C deficiency increases the lung pathology of influenza virus-infected gulo-/-mice. J. Nutr. 136(10):2611–2616. https://doi.org/10.1093/jn/136.10.2611.

Lima, H.J.D. and Souza, L.A.Z. (2018) Vitamin A in the diet of laying hens: enrichment of table eggs to prevent nutritional deficiencies in humans. Worlds Poult. Sci. J. 74(4):619–626. https://doi.org/10.1017/S004393391800065X.

Lin, C.F., Asghar, A., Gray, J.I., Buckley, D.J., Booren, A.M., Crackel, R.L. and Flegal, C.J. (1989a) Effects of oxidised dietary oil and antioxidant supplementation on broiler growth and meat stability. Br. Poult. Sci. 30(4):855–864. https://doi.org/10.1080/00071668908417212.

Lin, C.F., Gray, J.I., Asghar, A., Buckley, D.J., Booren, A.M. and Flegal, C.J. (1989b) Effects of dietary oils and α-tocopherol supplementation on lipid composition and stability of broiler meat. J. Food Sci. 54(6):1457–1460. https://doi.org/10.1111/j.1365-2621.1989.tb05134.x.

Lin, H., Du, R. and Zhang, Z.Y. (2000) The peroxidation in tissues of heat-stressed broilers. Aust. J. Anim. Sci. 13(10):1373–1376. https://doi.org/10.5713/ajas.2000.1373.

Lin, H., Wang, L.F., Song, J.L., Xie, Y.M. and Yang, Q.M. (2002) Effect of dietary supplemental levels of vitamin A on the egg production and immune responses of heat-stressed laying hens. Poult. Sci. 81(4):458–465. https://doi.org/10.1093/ps/81.4.458.

Lin, H., Buyse, J., Sheng, Q.K., Xie, Y.M. and Song, J.L. (2003) Effects of ascorbic acid supplementation on the immune function and laying hen performance of heat- stressed laying hens. J. Feed Agric. Environ. 1(2):103–107.

Lin, H., Jiao, H.C., Buyse, J. and Decuypere, E. (2006) Strategies for preventing heat stress in poultry. Worlds Poult. Sci. J. 62(1):71–86. https://doi.org/10.1079/WPS200585.

Lin, H.Y., Chung, T.K., Chen, Y.H., Walzem, R.L. and Chen, S.E. (2019) Dietary supplementation of 25-hydroxycholecalciferol improves livability in broiler breeder hens. Poult. Sci. 98(11):6108–6116. https://doi.org/10.3382/ps/pez330.

Lin, P., Lu, J., Lin, P.H. and Lu, J.J. (1997) The effects of different dietary nutrients levels and ascorbic acid supplementations on performances, eggshell quality and blood parameter of laying hens in a hot season in Taiwan. J. Chin. Soc. Anim. Sci. 26:395–408.

Lin, Y.F., Chang, S.J. and Hsu, A.L. (2004) Effects of supplemental vitamin E during the laying period on the reproductive performance of Taiwan native chickens. Br. Poult. Sci. 45(6):807–814. https://doi.org/10.1080/00071660400012717.

Lin, Y.F., Chang, S.J., Yang, J.R., Lee, Y.P. and Hsu, A.L. (2005a) Effects of supplemental vitamin E during the mature period on the reproduction performance of Taiwan native chicken cockerels. Br. Poult. Sci. 46(3):366–373. https://doi.org/10.1080/00071660500098186.

Lin, Y.F., Tsai, H.L., Lee, Y.C. and Chang, S.J. (2005b) Maternal vitamin E supplementation affects the antioxidant capability and oxidative status of hatching chicks. J. Nutr. 135(10):2457–2461. https://doi.org/10.1093/jn/135.10.2457.

Lindshield, B.L. and Erdman, J.W. (2006) Carotenoids. In Present knowledge in nutrition 9th ed Bowman, B.A. and Russell, R.M. (ed.). International Life Sciences Institute. (p. 184.197).

Linh, N.T., Guntoro, B. and Hoang Qui, N.H. (2021) Immunomodulatory, behavioral, and nutritional response of tryptophan application on poultry. Vet. World 14(8):2244–2250. https://doi.org/10.14202/vetworld.2021.2244-2250.

Liu, A. and Feng, L. (1992) Effect of supplementation of folic acid, ascorbic acid and cyanocobalamin on the performance of layers. Ningxia J. Agro-For. Sci. Technol. 6:40–42.

Liu, H., Zhang, J., Sorbara, J.O. and Hernandez, J.M. (2022) Effect of coccidiosis vaccine challenge on health growth performance and plasma vitamin absorption of broilers fed optimum dietary vitamins. Poster International Poultry Scientific Forum. Atlanta, GA, USA.

Liu, X., Byrd, J.A., Farnell, M. and Ruiz-Feria, C.A. (2014) Arginine and vitamin E improve the immune response after a salmonella challenge in broiler chicks. Poult. Sci. 93(4):882–890. https://doi.org/10.3382/ps.2013-03723.

Liu, Y., Shen, J., Yang, X., Sun, Q. and Yang, X. (2018) Folic acid reduced triglycerides deposition in primary chicken hepatocytes. J. Agric. Food Chem. 66(50):13162–13172. https://doi.org/10.1021/acs.jafc.8b05193.

Lofland Jr, H.B., Goodman, H.O., Clarkson, T.B. and Prichard, R.W. (1963) Enzyme studies in thiamine-deficient pigeons. J. Nutr. 79(2):188–194. https://doi.org/10.1093/jn/79.2.188.

Lotfi, S., Fakhraei, J. and Mansoori Yarahmadi, H.M. (2021) Dietary supplementation of pumpkin seed oil and sunflower oil along with vitamin E improves sperm characteristics and reproductive hormones in roosters. Poult. Sci. 100(9):101289. https://doi.org/10.1016/j.psj.2021.101289.

Lofton, J.T. and Soares, J.H. (1986) The effects of vitamin D_3 on leg abnormalities in broilers. Poult. Sci. 65(4):749–756. https://doi.org/10.3382/ps.0650749.

Lohakare, J.D., Kim, J.K., Ryu, M.H., Hahn, T.-W. and Chae, B.J. (2005a) Effects of vitamin C and vitamin D interaction on the performance, immunity, and bone characteristics of commercial broilers. J. Appl. Poult. Res. 14(4):670–678. https://doi.org/10.1093/japr/14.4.670.

Lohakare, J.D., Ryu, M.H., Hahn, T.-W., Lee, J.K. and Chae, B.J. (2005b) Effects of supplemental ascorbic acid on the performance and immunity of commercial broilers. J. Appl. Poult. Res. 14(1):10–19. https://doi.org/10.1093/japr/14.1.10.

Lopez, G.A., Phillips, R.W., Nockels, C.F. and Faulkner, L.C. (1973) Body water kinetics in vitamin A-deficient chickens. Proc. Soc. Exp. Biol. Med. 144(1):54–55. https://doi.org/10.3181/00379727-144-37525.

López-Bote, C.J., Gray, J.I., Gomaa, E.A. and Flegal, C.J. (1998a) Effect of dietary oat administration on lipid stability in broiler meat. Br. Poult. Sci. 39(1):57–61. https://doi.org/10.1080/00071669889402.

López-Bote, C.J., Gray, J.I., Gomaa, E.A. and Flegal, C.J. (1998b) Effect of dietary administration of oil extracts from rosemary and sage on lipid oxidation in broiler meat. Br. Poult. Sci. 39(2):235–240. https://doi.org/10.1080/00071669889187.

Lorenzoni, A.G. and Ruiz-Feria, C.A. (2006) Effects of vitamin E and L-arginine on cardiopulmonary function and ascites parameters in broiler chickens reared under subnormal temperatures. Poult. Sci. 85(12):2241–2250. https://doi.org/10.1093/ps/85.12.2241.

Lowry, K.R., Izquierdo, O.A. and Baker, D.H. (1987) Efficacy of betaine relative to choline as a dietary methyl donor. Poult. Sci. 66(1):135 (abstract).

Lu, J., Weil, J.T., Maharjan, P., Manangi, M.K., Cerrate, S. and Coon, C.N. (2021) The effect of feeding adequate or deficient vitamin B_6 or folic acid to breeders on methionine metabolism in 18-day-old chick embryos. Poult. Sci. 100(4):101008. https://doi.org/10.1016/j.psj.2020.12.075.

Luck, M.R., Jeyaseelan, I. and Scholes, R.A. (1995) Ascorbic acid and fertility. Biol. Reprod. 52(2):262–266. https://doi.org/10.1095/biolreprod52.2.262.

Luce, W.G., Peo, E.R. and Hudman, D.B. (1966) Availability of niacin in wheat for swine. J. Nutr. 88(1):39–44. https://doi.org/10.1093/jn/88.1.39.

Luce, W.G., Peo, E.R. and Hudman, D.B. (1967) Availability of niacin in corn and milo for swine. J. Anim. Sci. 26(1):76–84. https://doi.org/10.2527/jas1967.26176x.

Luo, L. and Huang, J. (1991) Effects of vitamin A and D supplementation on tibial dyschondroplasia in broilers. Anim. Feed Sci. Technol. 34(1–2):21–27. https://doi.org/10.1016/0377-8401(94)90188-0.

Lynch, M.P., Faustman, C., Chan, W.K.M., Kerry, J.P. and Buckley, D.J. (1998) A potential mechanism by which α-tocopherol maintains oxymyoglobin pigment through cytochrome b_5 mediated reduction. Meat Sci. 50(3):333–342. https://doi.org/10.1016/S0309-1740(98)00040-0.

Lyon, B.G. and Lyon, C.E. (2002) Color of uncooked and cooked broiler leg quarters associated with chilling temperature and holding time. Poult. Sci. 81(12):1916–1920. https://doi.org/10.1093/ps/81.12.1916.

Machlin, L.J. (1991) Vitamin E. In "Handbook of vitamins" 2nd edn. Machlin, L.J. (ed.). Marcel Dekker, New York.

Machlin, L.J. and Sauberlich, H.E. (1994) New views on the function and health effects of vitamins. Nutr. Today 29(1):25–29. https://doi.org/10.1097/00017285-199401000-00006.

Macklin, K.S., Norton, R.A., Hess, J.B. and Bilgili, S.F. (2000) The effect of vitamin E on cellulitisi in broiler chickens experiencing scratches in a challenge model. Avian Dis. 44(3):701–705. https://doi.org/10.2307/1593115.

Maeda, Y., Kawata, S., Inui, Y., Fukuda, K., Igura, T. and Matsuzawa, Y. (1996) Biotin deficiency decreases ornithine transcarbamylase activity and mRNA in rat liver. J. Nutr. 126(1):61–66. https://doi.org/10.1093/jn/126.1.61.

Maghoul, M.A., Moghadam, H., Kermanshahi, H. and Mesgaran, M. (2009) The effect of different levels of choline and betaine on broilers performance and carcass characteristics. J. Anim. Vet. Adv. 8(1):125–128.

Maharjan, P., Martinez, D.A., Weil, J., Suesuttajit, N., Umberson, C., Mullenix, G., Hilton, K.M., Beitia, A. and Coon, C.N. (2021) Review: physiological growth trend of current meat broilers and dietary protein and energy management approaches for sustainable broiler production. Animal 15(1) (suppl. 1):100284. https://doi.org/10.1016/j.animal.2021.100284.

Mahmood, F.A. and Ahmed, S.Kh. (2017) Effect of adding different levels of biotin to diet on some performance of broiler submitted to oxidative stress. Al-Anbar. J. Vet. Sci. 10(2):1–10.

Mahmoud, K.Z., Edens, F.W., Eisen, E. and Havenstein, G.B. (2004) Ascorbic acid decreases heat-shock protein 70 and plasma corticosterone response in broilers (*Gallus gallus domesticus*) subjected to cyclic heat stress. Comp. Biochem. Physiol. 137(1):35–42. https://doi.org/10.1016/j.cbpc.2003.09.013.

Mahmoudi, M., Azarfar, A. and Khosravinia, H. (2018) Partial replacement of dietary methionine with betaine and choline in heat-stressed broiler chickens. J. Poult. Sci. 55(1):28–37. https://doi.org/10.2141/jpsa.0170087.

Maini, S., Rastogi, S.K., Korde, J.P., Madan, A.K. and Shukla, S.K. (2007) Evaluation of oxidative stress and its amelioration through certain antioxidants in broilers during summer. J. Poult. Sci. 44(3):339–347. https://doi.org/10.2141/jpsa.44.339.

Maiorka, A., Laurentiz, A.C., Santin, E., Araújo, L.F. and Macari, M. (2002) Dietary vitamin or mineral mix removal during the finisher period on broiler chicken performance. J. Appl. Poult. Res. 11(2):121–126. https://doi.org/10.1093/japr/11.2.121.

Maiorka, A., Félix, A.P., Sorbara, J.O.B. and Lecznieski, J. (2010a) Broiler diets demand balanced vitamin supplementation. World Poult. Sci. 26(5):12–14.

Maiorka, A., Portella Félix, A., Sorbara, J.O.B. and Lecznieski, J. (2010b) Niveles vitamínicos para una producción moderna y eficiente de carne de pollo. Selecciones Avícolas.

Malan, D.D., Buyse, J. and Decuypere, E. (2001) Nutrition: an exogenous factor in broiler ascites Proc. 13th Eur. Symp. Poult. Nutr., Blankenberge, Belgium. (pp. 319–326).

Malczyk, E., Kopec, W. and Smolinska, T. (1999) Influence of oil and vitamin E (α-tocopherol) supplementation on lipid oxidation and flavour of poultry meat. 14th Eur. Symp. Quality Poult. Meat., Bologna, Italy.

Manley, J.M., Voitle, R.A. and Harms, R.H. (1978) The influence of hatchability of turkey eggs from the addition of 25-hydroxycholecalciferol to the diet. Poult. Sci. 57(1):290–292 https://doi.org/10.3382/ps.0570290.

Manson, O.H., El-Gendi, G.M. and Okasha, H.M. (2019) Effect of housing system and dietary biotin supplementation on productive performance, some blood constituents and economic efficiency of benha line chicken. Egypt Poult. Sci. 39(1):219–234. https://doi.org/10.21608/epsj.2019.29132.

Manthey, K.C., Griffin, J.B. and Zempleni, J. (2002) Biotin supply affects expression of biotin transporters, biotinylation of carboxylases and metabolism of interleukin-2 in Jurkat cells. J. Nutr. 132(5):887–892. https://doi.org/10.1093/jn/132.5.887.

Maraschiello, C., Sárraga, C. and García-Regueiro, J.A. (1999) Glutathione peroxidase activity, TBARS and α-tocopherol in meat from chickens fed different diets. J. Agric. Food Chem. 47(3):367–382. https://doi.org/10.1021/jf980824o.

March, B.E. (1981) Choline supplementation of layer diets containing soybean meal or rapeseed meal as protein supplement. Poult. Sci. 60(4):818–823. https://doi.org/10.3382/ps.0600818.

Marion, J.E., Harms, R.H. and Arafa, A.S. (1985) Effect of dicumarol and vitamin K source on blood loss and processed yields of broilers. Poult. Sci. 64(7):1306–1309. https://doi.org/10.3382/ps.0641306.

Marks, J. (1975) "A Guide to the vitamins. Their role in health and disease". Springer, Netherlands.

Marounek, M. and Pebriansyah, A. (2018) Use of carotenoids in feed mixtures for poultry: a review. Agric. Trop. Subtrop. 51(3):107–111. https://doi.org/10.2478/ats-2018-0011.

Marriott, B. P., Birt, F. D. , Stalling, V. A. and Yates, A. (2020) Present knowledge in nutrition: basic nutrition and metabolism 11th ed. Academic Press. https://doi.org/10.1016/C2018-0-02422-6.

Marron, L., Bedford, M.R. and McCracken, K.J. (2001) The effects of adding xylanase, vitamin C and copper sulphate to wheat-based diets on broiler performance. Br. Poult. Sci. 42(4):493–500. https://doi.org/10.1080/00071660120070569.

Martin, P.R., Singleton, C.K. and Hiller-Sturmhöfel, S. (2003) The role of thiamine deficiency in alcoholic brain disease. Alcohol Res. Health 27(2):134–142. PMID:15303623.

Martrenchar, A., Boilletot, E., Huonnic, D. and Pol, F. (2002) Risk factors for foot-pad dermatitis in chicken and turkey broilers in France. Prev. Vet. Med. 52(3–4):213–226. https://doi.org/10.1016/s0167-5877(01)00259-8.

Marusich, W.L., Ogrinz, E.F., Brand, M. and Mitrovic, M. (1970) Induction, prevention and therapy of biotin deficiency in turkey poults on semi-purified and commercial-type rations. Poult. Sci. 49(2):412–421. https://doi.org/10.3382/ps.0490412.

Marusich, W.L., Ogrinz, E.F. and Mitrovic, M. (1974) Laboratory model for the detection of poultry growth promotants. Br. Poult. Sci. 15(6):525–533. https://doi.org/10.1080/00071667408416143.

Marusich, W.L. (1984) Vitamin E as an *in vivo* lipid stabilizer and its effect on flavor and properties of milk and meat. In Vitamin E: a comprehensive treatise Machlin, L.J. (ed.). Marcel Dekker, Inc. (p. 445).

Massé, P.G., Pritzker, K.P.H., Mendes, M.G., Boskey, A.L. and Weiser, H. (1994) Vitamin B_6 deficiency experimentally induced bone and joint disorder: microscopic, radiographic and biochemical evidence. Br. J. Nutr. 71(6):919–932. https://doi.org/10.1079/bjn19940196.

Massé, P.G., Rimnac, C.M., Yamauchi, M., Coburn, S.P., Rucker, R.B., Howell, D.S. and Boskey, A.L. (1996) Pyridoxine deficiency affects biomechanical properties of chick tibial bone. Bone 18(6):567–574. https://doi.org/10.1016/8756-3282(96)00072-5.

Matthews, J.O., Ward, T.L. and Southern, L.L. (1997) Interactive effects of betaine and monensin in uninfected and *Eimeria acervulina* infected chicks. Poult. Sci. 76(7):1014–1019. https://doi.org/10.1093/ps/76.7.1014.

Mattila, P., Lehikoinen, K., Kiiskinen, T. and Piironen, V. (1999) Cholecalciferol and 25-hydroxycholecalciferol content of chicken egg yolk as affected by the cholecalciferol content of feed. J. Agric. Food Chem. 47(10):4089–4092. https://doi.org/10.1021/jf990183c.

Mattila, P., Rokka, T., Könkö, K., Valaja, J., Rossow, L. and Ryhänen, E.L. (2003) Effect of cholecalciferol-enriched hen feed on egg quality. J. Agric. Food Chem. 51(1):283–287. https://doi.org/10.1021/jf020743z.

Mattila, P., Valaja, J., Rossow, L., Venäläinen, E. and Tupasela, T. (2004) Effect of vitamin D_2 and D_3 enriched diets on egg vitamin D content, production, and bird condition during an entire production period. Poult. Sci. 83(3):433–440. https://doi.org/10.1093/ps/83.3.433.

Maurice, D.V. (1988) Use of high levels of vitamin B_3 in turkeys. Proc. 1988 Degussa Technical Symposium, Minneapolis, Minnesota Degussa Corp.

Maurice, D.V., Jones, J.E., Lightsey, S.F. and Rhoades, J.F. (1990a) Response of male poults to high levels of dietary niacinamide. Poult. Sci. 69(4):661–668. https://doi.org/10.3382/ps.0690661.

Maurice, D.V., Jones, J.E., Lightsey, S.F., Rhoades, J.F. and Hsu, K.T. (1990b) High dietary niacinamide and performance of male poults at 16 weeks of age. Br. Poult. Sci. 31(4):795–802. https://doi.org/10.1080/00071669008417310.

Maurice, D.V. (1996) Anabolic agents, vitamins, and fermentation co-products as growth promoters in poultry. Proc. 20th World's Poult. Congress, New Delhi, India. (p. 255).

Maurice, D.V. and Lightsey, S.F. (1995) Effect of three grade fats on performance and tissue vitamin E content of broiler chickens. Poult. Sci. 74(1):204.

Maurice, D.V. and Lightsey, S.F. (1996) Toxicity of coproducts of niacinamide synthesis and bioefficacy of niacin sources. Poult. Sci. 75(1):11.

Maurice, D.V., Lightsey, S.F. and Gaylord, T.C. (1993) Immunoenhancement in chickens fed excess dietary vitamin E is dependent on genotype and concentration. Poult. Sci. 72(1):55.

Maurya, V.K. and Aggarwal, M. (2017) Factors influencing the absorption of vitamin D in GIT: an overview. J. Food Sci. Technol. 54(12):3753–3765. https://doi.org/10.1007/s13197-017-2840-0.

Maynard, L.A., Loosli, J.K., Hintz, H.F. and Warner, R.G. (1979) Animal nutrition 7th ed. McGraw-Hill Book, Co.

Mayne, R.K., Else, R.W. and Hocking, P.M. (2007a) High dietary concentrations of biotin did not prevent foot pad dermatitis in growing turkeys and external scores were poor indicators of histopathological lesions. Br. Poult. Sci. 48(3):291–298. https://doi.org/10.1080/00071660701370509.

Mayne, R.K., Else, R.W. and Hocking, P.M. (2007b) High litter moisture alone is sufficient to cause footpad dermatitis in growing turkeys. Br. Poult. Sci. 48(5):538–545. https://doi.org/10.1080/00071660701573045.

Mbajiorgu, C.A., Ng`ambi, J.W. and Norris, D. (2007) Effect of time of initiation of feeding after hatching and influence of dietary ascorbic acid supplementation on productivity, mortality and carcass characteristics of Ross 308 broiler chickens in South Africa. Int. J. Poult. Sci. 6(8):583–591. https://doi.org/10.3923/ijps.2007.583.591.

McCance and Widdowson's (2002) "The composition of foods", 6th summary edition, Food Standards Agency. Royal Society of Chemistry, Cambridge.

McCann, M.E.E., McCracken, K.J., Hoey, L., Pentieva, K., McNulty, H. and Scott, J. (2004) Effect of dietary folic acid supplementation on the folate content of broiler chicken meat. Br. Poult. Sci. 45(1)(suppl. 1):S65-S66. https://doi.org/10.1080/00071660410001698399.

McCay, P.B., Gibson, D.D. and Hornbrook, K.R. (1981) Glutathione dependent inhibition of lipid peroxidation by a soluble heat-labile factor not glutathione peroxidase. Fed Proc. 40(2):199-205 PMID: 7461144.

McCollum, E.V. (1957) "A history of nutrition". Houghton Mifflin Co., Boston, MA.

McCormack, H.A., McTeir, L., Fleming, R.H. and Whitehead, C.C. (2002) Vitamin D requirements of broilers at different dietary concentrations of calcium, phosphorus, and vitamin A. Proc. 11th Eur. Poult. Conf.

McCormick, D.B. (1990) "Riboflavin". In Nutrition reviews, present knowledge in nutrition, Brown, M.L. (ed.), International Life Sci.

McCormick, C.C. and Parker, R.S. (2004) The cytotoxicity of vitamin E is both vitamer- and cell-specific and involves a selectable trait. J. Nutr. 134(12):3335–3342. https://doi.org/10.1093/jn/134.12.3335.

McCormick, D.B. (2006) Vitamin B_6. In Present knowledge in nutrition 9th ed. Bowman, B.A. and Russell, R.M. (ed.). International Life Sciences Institute. (pp. 269–277).

McDowell, L. (1989a) Vitamin supplementation is critical part of good animal nutrition. Feedstuffs 11:15–31.

McDowell, L. (1989b) Vitamins in animal nutrition, comparative aspects to human nutrition Cunha, T.J. (ed.). Academic Press, Inc.

McDowell, L.R. (1989c) Vitamins in animal nutrition 1st ed. Academic Press, New York.

McDowell, L.R. (1992) "Minerals in animal and human nutrition". Academic Press (report).

McDowell, L.R. (1996) Benefits of supplemental vitamin E including relationship to gossypol. University of Florida.

McDowell, L.R. (2000a) Vitamins in animal and human nutrition. Iowa State University Press, Ames, IA.

McDowell, L.R. (2000b) Re-evaluation of the metabolic essentiality of the vitamins. Asian. Australas J. Anim. Sci. 13(1):115–125. https://doi.org/10.5713/ajas.2000.115.

McDowell, L.R. (2004) Re-evaluation of the essentiality of the vitamins Calif. Anim. Nutr. Conference. 2004. (pp. 37–67).

McDowell, L.R. (2006) Vitamins and minerals functioning as antioxidants and vitamin and mineral supplementation considerations. ARPAS Calif. Chapter Conference Proc. (pp. 1–22).

McDowell, L.R. (2013) "Vitamin history, the early years". Design Publishing Inc., Sarasora, FL, USA.

McDowell, L.R. and Ward, N. (2008) Optimum vitamin nutrition for poultry. Int. Poult. Prod. 16(4):27–34.

McGhee, J.R., Mestecky, J., Dertzbaugh, M.T., Eldridge, J.H., Hirasawa, M. and Kiyono, H. (1992) The mucosal immune system: from fundamental concepts to vaccine development. Vaccine 10(2):75–88. https://doi.org/10.1016/0264-410x(92)90021-b.

McGinnis, C.H. (1986) Vitamin stability and activity of water-soluble vitamins as influenced by manufacturing processes and recommendations for the water-soluble vitamin. In "Bioavailability of nutrients in feed ingredients" National Feed Ingredient Association (NFIA), Des Moines, IA.

McGinnis, C.H. (1988) New concepts in vitamin nutrition. Proc. 1988 Georgia Nutrition Conference of the Feed Industry.

McIlroy, S.G., Goodall, E.A. and McMurray, C.H. (1987) A contact dermatitis of broilers: epidemiological findings. Avian Pathol. 16(1):93–105. https://doi.org/10.1080/03079458708436355.

McIlroy, S.G., Goodall, E.A., Rice, D.A., Mcnulty, M.S. and Kennedy, D.G. (1993) Improved performance in commercial broiler flocks with subclinical infectious bursal disease when fed diets containing increased concentrations of vitamin E. Avian Pathol. 22(1):81–94. https://doi.org/10.1080/03079459308418902.

McIntosh, G.H., Lawson, C.A., Bulman, F.H. and McMurchie, E.J. (1985) Vitamin E status affects platelet aggregation in the pig. Proc. Nutr. Soc. Australia 10:207.

McKee, J.S. and Harrison, P.C. (1995) Effects of supplemental ascorbic acid on the performance of broiler-chickens exposed to multiple concurrent stressors. Poult. Sci. 74(11):1772–1785. https://doi.org/10.3382/ps.0741772.

McKee, J.S. and Harrison, P.C. (1996) Ascorbic acid-induced reductions in the respiratory quotient of heat-stressed chicks may result from increased availability of fatty acids for energy purposes. Poult. Sci. J. 75(1):35.

McKee, J.S., Harrison, P.C. and Riskowski, G.L. (1997) Effects of supplemental ascorbic acid on the energy conversion of broiler chicks during heat stress and feed withdrawal. Poult. Sci. 76(9):1278–1286. https://doi.org/10.1093/ps/76.9.1278.

McKnight, W.F., Coelho, M.B. and McNaughton, J.L. (1995a) Turkey vitamin fortification. I. Commercial U.S. turkey vitamin survey. Poult. Sci. 74 (suppl. 1):185 (abstract).

McKnight, W.F., Coelho, M.B. and McNaughton, J.L. (1995b) Turkey vitamin fortification. II. Performance of turkeys fed industry levels of vitamins. Poult. Sci. 74 (suppl. 1):205 (abstract).

McKnight, W.F., Coelho, M. and McNaughton, J.L. (1996a) Effect of increased maternal vitamin E levels in combination with increased dietary antioxidant vitamins on poult performance. Poult. Sci. 75(1):129.

McKnight, W.F., Coelho, M. and McNaughton, J.L. (1996b) Effect of antioxidant vitamins on broiler meat quality. Poult. Sci. 75 (suppl. 1):129 (abstract).

McManus, E.C. and Judith, F.R. (1972) Effects of *Eimeria acervulina* infection on blood radioactivity following oral dosing with thiamine. Poult. Sci. 51:1835.

McMurchie, E.J. and McIntosh, G.H. (1986) Thermotropic interaction of vitamin E with dimyristoyl and dipalmitoyl phosphatidylcholine liposomes. J. Nutr. Sci. Vitaminol. (Tokyo) 32(5):551–558. https://doi.org/10.3177/jnsv.32.551.

McNaughton, J.L. and Murray, R. (1990) Effect of 25- hydroxycholecalciferol (25–OH-D_3) and vitamin D_3 on phosphorus requirement of broilers. Poult. Sci. 69(1):178.

Mehansho, H. and Henderson, L.M. (1980) Transport and accumulation of pyridoxine and pyridoxal by erythrocytes. J. Biol. Chem. 255(24):11901–11907. https://doi.org/10.1016/S0021-9258(19)70220-8.

Meldrum, J.B., Evans, R.D., Robertson, J.L., Watkins, K.L. and Novilla, M.N. (2000) Alterations in levels of various host antioxidant factors in turkey knockdown syndrome. Avian Dis. 44(4):891–895. https://doi.org/10.2307/1593062.

Meluzzi, A., Sirri, F., Tallarico, N. and Vandi, L. (1999) Dietary vitamin E eggs enriched with n-3 fatty acids Quality of eggs and egg products. 8th Eur. Symp. on the Quality of Egg and Egg Products, Budapest, Hungary. (pp. 153–159).

Mendonca, C.X.J., Guerra, E.M. and Oliveria, C.A. (1989) Choline supplementation in hisex brown and hisex white laying hens. 2. Deposition of lipids in liver and lipids in plasma. Braz. J. Vet. Res. Anim. Sci. 26(1):93–103. https://doi.org/10.11606/issn.2318-3659.v26i1p93-103.

Mendonça, C.X.J., Almeida, C.R.M., Mori, A.V. and Watanabe, C. (2002) Effect of dietary vitamin A on egg yolk retinol and tocopherol levels. J. Appl. Poult. Res. 11(4):373–378. https://doi.org/10.1093/japr/11.4.373.

Menten, J.F.M., Pesti, G.M. and Bakalli, R.I. (1997) A new method for determining the availability of choline in soybean meal. Poult. Sci. 76(9):1292–1297. https://doi.org/10.1093/ps/76.9.1292.

Mercier, Y., Gatellier, P., Viau, M., Remignon, H. and Renerre, M. (1998a) Effect of dietary fat and vitamin E on colour stability and on lipid and protein oxidation in turkey meat during storage. Meat Sci. 48(3–4):301–318. https://doi.org/10.1016/S0309-1740(97)00113-7.

Mercier, Y., Gatellier, P., Viau, M., Remignon, H. and Renerre, M. (1998b) Protein and lipid oxidation in turkey sartorius muscle during frozen storage as influenced by dietary fat sources and vitamin E supplementation. Proc. 41st Int. Congr. Meat Sci. Techn. (pp. 638–639).

Mercier, Y., Gatellier, P., Vincent, A. and Renerre, M. (2001) Lipid and protein oxidation in microsomal fraction from turkeys: influence of dietary fat and vitamin E supplementation. Meat Sci. 58(2):125–134. https://doi.org/10.1016/S0309-1740(00)00138-8.

Messikommer, R., Balzer, S. and Wenk, C. (2005) Impact of oregano essential oil on production data and lipid oxidation parameters in broiler chickens Proc. 15th Eur. Symp. Poult. Nutr., Balatonfured, Hungary. (pp. 298–303).

Meydani, M., Macauley, J.B. and Blumberg, J.B. (1988) Effect of dietary vitamin E and selenium on susceptibility of brain regions to lipid peroxidation. Lipids 23(5):405–409. https://doi.org/10.1007/BF02535510.

Meydani, N. and Han, S.N. (2006) Nutrient regulation of the immune response: the case of vitamin E. In Present knowledge in nutrition 9th ed Bowman, B.A. and Russell, R.M. (ed.). International Life Sciences Institute. (pp. 585–603).

Meydani, S.N., Ribaya-Mercado, J.D., Russell, R.M., Sahyoun, N., Morrow, F.D. and Gershoff, S.N. (1991) Vitamin B_6 deficiency impairs interleukin 2 production and lymphocyte proliferation in elderly adults. Am. J. Clin. Nutr. 53(5):1275–1280. https://doi.org/10.1093/ajcn/53.5.1275.

Michalczuk, M., Zdanowska-Sąsiadek, Ż, Damaziak, K. and Niemiec, J. (2016) Influence of indoor and outdoor systems on meat quality of slow-growing chickens. CyTA J. Food 15(1):1–6. https://doi.org/10.1080/19476337.2016.1196246.

Mielche, M.M. and Bertelsen, G. (1994) Approaches to the prevention of warmed-over flavour. Trends Food Sci. Technol. 5(10):322–327. https://doi.org/10.1016/0924-2244(94)90183-X.

Mielnik, M.B. and Skrede, G. (2003) Antioxidative properties of grape seed extract in cooked turkey meat. Proc. 16th Eur. Symp. Quality Poultry Meat, St.-Brieuc, France. (pp. 298–303).

Miles, R.D., Ruiz, N. and Harms, R.H. (1983) The interrelationship between methionine, choline, and sulfate in broiler diets. Poult. Sci. 62(3):495–498. https://doi.org/10.3382/ps.0620495.

Miles, R.D. and Harms, R.H. (1984) Effects of supplemental methionine and potassium sulfate on the choline requirement of the turkey poult. Poult. Sci. 63(7):1464–1466. https://doi.org/10.3382/ps.0631464.

Miles, R.D., Ruiz, N. and Harms, R.H. (1986) Response of laying hens to choline when fed practical diets devoid of supplemental sulfur amino acids. Poult. Sci. 65(9):1760–1764. https://doi.org/10.3382/ps.0651760.

Miles, R.D., Ruiz, N. and Harms, R.H. (1987) Dietary conditions necessary for a methyl donor response in broilers and laying hens fed a corn-soybean meal diet. Poult. Sci. 66(1):29–30.

Millar, R.I., Smith, L.T. and Wood, J.H. (1977) The study of the dietary vitamin D requirements of ring-necked pheasant chicks. Poult. Sci. 56:1739.

Miller, B.F. (1963) Pendulous crop in pyridoxine deficient chicks. Poult. Sci. 42(3):795–796. https://doi.org/10.3382/ps.0420795.

Miller, D.L. and Balloun, S.L. (1967) Folacin requirements of turkey breeder hens. Poult. Sci. 46(6):1502–1508. https://doi.org/10.3382/ps.0461502.

Miller, E.L. and Huang, Y.X. (1993) Improving the nutritional value of broiler meat through increased n-3 fatty acid and vitamin E content. 11th Eur. Symp. on the Quality of Poult. Meat, Tours, France. (pp. 404–411).

Miller, J.W., Rogerf, L.M. and Rucker, R.B. (2006) Pantothenic acid. In Present knowledge in nutrition 9th ed Bowman, B.A. and Russell, R.M. (ed.). International Life Sciences Institute. (pp. 327–339).

Min, Y.N., Niu, Z.Y., Sun, T.T., Wang, Z.P., Jiao, P.X., Zi, B.B., Chen, P.P., Tian, D.L. and Liu, F.Z. (2018) Vitamin E and vitamin C supplementation improves antioxidant status and immune function in oxidative stressed breeder roosters by up-regulating expression of GSH-Px gene. Poult. Sci. 97(4):1238–1244. https://doi.org/10.3382/ps/pex417.

Ministry of Agriculture of People's Republic of China (2004) Chicken feeding standards. China Agricultural Press, Beijing, China (in Chinese). (pp. 11–12).

Miranda, H.A.F., Lopes, I.M.G., Lima, M.Dd, Ferreira, F., Pereira, E.B., Silva, L.Fd and Costa, L.F. (2021) Efeitos da nutrição *in ovo* no desempenho de frangos de Corte: uma revisão. Res. Soc. Dev. 10(2):e38810212307. https://doi.org/10.33448/rsd-v10i2.12307.

Mireles, A. (1997) The impact of using 25-hydroxyvitamin D_3 on performance and the immune system of broilers. Mem. Jornada Int. Avicultura Carne Trouw Nutr. (pp. 30–38).

Mireles, A., Klasing, K.C. and Kim, S. (1999) Evidence that dietary 25-hydroxycholecalciferol (25-0H-D_3) supplementation affects commercial broiler performance by modification of their immune response. Poult. Sci. 78(1):50–56.

Mirfendereski, E. and Jahanian, R. (2015) Effects of dietary organic chromium and vitamin C supplementation on performance, immune responses, blood metabolites, and stress status of laying hens subjected to high stocking density. Poult. Sci. 94(2):281–288. https://doi.org/10.3382/ps/peu074.

Mirshekar, R., Dastar, B., Shabanpour, B. and Hassani, S. (2013) Effect of dietary nutrient density and vitamin premix withdrawal on performance and meat quality of broiler chickens. J. Sci. Food Agric. 93(12):2979–2985. https://doi.org/10.1002/jsfa.6127.

Mishra, B. and Jha, R. (2019) Oxidative stress in the poultry gut: potential challenges and interventions. Front. Vet. Sci. 6:60. https://doi.org/10.3389/fvets.2019.00060.

Misir, R. and Blair, R. (1984) Bioavailable biotin from cereal grains for broiler chicks as affected by added dietary fiber. Poult. Sci. 63(1):152.

Misir, R. and Blair, R. (1984) Effect of biotin supplementation on performance of biotin deficient sows. Vet. Sci. Res. J. 59(1):212–218. https://doi.org/10.1016/S0034-5288(18)30515-0.

Misir, R. and Blair, R. (1988) Biotin bioavailability of protein supplements and cereal grains for starting turkey poults. Poult. Sci. 67(9):1274–1280. https://doi.org/10.3382/ps.0671274.

Mitchell, R.D. and Edwards, H.M. (1996) Effects of phytase and 1,25-dihydroxycholecalciferol on phytate utilization and the quantitative requirement for calcium and phosphorus in young broiler chickens. Poult. Sci. 75(1):95–110. https://doi.org/10.3382/ps.0750095.

Mitchell, R.D., Edwards, H.M. and McDaniel, G.R. (1997a) The effects of ultraviolet light and cholecalciferol and its metabolites on the development of leg abnormalities in chickens genetically selected for a high and low incidence of tibial dyschondroplasia. Poult. Sci. 76(2):346–354. https://doi.org/10.1093/ps/76.2.346.

Mitchell, R.D., Edwards, H.M., McDaniel, G.R. and Rowland, G.N. (1997b) Dietary 1,25-dihydroxycholecalciferol has variable effects on the incidences of leg abnormalities, plasma vitamin D metabolites, and vitamin D receptors in chickens divergently selected for tibial dyschondroplasia. Poult. Sci. 76(2):338–345. https://doi.org/10.1093/ps/76.2.338.

Mochamat, N., Idrus, Z., Soleimani Farjam, A. and Hossain, M.A. (2017) Response to withdrawal of vitamin and trace mineral premixes from finisher diet in broiler chickens under the hot and humid tropical condition. Ital. J. Anim. Sci. 16(2):239–245. https://doi.org/10.1080/1828051X.2016.1268935.

Mock, D.M. (1990) Biotin. In “Nutrition reviews, present knowledge in nutrition” Olson, R.E. (ed.) Nutritional Foundation.

Mock, D.M. (2009) Marginal biotin deficiency is common in normal human pregnancy and is highly teratogenic in mice. J. Nutr. 139(1):154–157. https://doi.org/10.3945/jn.108.095273.

Mock, D.M. (2013) Biotin. In “Handbook of vitamins” 5th ed. Zempleni, J., Suttie, J., Gregory, J. and Stover P. J. (ed.). CRC Press, Taylor & Francis Group. (pp. 397–420).

Mock, D.M. and Malik, M.I. (1992) Distribution of biotin in human plasma: most of the biotin is not bound to protein. Am. J. Clin. Nutr. 56(2):427–432. https://doi.org/10.1093/ajcn/56.2.427.

Mock, N.I. and Mock, D.M. (1992) Biotin deficiency in rats: disturbances of leucine metabolism are detectable early. J. Nutr. 122(7):1493–1499. https://doi.org/10.1093/jn/122.7.1493.

Mohammed, A., Gibney, M.J. and Taylor, T.G. (1991) The effects of dietary levels of inorganic phosphorus, calcium and cholecalciferol on the digestibility of phytate-P by the chick. Br. J. Nutr. 66(2):251–259. https://doi.org/10.1079/bjn19910029.

Mol, B.W. and Zoll, M. (2015) Fertility preservation for age-related fertility decline. Lancet 385(9967):507. https://doi.org/10.1016/S0140-6736(15)60199-4.

Molitoris, B.A. and Baker, D.H. (1976) The choline requirement of broiler chicks during the seventh week of life. Poult. Sci. 55(1):220–224. https://doi.org/10.3382/ps.0550220.

Monsi, A. and Onitchi, D.O. (1991) Effects of ascorbic- acid (vitamin-C) supplementation on ejaculated semen characteristics of broiler breeder chickens under hot and humid tropical conditions. Anim. Feed Sci. Technol. 34(1–2):141–146. https://doi.org/10.1016/0377-8401(94)90197-X.

Mookerjea, S. (1969) Studies on the plasma glycoprotein synthesis by the isolated perfused liver: effect of early choline deficiency. Can. J. Biochem. 47(2):125–133. https://doi.org/10.1139/o69-021.

Moravej, H., Alahyari, S.M. and Shivazad, M. (2012) Effects of the reduction or withdrawal of the vitamin premix from the diet on chicken performance and meat quality. Rev. Bras. Cienc Avic 14(4):239–244. https://doi.org/10.1590/S1516-635X2012000400002.

Mori, A.V., Mendonça, C.X., Almeida, C.R.M. and Pita, M.C.G. (2003) Supplementing hen diets with vitamins A and E affects egg yolk retinol and α-tocopherol levels. J. Appl. Poult. Res. 12(2):106–114. https://doi.org/10.1093/japr/12.2.106.

Moriuchi, S. and Deluca, H.F. (1974) Metabolism of vitamin D_3 in chick embryo. Arch. Biochem. Biophys. 164(1):165–171. https://doi.org/10.1016/0003-9861(74)90018-6.

Morris, A. and Selvaraj, R.K. (2014) In vitro 25-hydroxycholecalciferol treatment of lipopolysaccharide-stimulated chicken macrophages increases nitric oxide production and mRNA of interleukin-1beta and 10. Vet. Immunol. Immunopathol. 161(3–4):265–270. https://doi.org/10.1016/j.vetimm.2014.08.008.

Morris, A., Shanmugasundaram, R., Lilburn, M.S. and Selvaraj, R.K. (2014) 25-Hydroxycholecalciferol supplementation improves growth performance and decreases inflammation during an experimental lipopolysaccharide injection. Poult. Sci. 93(8):1951–1956. https://doi.org/10.3382/ps.2014-03939.

Morris, A., Shanmugasundaram, R., McDonald, J. and Selvaraj, R.K. (2015) Effect of in vitro and in vivo 25-hydroxyvitamin D treatment on macrophages, T cells, and layer chickens during a coccidia challenge. J. Anim. Sci. 93(6):2894–2903. https://doi.org/10.2527/jas.2014-8866.

Morris, M.S., Sakakeeny, L., Jacques, P.F., Picciano, M.F. and Selhub, J. (2010) Vitamin B_6 intake is inversely related to, and the requirement is affected by, inflammation status. J. Nutr. 140(1):103–110. https://doi.org/10.3945/jn.109.114397.

Morrissey, P.A., Brandon, S., Buckley, D.J., Sheehy, P.J.A. and Frigg, M. (1997) Tissue content of α-tocopherol and oxidative stability of broiler receiving dietary α-tocopheryl acetate supplement for various periods preslaughter. Br. Poult. Sci. 38(1):84–88. https://doi.org/10.1080/00071669708417945.

Morrissey, P.A., Sheehy, P.J.A., Galvin, K., Kerry, J.P. and Buckley, D.J. (1998) Lipid stability in meat and meat products. Meat Sci. 49S1(1):S73-S86. https://doi.org/10.1016/s0309-1740(98)90039-0.

Moser, U. and Bendich, A. (1991) Vitamin C. In Handbook of vitamins 2nd ed Machlin, L.J. (ed.). Marcel Dekker, New York. (p. 195).

Moslehi, H., Irani, M. and Shivazad, M. (2004) Investigation in the optimum level of vitamin premix in broiler performance. Proc. 22nd World's Poult. Congress, Istanbul, Turkey.

Muduuli, D.S., Marquardt, R.R. and Guenter, W. (1982) Effect of dietary vicine and vitamin E supplementation on the productive performance of growing and laying chickens. Br. J. Nutr. 47(1):53–60. https://doi.org/10.1079/BJN19820008.

Muggli, R. (1994) Physiological requirements of vitamin E as a function of the amount and type of polyunsaturated fatty acid. World Rev. Nutr. Diet. 75:166–168. https://doi.org/10.1159/000423574.

Mugnai, C., Sossidou, E.N., Dal Bosco, A., Ruggeri, S., Mattioli, S. and Castellini, C. (2014) The effects of husbandry system on the grass intake and egg nutritive characteristics of laying hens. J. Sci. Food Agric. 94(3):459–467. https://doi.org/10.1002/jsfa.6269.

Muir, W.I., Husband, A.J. and Bryden, W.L. (2002) Dietary supplementation with vitamin E modulates avian intestinal immunity. Br. J. Nutr. 87(6):579–585. https://doi.org/10.1079/BJNBJN2002562.

Muralt, A. (1962) The role of thiamin in neurophysiology. Ann. N. Y. Acad. Sci. 98:499. https://doi.org/10.1111/j.1749-6632.1962.tb30571.x.

Mwalusanya, N.A., Katule, A.M., Mutayoba, S.K., Mtambo, M.M.A., Olsen J.E. and U.M. Minga (2002) Productivity of Local Chickens under Village Management ConditionsTropical Anim. Health Prod. (34):405–416. https://doi.org/10.1023/A:1020048327158.

Nääs, IdA., Baracho, MdS., Bueno, L.G.F., De Moura, D.J., Vercelino, RdA. and Salgado, D.D. (2012) Use of vitamin D to reduce lameness in broilers reared in harsh environments. Braz. J. Poult. Sci. 14(3):165–172. https://doi.org/10.1590/S1516-635X2012000300002.

Naber, E.C. (1993) Modifying vitamin composition of eggs: a review. J. Appl. Poult. Res. 2(4):385–393. https://doi.org/10.1093/japr/2.4.385.

Naber, E.C. and Squires, M.W. (1993a) Vitamin profiles of eggs as indicators of nutritional status in the laying hen: diet to egg transfer and commercial flock survey. Poult. Soc. 72(6):1046–1053. https://doi.org/10.3382/ps.0721046.

Naber, E.C. and Squires, M.W. (1993b) Research Note: early detection of the absence of a vitamin premix in layer diets by egg albumen riboflavin analysis. Poult. Sci. 72(10):1989–1993. https://doi.org/10.3382/ps.0721989.

Nabi, F., Arain, M.A., Rajput, N., Alagawany, M., Soomro, J., Umer, M., Soomro, F., Wang, Z., Ye, R. and Liu, J. (2020) Health benefits of carotenoids and potential application in poultry industry: a review. J. Anim. Physiol. Anim. Nutr. (Berl) 104(6):1809–1818. https://doi.org/10.1111/jpn.13375.

Nabokina, S.M., Kashyap, M.L. and Said, H.M. (2005) Mechanism and regulation of human intestinal niacin uptake. Am. J. Physiol. Cell Physiol. 289(1):C97-C103. https://doi.org/10.1152/ajpcell.00009.2005.

Nagaraj, R.Y., Wu, W.D. and Vesonder, R.F. (1994) Toxicity of corn culture material of *Fusarium proliferatum* M-7176 and nutritional intervention in chicks. Poult. Sci. 73(5):617–626. https://doi.org/10.3382/ps.0730617.

Nagy, G., Rice, M.E. and Adams, R.N. (1982) A new type of enzyme electrode: the ascorbic acid eliminator electrode. Life Sci. 31(23):2611–2616. https://doi.org/10.1016/0024-3205(82)90736-6.

Naidoo, D. (1956) The activity in sites of 5′nucleotidase, phosphomonoesterase and thiamin pyrophosphatase in vitamin B_1 deficient brain tissue. Acta psychiatr. neurol. scand. 31:20.

Nain, S., Laarveld, B., Wojnarowicz, C. and Olkowski, A.A. (2007a) Excessive dietary vitamin D supplementation as a risk factor for sudden death syndrome in fast growing commercial broilers. Comp. Biochem. Physiol. A Mol. Integr. Physiol. 148(4):828–833. https://doi.org/10.1016/j.cbpa.2007.08.023.

Nain, S.B., Laarveld B. and Olkowski, A.A. (2007b) Over-supplementation of vitamin D as a risk factor for chronic heart failure in fast growing commercial broilers. J. Anim. Sci. 85 (suppl. 1):128 (abstr.).

Nakagawa, K., Shibata, A., Yamashita, S., Tsuzuki, T., Kariya, J., Oikawa, S. and Miyazawa, T. (2007) In vivo angiogenesis is suppressed by unsaturated vitamin E, tocotrienol. J. Nutr. 137(8):1938–1943. https://doi.org/10.1093/jn/137.8.1938.

Nakano, H. and Gregory, J.F. (1995) Pyridoxine and pyridoxine-5′-β-D-glucoside exert different effects on tissue B_6 vitamers but similar effects on β-glucosidase activity in rats. J. Nutr. 125(11):2751–2762.

Nakano, H., McMahon, L.G. and Gregory, J.F. (1997) Pyridoxine-5′-beta-glucoside exhibits incomplete bioavailability as a source of vitamin B_6 and partially inhibits the utilization of co-ingested pyridoxine in humans. J. Nutr. 127(8):1508–1513. https://doi.org/10.1093/jn/127.8.1508.

Nakaya, T., Suzuki, S. and Watanabe, K. (1986) Effects of high dose supplementation of ascorbic acid on chicks. Jpn. Poult. Sci. 23(5):276–283. https://doi.org/10.2141/jpsa.23.276.

Nam, K.C. and Ahn, D.U. (2003) Use of double packaging and antioxidant combinations to improve color, lipid oxidation, and volatiles of irradiated raw and cooked turkey breast patties. Poult. Sci. 82(5):850–857. https://doi.org/10.1093/ps/82.5.850.

Nam, K.T., Lee, H.A., Min, B.S. and Kang, C.W. (1997) Influence of dietary supplementation with linseed and vitamin E on fatty acids, α-tocopherol, and lipid peroxidation in muscles of broiler chicks. Anim. Feed Sci. Technol. 66(1–4):149–158. https://doi.org/10.1016/S0377-8401(96)01108-X.

Nam, K.C., Min, B.R., Yan, H., Lee, E.J., Mendoça, A., Wesley, I. and Ahn, D.U. (2003) Effect of dietary vitamin E and irradiation on lipid oxidation, color, and volatiles of fresh and previously frozen turkey breast patties. Meat Sci. 65(1):513-21. https://doi.org/10.1016/S0309-1740(02)00243-7.

Narbaitz, R. (1987) Role of vitamin D in the development of the chick embryo. J. Exp. Zool. Suppl. 1:15–23.

Narciso-Gaytán, C., Shin, D., Sams, A.R., Bailey, C.A., Miller, R.K., Smith, S.B., Leyva-Ovalle, O.R. and Sánchez-Plata, M.X. (2010) Soybean, palm kernel, and animal-vegetable oils and vitamin E supplementation effect on lipid oxidation stability of sous vide chicken meat. Poult. Sci. 89(4):721–728. https://doi.org/10.3382/ps.2009-00241.

Nascimento, Gd, Murakami, A.E.I., Guerra, A.F.Q.M.I., Ospinas-Rojas, I.C.I., Ferreira, M.F.Z.I. and Fanhani, J.C.I. (2014) Effect of different vitamin D sources and calcium levels in the diet of layers in the second laying cycle. Rev. Bras. Cienc. Avic. 16(2):37–42. https://doi.org/10.1590/1516-635x160237-42.

Naseem, S., Younus, M., Anwar, B., Ghafoor, A., Aslam, A. and Akhter, S. (2005) Effect of ascorbic acid and acetylsalicylic acid supplementation on performance of broiler chicks exposed to heat stress. Int. J. Poult. Sci. 4(11):900–904. https://doi.org/10.3923/ijps.2005.900.904.

National Chicken Council USA (2022) https://www.nationalchickencouncil.org/industry/statistics/.

Nawab, A., Tang s., Liu, W., Wu, J., Ibtisham, F., Kang, K., Ghani, M. W., Birmani, M. W., Li, G., Sun, C., Zhao, Y., Xiao, M. and An, L. (2019) Vitamin E and fertility in the poultry birds; deficiency of vitamin E and its hazardous effects. Appro Poult Dairy & Vet Sci 6(1). https://doi.org/10.31031/APDV.2019.06.000626.

Nazir, A. and Memon, A.U., Akbar Khan, S., Kuthu, Z.H., Rasool, F., Ahmed, Z., Ahmed, I., Shamim, A. and Aziz, A. (2017) Study on the effects of antibiotic (Lincomycin) and feed additive (niacin) on the growth of broilers. Global Veterinaria 18 (5):335–342.

Nelsestuen, G.L., Zytkovicz, T.H. and Howard, J.B. (1974) The mode of action of vitamin K. Identification of gamma-carboxyglutamic acid as a component of prothrombin. J. Biol. Chem. 249(19):6347–6350. https://doi.org/10.1016/S0021-9258(19)42259-X.

Nelson, T.S. and Norris, L.C. (1960) Studies on the vitamin K requirement of the chick. I. Requirements of the chick for vitamin K_1, menadione and menadione sodium bisulfite. J. Nutr. 72:137–144. https://doi.org/10.1093/jn/72.2.137.

Nelson, T.S. and Norris, L.C. (1961) Studies on the vitamin K requirement of the chick. II. J. Nutr. 73(2):135–142. https://doi.org/10.1093/jn/73.2.135.

Neri, M. (2000) Use of 25–0H-D_3 in fowl diets. Riv. avicoltura 69:16–19.

Nesheim, M.C., Norvell, M.J., Ceballos, E. and Leach, R.M. (1971) The effect of choline supplementation of diets for growing pullets and laying hens. Poult. Sci. 50(3):820–831. https://doi.org/10.3382/ps.0500820.

Newbrey, J.W., Truitt, S.T., Roland, D.A., Frost, T.J. and Untawale, G.G. (1992) Bone histomorphometry in 1,25$(OH)_2D_3$- and vitamin D_3 treated aged laying hens. Avian Dis. 36(3):700–706. https://doi.org/10.2307/1591768.

Newman, S. and Leeson, S. (1999) The effect of dietary supplementation with 1,25-dihydroxycholecalciferol or vitamin C on the characteristics of the tibia of older laying hens. Poult. Sci. 78(1):85–90. https://doi.org/10.1093/ps/78.1.85.

Niki, E. (1993) Function of vitamin E as antioxidant in the membranes. In Vitamin E: its usefulness in health and curing diseases Mino, N., Nakamura, N., Diplock, A. and Kayden, H. (ed.). Japan Scientific Societies Press. (pp. 23–30). https://doi.org/10.1159/000422496.

Niu, Z.Y., Liu, F.Z., Yan, Q.L. and Li, W.C. (2009) Effects of different levels of vitamin E on growth performance and immune responses of broilers under heat stress. Poult. Sci. 88(10):2101–2107. https://doi.org/10.3382/ps.2009-00220.

Niu, Z.Y., Min, Y.N. and Liu, F.Z. (2018) Dietary vitamin E improves meat quality and antioxidant capacity in broilers by upregulating the expression of antioxidant enzyme genes. J. Appl. Anim. Res. 46(1):397–401. https://doi.org/10.1080/09712119.2017.1309321.

Nixey, C. (2005) The role of nutrition in tibial dyschondroplasia occurrence in turkeys. Proc. 15th Eur. symp. poultr. nutr., Balatonfured, Hungary. (pp. 166–178).

Njoku, P.C. (1984) The effect of ascorbic acid supplementation on broiler performance in a tropical environment. Poult. Sci. 63(1):156.

Njoku, P.C. (1986) Effect of dietary ascorbic acid (vitamin C) supplementation on the performance of broiler chickens in a tropical environment. Anim. Feed Sci. Technol. 16(1–2):17–24. https://doi.org/10.1016/0377-8401(86)90046-5.

Njoku, P.C. and Nwazota, A.O.U. (1989) Effects of dietary inclusion of ascorbic acid and palm oil on the performance of laying hens in a tropical environment. Br. Poult. Sci. 30(4):831–840. https://doi.org/10.1080/00071668908417209.

Nobakht, A. (2014) Effect of different levels of mineral and vitamin premix on laying hens performance during the first laying phase. Iran. J. Appl. Anim. Sci. 4(4):883–886.

Nobakht, A., Tabatbaei, S. and Khodaei, S. (2011) Effects of different sources and levels of vegetable oils on performance, carcass traits and accumulation of vitamin E in breast meat of broilers. Curr. Res. J. Biol. Sci. 3(6):601–605.

Nockels, C.F. (1988) The role of vitamins in modulating disease resistance. Vet. Clin. North Am. Food Anim. Pract. 4(3):531–542. https://doi.org/10.1016/S0749-0720(15)31030-6.

Nockels, C.F. (1990) Mineral alterations associated with stress, trauma and infection and the effect on immunity. Cont. Educ. Pract. Vet. 12(8):1133–1139.

Noel, K. and Brinkhaus, F. (1998) Vitamin A retention of a high pigment broiler growing feed treated with endox or ethoxyquin. Poult. Sci. 77(1):144.

Nofal, M.E., Samak, H.R., Alderey, A.A. and Nasr, A.M.E. (2018) Effect of dietary folic acid supplementation to diets of low levels of energy and methionine of developed laying hens in summer season on performance, physiological status and immune response. Anim. J. Poult. Prod. 9(12):471–480. https://doi.org/10.21608/jappmu.2018.41163.

Noll, S.L. (1997) (2006) Vitamin C for turkey breeders. Proc. of the Arkansas Nutr. Conf., Arkansas Poultry Federation.

Norman, A.W. (2006) Vitamin D receptor: new assignments for an already busy receptor. Endocrinology 147(12):5542–5548. https://doi.org/10.1210/en.2006-0946.

Norman, A.W. and Henry, H.C. (2007) Vitamin D. In Handbook of vitamins 4th ed. Zempleni, J., Rucker, R.B., McCormick, D.B. and Suttle, J.W. (ed.). CRC Press, Boca Raton. (pp. 47–99).

Norman, A.W. and Hurwitz, S. (1993) The role of the vitamin-D endocrine system in avian bone biology. J. Nutr. 123(2) (suppl.):310–316. https://doi.org/10.1093/jn/123.suppl_2.310.

North, M. O. (1984) Commercial chicken production manual. 3rd ed. AVI. Publ. Co. Ltd.

Norvell, M.J. and Nesheim, M.C. (1969) Studies of choline biosynthesis in chicks. Poult. Sci. 48:1852.

Nouri, S., Ghalehkandi, J.G., Hassanpour, S. and Aghdam-Shahryar, H. (20188) Effect of *in ovo* feeding of folic acid on subsequent growth performance and blood constituents levels in broilers. Int. J. Pept. Res. Ther. 24:463–470. https://doi.org/10.1007/s10989-017-9629-x.

Novogen (2020) Nutrition guide. https://novogen-layers.com/wp-content/uploads/2020/12/202007-Guide-Nutrition-CS_PS-EN.pdf.

Nowaczewski, S., Kontecka, H. and Krystianiak, S. (2012) Effect of in ovo injection of vitamin C during incubation on hatchability of chickens and ducks. Folia biol. 60(1–2):93–97. https://doi.org/10.3409/fb60_1-2.93-97.

NRC (1987) Vitamin tolerance of animals. National Academy of Sciences. National Research Council. https://doi.org/10.17226/949.

NRC (1994) Nutrient requirement of poultry 9th rev. ed. National Academy Press. https://doi.org/10.17226/2114.

Nys, Y. (2000) Dietary carotenoids and egg yolk coloration a review arch. Geflugelk 64(2):45–54.

Odabaşi, A.Z., Miles, R.D., Balaban, M.O., Portier, K.M. and Sampath, V. (2006) Vitamin C overcomes the detrimental effect of vanadium on brown eggshell pigmentation. J. Appl. Poult. Res. 15(3):425–432. https://doi.org/10.1093/japr/15.3.425.

O'Dell, B.L. and Hogan, A.G. (1943) Additional observations on the chick antianemia vitamin. J. Biol. Chem. 149(2):323–337. https://doi.org/10.1016/S0021-9258(18)72179-0.

Oduho, G.W. and Baker, D.H. (1993) Quantitative efficacy of niacin sources for chicks: nicotinic acid, nicotinamide, NAD and tryptophan. J. Nutr. 123(12):2201–2206. https://doi.org/10.1093/jn/123.12.2201.

Oduho, G.W., Chung, T.K. and Baker, D.H. (1993) Menadione nicotinamide bisulfite is a bioactive source of vitamin K and niacin activity for chicks. J. Nutr. 123(4):737–743. https://doi.org/10.1093/jn/123.4.737.

Oduho, G.W., Han, Y.M. and Baker, D.H. (1994) Iron deficiency reduces the efficacy of tryptophan as a niacin precursor. J. Nutr. 124(3):444–450. https://doi.org/10.1093/jn/124.3.444.

Ogbuinya, P. (1991) Vitamin C increased broiler body weight. Poult. Int. 91:24.

Ognik, K. and Wertelecki, T. (2012) Effect of different vitamin E sources and levels on selected oxidative status indices in blood and tissues as well as on rearing performance of slaughter turkey hens. J. Appl. Poult. Res. 21(2):259–271. https://doi.org/10.3382/japr.2011-00366.

Ogunmodede, B.K. (1977) Riboflavin requirement of starting chickens in a tropical environment. Poult. Sci. 56(1):231–234. https://doi.org/10.3382/ps.0560231.

Oikeh, I., Sakkas, P., Blake, D.P. and Kyriazakis, I. (2019) Interactions between dietary calcium and phosphorus level, and vitamin D source on bone mineralization, performance and intestinal morphology of coccidia-infected broilers. Poult. Sci. 98(11):5679–5690. https://doi.org/10.3382/ps/pez350.

Okasha, H.M.A., El Garhy, O.H.M. and El-Gendi, G.M. (2019) Effect of housing system and dietary biotin supplementation on 2-Egg quality traits and some blood constituents. Anim. Biotechnol. 91(98):91. https://doi.org/10.21608/assjm.2018.57338.

Okolelova, T.M., Grigorieva, E.N., Posviryakobao, A., Papzyan, T.T. and Nollet, L. (2006) The vitamin E improvement of broiler performance depends also on the form of Se administration. Proc. 12th Eur. Poult. Nutr., Verona, Italy. (p. 237).

Okoye, J.O.A., Okwor, L.J.E., Ezema, W.S., Okosi, L.I., Chiwuba, A.R.S., Adeyeye, O.V. and Amadi, C.H. (2000) Effect of ascorbic acid supplementation on body weight gain, antibody response and resistance to infectious bursal disease. Proc. 21st world poult. conf. Montreal, Canada.

Olcese, O., Couch, J.R., Quisenberry, J.H. and Pearson, P.B. (1950) Congenital anomalies in the chick due to vitamin B_{12} deficiency. J. Nutr. 41(3):423–431. https://doi.org/10.1093/jn/41.3.423.

Oldfield, J.E. (1987) History of nutrition: development of the concept of antimetabolites. Introduction. J. Nutr. 117(7):1322–1323. https://doi.org/10.1093/jn/117.7.1322.

Olivares, M., Pizarro, F., Pineda, O., Name, J.J., Hertrampf, E. and Walter, T. (1997) Milk inhibits and ascorbic acid favors ferrous bis-glycine chelate bioavailability in humans. J. Nutr. 127(7):1407–1411. https://doi.org/10.1093/jn/127.7.1407.

Olivo, R., Soares, A.L., Ida, E.I. and Shimokomaki, M. (2007) Dietary vitamin E inhibits poultry PSE and improves meat functional properties. J. Food Biochem. 25(4):271–283. https://doi.org/10.1111/j.1745-4514.2001.tb00740.x.

Olkowski, A.A. and Classen, H.L. (1996) The study of thiamine requirement in broiler chickens. Int. J. Vitam. Nutr. Res. 66(4):332–341. PMID:8979162.

Olkowski, A.A. and Classen, H.L. (1998) The study of riboflavin requirement in broiler chickens. Int. J. Vitam. Nutr. Res. 68(5):316–327. PMID:9789764.

Olkowski, A.A. and Classen, H.L. (1999) The effect of maternal thiamine nutrition on thiamine status of the offspring in broiler chickens. Int. J. Vitam. Nutr. Res. 69(1):32–40. https://doi.org/10.1024/0300-9831.69.1.32.

Oloyo, R.A. (1991) Responses of broilers fed Guinea corn/palm kernel meal based ration to supplemental biotin. J. Sci. Food Agric. 55(4):539–550. https://doi.org/10.1002/jsfa.2740550406.

Oloyo, R.A. (1994) Studies on the biotin requirement of broilers fed sunflower seed meal-based diets. Arch. Tierernahr. 45(4):345–353. https://doi.org/10.1080/17450399409386109.

Oloyo, R.A. (1997) Effect of Guinea corn/palm kernel-meal based diet with niacin supplementation on the performance of broilers. Indian J. Anim. Sci. 67(5):422–425.

Oloyo, R.A. (2000) Niacin requirement of broilers fed maize – palm kernel meal-based diets. Nig. J. Anim. Prod. 29(1):27–33. https://doi.org/10.51791/njap.v29i1.1499.

Olson, J.A. (1984) Vitamin A. In “Handbook of vitamins” Machlin, L.J. (ed.). Marcel Dekker, Inc.

Olson, R.E. (1990) Pantothenic acid. In “Nutrition reviews, present knowledge in nutrition” Olson, R.E. (ed.). Nutrition Foundation.

O’Neill, L.M., Galvin, K., Morrissey, P.A. and Buckley, D.J. (1998a) Comparison of effects of dietary olive oil, tallow and vitamin E on the quality of broiler meat and meat products. Br. Poult. Sci. 39(3):365–371. https://doi.org/10.1080/00071669888917.

O’Neill, L.M., Galvin, K., Morrissey, P.A. and Buckley, D.J. (1998b) Inhibition of lipid oxidation in chicken by carnosine and dietary α-tocopherol supplementation and its determination by derivative spectrophotometry. Meat Sci. 50(4):479–488. https://doi.org/10.1016/S0309-1740(98)00061-8.

O’Neill, L.M., Galvin, K., Morrissey, P.A. and Buckley, D.J. (1999) Effect of carnosine, salt and dietary vitamin E on the oxidative stability of chicken meat. Meat Sci. 52(1):89–94. https://doi.org/10.1016/S0309-1740(98)00152-1.

Onwudike, O.C. and Adegbola, A.A. (1984) Riboflavin requirement of laying hens for egg production and reproduction in the humid tropics. Trop. Agric. 61(3):205–207.

Orban, J.I., Roland, D.A., Cummins, K. and Lovell, R.T. (1993) Influence of large doses of ascorbic acid on performance, plasma calcium, bone characteristics, and eggshell quality in broilers and leghorn hens. Poult. Sci. 72(4):691–700. https://doi.org/10.3382/ps.0720691.

Oruwari, B.M., Mbere, O.O. and Sese, B.T. (1995) Ascorbic acid as a supplement for Babcock hen in a tropical condition. J. Appl. Anim. Res. 8(2):121–128. https://doi.org/10.1080/09712119.1995.9706087.

O’Sullivan, S.M., E Ball, M.E., McDonald, E., Hull, G.L.J., Danaher, M. and Cashman, K.D. (2020) Biofortification of chicken eggs with vitamin K – nutritional and quality improvements. Foods 9(11):1619. https://doi.org/10.3390/foods9111619.

Ouart, M.D., Harms, R.H. and Wilson, H.R. (1987) Effect of graded levels of niacin in corn- soy and wheat-soy diets on laying hens. Poult. Sci. 66(3):467–470. https://doi.org/10.3382/ps.0660467.

Owens, G.M. and Ledoux, D.R. (2000) Effects of 25-hydroxycholecalciferol and vitamin D on phosphorus utilization by turkey poults fed a typical corn-soybean meal diet. Poult. Sci. 79 (suppl. 1):113 (abstract).

Owens, G.M. and Ledoux, D.R. (2001) Effects of 25-hydroxyvitamin D_3, vitamin D_3, low phytic acid corn, and phytase on phosphorus utilization by turkey poults fed dietary treatments from hatch to six weeks of age. Poult. Sci. 80 (suppl. 1):1981 (abstract).

Ozkan, S., Malayoğlu, H.B., Yalçin, S., Karadas, F., Koçtürk, S., Cabuk, M., Oktay, G., Ozdemir, S., Ozdemir, E. and Ergül, M. (2007) Dietary vitamin E (α-tocopherol acetate) and selenium supplementation from different sources: performance, ascites-related variables and antioxidant status in broilers reared at low and optimum temperatures. Br. Poult. Sci. 48(5):580–593. https://doi.org/10.1080/00071660701593951.

Padh, H. (1991) Vitamin C: newer insights into its biochemical functions. Nutr. Rev. 49(3):65–70. https://doi.org/10.1111/j.1753-4887.1991.tb07407.x.

Padhi, P. and Combs, G. (1965) Effect of dietary thiamine intake on red blood cell transketolase activity in laying hens. Poult. Sci. 44:1405.
PagazaurtundúaPagazaurtundúa, A. and Warriss, P.D. (2006) Levels of foot pad dermatitis in broiler chickens reared in 5 different systems. Br. Poult. Sci. 47(5):529–532. https://doi.org/10.1080/00071660600963024.
Palagina, N.K., Meledina, T.V. and Karpisheva, I.A. (1990) Simplified method for determining pantothenic acid in molasses. Appl. Biochem. Microbiol. 26:688.
Panagabko, C., Morley, S., Neely, S., Lei, H., Manor, D. and Atkinson, J. (2002) Expression and refolding of recombinant human alpha-tocopherol transfer protein capable of specific alpha-tocopherol binding. Protein Expr. Purif. 24(3):395–403. https://doi.org/10.1006/prep.2001.1576.
Panda, A.K. and Cherian, G. (2014) Role of vitamin E in counteracting oxidative stress in poultry. J. Poult. Sci. 51(2):109–117. https://doi.org/10.2141/jpsa.0130134.
Panda, A.K., Rama Rao, S.V., Raju, M.V.L.N., Niranjan, M. and Reddy, B.L.N. (2006) Influence of supplemental vitamin D_3 on production performance of aged white leghorn layer breeders and their progeny. Asian. Australas. J. Anim. Sci. 19(11):1638–1642. https://doi.org/10.5713/ajas.2006.1638.
Panda, A.K., Ramarao, S.V.R., Raju, M.V.L.N. and Chatterjee, R.N. (2008) Effect of dietary supplementation with vitamins E and C on production performance, immune responses and antioxidant status of white leghorn layers under tropical summer conditions. Br. Poult. Sci. 49(5):592–599. https://doi.org/10.1080/00071660802337233.
Panda, A.K., Rama-Rao, S.V., Raju, M.V.L.N. and Reddy, M.R. (2009) Vitamin supplementation could lower feed costs, reduce environmental risks. Watt Poultry.com. https://www.wattagnet.com/articles/404-vitamin-supplementation-could-lower-feed-costs-reduce-environmental-risks.
Panganamala, R.V. and Cornwell, D.G. (1982) The effects of vitamin E on arachidonic acid metabolism. Ann. N. Y. Acad. Sci. 393:376–391. https://doi.org/10.1111/j.1749-6632.1982.tb31277.x.
Panic, B., Stosic, D., Hristic, V., Cuperlovic, M. and Pesevska-Stoirova, M. (1970) Potrebl priploduih kokosi za vitamoni B_{12}. Pojoprivredne Nauk. 23:109–114.
Papesova, L. and Fucikova, A. (2000) Acute and long-term toxicity of coated vitamin D_3. Proc. 21st World's Poult. Congr., Montreal, Canada.
Papesova, L., Fucikova, A., Pipalova, M. and Tupy, P. (2008) The synergic effect of vitamin D_3 and 25-hydroxycholcalciferol in broiler fattening. Proc. 23rd World's Poult. Congr., Brisbane, Australia.
Pappu, A.S., Fatterpaker, P. and Sreenivasan, A. (1978) Possible interrelationship between vitamins E and B_{12} in the disturbance in methylmalonate metabolism in vitamin E deficiency. Biochem. J. 172(1):115–121. https://doi.org/10.1042/bj1720115.
Pardue, S.L. (1989) Ascorbic acid: adrenal functions, stress and supplementation. The role of vitamin C in poultry stress management. Animal health and nutrition. Hoffmann- La Roche Inc: 1-15.
Pardue, S.L. and Thaxton, J.P. (1982) Enhanced livability and improved immunological responsiveness in ascorbic acid supplemented cockerels during acute heat stress. Poult. Sci. 61(1):1522.
Pardue, S.L. and Thaxton, J.P. (1984) Evidence for amelioration of steroid-mediated immunosuppression by ascorbic acid. Poult. Sci. 63(6):1262–1268. https://doi.org/10.3382/ps.0631262.
Pardue, S.L. and Thaxton, J.P. (1986) Ascorbic acid in poultry: a review. Worlds Poult. Sci. J. 42(2):107–123. https://doi.org/10.1079/WPS19860009.
Pardue, S.L. and Williams, S.H. (1990) Ascorbic acid dynamics in avian neonates during stress. Ascorbic Acid Domest. Anim. Proc. 2nd Symp.
Pardue, S.L., Thaxton, J.P. and Brake, J. (1984) Plasma ascorbic acid concentration following ascorbic acid loading in chicks. Poult. Sci. 63(12):2492–2496. https://doi.org/10.3382/ps.0632492.
Pardue, S.L., Thaxton, J.P. and Brake, J. (1985) Influence of supplemental ascorbic acid on broiler performance following exposure to high environmental temperature. Poult. Sci. 64(7):1334–1338. https://doi.org/10.3382/ps.0641334.
Pardue, S.L., Uhf, W.E., Kubena, L.F. and Harvey, R.B. (1987) Influence of ascorbic acid on aflatoxicosis in broiler cockerels. Poult. Sci. 66(1):156.
Pardue, S.L., Brake, J., Seib, P.A. and Wang, X.Y. (1993) Relative bioavailability of L-ascorbyl-2-polyphosphate in broiler chickens. Poult. Sci. 72(7):1330–1338. https://doi.org/10.3382/ps.0721330.

Park, I.K., Shin, S. and Marquardt, R.R. (1991) Effects of niacin deficiency on the relative turnover rates of proteins in various tissues of Japanese quail. Int. J. Biochem. 30(8):943–953. https://doi.org/10.1016/s1357-2725(98)00027-2.

Park, S.W., Namkung, H., Ahn, H.J. and Paik, I.K. (2005) Enrichment of vitamins D_3, K and iron in eggs of laying hens. Asian. Australas. J. Anim. Sci. 18(2):226–229. https://doi.org/10.5713/ajas.2005.226.

Parkinson, G.B. and Cransberg, P.H. (2004) Effect of casein phosphopeptide and 25-hydroxycholecalciferol on tibial dyschondroplasia in growing broiler chickens. Br. Poult. Sci. 45(6):802–806. https://doi.org/10.1080/00071660400012733.

Parnian, A., Navidshad, B., Mirzaei, F., Behmaram, R. and Deldar, H. (2019) Effect of *in ovo* injection of nicotonic acid, pantothenic acid or folic acid on immune system and growth of broiler chickens. Iran. J. Vet. Res. 13(4):411–420. https://doi.org/10.22059/ijvm.2019.278345.1004976.

Parolini, M., Khoriauli, L., Possenti, C.D., Colombo, G., Caprioli, M., Santagostino, M., Nergadze, S.G., Milzani, A., Giulotto, E. and Saino, N. (2017) Yolk vitamin E prevents oxidative damage in gull hatchlings. R. Soc. Open Sci. 4(5):170098. https://doi.org/10.1098/rsos.170098.

Parsons, C.M. and Leeper, R.W. (1984) Choline and methionine supplementation of layer diets varying in protein content. Poult. Sci. 63(8):1604–1609. https://doi.org/10.3382/ps.0631604.

Parsons, J.L. and Klostermann, H.J. (1967) Dakota scientists report new antibiotic found in flaxseed. Feedstuffs 39(45):74.

Patel, K.P., Edwards, H.M. and Baker, D.H. (1997) Removal of vitamin and trace mineral supplements from broiler finisher diets. J. Appl. Poult. Res. 6(2):191–198. https://doi.org/10.1093/japr/6.2.191.

Patel, M.B. and McGinnis, J. (1977) The effect of levels of protein and vitamin B_{12} in hen diets on egg production and hatchability of eggs and on livability and growth of chicks. Poult. Sci. 56(1):45–53. https://doi.org/10.3382/ps.0560045.

Patel, M.B. and McGinnis, J. (1980) The effect of vitamin B_{12} on the tolerance of chicks for high levels of dietary fat and carbohydrate. Poult. Sci. 59(10):2279–2286. https://doi.org/10.3382/ps.0592279.

Pearson, P.B., Struglia, L. and Lindahl, I.L. (1953) The fecal and urinary excretion of certain B vitamins by sheep fed hay and semi-synthetic rations. J. Anim. Sci. 12(1):213–218. https://doi.org/10.2527/jas1953.121213x.

Peebles, E.D. (2018) In ovo applications in poultry: a review. Poult. Sci. 97(7):2322–2338. https://doi.org/10.3382/ps/pey081.

Peebles, E.D. and Brake, J. (1985) Relationship of dietary ascorbic acid to broiler breeder performance. Poult. Sci. 64(11):2041–2048. https://doi.org/10.3382/ps.0642041.

Peebles, E.D., Miller, E.H., Brake, J.D. and Schultz, C.D. (1992) Effects of ascorbic acid on plasma thyroxine concentrations and eggshell quality of leghorn chickens treated with dietary thiouracil. Poult. Sci. 71(3):553–559. https://doi.org/10.3382/ps.0710553.

Perek, M. and Snapir, N. (1963) Seasonal variations in semen production of different breeds of cocks and the effect of vitamin C feed supplementation upon the semen of white rocks. Br. Poult. Sci. 4(1):19–26. https://doi.org/10.1080/00071666308415478.

Perez, D.M., Richards, M.P., Parker, R.S., Berres, M.E., Wright, A.T., Sifri, M., Sadler, N.C., Tatiyaborworntham, N. and Li, N. (2016) Role of cytochrome P450 hydroxylase in the decreased accumulation of vitamin E in muscle from turkeys compared to that from chickens. J. Agric. Food Chem. 64(3):671–680. https://doi.org/10.1021/acs.jafc.5b05433.

Perez-Carbajal, C., Caldwell, D., Farnell, M., Stringfellow, K., Pohl, S., Casco, G., Pro-Martinez, A. and Ruiz-Feria, C.A. (2010) Immune response of broiler chickens fed different levels of arginine and vitamin E to a coccidiosis vaccine and Eimeria challenge. Poult. Sci. 89(9):1870–1877. https://doi.org/10.3382/ps.2010-00753.

Pérez-Vendrell, A.M. and Weber, G.M. (2007) The effects of elevated dietary vitamins (OVN™) combined with Hy D (25- hydroxycholecalciferol) on performance, health and processing yield of broilers. Proc. 16th Eur. Symp. Poult. Nutr., Strasbourg, France. (pp. 213–216).

Pérez-Vendrell, A.M., Hernandez, J.M., Llauradó, Ll. and Brufau, J. (2002) Effect of optimum vitamin levels in broiler diets on performance and meat quality parameters. Poster Eur. Conf. Poultr. Nutr.

Pérez-Vendrell, A.M., Hernández, J.M., Llauradó, L. and Brufau, J. (2003) Improving the nutritive value of

broiler meat by feeding optimum vitamin nutrition (OVN™). Proc. 16th Eur. symp. qual. poult. Meat, St.-Brieuc, France. (pp. 185–189).
Perry, R.W., Rowland, G.N., Foutz, T.L. and Glisson, J.R. (1991) Poult malabsorption syndrome. III. Skeletal lesions in market-age turkeys. Avian Dis. 35(4):707–713. https://doi.org/10.2307/1591599.
Perry, S.C. (1978) Vitamin allowances for animal feeds. In "Vitamin nutrition update – seminar series 2", RCD 5483/1078, Hoffmann-La Roche.
Persia, M.E., Higgins, M., Wang, T., Trample, D. and Bobeck, E.A. (2013) Effects of long-term supplementation of laying hens with high concentrations of cholecalciferol on performance and egg quality. Poult. Sci. 92(11):2930–2937. https://doi.org/10.3382/ps.2013-03243.
Pesti, G.M. and Rowland, G.N. (1989) The influence of folic acid supplementation to corn and soybean meal-based diets in broiler growth. Poult. Sci. 68(1):198.
Pesti, G.M., Harper, A.E. and Sunde, M.L. (1980) Choline/methionine nutrition of starting broiler chicks. Three models for estimating the choline requirement with economic considerations. Poult. Sci. 59(5):1073–1081. https://doi.org/10.3382/ps.0591073.
Pesti, G.M., Rowland, G.N. and Ryu, K.S. (1991) Folate deficiency in chicks fed diets containing practical ingredients. Poult. Sci. 70(3):600–604. https://doi.org/10.3382/ps.0700600.
Pesti, G.M. and Shivaprasad, H.L. (2010) The influence of excessive levels of 1a-hydroxycholecalciferol on the growth and tissue appearance of market weight chickens. J. Appl. Poult. Res. 19(4):349–353. https://doi.org/10.3382/japr.2010-00193.
Pesut, O., Jovanivic, I., Noller, L. and Tucker, L. (2005) Effect of Se (Sel-Plex®) in combination with α-tocopherol on GSH-Px activity and TBARS in plasma of broilers. Proc. 15th Eur. Symp. Poult. Nutr., Balatonfured, Hungary. (pp. 502–504).
Petek, M., Sönmez, G., Yildiz, H. and Baspinar, H. (2005) Effects of different management factors on broiler performance and incidence of tibial dyschondroplasia. Br. Poult. Sci. 46(1):16–21. https://doi.org/10.1080/00071660400023821.
Petracci, M., Mudalal, S., Soglia, F. and Cavani, C. (2015) Meat quality in fast-growing broiler chickens. Worlds Poult. Sci. J. 71(2):363–374. https://doi.org/10.1017/S0043933915000367.
Petracci, M., Soglia, F., Madruga, M., Carvalho, L., Ida, E. and Estévez, M. (2019) Wooden-breast, white striping, and spaghetti meat: causes, consequences and consumer perception of emerging broiler meat abnormalities. Compr. Rev. Food Sci. Food Saf. 18(2):565–583. https://doi.org/10.1111/1541-4337.12431.
Philips, P., Aureli, R., Weber, G. and Klünter, A.M. (2005) Effects of 25-hydroxycholecalciferol (Hy-D) at doses from 35 to 560 μg per kg feed on the performance of broiler chickens fed a diet based on maize, wheat and soybean meal. Proc. 15th Eur. Symp. Poult. Nutr., Balatonfured, Hungary. (pp. 189–191).
Philips, P., Aureli, R., Fru, F. and Weber, G. (2008) Effects of 25-hydroxycholecalciferol and a *Peniophora lycii* phytase on the growth performance and the apparent utilization of Ca and P in broiler chickens fed basal diets low in phosphorus and with different levels of vitamin D_3. Proc. 16th Eur. Symp. Poult. Nutr., Strasbourg, France. (pp. 609–612).
Pierson, F.W. and Hester, P.Y. (1982) Factors influencing leg abnormalities in poultry: a review. Worlds Poult. Sci. J. 38(1):5–17. https://doi.org/10.1017/WPS19820001.
Pikul, J., Holownia, K. and Plewinsky, A. (1997) Influence of dietary α- tocopheryl acetate on lipid oxidation in chicken meat. 13th Eur. Symp. Poult. Meat Qual., Poznań, Poland. (pp. 223–229).
Pillai, P.B., Fanatico, A.C., Beers, K.W., Blair, M.E. and Emmert, J.L. (2006a) Homocysteine remethylation in young broilers fed varying levels of methionine, choline and betaine. Poult. Sci. 85(1):90–95. https://doi.org/10.1093/ps/85.1.90.
Pillai, P.B., Fanatico, A.C., Blair, M.E. and Emmert, J.L. (2006b) Homocysteine remethylation in broilers fed surfeit choline or betaine and varying levels and sources of methionine from eight to twenty-two days of age. Poult. Sci. 85(10):1729–1736. https://doi.org/10.1093/ps/85.10.1729.
Pines, M., Hasdai, A.M. and Monsonego-Ornan, E. (2005) Tibial dyschondroplasia–tools, new insights and future prospects. World's Poult. Sci. 61(2):285–297. https://doi.org/10.1079/WPS200454.
Pinto, J.T. and Rivlin, R.S. (2013) Riboflavin (vitamin B_2). In "Handbook of vitamins" 5th ed. Zempleni, J., Suttie, J., Gregory, J. and Stover P.J. (ed.). CRC Press, Taylor & Francis Group. (pp. 191–266).

Plaimast, H. and Punyaphat, S.K. (2015) Effects of vitamin D_3 and calcium on productive performance, egg quality and vitamin D_3 content in egg of second production cycle hens. Thai J. Vet. Med. 45(2):189–195.

Podda, M. and Grundmann-Kollmann, M. (2001) Low molecular weight antioxidants and their role in skin ageing. Clin. Exp. Dermatol. 26(7):578–582. https://doi.org/10.1046/j.1365-2230.2001.00902.x.

Polak, D.M., Elliot, J.M. and Haluska, M. (1979) Vitamin B_{12} binding proteins in bovine serum. J. Dairy Sci. 62(5):697–701. https://doi.org/10.3168/jds.S0022-0302(79)83312-3.

Polin, D., Wynosky, E.R. and Porter, C.C. (1962) Amprolium 10: influence of egg yolk thiamine concentration on chick embryo mortality. Proc. Soc. Exp. Biol. Med. 110:844–846. https://doi.org/10.3181/00379727-110-27667.

Polin, D., Ott, W.H., Wynosky, E.R. and Porter, C.C. (1963) Estimation of thiamine requirement for optimum hatchability from the relationship between dietary and yolk levels of the vitamin. Poult. Sci. 42(4):925–928. https://doi.org/10.3382/ps.0420925.

Pollard, W.O. and Creek, R.D. (1964) Histological effects of certain nutrient deficiencies in the chick bone development. Poult. Sci. 43(6):1415–1420. https://doi.org/10.3382/ps.0431415.

Pompeu, M.A., Cavalcanti, L.F.L. and Toral, F.L.B. (2018) Effect of vitamin E supplementation on growth performance, meat quality, and immune response of male broiler chickens: a meta-analysis. Livest. Sci. 208:5–13. https://doi.org/10.1016/j.livsci.2017.11.021.

Portsmouth, J. (1996) Requerimientos vitamínicos de los broilers y las reproductoras pesadas (Vitamin requirements of heavy broilers and breeders) Proc. 33rd symp. WPSA's Spanish Branch, Toledo, Spain. (pp. 115–137).

Pourreza, J. and Smith, W.K. (1988) Performance of laying hens fed on low sulphur amino acids diets supplemented with choline and methionine. Br. Poult. Sci. 29(3):605–611. https://doi.org/10.1080/00071668808417087.

Powers, H.J., Weaver, L.T., Austin, S., (1991) Riboflavin deficiency in the rat: effects on iron utilization and loss. Br. J. Nutr. 65(3):487–496. https://doi.org/10.1079/BJN19910107.

Powers, H.J., Weaver, L.T., Austin, S. and Beresford, J.K. (1993) A proposed intestinal mechanism for the effect of riboflavin deficiency on iron loss in the rat. Br. J. Nutr. 69(2):553–561. https://doi.org/10.1079/bjn19930055.

Prabakar, G., Gopi, M., Tyagi, J.S. and Mohan, J. (2018) Combination of synthetic carotenoids on enhanced the haematological attributes in broiler breeders. Int. J. Chem. Stud. 6(5):3393–3395.

Praslickova, D., Sharif, S., Sarson, A., Abdul-Careem, M.F., Zadworny, D., Kulenkamp, A., Ansah, G. and Kuhnlein, U. (2008) Association of a marker in the vitamin D receptor gene with Marek's disease resistance in poultry. Poult. Sci. 87(6):1112–1119. https://doi.org/10.3382/ps.2008-00006.

Preisinger, R. (2018) Innovative layer genetics to handle global challenges in egg production. Br. Poult. Sci. 59(1):1–6. https://doi.org/10.1080/00071668.2018.1401828.

Premkumar, V.G., Yuvaraj, S., Shanthi, P. and Sachdanandam, P. (2008) Co-enzyme Q10, riboflavin and niacin supplementation on alteration of DNA repair enzyme and DNA methylation in breast cancer patients undergoing tamoxifen therapy. Br. J. Nutr. 100(6):1179–1182. https://doi.org/10.1017/S0007114508968276.

Price, F. (1968) The effect of vitamin E deficiency on fertility of *Coturnix coturnix*. Poult. Sci. 47(3):1037–1038. https://doi.org/10.3382/ps.0471037.

Prisco, F., De Biase, D., Piegari, G., d'Aquino, I., Lama, A., Comella, F., Mercogliano, R., Dipineto, L., Papparella, S. and Paciello, O. (2021) Pathologic characterization of white striping myopathy in broiler chickens. Poult. Sci. 100(7):101150. https://doi.org/10.1016/j.psj.2021.101150.

Puchal, F. (1989) Broiler nutrition and heat stress. Proc. 7th Eur. Symp. Poult. Nutr., Lloret de Mar, Spain. (pp. 65–81).

Puron, D., Santamaria, R. and Segura, J.C. (1994) Effects of sodium bicarbonate, acetylsalicylic, and ascorbic acid on broiler performance in a tropical environment. J. Appl. Poult. Res. 3(2):141–145. https://doi.org/10.1093/japr/3.2.141.

Puthpongsiriporn, U., Scheideler, S.E., Sell, J.L. and Beck, M.M. (2001) Effects of vitamin E and C supplementation on performance, in vitro lymphocyte proliferation and antioxidant status of laying hens during heat stress. Poult. Sci. 80(8):1190–1200. https://doi.org/10.1093/ps/80.8.1190.

Putnam, M. (1983) Composición de los alimentos y estabilidad vitamínica. Reunión de la sociedad de técnicos en alimentación, York, Inglaterra. Reimpresión Roche Inf. Serv. Anim. Nutr. Dept.

Putnam, M. and Taylor, A. (1997) Vitaminas en alimentos animales: los factores críticos. Avicultura Profesional. (pp.24–28).

Qazi, I.H., Cao, Y., Yang, H., Angel, C., Pan, B., Zhou, G. and Han, H. (2021) Impact of dietary selenium on modulation of expression of several non-selenoprotein genes related to key ovarian functions, female fertility, and proteostasis: a transcriptome-based analysis of the aging mice ovaries. Biol. Trace Elem. Res. 199(2):633–648. https://doi.org/10.1007/s12011-020-02192-x.

Qi, G.H. and Sim, J.S. (1998) Natural tocopherol enrichment and its effect in n-3 fatty acid modified chicken eggs. J. Agric. Food Chem. 46(5):1920–1926. https://doi.org/10.1021/jf9707804.

Qian, H., Kornegay, E.T. and Denbow, D.M. (1997) Utilization of phytate phosphorus and calcium as influenced by microbial phytase, cholecalciferol, and the calcium: total phosphorus ratio in broiler diets. Poult. Sci. 76(1):37–46. https://doi.org/10.1093/ps/76.1.37.

Quackenbush, F.W. (1963) Corn carotenoids: effect of temperature and moisture on losses during storage. Cereal Chem. 40:266.

Quadros, T.C.Od, Sgavioli, S., Castiblanco, D.M.C., Santos, E.T., Andrade, G.Md, Borges, L.L., Almeida, A.R. and Baraldi-Artoni, S.M. (2021) *In ovo* feeding with 25-hydroxycholecalciferol influences bone mineral density of chicks. R. Bras. Zootec. 50. https://doi.org/10.37496/rbz5020200050.

Quant, A.D., Pescatore, A.J., Pierce, J.L., McClelland, K.M., Rentfrow, G.R., Cantor, A.H., Ford, M.J. and King, W.D. (2010) Effect of dietary selenium yeast (Sel-Plex®) and vitamin E supplementation to broilers on meat quality characteristics of raw and marinated breast fillets. J. Dairy Sci. 93:276. https://doi.org/066251152.php.

Quarantelli, A., Cacchioli, A., Romanelli, S., Righi, F., Alpigiani, I. and Gabbi, C. (2007) Effects of different levels of dietary biotin on the performance and bone structure of broilers. Ital. J. Anim. Sci. 6(1):5–7.

Quarles, C.L. and Adrian, W.J. (1989) Evaluation of ascorbic acid for increasing carcass yield in broiler chickens. In "The role of vitamin C in poultry stress management", Animal health and nutrition. Hoffmann–La Roche, Inc.

Quillin, E.C., Combs, G.F., Creek, R.D. and Romoser, G.L. (1961) Effect of choline on the methionine requirements of broiler chickens. Poult. Sci. 40(3):639–645. https://doi.org/10.3382/ps.0400639.

Qureshi, M.A., Ferket, P.R. and Garlich, J.D. (1993) Effect of dietary supplementation of vitamin E on the immune function of turkey poults. Poult. Sci. 72 (suppl. 1):89 (abstract).

Qureshi, M.A. and Gore, A.B. (1997) Vitamin E exposure modulates prostaglandin and thromboxane production by avian cells of the mononuclear phagocytic system. Immunopharmacol. Immunotoxicol. 19(4):473–487. https://doi.org/10.3109/08923979709007669.

Qureshi, M.A., Vanhooser, S.L. and Teeter, R.G. (2000) Dietary vitamin E, vitamin C and drinking water electrolyte effects on broiler performance and immunity during exposure to high cycling ambient temperature. Poult. Sci. 79 (suppl. 1):89.

Qureshi, A.A., Salser, W.A., Parmar, R. and Emeson, E.E. (2001) Novel tocotrienols of rice bran inhibit atherosclerotic lesions in C57BL/6 apoE-deficient mice. J. Nutr. 131(10):2606–2618. https://doi.org/10.1093/jn/131.10.2606.

Raederstorff, D., Wyss, A., Calder, P.C., Weber, P. and Eggersdorfer, M. (2015) Vitamin E function and requirements in relation to PUFA. Br. J. Nutr. 114(8):1113–1122. https://doi.org/10.1017/S000711451500272X.

Raeisi-Zeydabad, S., Mirmahmoudi, R., Esmaeilipour, O. and Mazhari, M. (2017) Effects of coenzyme Q_{10} and vitamin C on growth performance and blood components in broiler chickens under heat stress. Poult. Sci. 5(2):145–152. https://doi.org/10.22069/psj.2017.13733.1272.

Rajabi, M. and Torki, M. (2021) Effect of dietary supplemental vitamin C and zinc sulfate on productive performance, egg quality traits and blood parameters of laying hens reared under cold stress condition. J. Appl. Anim. Res. 49(1):309–317. https://doi.org/10.1080/09712119.2021.1949999.

Rajkhowa, T.K., Katiyar, A.K. and Vegad, J.L. (1996) Effect of ascorbic acid on the inflammatory-reparative response in the punched wounds of the chicken skin. Indian J. Anim. Sci. 66:120–125.

Rajmane, B.V. and Ranade, A.S. (1992) Remedial measures to control high mortality during summer season in tropical countries. Proc. 19th world's poultry congress, Amsterdam, the Netherlands. (pp. 343–345).

Rall, L.C. and Meydani, S.N. (1993) Vitamin B_6 and immune competence. Nutr. Rev. 51(8):217–225. https://doi.org/10.1111/j.1753-4887.1993.tb03109.x.

Rama Rao, S.V., Sunder, G.S., Reddy, M.R., Praharaj, N.K., Raju, M.V.L.N. and Panda, A.K. (2001) Effect of supplementary choline on the performance of broiler breeders fed on different energy sources. Br. Poult. Sci. 42(3):362–367. https://doi.org/10.1080/00071660120055340.

Rama-Rao, S.V., Raju, M.V.L.N., Sharma, R.P., Nagalakshmi, D. and Reddy, M.R. (2003) Lameness in chickens: alleviation by dietary manipulation. Poult. Int.:53–61.

Rama-Rao, S.V., Raju, M.V.L.N., Panda, A.K., Sunder, G.S. and Sharma, R.P. (2006) Effect of high concentration of cholecalciferol on growth, bone mineralization, and mineral retention in broiler chicks fed suboptimal concentrations of calcium and non-phytate phosphorus. J. Appl. Poult. Res. 15(4):493–501. https://doi.org/10.1093/japr/15.4.493.

Rama-Rao, S.V., Raju, M.V.L.N., Panda, A.K., Shaharai, P.N., Reddy, M.R., Sunder, G.S. and Sharma, R.P. (2008) Effect of surfeit concentrations of vitamin D_3 on performance, bone mineralization, and mineral retention in commercial broiler chicks. The J. Poult. Sci. 45(1):25–30. https://doi.org/10.2141/jpsa.45.25.

Rao, C.V., Hirose, Y., Indranie, C. and Reddy, B.S. (2001) Modulation of experimental colon tumorigenesis by types and amounts of dietary fatty acids. Cancer Res. 61(5): 1927–1933.

Rath, N.C., Huff, G.R., Huff, W.E. and Balog, J.M. (2000) Factors regulating bone maturity and strength in poultry. Poult. Sci. 79(7):1024–1032. https://doi.org/10.1093/ps/79.7.1024.

Rath, N.C., Huff, G.R. and Huff, W.E. (2006) Thiram-induced tibial dyschondroplasia: a model to study its pathogenesis and prevention. Proc. 12th Eur. Poult. Nutr. Verona, Italy.

Rawling, J.M., Jackson, T.M., Driscoll, E.R. and Kirkland, J.B. (1994) Dietary niacin deficiency lowers tissue poly (ADP-ribose) and NAD+ concentrations in Fischer-344 rats. J. Nutr. 124(9):1597–1603. https://doi.org/10.1093/jn/124.9.1597.

Raza, A., Sharif, M., Ahmad, F., Kamboh, A.A., Saeed, M., Ashraf, M. and Hayder, A.U. (2022) Effect of vitamin D and phytase on growth, blood mineral level and slaughter parameters of broilers. Pak. J. Zool. 54(3):(1–4). https://doi.org/10.17582/journal.pjz/20200519070540.

Rebel, J.M.J., van Dam, J.T.P., Zekarias, B., Balk, F.R.M., Post, J., Flores Miñambres, A. and ter Huurne, A.A.H.M. (2004) Vitamin and trace mineral content in feed of breeders and their progeny: effects of growth, feed conversion and severity of malabsorption syndrome of broilers. Br. Poult. Sci. 45(2):201–209. https://doi.org/10.1080/00071660410001715803.

Rebolé, A., Rodríguez, M.L., Ortiz, L.T., Alzueta, C., Centeno, C., Viveros, A., Brenes, A. and Arija, I. (2006) Effect of dietary high- oleic acid sunflower seed, palm oil and vitamin E supplementation on broiler performance, fatty acid composition and oxidation susceptibility of meat. Br. Poult. Sci. 47(5):581–591. https://doi.org/10.1080/00071660600939727.

Reboul, E. and Borel, P. (2011) Proteins involved in uptake, intracellular transport and basolateral secretion of fat-soluble vitamins and carotenoids by mammalian enterocytes. Prog. Lipid Res. 50(4):388–402. https://doi.org/10.1016/j.plipres.2011.07.001.

Reddy, M.U. and Pushpamma, P. (1986) Effect of storage and insect infestation on thiamin and niacin content in different varieties of rice, sorghum, and legumes. Nutr. Rep. Int. 34:393–401.

Rehman, Z.U. et al. (2018) Supplementation of vitamin E protects chickens from Newcastle disease virus-mediated exacerbation of intestinal oxidative stress and tissue damage. Cell. Physiol. Biochem. 47(4):1655–1666. https://doi.org/10.1159/000490984.

Reinhardt, T.A. and Hustmeyer, F.G. (1987) Role of vitamin D in the immune system. J. Dairy Sci. 70(5):952–962. https://doi.org/10.3168/jds.S0022-0302(87)80099-1.

Remus, J.C. and Firman, J.D. (1989) Effect of thiamine-deficient anorexia on biogenic amines in the turkey brain. Poult. Sci. 68(suppl. 1):120. https://doi.org/10.3382/ps.0702345.

Remus, J.C. and Firman, J.D. (1990) Effect of thiamine deficiency on energy metabolites in the turkey. J. Nutr. Biochem. 1(12):636–639. https://doi.org/10.1016/0955-2863(90)90023-E.

Remus, J.C. and Firman, J.D. (1991a) Efficacy of lateral ventricular injection of epinephrine, cyproheptadine, or adenosine triphosphate on feed intake in thiamine-deficient turkeys. Poult. Sci. 70(11):2340–2344. https://doi.org/10.3382/ps.0702340.

Remus, J.C. and Firman, J.D. (1991b) The effect of thiamin deficiency on amino acids in the brain, liver, and plasma of the turkey. Poult. Sci. 70(11):2345–2353. https://doi.org/10.3382/ps.0702345.

Rengaraj, D. and Hong, Y.H. (2015) Effects of dietary vitamin E on fertility functions in poultry species. Int. J. Mol. Sci. 16(5):9910–9921. https://doi.org/10.3390/ijms16059910.

Rennie, J.S. (1994) Vitamin D metabolites and the prevention of tibial dyschondroplasia. Proc. 9th Eur. poultry conf. (pp. 207–210).

Rennie, S. (1995) Vitamin D, ascorbic acid and tibial dyschondroplasia. Poult. Int. 95:50–52.

Rennie, J.S. and Whitehead, C.C. (1996) Effectiveness of dietary 25- and 1-hydroxycholecalciferol in combating tibial dyschondroplasia in broiler chickens. Br. Poult. Sci. 37(2):413–421. https://doi.org/10.1080/00071669608417872.

Rennie, J.S., Whitehead, C.C. and Thorp, B.H. (1993) The effect of dietary 1,25-dihydroxycholecalciferol in preventing tibial dyschondroplasia in broilers fed on diets imbalanced in calcium and phosphorus. Br. J. Nutr. 69(3):809–816. https://doi.org/10.1079/bjn19930081.

Rennie, J.S., McCormack, H.A., Farquharson, C., Berry, J.L., Mawer, E.B. and Whitehead, C.C. (1995) Interaction between dietary 1,25-dihydroxycholecalciferol and calcium and effects of management on the occurrence of tibial dyschondroplasia, leg abnormalities and performance in broiler chickens. Br. Poult. Sci. 36(3):465–477. https://doi.org/10.1080/00071669508417792.

Rennie, J.S., Fleming, R.H., McCormack, H.A., Mccorquodale, C.C. and Whitehead, C.C. (1997) Studies on effects of nutritional factors on bone structure and osteoporosis in laying hens. Br. Poult. Sci. 38(4):417–424. https://doi.org/10.1080/00071669708418012.

Reyes, J.B.D., Kim, J.H., Han, G.P., Won, S.Y. and Kil, D.Y. (2021) Effects of dietary supplementation of vitamin C on productive performance, egg quality, tibia characteristics and antioxidant status of laying hens. Livest. Sci. 248:(104502). https://doi.org/10.1016/j.livsci.2021.104502.

Rhee, K.S., Anderson, L.M. and Sams, A.R. (1996) Lipid oxidation potential of beef, chicken, and pork. J. Food Sci. 61(1):8–12. https://doi.org/10.1111/j.1365-2621.1996.tb14714.x.

Riaz Rajoka, M.S., Thirumdas, R., Mehwish, H.M., Umair, M., Khurshid, M., Hayat, H.F., Phimolsiripol, Y., Pallarés, N., Martí-Quijal, F.J. and Barba, F.J. (2021) Role of food antioxidants in modulating gut microbial communities: novel understandings in intestinal oxidative stress damage and their impact on host health. Antioxidants (Basel) 10(10):1563. https://doi.org/10.3390/antiox10101563.

Rice, D.A. and McIlroy, S.G. (1988) The use of a computerised management and disease information system for large scale trials on micronutrients in broilers and broiler breeders. In: Proceedings, The Roche Symposium (Welwyn Garden City, Roche Products Limited).

Richter, G., Rödel, I., Wunderlich, E. and Marckwardt, E. (1985) Evaluation of laying-hen feed with varied vitamin E and antioxidant supplementation. Arch. Tierernahr. 35(10):707–714. https://doi.org/10.1080/17450398509425226.

Richter, G., Marckwardt, E., Hennig, A. and Steinbach, G. (1986) Vitamin E requirements of laying hens. Arch. Tierernahr. 36(12):1133–1143. https://doi.org/10.1080/17450398609434360.

Richter, G., Lemser, A., Jahreis, G. and Steinbach, G. (1987) Vitamin E requirement of chicks and young hens. Arch. Tierernahr. 37(11):1029–1039. https://doi.org/10.1080/17450398709428270.

Richter, G., Hennig, A. and Jeroch, H. (1989) The vitamin A supply of laying hens including during rearing. 1. Testing of mixed feed with a varied vitamin A supplementation in chicks and young hens. Arch. Tierernahr. 39(12):1053–1064. https://doi.org/10.1080/17450398909434381.

Richter, G., Sitte, E. and Petzold, M. (1990) The vitamin A supply of laying hens including during rearing. 2. Effect of varied vitamin A supplementation of mixed feed in rearing on production in the laying period. Arch. Tierernahr. 40(3):221–227. https://doi.org/10.1080/17450399009428397.

Richter, G., Lemser, A., Jahreis, G., Wanka, U., Matthey, M., Schubert, K. and Steinbach, G. (1996a) Studies in vitamin A requirement and recommendations for chicken and pullets. Archiv. Geflügelk 60(5):193–202.

Richter, G., Lemser, A. and Bargholz, J. (1996b) Is vitamin A supply of laying hens sufficient? Muhle Mischfuttertechnik 133:49–50. https://doi.org/10.1080/17450399609381884.

Richter, G., Lemser, A., Ludke, C., Steinbach, G. and Mockel, P. (1996c) Studies on the vitamin A requirements and recommendations for laying hens. Arch. geflugelkunde 60(4):174–180.

Ricks, C.A., Avakian, A., Bryan, T., Gildersleeve, R., Haddad, E., Ilich, R., King, S., Murray, L., Phelps, P., Poston, R., Whitfill, C. and Williams, C. (1999) *In ovo* vaccination technology. Adv. Anim. Vet. Sci. 41:495–515. https://doi.org/10.1016/S0065-3519(99)80037-8.

Riddell, C. (2000) Management of skeletal disease. Proc. 21st World's Poult. Congress, Montreal, Canada.

Rifici, V.A. and Khachadurian, A.K. (1993) Dietary supplementation with vitamins C and E inhibits in vitro oxidation of lipoproteins. J. Am. Coll. Nutr. 12(6):631–637. https://doi.org/10.1080/07315724.1993.10718353.

Ringrose, R.C., Manoukas, A.G., Hinkson, R. and Teerie, A. (1965) The niacin requirement of the hen. Poult. Sci. 44(4):1053–1065. https://doi.org/10.3382/ps.0441053.

Rings, B., Hoerr, F. and Halley, J. (2011) Toxicity effects of feeding 1-alpha hydroxy D_3 to broiler breeding hens. Proc. American Association of Avian Pathologists, St. Louis, Poultry science. 90:E-supplement 1.

Ristic, M. and Lidner, H. (1992) Influence of vitamin E supplementation on the meat quality and storage capability of broilers. 19th World's Poult. Congress. The Netherland, Amsterdam. (p. 146).

Rivlin, R.S. (2006) Riboflavin. In "Present knowledge in nutrition" 9th ed Bowman, B.A. and Russell, R.M. (ed.). International Life Sciences Institute. (pp. 250–259).

Robel, E.J. (1983) The effect of age of breeder hen on the level of vitamins and minerals in turkey eggs. Poult. Sci. 62(9):1751–1756. https://doi.org/10.3382/ps.0621751.

Robel, E.J. (1989) Increasing hatchability with biotin. Int. Hatch Pract. 4:47–51.

Robel, E.J. (1991) The value of supplemental biotin for increasing hatchability of turkey eggs. Poult. Sci. 70(8):1716–1722. https://doi.org/10.3382/ps.0701716.

Robel, E.J. (1992) Effect of dietary supplemental pyridoxine levels on the hatchability of turkey eggs. Poult. Sci. 71(10):1733–1738. https://doi.org/10.3382/ps.0711733.

Robel, E.J. (1993a) Evaluation of egg injection of folic acid and effect of supplemental folic acid on hatchability and poult weight. Poult. Sci. 72(3):546–553. https://doi.org/10.3382/ps.0720546.

Robel, E.J. (1993b) Evaluation of egg injection method of pantothenic acid in turkey eggs and effect of supplemental pantothenic acid on hatchability. Poult. Sci. 72(9):1740–1745. https://doi.org/10.3382/ps.0721740.

Robel, E.J. (2002) Assessment of dietary and egg injected D-biotin, pyridoxine and folic acid on turkey hatchability: folic acid and poult weight. Worlds Poult. Sci. J. 58(3):305–315. https://doi.org/10.1079/WPS20020024.

Robel, E.J. and Christensen, V.L. (1987) Increasing hatchability of turkey eggs with biotin egg injections. Poult. Sci. 66(9):1429–1430. https://doi.org/10.3382/ps.0661429.

Robel, E.J. and Christensen, V.L. (1991) Increasing hatchability of turkey eggs by injecting eggs with pyridoxine. Br. Poult. Sci. 32(3):509–513. https://doi.org/10.1080/00071669108417375.

Roberson, K.D. (1999) 25-Hydroxycholecalciferol fails to prevent tibial dyschondroplasia in broiler chicks raised in battery brooders. J. Appl. Poult. Res. 8(1):54–61. https://doi.org/10.1093/japr/8.1.54.

Roberson, K.D. and Edwards, H.M. (1994) Effects of ascorbic acid and 1,25-dihydroxycholecalciferol on alkaline phosphatase and tibial dyschondroplasia in broiler chickens. Br. Poult. Sci. 35(5):763–773. https://doi.org/10.1080/00071669408417741.

Roberson, K.D. and Edwards, H.M. (1996) Effect of dietary 1,25-dihydroxycholecalciferol level on broiler performance. Poult. Sci. 75(1):90–94. https://doi.org/10.3382/ps.0750090.

Roberson, K.D., Ledwaba, M.F. and Charbeneau, R.A. (2005) Studies on the efficacy of twenty-five-hydroxycholecalciferol to prevent tibial dyschondroplasia in Ross broilers fed marginal calcium diet. Int. J. Poult. Sci. 4(2):85–90. https://doi.org/10.3923/ijps.2005.85.90.

Roch, G., Boulianne, M. and De Roth, L. (2000a) Effects of dietary vitamin E and selenium on incidence of ascites, growth performances and blood parameters in cold stressed broilers. Poult. Sci. 79(suppl. 1):41–45.

Roch, G., Boulianne, M. and Roth, L. (2000b) Dietary antioxidants reduce ascites in broilers. World Poult. 16(11):18–22. ISSN: 1388–3119.

Rocha, J.S.R., Lara, L.J.C., Baião, N.C., Vasconcelos, R.J.C., Barbosa, V.M., Pompeu, M.A. and Fernandes, M.N.S. (2010) Antioxidant properties of vitamins in nutrition of broiler breeders and laying hens. Worlds Poult. Sci. J. 66(2):261–270. https://doi.org/10.1017/S0043933910000310.

Roche (1979) "Optimum vitamin nutrition". Hoffmann-La Roche, Nutley, NJ, USA.

Rodriguez-Lecompte, J.C., Yitbarek, A., Cuperus, T., Echeverry, H. and van Dijk, A. (2016) The immunomodulatory effect of vitamin D in chickens is dose-dependent and influenced by calcium and phosphorus levels. Poult. Sci. 95(11):2547–2556. https://doi.org/10.3382/ps/pew186.

Rodríguez-Meléndez, R., Cano, S., Méndez, S.T. and Velázquez, A. (2001) Biotin regulates the genetic expression of holocarboxylase synthetase and mitochondrial carboxylases in rats. J. Nutr. 131(7):1909–1913. https://doi.org/10.1093/jn/131.7.1909.

Rodríguez-Meléndez, R. and Zempleni, J. (2003) Regulation of gene expression by biotin [review]. J. Nutr. Biochem. 14(12):680–690. https://doi.org/10.1016/j.jnutbio.2003.07.001.

Rosa, A.P., Scher, A., Sorbara, J.O.B., Boemo, L.S., Forgiarini, J. and Londero, A. (2012) Effects of canthaxanthin on the productive and reproductive performance of broiler breeders. Poult. Sci. 91(3):660–666. https://doi.org/10.3382/ps.2011-01582.

Rosa, A.P., Bonilla, C.E.V., Londero, A., Giacomini, C.B.S., Orso, C., Fernandes, M.O., Moura, J.S. and Hermes, R. (2017) Effect of broiler breeders fed with corn or sorghum and canthaxanthin on lipid peroxidation, fatty acid profile of hatching eggs, and offspring performance. Poult. Sci. 96(3):647–658. https://doi.org/10.3382/ps/pew294.

Rose, R. (1990) Vitamin absorption. In Proc. national feed Ingr. Ass., Nutr. Inst. "Developments in vitamin nutrition and health applications", Kansas City. National Feed Ingredients Association, Missouri.

Rose, R.C., McCorrmick, D.B., Li, T.K., Lumeng, L., Haddad, J.G. and Spector, R. (1986) Transport and metabolism of vitamins. Fed. Proc. 45(1):30–39. PMID:3000833.

Rose, S.P. and Peter, J.S. (2000) Dietary ascorbic acid and tocopherol acetate supplements for broiler chickens kept at high temperatures. Proc. 21st World's Poult. Congress, Montreal, Canada.

Rosenberg, I.H. and Neumann, H. (1974) Multi-step mechanism in the hydrolysis of pteroyl polyglutamates by chicken intestine. J. Biol. Chem. 249(16):5126–5130. https://doi.org/10.1016/S0021-9258(19)42336-3.

Ross, A.C. (1992) Vitamin A status: relationship to immunity and the antibody response. Proc. Soc. Exp. Biol. Med. 200(3):303–320. https://doi.org/10.3181/00379727-200-43436A.

Ross, A.C. (1993) Overview of retinoid metabolism. J. Nutr. 123(2)(suppl.):346–350. https://doi.org/10.1093/jn/123.suppl_2.346.

Ross, A.C. and Harrison, E.H. (2013) Vitamin A: nutritional aspects of retinoids and carotenoids. In "Handbook of vitamins" 5th ed. Zempleni, J., Suttie, J., Gregory, J. and Stover P.J. (ed.). CRC Press, Taylor & Francis Group, LLC. (pp. 1–50).

Rostagno H.S., Albino L.F.T., Hannas M.I., Donzele J.L., Sakomura N.K., Perazzo F.G., Saraiva A., Abreu M.L.T. De, Rodrigues P.B., Oliveira R.F. De, Barreto S.L.T. and Brito C.O. (2017) "Brazilian tables for poultry and swine: composition of feedstuffs and nutritional requirements", 4th ed. Viçosa: Departamento de Zootecnia, Univesidade Federal de Vicosa.

Roth-Maier, D.A. and Paulicks, B.R. (2002) Effects of a suboptimal dietary intake of particular B-vitamins on the growth of fattening chicken. Arch. Geflügelk 66:201–205. ISSN 0003–9098.

Roussan, D.A., Khwaldeh, G.Y., Haddad, R.R., Shaheen, I.A., Salameh, G. and Al Rifai, R. (2008) Effect of ascorbic acid, acetylsalicylic acid, sodium bicarbonate, and potassium chloride supplementation in water on the performance of broiler chickens exposed to heat stress. J. Appl. Poult. Res. 17(1):141–144. https://doi.org/10.3382/japr.2007-00087.

Rucker, R.B. and Bauerly, K. (2013) Pantothenic acid. In "Handbook of vitamins" 5th ed. Zempleni, J., Suttie, J., Gregory, J. and Stover P.J. (ed.). CRC Press, Taylor & Francis Group, LLC ISBN 9781466515567. (pp. 289–313).

Ruiz, J.A., Perez-Vendrell, A.M. and Esteve-Garcia, E. (1998) Antioxidant properties of β-carotene in poultry meat as affected by its concentration in feed during storage. Proc. 44th Int. Conf. Meat Sci. Tech, Barcelona, Spain. (pp. 642–643).

Ruiz, J.A., Pérez-Vendrell, A.M. and Esteve-García, E. (1999) Effect of beta-carotene and vitamin E on oxidative stability in leg meat of broilers fed different supplemental fats. J. Agric. Food Chem. 47(2):448–454. https://doi.org/10.1021/jf980825g.

Ruiz, J.A., Guerrero, L., Arnau, J., Guardia, M.D. and Esteve-Garcia, E. (2001) Descriptive sensory analysis of meat from broilers fed diets containing vitamin E or β-carotene as antioxidants and different supplemental fats. Poult. Sci. 80(7):976–982. https://doi.org/10.1093/ps/80.7.976.

Ruiz, N. and Harms, R.H. (1987) The niacin requirement of broiler chickens fed a corn-soybean meal diet from three to seven weeks of age. Poult. Sci. 66(suppl. 1):37.

Ruiz, N. and Harms, R.H. (1988a) Riboflavin requirement of broiler chicks fed a corn-soybean meal diet. Poult. Sci. 67(5):794–799. https://doi.org/10.3382/ps.0670794.

Ruiz, N. and Harms, R.H. (1988b) Niacin requirement of turkey poults fed a corn-soybean meal diet from 1 to 21 days of age. Poult. Sci. 67(5):760–765. https://doi.org/10.3382/ps.0670760.

Ruiz, N. and Harms, R.H. (1988c) Comparison of the biopotencies of nicotinic acid and nicotinamide for broiler chicks. Br. Poult. Sci. 29(3):491–498. https://doi.org/10.1080/00071668808417075.

Ruiz, N. and Harms, R.H. (1989a) Riboflavin requirement of turkey poults fed a corn-soybean meal diet from 1 to 21 days of age. Poult. Sci. 68(5):715–718. https://doi.org/10.3382/ps.0680715.

Ruiz, N. and Harms, R.H. (1989b) Pantothenic studies with turkey poults. Nutr. rept int. 40:639–642.

Ruiz, N., Harms, R.H. and Linda, S.B. (1990a) Niacin requirement of broiler chickens fed a corn-soybean meal diet from 1 to 21 days of age. Poult. Sci. 69(3):433–439. https://doi.org/10.3382/ps.0690433.

Ruiz, N. and Harms, R.H. (1990b) The lack of response of broiler chickens to supplemental niacin when fed a corn-soybean meal diet from 3 to 7 weeks of age. Poult. Sci. 69(12):2231–2234. https://doi.org/10.3382/ps.0692231.

Ruiz, N., Miles, R.D. and Harms, R.H. (1983) Choline, methionine and sulphate interrelationships in poultry nutrition a review. World's. Poult. Sci. 39(3):185–198. https://doi.org/10.1079/WPS19830017.

Ruksomboonde, A. and Sullivan, T.W. (1985) Vitamins A, D_3, and K interactions in broiler chicks and turkey poults. Poult. Sci. 64(suppl. 1):175.

Rush, J.K., Angel, C.R., Banks, K.M., Thompson, K.L. and Applegate, T.J. (2005) Effect of dietary calcium and vitamin D_3 on calcium and phosphorus retention in white Pekin ducklings. Poult. Sci. 84(4):561–570. https://doi.org/10.1093/ps/84.4.561.

Rutz, F., Cantor, A.H., Pescatore, A.J., Johnsson, T.H. and Pfaff, W.K. (1989) Effect of dietary riboflavin and selenium on metabolism and performance of young broiler chicks. Poult. Sci. 68(suppl. 1):202.

Ryu, K.S. and Pesti, G.M. (1993) Effects of supplemental folic acid on the performance of starting broiler chicks. Poult. Sci. 72(suppl. 1):118.

Ryu, K.S., Pesti, G.M. and Edwards, H.M. (1994) Folic acid and methionine requirements of broiler chicks. Poult. Sci. 73(suppl. 1):73.

Ryu, K.S., Roberson, K.D., Pesti, G.M. and Eitenmiller, R.R. (1995) The folic acid requirements of starting broiler chicks fed diets based on practical ingredients: 1. Interrelationships with dietary choline. Poult. Sci. 74(9):1447–1455. https://doi.org/10.3382/ps.0741447.

Ryu, Y.C., Rhee, M.S., Lee, K.M. and Kim, B.C. (2005) Effects of different levels of dietary supplemental selenium on performance, lipid oxidation, and color stability of broiler chicks. Poult. Sci. 84(5):809–815. https://doi.org/10.1093/ps/84.5.809.

Safari Asl, R., Shariatmadari, F., Sharafi, M., Karimi Torshizi, M.A. and Shahverdi, A. (2018) Improvements in semen quality, sperm fatty acids, and reproductive performance in aged Ross breeder roosters fed a diet supplemented with a moderate ratio of n-3: n-6 fatty acids. Poult. Sci. 97(11):4113–4121. https://doi.org/10.3382/ps/pey278.

Safonova, I., Darimont, C., Amri, E.Z., Grimaldi, P., Ailhaud, G., Reichert, U. and Shroot, B. (1994) Retinoids are positive effectors of adipose cell differentiation. Mol. Cell. Endocrinol. 104(2):201–211. https://doi.org/10.1016/0303-7207(94)90123-6.

Sahin, K. and Sahin, N. (2002) Effects of chromium picolinate and ascorbic acid dietary supplementation on nitrogen and mineral excretion of laying hens reared in a low ambient temperature (7 degrees C). Acta vet. Brno 71(2):183–189. https://doi.org/10.2754/avb200271020183.

Sahin, K. and Önderci, M (2002) Optimal dietary concentrations of vitamin C and chromium for alleviating the effect of low ambient temperature on serum insulin, corticosterone, and some blood metabolites in laying hens J. Trace elements Exp. Med. 15:153-161. https://doi.org/10.1002/jtra.10014.

Sahin, K., Sahin, N., Onderci, M., Yaralioglu, S. and Kucuk, O. (2001) Protective role of supplemental vitamin E on lipid peroxidation, vitamins E, A and some mineral concentrations of broilers reared under heat stress. Veterinarni. Medicina. 46(5):140–144. https://doi.org/10.17221/7870-VETMED.

Sahin, K., Sahin, N., Sarı, M. and Gursu, M.F. (2002a) Effects of vitamins E and A supplementation on lipid peroxidation and concentration of some mineral in broilers reared under heat stress (32°C). Nutr. Res. 22(6):723–731. https://doi.org/10.1016/S0271-5317(02)00376-7.

Sahin, K., Kucuk, O., Sahin, N. and Gurso, M.F. (2002b) Optimal dietary concentration of vitamin E for alleviating the effect of heat stress on performance, thyroid status, ACTH and some serum metabolite and mineral concentrations in broilers. Vet. Med. 47:110–116. https://doi.org/10.17221/5813-VETMED.

Sahin, K., Sahin, N. and Kucuk, O. (2003) Effects of chromium, and ascorbic acid supplementation on growth, carcass traits, serum metabolites, and antioxidant status of broiler chickens reared at a high ambient temperature (32°C). Nutr. Res. 23(2):225–238. https://doi.org/10.1016/S0271-5317(02)00513-4.

Sahin, N., Sahin, K. and Küçük, O. (2001) Effects of vitamin E and vitamin A supplementation on performance, thyroid status and serum concentrations of some metabolites and minerals in broilers reared under heat stress (32°C). Veterinarni. Medicina. 46(11–12):286–292. https://doi.org/10.17221/7894-VETMED.

Sahota, A.W. and Gillani, A.H. (1995) Effect of ascorbic acid supplementation on performance and cost of production in layers maintained under high ambient temperatures. Pak. Vet. J. 15(4):155–158.

Said, H.M. (2011) Intestinal absorption of water-soluble vitamins in health and disease. Biochem. J. 437(3):357–372. https://doi.org/10.1042/BJ20110326.

Said, H.M. and Derweesh, I. (1991) Carrier-mediated mechanism for biotin transport in rabbit intestine: studies with brush-border membrane vesicles. Am. J. Physiol. 261(1 Pt 2):R94-R97. https://doi.org/10.1152/ajpregu.1991.261.1.R94.

Said, H.M., Hoefs, J., Mohammadkhani, R. and Horne, D.W. (1992) Biotin transport in human liver basolateral membrane vesicles: a carrier-mediated, Na+ gradient-dependent process. Gastroenterology 102(6):2120–2125. https://doi.org/10.1016/0016-5085(92)90341-u.

Said, H.M., Redha, R. and Nylander, W. (1988) Biotin transport in the human intestine: site of maximum transport and effect of pH. Gastroenterology 95(5):1312–1317. https://doi.org/10.1016/0016-5085(88)90366-6.

Sakkas, P., Smith, S., Hill, T.R. and Kyriazakis, I. (2019) A reassessment of the vitamin D requirements of modern broiler genotypes. Poult. Sci. 98(1):330–340. https://doi.org/10.3382/ps/pey350.

Sakurai, T., Asakura, T., Mizuno, A. and Matsuda, M. (1992) Absorption and metabolism of pyridoxamine in mice. II. Transformation of pyridoxamine to pyridoxal in intestinal tissues. J. Nutr. Sci. Vitaminol. (Tokyo) 38(3):227–233. https://doi.org/10.3177/jnsv.38.227.

Salami, S.A., Oluwatosin, O.O., Oso, A.O., Fafiolu, A.O., Sogunle, O.M., Jegede, A.V., Bello, F.A. and Pirgozliev, V. (2016) Bioavailability of Cu, Zn and Mn from mineral chelates or blends of inorganic salts in growing turkeys fed with supplemental riboflavin and/or pyridoxine. Biol. Trace Elem. Res. 173(1):168–176. https://doi.org/10.1007/s12011-016-0618-2.

Salary, J., Sahebi-Ala, F., Kalantar, M. and Matin, H.R.H. (2014) *In ovo* injection of vitamin E on post-hatch immunological parameters and broiler chicken performance. Asian Pac. J. Trop. Biomed. 4(suppl. 2):S616-S619. https://doi.org/10.12980/APJTB.4.2014APJTB-2014-0088.

Sallmann, H.-P., Fuhrmann, H. and Götzke, S. (1998) The effect of the vitamins A and E and dietary fat on the oxidative stability of turkey muscle in vivo. J. Anim. Physiol. Anim. Nutr. 80(1–5):226–231. https://doi.org/10.1111/j.1439-0396.1998.tb00532.x.

Sanders, A.M. and Edwards Jr, H.M. (1991) The effects of 1,25-dihydroxycholecalciferol on performance and bone development in the turkey poult. Poult. Sci. 70(4):853–866. https://doi.org/10.3382/ps.0700853.

San Martin Diaz, V.E. (2018) "Effects of 1-alpha-hydroxycholecaciferol and other vitamin D analogs on live performance, bone development, meat yield and quality, and mineral digestibility on broilers". MS thesis. North Carolina State University.

Santé, V., Renerre, M. and Lacourt, A. (1992) Effect of dietary vitamin E supplementation on color stability and lipid oxidation in turkey meat. Proc. 38th Int. Conf. Meat Sci. Tech. Clermont-Ferrand, France. (pp. 591–594).

Santé, V.S. and Lacourt, A. (1994) The effect of dietary α-tocopherol supplementation and antioxidant spraying on colour stability and lipid oxidation of turkey meat. J. Sci. Food Agric. 65(4):503–507. https://doi.org/10.1002/jsfa.2740650419.

Santos, Y. and Soto-Salanova, M.F. (2005) Effect of HyD® addition on performance and slaughter results of broilers. Proc. 15th Eur. Symp. Poult. Nutr. Balatonfured, Hungary. (pp. 219–221).

Sárraga, C. and García-Regueiro, J.A. (1999) Membrane lipid oxidation and proteolytic activity in thigh muscles from broilers fed different diets. Meat Sci. 52(2):213–219. https://doi.org/10.1016/s0309-1740(98)00170-3.

Sárraga, C., Carreras, I., García-Regueiro, J.A., Guàrdia, M.D. and Guerrero, L. (2006) Effects of α-tocopheryl acetate and β-carotene dietary supplementation on the antioxidant enzymes, TBARS and sensory attributes of turkey meat. Br. Poult. Sci. 47(6):700–707. https://doi.org/10.1080/00071660601038750.

Sárraga, C., Guàrdia, M.D., Díaz, I., Guerrero, L. and Arnau, J. (2008) Nutritional and sensory qualities of raw meat and cooked brine-injected turkey breast as affected by dietary enrichment with docosahexaenoic acid (DHA) and vitamin E. J. Sci. Food Agric. 88(8):1448–1454. https://doi.org/10.1002/jsfa.3238.

Sashidhar, R.B., Jaya-Rao, K.S. and Rao, N. (1988) Effect of dietary aflatoxins on tryptophan-niacin metabolism. Nutr. Rep. Int. 37(3):515–521.

Satterlee, D.G., Aguilera-Quintana, I. and Munn, B.J. (1989) Vitamin C reduces stress responses associated with preslaughter management practices in broiler chickens. In "The Role of Vitamin C in poultry stress management". Anim. Health Nutr. (pp. 16–36).

Satterlee, D.G., Ryder, F.H. and Godber, J.S. (1991) Effect of ascorbic acid on plasma aldosterone and electrolyte levels in broiler chickens being prepared for slaughter. Poult. Sci. 70(1):181.

Sauberlich, H.E. (1985) Bioavailability of vitamins. Prog. Food Nutr. Sci. 9(1–2):1–33. PMID:3911266.

Sauberlich, H.E. (1999). "Laboratory tests for the assessment of nutritional status" 2nd ed. Routledge. https://doi.org/10.1201/9780203749647.

Saunders-Blades, J.L. and Korver, D.R. (2006) HyD® and poultry: bones and beyond. Proc. DSM satellite meeting, 12th Eur. Poult. Nutrerence. (pp. 1–11).

Saunders-Blades, J.L. and Korver, D.R. (2008) Effect of maternal and dietary 25-OH on broiler production and immunity. Proc. 23rd World's Poult. Congress, Brisbane, Australia.

Saunders-Blades, J.L. and Korver, D.R. (2014) The effect of maternal vitamin D source on broiler hatching egg quality, hatchability, and progeny bone mineral density and performance. J. Appl. Poult. Res. 23(4):773–783. https://doi.org/10.3382/japr.2014-01006.

Saunders-Blades, J.L. and Korver, D.R. (2015) Effect of hen age and maternal vitamin D source on performance, hatchability, bone mineral density, and progeny in vitro early innate immune function. Poult. Sci. 94(6):1233–1246. https://doi.org/10.3382/ps/pev002.

Sauveur, B. (1984) Dietary factors as causes of leg abnormalities in poultry: a review. Worlds Poult. Sci. J. 40(3):195–206. https://doi.org/10.1079/WPS19840015.

Sauveur, B. (1988) Lésions osseuses et articulaires des pattes des volailles: roles de l'alimentation. INRA Prod. Anim. 1(1):35–45. Sauveur, B. prod Lésions osseuses et articulaires des pattes des volailles: rôles de l'alimentation. INRA Prod. Anim. 1(1):35–45. https://doi.org/10.20870/productions-animales.1988.1.1.4433.

Savage, D.G. and Lindenbaum, J. (1995) Folate-cobalamin interactions. In "Folate in health and disease" Bailey, L.B. (ed.). (p. 237).

Savaris, V.D.L., Souza, C., Wachholz, L., Broch, J., Polese, C., Carvalho, P.L.O. and Nunes, R.V. (2021) Interactions between lipid source and vitamin A on broiler performance, blood parameters, fat and protein deposition rate, and bone development. Poult. Sci. 100(1):17–185. https://doi.org/10.1016/j.psj.2020.09.001.

Saxena, H.C. (1996) Need for reappraisal: practical aspects of calcium, phosphorus and vitamin D_3 nutrition for broilers. World Poult. 12(10):52.

Saxena, S.P., Fan, T., Li, M., Israels, E.D. and Israels, L.G. (1997) A novel role for vitamin K_1 in a tyrosine phosphorylation cascade during chick embryogenesis. J. Clin. Invest. 99(4):602–607. https://doi.org/10.1172/JCI119202.

Schaffer, S., Müller, W.E. and Eckert, G.P. (2005) Tocotrienols: constitutional effects in aging and disease. J. Nutr. 135(2):151–154. https://doi.org/10.1093/jn/135.2.151.

Scheideler, S.E. (1998) Vitamin E and heat stress in layers. Proc. of the multi-state poultry Meeting. Purdue Univ. Press.

Scheideler, S.E. and Froning, G.W. (1996) The combined influence of dietary flaxseed variety, level, form, and storage conditions on egg production and composition among vitamin E-supplemented hens. Poult. Sci. 75(10):1221–1226. https://doi.org/10.3382/ps.0751221.

Scheideler, S.E., Weber, P. and Monsalve, D. (2010) Supplemental vitamin E and selenium effects on egg production, egg quality, and egg deposition of α-tocopherol and selenium. J. Appl. Poult. Res. 19(4):354–360. https://doi.org/10.3382/japr.2010-00198.

Schenker, S., Johnson, R.F., Mahuren, J.D., Henderson, G.I. and Coburn, S.P. (1992) Human placental vitamin B_6 (pyridoxali) transport: normal characteristics and effects of ethanol. Am. J. Physiol. 262(6 Pt 2):R966-R974. https://doi.org/10.1152/ajpregu.1992.262.6.R966.

Schexnailder, R. and Griffith, M. (1973) Liver fat and egg production of laying hens as influenced by choline and other nutrients. Poult. Sci. 52(3):1188–1194. https://doi.org/10.3382/ps.0521188.

Schiavone, A. and Barroeta, A.C. (2011) Egg enrichment in vitamins and minerals. In "Improving egg and egg product safety and quality" Nys, Y., Bain, M. and Van-Immerseel, F. (ed.). Woodhead Publishing Ltd.

Schneider, J. (1986) Vitamin stability and activity of fat-soluble vitamins as influenced by manufacturing processes. In Proc. "National feed Ingred. assoc. nutr." 1986. Inst. "Bioavailability of vitamins in feed ingredients,", Chicago, Illinois. National Feed Ingredients Association (NFIA), Des Moines, Iowa.

Schulde, M. (1986) Extrusion technology for the food industry. In "The stability of vitamin in extrusion cooking". Elsevier Appl. Sci. London, UK. (pp. 22–34).

Schurgers, L.J. and Vermeer, C. (2002) Differential lipoprotein transport pathways of K-vitamins in healthy subjects. Biochim. Biophys. Acta 1570(1):27–32. https://doi.org/10.1016/S0304-4165(02)00147-2.

Schwean, K. and Classen, H.L. (1995) The effects of high dietary pyridoxine on broiler productivity and tonic immobility. Poult. Sci. 74(1):94 (abstract).

Schweigert, B.S., German, H.L., Pearson, P.B. and Sherwood, R.M. (1948) Effect of the pteroylglutamic acid intake on the performance of turkeys and chickens. J. Nutr. 35(1):89–102. https://doi.org/10.1093/jn/35.1.89.

Scott, C.G., Cohen, N., Riggio, P.P. and Weber, G. (1982) Gas chromatographic assay of the diastereomeric composition of all-rac-α-tocopheryl acetate. Lipids 17(2):97–101. https://doi.org/10.1007/BF02535182.

Scott, H.M., Singsen, E.P. and Matterson, L.D. (1946) The influence of nicotinic acid on the response of chicks receiving a diet high in corn. Poult. Sci. 25(3):303–304. https://doi.org/10.3382/ps.0250303.

Scott, M.L., Holm, E.R. and Reynolds, R.E. (1964) Studies on the pantothenic acid and unidentified factor requirements of young ringnecked pheasants and bobwhite quail. Poult. Sci. 43(6):1534–1539. https://doi.org/10.3382/ps.0431534.

Scott, M.L. (1981) Importance of biotin for chickens and turkeys. Feedstuffs 53(8):59.

Scott, M. L., Nesheim, M. C., and Young, R. J. (1982). Nutrition of the Chicken, 3rd ed., pp. 490–493. M. L. Scott and Associates, Ithaca, New York.

Sebrell, W.H. and Harris, R.S. (ed.) "The vitamins". Academic Press, New York.

Seeman, V. and Hazijah, H. (1985) Effects of nutrition on the strength of acquired immunity against Newcastle disease. Veterinarski Arhiv 55(1):1.

Seemann, M. (1991) Is vitamin C essential in poultry nutrition? World Poult.7:(17–19).

Seemann, S. (1992) Effect on laying performance and eggshell quality of vitamin C and $1,25OH_2D_3$ in old layers. Ludwig Maximilians University, Munich, Germany.

Seerley, R.W., et al. (1976) Southern, L.L., and Baker, D.H. 1981. J. Anim. Sci. 53(42):599. https://doi.org/10.2527/jas1976.423599x.

Seetharam, B. and Alpers, D.H. (1982) Absorption and transport of cobalamin (vitamin B_{12}). Annu. Rev. Nutr. 2:343–369. https://doi.org/10.1146/annurev.nu.02.070182.002015.

Selim, S.A., Gaafar, K.M. and El-Ballal, S.S. (2012) Influence of *in-ovo* administration with vitamin E and ascorbic acid on the performance of Muscovy ducks. Emir. J. Food Agric. 24(3):264–271. https://doi.org/10.5285/ecb17680-da2e-49ae-b250-2d04a6a08d2a.

Sell, J.L. (1996) Physiological limitations and potential for improvement in gastrointestinal tract function of poultry. J. Appl. Poult. Res. 5(1):96–101. https://doi.org/10.1093/japr/5.1.96.

Sell, J.L., Soto-Salanova, M., Jeffrey, M., Ahn, D. and Palo, P.E. (1995) Further evaluation of the dietary vitamin E requirement of growing turkeys. Poult. Sci. 74(suppl. 1):149 (abstract).

Sell, J.L., Soto-Salanova, M., Palo, P.E. and Jeffrey, M., (1995) Influence of supplementing corn-soybean meal diets with vitamin E on performance and selected physiological traits of male turkeys Poult. Sci. 76(10):1405–1417. https://doi.org/10.1093/ps/76.10.1405.

Sell, J.L., Jin, S. and Jeffrey, M. (2001) Metabolizable energy value of conjugated linoleic acid for broiler chicks and laying hens. Poult. Sci. 80(2):209–214. https://doi.org/10.1093/ps/80.2.209.

Seo, E.G., Einhorn, T.A. and Norman, A.W. (1997) 24R,25-Dihydroxyvitamin D_3: an essential vitamin D_3 metabolite for both normal bone integrity and healing of tibial fracture in chicks. Endocrinology 138(9):3864–3872. https://doi.org/10.1210/endo.138.9.5398.

Seokand, B.S. and Singh, R.A. (1996) Effect of ascorbic acid supplementation during summer and winter months on performance of broilers. Proc. 20th World's Poult. Congress, Delhi, India. (p. 258).

Serman, V. and Mazija, V. (1985) Effects of nutrition on the strength of acquired immunity against Newcastle disease. IV. Role Vitam. Vet. Arch. 55(1):1.

Sergeev, I.N., Arkhapchev, Y.P. and Spirichev, V.B. (1990) The role of vitamin E in the metabolism and reception of vitamin E. Biokhimiya-Engl. TR 55(11):1483.

Seuss-Baum, I., Nau, F. and Guérin-Dubard C. (2011) The nutritional quality of eggs, in Nys Y., Bain M. and Van Immersel F. (ed.) "Improving the Safety and Quality of Eggs and Egg Products – vol Woodhead Publishing Series in Food Science, Technology and Nutrition II – Egg Safety and Nutritional Quality" (pp.201–236).

Seven, P.T. (2008) The effects of dietary Turkish propolis and vitamin C on performance, digestibility, egg production and egg quality in laying hens under different environmental temperatures. Asian-Australas. J. Anim. Sci. 21(8):1164–1170. https://doi.org/10.5713/ajas.2008.70605.

Shabani, S., Mehri, M., Shirmohammad, F. and Sharafi, M. (2022) Enhancement of sperm quality and fertility-related parameters in Hubbard grandparent rooster fed diets supplemented with soybean lecithin and vitamin E. Poult. Sci. 101(3):101635. https://doi.org/10.1016/j.psj.2021.101635.

Shafey, T.M., McDonald, M.W. and Pym, R.A.E. (1990) Effects of dietary calcium, available phosphorus and vitamin D on growth rate, food utilisation, plasma and bone constituents and calcium and phosphorus retention of commercial broiler strains. Br. Poult. Sci. 31(3):587–602. https://doi.org/10.1080/00071669008417290.

Shakeri, M., Oskoueian, E., Le, H.H. and Shakeri, M. (2020) Strategies to combat heat stress in broiler chickens: unveiling the roles of selenium, vitamin E and vitamin C. Vet. Sci. 7(2):71. https://doi.org/10.3390/vetsci7020071.

Shanker, A. (2006) Nutritional modulation of immune function and infectious disease. In "Present knowledge in nutrition" 9th ed Bowman, B.A. and Russell, R.M. (ed.). International Life Sciences Institute. (pp. 604–624).

Shanmugasundaram, R. and Selvaraj, R.K. (2012) Vitamin D-1α-hydroxylase and vitamin D-24-hydroxylase mRNA studies in chickens. Poult. Sci. 91(8):1819–1824. https://doi.org/10.3382/ps.2011-02129.

Shanmugasundaram, R., Morris, A. and Selvaraj, R.K. (2019) Effect of 25-hydroxycholecalciferol supplementation on turkey performance and immune cell parameters in a coccidial infection model. Poult. Sci. 98(3):1127–1133. https://doi.org/10.3382/ps/pey480.

She, R.P., Xia, Z.F., Zhang, J.L., Meng, Y., Ma, X. and Liu, F. (1997) Toxic effects of excessive vitamin A and K on the immune system of chickens. Poult. Sci. 76(suppl. 1):78 (abstract).

Shearer, M.J., Barkhan, P. and Webster, G.R. (1970) Absorption and excretion of an oral dose of tritiated vitamin K_1 in man. Br. J. Haematol. 18(3):297–308. https://doi.org/10.1111/j.1365-2141.1970.tb01444.x.

Sheehy, P.J.A., Morrissey, P.A. and Flynn, A. (1991) Influence of dietary α-tocopherol on tocopherol concentrations in chick tissues. Br. Poult. Sci. 32(2):391–397. https://doi.org/10.1080/00071669108417364.

Sheehy, P.J.A., Morrissey, P.A. and Flynn, A. (1993) Influence of heated vegetable oils and α-tocopheryl acetate supplementation on α-tocopherol, fatty acids and lipid peroxidation in chicken muscle. Br. Poult. Sci. 34(2):367–381. https://doi.org/10.1080/00071669308417592.

Sheehy, P.J.A., Morrissey, P.A. and Buckley, D.J. (1995) Advances in research and application of vitamin E as an antioxidant for poultry meat. Proc. 12th Eur. Symp. on the Quality of Poultry Meat, Zaragoza, Spain. (pp. 425–436).

Sheehy, P.J.A., Morrissey, P.A. and Buckley, D.J. (1997) Influence of vegetable oils and alpha-tocopheryl acetate supplementation in lipid peroxidation in chick muscle. Proc. 47th Int. Cong. Meat Sci. Tech. (pp. 1285–1289).

Sheffy, B.E. and Schultz, R.D. (1979) Influence of vitamin E and selenium on immune response mechanisms. Fed. Proc. 38(7):2139–2143.

Shekhu, N.A., M'Sadeq, S.A., Beski, S.S.M. and Sulaiman, K. (2019) Effects of different levels of dietary biotin on the performance, apparent digestibility and carcass characteristics of broilers. J. Univ. Duhok 22(2):124–130. https://doi.org/10.26682/cajuod.2020.22.2.14.

Sheldon, B.W. (1984) Effect of dietary tocopherol on the oxidative stability of turkey meat. Poult. Sci. 63(4):673–681. https://doi.org/10.3382/ps.0630673.

Sheldon, B.W., Curtis, P.A., Dawson, P.L. and Ferket, P.R. (1997) Effect of dietary vitamin E on the oxidative stability, flavor, color, and volatile profiles of refrigerated and frozen turkey breast meat. Poult. Sci. 76(4):634–641. https://doi.org/10.1093/ps/76.4.634.

Shen, H., Summers, J.D. and Leeson, S. (1981) Egg production and shell quality of layers fed various levels of vitamin D_3. Poult. Sci. 60(7):1485–1490. https://doi.org/10.3382/ps.0601485.

Sherwood, T.A., Alphin, R.L., Saylor, W.W. and White, H.B. (1993) Folate metabolism and deposition in eggs by laying hens. Arch. Biochem. Biophys. 307(1):66–72. https://doi.org/10.1006/abbi.1993.1561.

Shideler, C.E. (1983) Vitamin B_6: an overview. Am. J. Med. Technol. 49(1):17–22. https://doi.org/10.1017/S0021875800017783.

Shields, R.G., Campbell, D.R., Huges, D.M. and Dillingham, D.A. (1982) Researchers study vitamin A stability in feeds. Feedstuffs 54(47):22.

Shim, M.Y., Pesti, G.M., Bakalli, R.I. and Edwards, H.M. (2008) The effect of breeder age and egg storage time on phosphorus utilization by broiler progeny fed a phosphorus deficiency diet with 1α- OH vitamin D_3. Poult. Sci. 87(6):1138–1145. https://doi.org/10.3382/ps.2007-00378.

Shin, D.J. and McGrane, M.M. (1997) Vitamin A regulates genes involved in hepatic gluconeogenesis in mice: phosphoenolpyruvate carboxykinase, fructose-1,6-bisphosphatase and 6-phosphofructo-2-kinase/fructose-2,6-bisphosphatase. J. Nutr. 127(7):1274–1278. https://doi.org/10.1093/jn/127.7.1274.

Shirley, R.B., Davis, A.J., Compton, M.M. and Berry, W.D. (2003) The expression of calbindin in chicks that are divergently selected for low or high incidence of tibial dyschondroplasia. Poult. Sci. 82(12):1965–1973. https://doi.org/10.1093/ps/82.12.1965.

Shojadoost, B., Yitbarek, A., Alizadeh, M., Kulkarni, R.R., Astill, J., Boodhoo, N. and Sharif, S. (2021) Centennial review: effects of vitamins A, D, E, and C on the chicken immune system. Poult. Sci. 100(4):100930. https://doi.org/10.1016/j.psj.2020.12.027.

Siddons, R.C. (1978) Nutrient deficiencies in animals – folic acid. In "Nutritional Disorders", Rechcigl, M. (ed.). CRC Press, Baton Rouge, FL.

Siegel, P.B., Larsen, C.T., Emmerson, D.A., Gereart, P.A. and Picard, M. (2000) Feeding regimen, dietary vitamin E, and genotype influences on immunological and production traits of broilers. J. Appl. Poult. Res. 9(2):269–278. https://doi.org/10.1093/japr/9.2.269.

Siegel, P.B., Price, S.E., Meldrum, B., Picard, M. and Geraert, P.A. (2001) Performance of pureline broiler breeders fed two levels of vitamin E. Poult. Sci. 80(9):1258–1262. https://doi.org/10.1093/ps/80.9.1258.

Siegel, P.B., Blair, M., Gross, W.B., Meldrum, B., Larsen, C., Boa-Amponsem, K. and Emmerson, D.A. (2006) Poult performance as influenced by age of dam, genetic line, and dietary vitamin E. Poult. Sci. 85(5):939–942. https://doi.org/10.1093/ps/85.5.939.

Siegert, W., Ahmadi, H., Helmbrecht, A. and Rodehutscord, M. (2015) A quantitative study of the interactive effects of glycine and serine with threonine and choline on growth performance in broilers. Poult. Sci. 94(7):1557–1568. https://doi.org/10.3382/ps/pev109.

Sijtsma, S.R., West, C.E., Rombout, J.H. and Van Der Zijpp, A.J. (1989) The interaction between vitamin A status and Newcastle disease virus infection in chickens. J. Nutr. 119(6):932–939. https://doi.org/10.1093/jn/119.6.932.

Sijtsma, S.R., Rombout, J.H.W.M., West, C.E. and Van Der Zijpp, A.J. (1990) Vitamin A deficiency impairs cytotoxic T lymphocyte activity in Newcastle disease virus-infected chickens. Vet. Immunol. Immunopathol. 26(2):191–201. https://doi.org/10.1016/0165-2427(90)90067-3.

Sijtsma, S.R., Rombout, J.H.W.M., Dohmen, M.J.W., West, C.E. and Van Der Zijpp, A.J. (1991) Effect of vitamin A deficiency on the activity of macrophages in Newcastle disease virus-infected chickens. Vet. Immunol. Immunopathol. 28(1):17–27. https://doi.org/10.1016/0165-2427(91)90039-F.

Silva, Id, Ribeiro, A.M.L., Canal, C.W., Vieira, M.M., Pinheiro, C.C., Gonçalves, T., de Moraes, M.L. and Ledur, V.S. (2011) Effect of vitamin E levels on the cell-mediated immunity of broilers vaccinated against coccidiosis. Rev. Bras. cienc. avic. 13(1):53–56. https://doi.org/10.1590/S1516-635X2011000100008.

Simon, J. (1999) Choline, betaine and methionine interactions in chickens, pigs and fish (including crustaceans). Worlds Poult. Sci. J. 55(4):353–374. https://doi.org/10.1079/WPS19990025.

Singh, H., Sodhi, S. and Kaur, R. (2006) Effects of dietary supplements of selenium, vitamin E or combinations of the two on antibody responses of broilers. Br. Poult. Sci. 47(6):714–719. https://doi.org/10.1080/00071660601040079.

Sirri, F. and Barroeta, A.C. (2007) Enrichment in vitamin. In "Bioactive egg compounds" Huopalahti, R., López-Fandiño, R., Anton, M. and Schade, R. (ed.). Springer-Verlag, Berlin, Heidelberg. (pp. 171–182). https://doi.org/10.1007/978-3-540-37885-3_21.

Sitara, D., Razzaque, M.S., St-Arnaud, R., Huang, W., Taguchi, T., Erben, R.G. and Lanske, B. (2006) Genetic ablation of vitamin D activation pathway reverses biochemical and skeletal anomalies in Fgf-23-null animals. Am. J. Pathol. 169(6):2161–2170. https://doi.org/10.2353/ajpath.2006.060329.

Sitrin, M.D., Lieberman, F., Jensen, W.E., Noronha, A., Milburn, C. and Addington, W. (1987) Vitamin E deficiency and neurologic disease in adults with cystic fibrosis. Ann. Intern. Med. 107(1):51–54. Sitrin, M.D., Lieberman, F., Jensen, W.E., Noronha, A., Milburn, C. and Addington, W. Short Papers (1987) Vitamin E deficiency and neurologic disease in adults with cystic fibrosis. Ann. Intern. Med. 107(1):51–54. https://doi.org/10.7326/0003-4819-107-1-51.

Skinner, J.L., Quisenberry, J. and Couch, J. (1951) High efficiency and APF concentrates in the ration of the laying fowl. Poult. Sci. 30(3):319–324. https://doi.org/10.3382/ps.0300319.

Skinner, J.T., Waldroup, A.L. and Waldroup, P.W. (1992) Effects of removal of vitamin and trace mineral supplements from grower and finisher diets on live performance and carcass composition of broilers. J. Appl. Poult. Res. 1(3):280–286. https://doi.org/10.1093/japr/1.3.280.

Sklan, D., Bartov, I. and Hurwitz, S. (1982) Tocopherol absorption and metabolism in the chick and turkey. J. Nutr. 112(7):1394–1400. https://doi.org/10.1093/jn/112.7.1394.

Sklan, D., Melamed, D. and Friedman, A. (1994) The effect of varying levels of dietary vitamin A on immune response in the chick. Poult. Sci. 73(6):843–843. https://doi.org/10.3382/ps.0730843.

Sklan, D., Melamed, D. and Friedman, A. (1995) The effect of varying dietary concentrations of vitamin A on immune response in the turkey. Br. Poult. Sci. 36(3):385–385. https://doi.org/10.1080/00071669508417785.

Skřivan, M., Marounek, M., Dlohuá, G. and Sevcíkova, S. (2008) Dietary selenium increases vitamin E contents of egg yolk and chicken meat. Br. Poult. Sci. 49(4):482–486. https://doi.org/10.1080/00071660802236021.

Skřivan, M., Bubancová, I., Marounek, G. and Dlouhá, G. (2010) Selenium and α-tocopherol content in eggs produced by hens that were fed diets supplemented with selenomethionine, sodium selenite and vitamin E. Czech J. Anim. Sci. 55(9):388–397. https://doi.org/10.17221/92/2010-CJAS.

Skřivan, M., Marounek, M., Englmaierová, M. and Skřivanová, E. (2012) Influence of dietary vitamin C and selenium, alone and in combination, on the composition and oxidative stability of meat of broilers. Food Chem. 130(3):660–664. https://doi.org/10.1016/j.foodchem.2011.07.103.

Skřivan, M., Marounek, M., Englmaierová, M. and Skrivanova, V. (2013) Influence of dietary vitamin C and selenium, alone and in combination, on the performance of laying hens and quality of eggs. Czech J. Anim. Sci. 58(2):91–97. https://doi.org/10.17221/6619-CJAS.

Sljivovacki, K., Jokic, Z. and Popov, D. (1988) Effect of the concentration of methionine and choline in the diet on productive performance of laying hens. Vet. Glas. 42:315–321.

Smet, K., Raes, K., Huyghebaert, G. and Haak, L. (2005) Influence of feed enriched with natural antioxidants and the oxidative stability of broiler meat. Proc. 17th Eur. Symp. Quality Poult. Meat. Doorwerth, The Netherlands. (pp. 99–106).

Smith, P.J., Tappel, A.L. and Chow, C.K. (1974) Glutathione peroxidase activity as a function of dietary selenomethionine. Nature 247(5440):392. https://doi.org/10.1038/247392a0.

Snow, J.L., Baker, D.H. and Parsons, C.M. (2004) Phytase, citric acid, and 1-α-hydroxycholecalciferol improve phytate phosphorus utilization in chicks fed a corn-soybean meal diet. Poult. Sci. 83(7):1187–1192. https://doi.org/10.1093/ps/83.7.1187.

Snow, J.L., Baker, D.H., Parsons, J.H. and Lofton, J.T. (1986) Recent studies on vitamin D and skeletal problems in broilers. Proc. Maryland Nutr. Conference. (pp. 1–6).

Soares, J.H. and Lofton, J.T. (1986) Recent studies on vitamin D and skeletal problems in broilers. Proc. Maryland Nutr. Conf. (pp. 1–6).

Soares, J.H., Kerr, J.M. and Gray, R.W. (1995) 25-Hydroxycholecalciferol in poultry nutrition. Poult. Sci. 74(12):1919–1919. https://doi.org/10.3382/ps.0741919.

Solomons, N.W. (2006) Vitamin A. In "Present knowledge in nutrition" 9th ed Bowman, B. and Russell, R. (ed.). International Life Sciences Institute. (pp. 157–183). https://doi.org/10.1017/S0007114507708838.

Sossidou, E.N., Dal-Bosco, A., Elson, H.A. and Fontes, C.M.G.A. (2011) Pasture-based systems for poultry production: implications and perspectives. Poult. Sci. 67(1):47–58. https://doi.org/10.1017/S0043933911000043.

Soto-Salanova, M.F. and Sell, J.L. (1995) Influence of supplemental dietary fat on changes in vitamin E concentration in livers of poults. Poult. Sci. 74(1):201–201. https://doi.org/10.3382/ps.0740201.

Soto-Salanova, M.F. and Sell, J.L. (1996) Efficacy of dietary and injected vitamin E for poults. Poult. Sci. 75(11):1393–1393. https://doi.org/10.3382/ps.0751393.

Soto-Salanova, M.F., Sell, J.L., Mallarino, E.G., Piquer, J., Barker, D., Palo, P. and Ewan, R.C. (1991) Unalleviated depletion of vitamin E in poults. Poult. Sci. 70(suppl. 1):116 (abstract).

Soto-Salanova, M.F., Sell, J.L., Mallarino, E.G., Piquer, F.J., Barker, D.L., Palo, P.E. and Ewan, R.C. (1993) Research note: vitamin E status of turkey poults as influenced by different dietary vitamin E sources, a bile salt, and an antioxidant. Poult. Sci. 72(6):1184–1184. https://doi.org/10.3382/ps.0721184.

Souci, S.W., Fachman, W. and Kraut, H. (1989) "Food composition and nutrition tables" 4th ed. (pp. 1989–1990).

Southern, L.L. and Baker, D.H. (1981) Bioavailable pantothenic acid in cereal grains and soybean meal. J. Anim. Sci. 53(2):403–408. https://doi.org/10.2527/jas1981.532403x.

Souza, R.A., Souza, P.A., Souza, R.C. and Neves, A.C.R.S. (2008) Efeito da utilização de Carophyll Red nos índices reprodutivos de matrizes de frangos de Corte. Rev. Bras. Cienc. 10:32.

Souza, C., Santos, T.C., Murakami, A.E., Iwaki, L.C.V. and Mello, J.F. (2017) Influence of graded levels of calcium and vitamin K in the diets of laying hens during the growing phase and their effects on the laying phase. J. Anim. Physiol. Anim. Nutr. (Berl) 101(5):974–983. https://doi.org/10.1111/jpn.12533.

Sozen, E., Karademir, B. and Ozer, N.K. (2015) Basic mechanisms in endoplasmic reticulum stress and relation to cardiovascular diseases. Free Radic. Biol. Med. 78:30–30. https://doi.org/10.1016/j.freeradbiomed.2014.09.031.

Spasevski, N.J., Vukmirovic, D., Levic, J. and Kokic, B. (2015) Influence of pelleting process and material particle size on the stability of retinol acetate. Arch. Zootech. 18(2):67–72.

Speake, B.K., Surai, P.F., Gaal, T., Mezes, M. and Noble, R.C. (1996) Tissue-specific development of antioxidant systems during avian embryogenesis. Biochem. Soc. Trans. 24(2):182S. https://doi.org/10.1042/bst024182s.

Spencer, R., Purdy,P. S., Hoeldtke, R., Bow, T. M. and Markulis, M. A. (1963) Studies on intestinal absorption of L-ascorbic acid-1-C14. Gastroenterology 44:768 PMID: 13990035.

Spires, H.R., Botts, R.L. and King, B.D. (1982) Methionine and choline supplementation of broiler diets for maximum profitability. Syntax. Res [report]. Series. (A.1).

Squires, M.W. and Naber, E.C. (1992) Vitamin profiles of eggs as indicators of nutritional status in the laying hen: vitamin B_{12} study. Poult. Sci. 71(12):2075–2075. https://doi.org/10.3382/ps.0712075.

Squires, M.W. and Naber, E.C. (1993a) Vitamin profiles of eggs as indicators of nutritional status in the laying hen: vitamin A study. Poult. Sci. 72(1):154–164. https://doi.org/10.3382/ps.0720154.

Squires, M.W. and Naber, E.C. (1993b) Vitamin profiles of eggs as indicators of nutritional status in the laying hen: riboflavin study. Poult. Sci. 72(3):483–494. https://doi.org/10.3382/ps.0720483.

Stabler, S.P. (2006) Vitamin B_{12}. In "Present knowledge in nutrition" 9th ed, Bowman, B.A. and Russell, R.M. (ed.). International Life Sciences Institute. (pp. 302–313).

Stahl, W., Schwarz, W., Von Laar, J. and Sies, H. (1995) All-trans beta-carotene preferentially accumulates in human chylomicrons and very low density lipoproteins compared with the 9-cis geometrical isomer. J. Nutr. 125(8):2128–2133. https://doi.org/10.1093/jn/125.8.2128.

Stanley, V.G., Chukwu, H., Thompson, D., Jones, G. and Gray, C. (1997) Singly and combined effects of organic selenium (Se- yeast) and vitamin E on ascites reduction in broilers. Poult. Sci. 76(1):28. https://doi.org/10.1093/ps/76.2.306.

Steenbock, H. (1924) The induction of growth promoting and calcifying properties in a ration by exposure to light. Science 60(1549):224–224. https://doi.org/10.1126/science.60.1549.224.

Stein, J., Daniel, H., Whang, E., Wenzel, U., Hahn, A. and Rehner, G. (1994) Rapid postabsorptive metabolism of nicotinic acid in rat small intestine may affect transport by metabolic trapping. J. Nutr. 124(1):61–61. https://doi.org/10.1093/jn/124.1.61.

Stephensen, C., Moldoveanu, Z. and Gangopadhyay, N.N. (1996) Vitamin A deficiency diminishes the salivary immunoglobulin A response and enhances the serum immunoglobulin G response to influenza A virus infection in BALB/c mice. J. Nutr. 126(1):94–94. https://doi.org/10.1093/jn/126.1.94.

Stilborn, H.L., Harris, G.C., Botje, W.G. and Waldroup, P.W. (1988) Ascorbic acid and acetylsalicylic acid (aspirin) in the diet of broilers maintained under heat stress conditions. Poult. Sci. 67(8):1183–1183. https://doi.org/10.3382/ps.0671183.

Stoianov, P. and Zhekov, R. (1982) Causes of disorders affecting the hatching and viability of broiler chicks. Vet. Med Nauki 19(1):47–47.

Sturkie, P.D., Singsen, E.P., Matterson, L.D., Kozeff, A. and Jungherr, E.L. (1954) The effects of dietary deficiencies of vitamin E and the B complex vitamins on the electrocardiogram of chickens. Am. J. Vet. Res. 15(56):457–462.

Suckeveris, D.I., Burin Jr, A.I., Oliveira, A.B.I., Nascimento, M.A.I., Pereira, R.I., Luvizotto Jr, J.M., Bittencourt, L.C., Hermes, R.G. and Menten, J.F. (2020) Supra-nutritional levels of selected B vitamins in animal or vegetable diets for broiler chicken. Braz. J. Poult. Sci. 22(3):001–010. https://doi.org/10.1590/1806-9061-2019-1024.

Summers, J.D., Shen, H., Leeson, S. and Julian, R.J. (1984) Influence of vitamin deficiency and level of dietary protein on the incidence of leg problems in broiler chickens. Poult. Sci. 63(6):1115–1121. https://doi.org/10.3382/ps.0631115.

Sun, D., Jin, Y., Zhao, Q., Tang, C., Li, Y., Wang, H., Qin, Y. and Zhang, J. (2021) Modified EMR-lipid method combined with HPLC-MS/MS to determine folates in egg yolks from laying hens supplemented with different amounts of folic acid. Food Chem. 337(1):127767. https://doi.org/10.1016/j.foodchem.2020.127767.

Sun, L., Huang, J.Q., Deng, J. and Lei, X.G. (2019) Avian selenogenome: response to dietary Se and vitamin E deficiency and supplementation. Poult. Sci. 98(10):4247–4247. https://doi.org/10.3382/ps/pey408.

Sun, M.K. and Alkon, D.L. (2008) Synergistic effects of chronic bryostatin-1 and α-tocopherol on spatial learning and memory in rats. Eur. J. Pharmacol. 584(2–3):328–337. https://doi.org/10.1016/j.ejphar.2008.02.014.

Sun, Z.W., Yan, L., G., Y.Y., Zhao, J.P., Lin, H. and Guo, Y.M. (2013) Increasing dietary vitamin D_3 improves the walking ability and welfare status of broiler chickens reared at high stocking densities. Poult. Sci. 92(12):3071–3071. https://doi.org/10.3382/ps.2013-03278.

Sun, Z.W., Fan, Q.H., Wang, X.X., Guo, Y.M., Wang, H.J. and Dong, X. (2017) High dietary biotin levels affect the footpad and hock health of broiler chickens reared at different stocking densities and litter conditions. J. Anim. Physiol. Anim. Nutr. (Berl) 101(3):521–521. https://doi.org/10.1111/jpn.12465.

Sunde, M.L., Turk, C.M. and DeLuca, H.F. (1978) The essentiality of vitamin D metabolites for embryonic chick development. Science 200(4345):1067–1067. https://doi.org/10.1126/science.206963.

Sunder, A. and Flachowsky, G. (2001) Influence of high vitamin E dosages on retinol and carotinoid concentration in body tissues and eggs of laying hens. Arch. Tierernahr. 55(1):43–52. https://doi.org/10.1080/17450390109386181.

Surai, P.F. (1992) Vitamin E feeding of poultry males. World Poult. Congress, Amsterdam. (pp. 575–577).

Surai, P.F. (1999a) Vitamin E in avian reproduction. Avian Poult. Biol. Rev. 10(1):1–60.

Surai, P.F. (1999b) Tissue-specific changes in the activities of antioxidant enzymes during the development of the chicken embryo. Br. Poult. Sci. 40(3):397–397. https://doi.org/10.1080/00071669987511.

Surai, P.F. (2000) Effect of selenium and vitamin E content of the maternal diet on the antioxidant system of the yolk and the developing chick. Br. Poult. Sci. 41(2):235–235. https://doi.org/10.1080/713654909.

Surai, P.F. (2003). "Natural antioxidants in avian nutrition and reproduction". Nottingham University Press.

Surai, P.F. (2015) Antioxidant systems in poultry biology: superoxide dismutase. J. Anim. Res. Nutr. 01(1):8. https://doi.org/10.21767/2572-5459.100008.

Surai, P.F. and Kuklenko, T.V. (2000) Effects of vitamin A on the antioxidant systems of the growing chicken. Asian. Australas. J. Anim. Sci. 13(9):1290–1295. https://doi.org/10.5713/ajas.2000.1290.

Surai, P.F. and Speake, B.K. (2000) Antioxidant systems and avian embryonic development. Proc. World Poult. 38(1):1–27. https://doi.org/10.2141/jpsa.38.1.

Surai, P.F. and Sparks, N.H.C. (2001a) Comparative evaluation of the effect of two maternal diets on fatty acids, vitamin E and carotenoids in the chick embryo. Br. Poult. Sci. 42(2):252–252. https://doi.org/10.1080/00071660120048519.

Surai, P.F. and Sparks, N.H.C. (2000) Tissue-specific fatty acid and α-tocopherol profiles in male chickens depending on dietary tuna oil and vitamin E provision. Poult. Sci. 79(8):1132–1142. https://doi.org/10.1093/ps/79.8.1132.

Surai, P.F., Ionov, I.A., Sakhatsy, N.I. and Kuklenko, T.V. (1993) Vitamins A and E content in poultry meat and its quality. Proc. 11th Eur. Symp. on the Quality of Poult. Meat, Tours, France. (pp. 455–460).

Surai, P.F., Ionov, I.A. and Buzhina, N. (1995) Vitamin E and egg quality: egg and egg products quality. Proc. 6th Eur. Symp. Quality of Eggs and Egg Products. (pp. 387–394).

Surai, P.F., Noble, R.C. and Speake, B.K. (1996) Tissue-specific differences in antioxidant distribution and susceptibility to lipid peroxidation during development of the chick embryo. Biochim. Biophys. Acta 1304(1):1–1. https://doi.org/10.1016/s0005-2760(96)00099-9.

Surai, P.F., Kutz, E., Wishart, G.J., Noble, R.C. and Speake, B.K. (1997a) The relationship between the dietary provision of α-tocopherol and the concentration of this vitamin in the semen of chicken: effects on lipid composition and susceptibility to peroxidation. J. Reprod. Fertil. 110(1):47–51. https://doi.org/10.1530/jrf.0.1100047.

Surai, P.F., Gaal, T., Noble, R.C. and Speake, B.K. (1997b) The relationship between the α-tocopherol content of the yolk and its accumulation in the tissues of the newly hatched chick. J. Sci. Food Agric. 75(2):212–216. https://doi.org/10.1002/(SICI)1097-0010(199710)75:2<212::AID-JSFA866>3.0.CO;2-W.

Surai, P.E., Ionov, I.A., Kuklenko, T.V., Kostjuk, I.A., Macpherson, A., Speake, B.K., Noble, R.C. and Sparks, N.H.C. (1998a) Effect of supplementing the hen's diet with vitamin A on the accumulation of vitamins A and E, ascorbic acid and carotenoids in the egg yolk and in the embryonic liver. Br. Poult. Sci. 39(2):257–263. https://doi.org/10.1080/00071669889222.

Surai, P., Kostjuk, I., Wishart, G., Macpherson, A., Speake, B., Noble, R., Ionov, I. and Kutz, E. (1998b) Effect of vitamin E and selenium supplementation of cockerel diets on glutathione peroxidase activity and lipid peroxidation susceptibility in sperm, testes, and liver. Biol. Trace Elem. Res. 64(1–3):119–119. https://doi.org/10.1007/BF02783329.

Surai, P.F., Ionov, I.A., Kuchmistova, E.F., Noble, R.C., Speake, B.K., Sakhatsy, N.I. and Kuklenko, T.V. (1998c) The relationship between the levels of α-tocopherol and carotenoids in the maternal feed, yolk and neonatal tissues: comparison between the chicken, turkey, duck, and goose. J. Sci. Food Agric. 76(4):593–598. https://doi.org/10.1002/(SICI)1097-0010(199804)76:4<593::AID-JSFA993>3.0.CO;2-R.

Surai, P.F., Blesbois, E., Grasseau, I., Chalah, T., Brillard, J.P., Wishart, G.J., Cerolini, S. and Sparks, N.H. (1998d) Fatty acid composition, glutathione peroxidase and superoxide dismutase activity and total antioxidant activity of avian semen. Comp. Biochem. Physiol. B Biochem. Mol. Biol. 120(3):527–527. https://doi.org/10.1016/s0305-0491(98)10039-1.

Surai, P.F., Speake, B.K., Noble, R.C. and Sparks, N.H.C. (1999a) Tissue-specific antioxidant profiles and susceptibility to lipid peroxidation of the newly hatched chick. Biol. Trace Elem. Res. 68(1):63–63. https://doi.org/10.1007/BF02784397.

Surai, P.F., Noble, R.C. and Speake, B.K. (1999b) Relationship between vitamin E content and susceptibility to lipid peroxidation in tissues of the newly hatched chick. Br. Poult. Sci. 40(3):406–406. https://doi.org/10.1080/00071669987520.

Surai, P.F., Noble, R.C., Sparks, N.H. and Speake, B.K. (2000) Effect of long-term supplementation with arachidonic or docosahexaenoic acids on sperm production in the broiler chicken. J. Reprod. Fertil. 120(2):257–257. https://doi.org/10.1530/reprod/120.2.257.

Surai, P.F., Speake, B.K. and Sparks, N.H.C. (2001) Carotenoids in avian nutrition and embryonic development. 1. Absorption, availability and levels in plasma and egg yolk. Jpn. Poult. Sci. 38(1):1–27. https://doi.org/10.2141/jpsa.38.1.

Surai, A.P., Surai, P.F., Steinberg, W., Wakeman, W.G., Speake, B.K. and Sparks, N.H.C. (2003) Effect of canthaxanthin content of the maternal diet on the antioxidant system of the developing chick. Br. Poult. Sci. 44(4):612–612. https://doi.org/10.1080/0007166031000161620 0.

Surai, P.F., Fisinin, V.I. and Karadas, F. (2016) Antioxidant systems in chick embryo development. Part 1. Vitamin E, carotenoids and selenium. Anim. Nutr. 2(1):1–11. https://doi.org/10.1016/j.aninu.2016.01.001.

Surai, P.F., Kochish, I.I., Romanov, M.N. and Griffin, D.K. (2019) Nutritional modulation of the antioxidant capacities in poultry: the case of vitamin E. Poult. Sci. 98(9):4030–4030. https://doi.org/10.3382/ps/pez072.

Suryawan, A. and Hu, C.Y. (1997) Effect of retinoic acid on differentiation of cultured pig preadipocytes. J. Anim. Sci. 75(1):112–112. https://doi.org/10.2527/1997.751112x.

Sushil, P., Aggarwal, C.K. and Chopra, S.K. (1998a) Effect of feeding antistress agents on the performance of egg type pullets housed in cages during summer. Indian J. Poult. Sci. 33(1):7.

Sushil, P., Aggarwal, C.K. and Chopra, S.K. (1998b) Effect of supplementation of antistress agents in the ration on egg quality of pullets during summer. Indian J. Anim. Sci. 68(7):667–668.

Suter, C. (1990) Vitamins at the molecular level. In Proc. "National feed Ingr. ass. nutr. inst.": "Developments in vitamin nutrition and health applications" Kansas City, Missouri. 1990. National Feed Ingredients Association (NFIA), Des Moines, Iowa, USA.

Suttie, J.W. (2013) Vitamin K. In "Handbook of vitamins" 5th ed. Zempleni, J., Suttie, J., Gregory, J. and Stover P. J. (ed.). CRC Press, Taylor & Francis Group, LLC. (pp. 89–124).

Suttie, J.W. and Jackson, C.M. (1977) Prothrombin structure, activation, and biosynthesis. Physiol. Rev. 57(1):1–1. https://doi.org/10.1152/physrev.1977.57.1.1.

Suttie, J.W. and Olson, R.E. (1990) Vitamin K. In "Nutrition reviews, present knowledge in nutrition" 6th ed. Olson, R.E. (ed.) Int. Life Science Institute Nutrition Foundation.

Sutton, R.A.L. and Dirks, J.H. (1978) Renal handling of calcium. Fed. Proc. 37(8):2112.

Suzuki, Y. and Okamoto, M. (1997) Production of hen's eggs rich in vitamin K. Nutr. Res. 17(10):1607–1615. https://doi.org/10.1016/S0271-5317(97)00155-3.

Svendsen, O.L. and Weber, G.M. (2001). "Optimum vitamin nutrition (OVN) for poultry". Hoffmann La Roche Ltd.

Svihus, B. and Zimonja, O. (2011) Chemical alterations with nutritional consequences due to pelleting animal feeds: a review. Anim. Prod. Sci. 51(7):590–596. https://doi.org/10.1071/AN11004.

Swank, R.L. (1940) Avian thiamin deficiency: a correlation of the pathology and clinical behavior. J. Exp. Med. 71(5):683–683. https://doi.org/10.1084/jem.71.5.683.

Sweeney, G., Morrissey, P.A. and Buckley, D.J. (1992) Effect of dietary α-tocopheryl acetate supplementation on α-tocopherol levels in broiler tissues and on lipid oxidation. 19th World´s Poultr. Congress, Amsterdam, The Netherlands. (pp. 582–585).

Świątkiewicz, S., Arczewska-Włosek, A., Bederska-Lojewska, D. and Józefiak, D. (2017) Efficacy of dietary vitamin D and its metabolites in poultry – review and implications of the recent studies. Worlds Poult. Sci. J. 73(1):57–68. https://doi.org/10.1017/S0043933916001057.

Swierczewska, E., Skomial, J., Smolinska, T. and Kopowski, J. (2005) The quality of meat of broiler chickens fed with doubled amount of vitamins B group and fat- mineral preparation. Proc. 17th Eur. Symp. Quality Poult. Meat, Doorwerth, The Netherlands. (pp. 185–118).

Tactacan, G.B., Jing, M., Thiessen, S., Rodriguez-Lecompte, J.C., O'Connor, D.L., Guenter, W. and House, J.D. (2010a) Characterization of folate-dependent enzymes and indices of folate status in laying hens supplemented with folic acid or 5-methyltetrahydrofolate. Poult. Sci. 89(4):688–696. https://doi.org/10.3382/ps.2009-00417.

Tactacan, G.B., Guenter, W. and House, J.D. (2010b) Functional characterization of folic acid transport in the intestine of the laying hen. Poult. Sci. 89(E-Suppl.1):561 (abstr.).

Tactacan, G.B., Rodriguez-Lecompte, J.C. and House, J.D. (2012) The adaptive transport of folic acid in the intestine of laying hens with increased supplementation of dietary folic acid. Poult. Sci. 91(1):121–128. https://doi.org/10.3382/ps.2011-01711.

Tagar, M.A. (2005). Effect of pyridoxine (vitamin B_6) as supplement on the growth and carcass yield of broiler. Thesis. Sindh Agriculture Univ.

Taheri, H.R. and Mirisakhani, L. (2020) Effect of citric acid, vitamin D_3 and high dose phytase on performance of broiler chicken fed diet severely limited in non-phytate phosphorus. Livest. Sci. 241:104223. https://doi.org/10.1016/j.livsci.2020.104223.

Takahashi, K., Akiba, Y. and Horiguchi, M. (1991) Effects of supplemental ascorbic acid on performance, organ weight and plasma cholesterol concentration in broilers treated with propylthiouracil. Br. Poult. Sci. 32(3):545–554. https://doi.org/10.1080/00071669108417379.

Tanaka, K., Hashimoto, T., Tokumaru, S., Iguchi, H. and Kojo, S. (1997) Interactions between vitamin C and vitamin E are observed in tissues of inherently scorbutic rats. J. Nutr. 127(10):2060–2064. https://doi.org/10.1093/jn/127.10.2060.

Tang, F.I. and Wei, I.L. (2004) Vitamin B_6 deficiency prolongs the time course of evoked dopamine release from rat striatum. J. Nutr. 134(12):3350–3354. https://doi.org/10.1093/jn/134.12.3350.

Tang, K.N., Rowland, G.N. and Veltmann, J.R. (1985) Vitamin A toxicity: comparative changes in bone of the broiler and Leghorn chicks. Avian Dis. 29(2):416–429. https://doi.org/10.2307/1590503.

Tang, S.Z., Kerry, J.P., Sheehan, D., Buckley, D.J. and Morrissey, P.A. (2001) Antioxidative effect of dietary tea catechins on lipid oxidation of long-term frozen stored chicken meat. Meat Sci. 57(3):331–336. https://doi.org/10.1016/s0309-1740(00)00112-1.

Tani, M. and Iwai, K. (1984) Some nutritional effects of folate-binding protein in bovine milk on the bioavailability of folate to rats. J. Nutr. 114(4):778–785. https://doi.org/10.1093/jn/114.4.778.

Taniguchi, A. and Watanabe, T. (2007) Roles of biotin in growing ovarian follicles and embryonic development in domestic fowl. J. Nutr. Sci. Vitaminol. (Tokyo) 53(6):457–463. https://doi.org/10.3177/jnsv.53.457.

Tanphaichair, V. (1976) Thiamine. In "Nutrition reviews present knowledge in nutrition" 4th ed Hegsted, D.M., Chichester, C.O., Darby, W.J., McNutt, K.W., Stalvey, R.M. and Stotz, E.H. (ed.). Nutrition Foundation Inc.

Tanumihardjo, S.A. (2011) Vitamin A: biomarkers of nutrition for development. Am. J. Clin. Nutr. 94(2):658S–665S. https://doi.org/10.3945/ajcn.110.005777.

Tanumihardjo, S.A. and Howe, J.A. (2005) Twice the amount of alpha-carotene isolated from carrots is as effective as beta-carotene in maintaining the vitamin A status of Mongolian gerbils. J. Nutr. 135(11):2622–2626. https://doi.org/10.1093/jn/135.11.2622.

Tanumihardjo, S.A., Russell, R.M., Stephensen, C.B., Gannon, B.M., Craft, N.E., Haskell, M.J., Lietz, G., Schulze, K. and Raiten, D.J. (2016) Biomarkers of nutrition for development (BOND)—vitamin A review. J. Nutr. 146(9):1816S–1848S. https://doi.org/10.3945/jn.115.229708.

Tapia Romero, E., Rojas, R.E., Arias, L.E. and Avila, G. (1985) In Resumenes ALPA 85 (Abstr.). Acapulco, Mexico.

Taranu, I. (1999) Optimizing vitamin supplementation in broilers. Poult. Int. 99:104–105.

Taranu, I., Criste, R.D., Burlacu, R., Olteanu, M. and Burlacu, G. (1995) Influence of vitamin and mineral nutrition and of low ambient temperature on broiler performance and quality of body composition. Proc. 12th Eur. Symp. Poult. Meat Quality, Zaragoza, Spain. (pp. 83–90).

Tavakoli, M., Bouyeh, M. and Seidavi, A. (2020) Effects of dietary vitamin C supplementation on fatty acid profile in breast meat of broiler chickens. MESO Prvi Hrvatski Cas. Mesu 22(4):268–273. https://doi.org/10.31727/m.22.4.4.

Tavakoli, M., Bouyeh, M. and Seidavi, A. (2021) Effects of dietary vitamin C supplementation on growth performance, carcass characteristics, gastrointestinal organs, liver enzymes, abdominal fats, immune response and cecum microflora of broiler chickens. Iran. J. Anim. Sci. 31(1):67–78. https://doi.org/10.22034/AS.2021.42573.1589.

Taylor, L.W. (1947) The effect of folic acid on egg production and hatchability. Poult. Sci. 26(4):372–376. https://doi.org/10.3382/ps.0260372.

Taylor, S.L., Lamden, M.P. and Tappel, A.L. (1976) Sensitive fluorometric method for tissue tocopherol analysis. Lipids 11(7):530–538. https://doi.org/10.1007/BF02532898.

Taylor, T., Hawkins, D.R., Hathway, D.E. and Partington, H. (1972) A new urinary metabolite of pantothenate in dogs. Br. Vet. J. 128(10):500–505. https://doi.org/10.1016/s0007-1935(17)36734-9.

Teeter, R.G. and Belay, T. (1996) Broiler management during acute heat stress. Anim. Feed Sci. Technol. 58(1–2):127–142. https://doi.org/10.1016/0377-8401(95)00879-9.

Teeter, R. and Deyhim, F. (1993). "Broiler vitamin nutrition". BASF Technical Seminary.

Tengerdy, R.P. (1980) Disease resistance: immune response. In "Vitamin E: a comprehensive treatise (Basic & Clinical Nutrition Series) Marcel" Machlin, L.J. (ed.). Dekker Inc.

Tengerdy, R.P. and Brown, J.C. (1977) Effect of vitamin E and A on humoral immunity and phagocytosis on *E. coli* infected chickens. Poult. Sci. 56(3):957–963. https://doi.org/10.3382/ps.0560957.

Tengerdy, R.P. and Nockels, C.F. (1973) Effect of vitamin E on egg production, hatchability and humoral immune response of chickens. Poult. Sci. 52(2):778–783. https://doi.org/10.3382/ps.0520778.

Tengerdy, R.P. and Nockels, C.F. (1975) Vitamin E or vitamin A protects chickens against *E. coli* infection. Poult. Sci. 54(4):1292–1296. https://doi.org/10.3382/ps.0541292.

Tengerdy, R.P., Lacetera, N.G. and Nockels, C.F. (1990) Effect of beta carotene on disease protection and humoral immunity in chickens. Avian Dis. 34(4):848–854. https://doi.org/10.2307/1591372.

Terry, M., Lanenga, M., McNaughton, J.L. and Stark, L.E. (1999) Safety of 25-hydroxyvitamin D_3 as a source of vitamin D_3 in layer poultry feed. Vet. Hum. Toxicol. 41(5):312–316.

Teymouri, B., Ghiasi Ghalehkandi, J.G., Hassanpour, S. and Aghdam-Shahryar, H. (2020) Effect of *in ovo* feeding of the vitamin B_{12} on hatchability, performance and blood constitutes in broiler chicken. Int. J. Pept. Res. Ther. 26(1):381–387. https://doi.org/10.1007/s10989-019-09844-0.

Thierry, M.J., Hermodson, M.A. and Suttie, J.W. (1970) Vitamin K and warfarin distribution and metabolism in the warfarin-resistant rat. Am. J. Physiol. 219(4):854–859. https://doi.org/10.1152/ajplegacy.1970.219.4.854.

Thomas, R.A., Izat, A.L. and Waldroup, P.W. (1988) Effects of high levels of vitamin E on finisher diets on quality of broiler meat. Poult. Sci. (Suppl. 1).

Thornton, P.A. and Shutze, J.V. (1960) The influence of dietary energy level, energy source and breed on the thiamine requirement of chicks. Poult. Sci. 39(1):192–199. https://doi.org/10.3382/ps.0390192.

Thorp, B.H. (1994) Skeletal disorders in the fowl: a review. Avian Pathol. 23(2):203–236. https://doi.org/10.1080/03079459408418991.

Thorp, B.H., Ducro, B., Whitehead, C.C., Farquharson, C. and Sorensen, P. (1993) Avian tibial dyschondroplasia: the interaction of genetic selection and dietary 1, 25-dihydroxycholecalciferol. Avian Pathol. 22(2):311–324. https://doi.org/10.1080/03079459308418923.

Tian, X.Q., Chen, T.C., Lu, Z., Shao, Q. and Holick, M.F. (1994) Characterization of the translocation process of vitamin D_3 from the skin into the circulation. Endocrinology 135(2):655–661. https://doi.org/10.1210/endo.135.2.8033813.

Tillman, B. and Pesti, G.M. (1985) Response from male broilers to L-methionine and choline supplementation in a corn- soybean meal diet. Poult. Sci. 64(suppl. 1):44.

Tobias, S., Rajíc, I. and Ványi, A. (1992) Effect of T-2 toxin on egg production and hatchability in laying hens. Acta Vet. Hung. 40(1–2):47–54.

Toghyani, M., Zia, M.A., Tabeidian, S.A., Ghalamkari, G. and Gheisari, A. (2015) Effect of vitamin C, shackling and crating stress on tonic immobility reactions of broiler chickens in preslaughter. Int. J. Poult. Sci. 14(2):72–75. https://doi.org/10.3923/ijps.2015.72.75.

Tollersrud, S. (1973) Changes in the enzymatic profile in blood and tissues in preclinical and clinical vitamin E deficiency in pigs. Acta Agric. Scand. suppl. 19:124.

Torki, M., Zangeneh, S. and Habibian, M. (2014) Performance, egg quality traits, and serum metabolite concentrations of laying hens affected by dietary supplemental chromium picolinate and vitamin C under a heat-stress condition. Biol. Trace Elem. Res. 157(2):120–129. https://doi.org/10.1007/s12011-013-9872-8.

Torres, C.A., Vieria, S.L., Reis, R.N., Ferreira, A.K., Da-Silva, F.A. and Furtado, F.V.F. (2009) Productive performance of broiler breeder hens fed 25-hydroxycholecalciferol. Braz. J. Anim. 38(7):1286–1290. https://doi.org/10.1590/S1516-35982009000700018.

Toussant, M.J. and Latshaw, J.D. (1994) Evidence of multiple metabolic routes in vanadium's effects on layers. Ascorbic acid differential effects on prepeak egg production parameters following prolonged vanadium feeding. Poult. Sci. 73(10):1572–1580. https://doi.org/10.3382/ps.0731572.

Traber, M.G., Rader, D., Acuff, R.V., Ramakrishnan, R., Brewer, H.B. and Kayden, H.J. (1998) Vitamin E dose–response studies in humans using deuterated RRR-a-tocopherol. Am. J. Clin. Nutr. 68(4):847–853. https://doi.org/10.1093/ajcn/68.4.847.

Traber, M.G. (2006) Vitamin E. In "Present knowledge in nutrition" 9th ed. Bowman, B.A. and Russell, R.M. Intl Life Science Inst. (pp. 211–219).

Traber, M.G. (2013) Vitamin E. In "Handbook of vitamins" 5th ed. Zempleni, J., Suttie, J., Gregory, J. and Stover P. J. (ed.). CRC Press, Taylor & Francis Group, LLC. (pp. 125–148).

Troescher, A.H.A. and Coelho, M.B. (1996) Vitamins levels in the US feeds and effect of graded vitamin levels on stress challenged broiler. 20th World´s Poult. Congr., New Delhi, India.

Trzeciak, K.B., Lis, M.W., Sechman, A., Płytycz, B., Rudolf, A., Wojnar, T. and Niedziolka, J.W. (2014) Course of hatch and developmental changes in thyroid hormone concentration in blood of chicken embryo following in ovo riboflavin supplementation. Turk. J. Vet. Anim. Sci. 38(3):230–237. https://doi.org/10.3906/vet-1307-43.

Tsang, C.P.W. (1992) Research Note: Calcitriol reduces egg breakage. Poult. Sci. 71(1):215–217. https://doi.org/10.3382/ps.0710215.

Tsang, C.P. and Daghir, N.J. (1990) The effect of 1-alpha, 25-dihydroxyvitamin D_3 added to a layer diet containing adequate amounts of vitamin D_3 on the performance of layers. Poult. Sci. 69(10):1822–1825. https://doi.org/10.3382/ps.0691822.

Tsang, C.P. and Grunder, A.A. (1993) Effect of dietary contents of cholecalciferol, 1α, 25-dihydroxycholecalciferol and 24,25-dihydroxycholecalciferol on blood concentrations of 25-dihydroxycholecalciferol, 1α, 25-dihydroxycholecalciferol, total calcium and eggshell quality. Br. Poult. Sci. 34(5):1021–1027. https://doi.org/10.1080/00071669308417661.

Tsang, C.P., Grunder, A.A. and Narbaitz, R. (1990a) Optimal dietary level of 1-alpha, 25-dihydroxycholecalciferol for eggshell quality in laying hens. Poult. Sci. 69(10):1702–1712. https://doi.org/10.3382/ps.0691702.

Tsang, C.P., Grunder, A.A., Soares, J.H. and Narbaitz, R. (1990b) Effect of 1-alpha, 25-dihydroxycholecalciferol on eggshell quality and egg production. Br. Poult. Sci. 31(2):241–247. https://doi.org/10.1080/00071669008417253.

Tsiagbe, V.K., Kang, C.W. and Sunde, M.L. (1982) The effect of choline supplementation in growing pullet and laying hen diets. Poult. Sci. 61(10):2060–2064. https://doi.org/10.3382/ps.0612060.

Tsiagbe, V.K., Straub, R.J., Cook, M.E., Harper, A.E. and Sunde, M.L. (1987) Critical vitamin supplementation of broiler diets high in alfalfa juice protein. Poult. Sci. 66(11):1771–1778. https://doi.org/10.3382/ps.0661771.

Tsiagbe, V.K., Cook, M.E., Harper, A.E. and Sunde, M.L. (1987) Enhanced immune responses in broiler chicks fed methionine- supplemented diets. Poult. Sci. 66(7):1147–1154. https://doi.org/10.3382/ps.0661147.

Tsiagbe, V.K., Cook, M.E., Harper, A.E. and Sunde, M.L. (1988) Alterations in phospholipid composition of egg yolks from laying hens fed choline and methionine-supplemented diets. Poult. Sci. 67(12):1717–1724. https://doi.org/10.3382/ps.0671717.

Tuan, R.S. and Suyama, E. (1996) Developmental expression and vitamin D regulation of calbindin-D-28K in chick embryonic yolk sac endoderm. J. Nutr. 126(4)(suppl.):1308S-1316S. https://doi.org/10.1093/jn/126.suppl_4.1308S.

Tudor, D. and Bunaciu, P. (2001) Can vitamin C help fight aflatoxicosis? Poult. Int.1:10–14.

Tufarelli, V. and Laudadio, V. (2016) Antioxidant activity of vitamin E and its role in avian reproduction. J. Exp. Biol. Agric. Sci. 4(3s):267–272. https://doi.org/10.18006/2016.4(3S).266.272.

Tufarelli, V., Ghane, F., Shahbazi, H.R., Slozhenkina, M., Gorlov, I., Viktoronova, F.M., Seidavi, A. and Laudadio, V. (2022) Effect of *in ovo* injection of some B-group vitamins on performance of broiler breeders and their progeny. Worlds Poult. Sci. J. 78(1):125–138. https://doi.org/10.1080/00439339.2022.2003169.

Tuite, P.J. and Austic, R.E. (1974) Studies on a possible interaction between riboflavin and vitamin B_{12} as it affects hatchability of the hen's egg. Poult. Sci. 53(6):2125–2136. https://doi.org/10.3382/ps.0532125.

Turley, C.P. and Brewster, M.A. (1993) α-tocopherol protects against a reduction in adenosylcobalamin in oxidatively stressed human cells. J. Nutr. 123(7):1305–1312. https://doi.org/10.1093/jn/123.7.1305.

Tyczkowski, J.K. and Hamilton, P.B. (1987) Altered metabolism of carotenoids during aflatoxicosis in young chickens. Poult. Sci. 66(7):1184–1188. https://doi.org/10.3382/ps.0661184.

Ullrey, D.E. (1981) Vitamin E for swine. J. Anim. Sci. 53(4):1039–1056. https://doi.org/10.2527/jas1981.5341039x.

Underwood, G., Andrews, D. and Phung, T. (2021) Advances in genetic selection and breeder practice improve commercial layer hen welfare. Anim. Prod. Sci. 61(10):856–866. https://doi.org/10.1071/AN20383.

Uni, Z., Zaiger, G. and Reifen, R. (1998) Vitamin A deficiency induces morphometric changes and decreased functionality in chicken small intestine. Br. J. Nutr. 80(4):401–407. https://doi.org/10.1017/S0007114500070008.

United States Pharmacopeia (1980) 20th edn. Mack Printing Comp., Easton, Pennsylvania.

Uribe-Diaz, S., Nazeer, N., Jaime, J., Vargas-Bermúdez, D.S., Yitbarek, A., Ahmed, M. and Rodríguez-Lecompte, J.C. (2022) Folic acid enhances proinflammatory and antiviral molecular pathways in chicken B-lymphocytes infected with a mild infectious bursal disease virus. Br. Poult. Sci. 63(1):1–13. https://doi.org/10.1080/00071668.2021.1958298.

Urso, U.R.A., Dahlke, F., Maiorka, A., Bueno, I.J.M., Schneider, A.F., Surek, D. and Rocha, C. (2015) Vitamin E and selenium in broiler breeder diets: effect on live performance, hatching process, and chick quality. Poult. Sci. 94(5):976–983. https://doi.org/10.3382/ps/pev042.

USDA (United States Department of Agriculture) (2009) National nutrient database for standard reference-release 22. Nutrient Data Laboratory.

Utno, L. and Klieste, E. (1971) The influence of D- and DL-pantothenate on the hen productivity chick hatching rate and viability. Latv. PSR Zinat/Nu Akademijas Vestis Izdevums 6:72–79.

Utomo, D.B., Mitchell, M.A. and Whitehead, C.C. (1994) Effects of alpha-tocopherol supplementation on plasma egg yolk precursor concentrations in laying hens exposed to heat stress. Br. Poult. Sci. 35(5):828–829.

Uzochukwu, I.E., Amaefule, B.C. and Ugwu, S.O.C. (2020) Effect of dietary supplementation of vitamins C and E on the semen quality of local turkeys. Agro-Science J. Trop. Agric. Food Environ. Ext 18(3):25–30. https://doi.org/10.4314/as.v19i1.4.

Vaccaro, L.A., Porter, T.E. and Ellestad, L.E. (2022) Effects of genetic selection on activity of corticotropic and thyrotropic axes in modern broiler chickens. Domest. Anim. Endocrinol. 78:106649. https://doi.org/10.1016/j.domaniend.2021.106649.

Vaiano, S.A., Azuolas, J.K., Parkinson, G.B. and Scott, P.C. (1994) Serum total calcium, phosphorus, 1,25-dihydroxycholecalciferol and endochondral ossification defects in commercial broiler chickens. Poult. Sci. 73(8):1296–1305. https://doi.org/10.3382/ps.0731296.

Valaja, J., Pertilla, S., Tupasela, T. and Helander, E. (2001) Effect of high-oil oats and vitamin E supplementation on broiler production. Proc. 13th Eur. Symp. Poult. Nutr., Paris, France. (pp. 33–34).

Van den Ouweland, J.M.W. (2016) Analysis of vitamin D metabolites by liquid chromatography-tandem mass spectrometry, TrAC Trends Anal. Chem. 84(part B):117-130. https://doi.org/10.1016/j.trac.2016.02.005.

Van Dyck, S.M.O. and Adams, C.A. (2003) Dietary antioxidants-antiradical active nutricines. Int. Poult. Prod. 11(6):15–19.

Van Emous, R.A., Mens, A.J.W. and Winkel, A. (2021) Effects of diet density and feeding frequency during the rearing period on broiler breeder performance. Br. Poult. Sci. 62(5):686–694. https://doi.org/10.1080/00071668.2021.1918634.

Van Niekerk, T., Garber, T.K., Dunnington, E.A., Gross, W.B. and Siegel, P.B. (1989) Response of White Leghorn chicks fed ascorbic acid and challenged with Escherichia coli or corticosterone. Poult. Sci. 68(12):1631–1636. https://doi.org/10.3382/ps.0681631.

Vanderschueren, D., Gevers, G., Raymaekers, G., Devos, P. and Dequeker, J. (1990) Sex- and age-related changes in bone and serum osteocalcin. Calcif. Tiss. Int. 46(3):179–182. https://doi.org/10.1007/BF02555041.

Vara-Ubol, S. and Bowers, J.A. (2001) Effect of α-tocopherol, β-carotene, and sodium tripolyphosphate on lipid oxidation of refrigerated cooked ground turkey and ground pork. J. Food Sci. 66(5):662–667. https://doi.org/10.1111/j.1365-2621.2001.tb04618.x.

Vazquez, J.R., Gómez, G.V., López, C.C., Cortés, A.C., Díaz, A.C., Fernández, S.R.T., Rosales, E.M. and Avila, A.G. (2018) Effects of 25-hydroxycholecalciferol with two D_3 vitamin levels on production and immunity parameters in broiler chickens. J. Anim. Physiol. Anim. Nutr. (Berl) 102(1):e493-e497. https://doi.org/10.1111/jpn.12715.

Veltmann Jr., J.R. and Jensen, L.S. (1986) Vitamin A toxicosis in the chick and turkey poults. Poult. Sci. 65(3):538–545. https://doi.org/10.3382/ps.0650538.

Veltmann Jr., J.R., Jensen, L.S. and Rowland, G.N. (1986) Excess dietary vitamin A in the growing chick: effect of fat source and vitamin D. Poult. Sci. 65(1):153–163. https://doi.org/10.3382/ps.0650153.

Verbeeck, J. (1975) Vitamin behaivior in premixes. Feedstuffs 47:45–48.

Vérice, E., Budowski, P. and Crawford, M.A. (1991) Chick nutritional encephalomalacia and prostanoid formation. J. Nutr. 121(7):966–969. https://doi.org/10.1093/jn/121.7.966.

Vermeer, C. (1986) Comparison between hepatic and nonhepatic vitamin K-dependent carboxylase. Haemostasis 16(3–4):239–245. https://doi.org/10.1159/000215296.

Viau, M., Métro, B., Genot, C., Rémignon, E. and Gandemer, G. (1998) Vitamin E status of muscle as related to vitamin E supply and dietary fat in the turkey. Proc. 44th int. cong. Meat Sci. Tech., Barcelona, Spain. (pp. 640–641).

Vieira, S.L. (2007) Chicken embryo utilization of egg micronutrients. Rev. Bras. Cienc Avic 9(1):1–8. https://doi.org/10.1590/S1516-635X2007000100001.

Vieira, A.V., Kuchler, K. and Schneider, W.J. (1995) Retinol in avian oogenesis: molecular properties of the carrier protein. DNA Cell Biol. 14(5):403–410. https://doi.org/10.1089/dna.1995.14.403.

Vieira, V., Marx, F.O., Bassi, L.S., Santos, M.C., Oba, A., de Oliveira, S.G. and Maiorka, A. (2021) Effect of age and different doses of dietary vitamin E on breast meat qualitative characteristics of finishing broilers. Anim. Nutr. 7(1):163–167. https://doi.org/10.1016/j.aninu.2020.08.004.

Vignale, K., Greene, E.S., Caldas, J.V., England, J.A., Boonsinchai, N., Sodsee, P., Pollock, E.D., Dridi, S. and Coon, C.N. (2015) 25-Hydroxycholecalciferol enhances male broiler breast meat yield through the mTOR pathway. J. Nutr. 145(5):855–863. https://doi.org/10.3945/jn.114.207936.

Villamide, M.J. and Fraga, M.J. (1999) Composition of vitamin supplements in Spanish poultry diets. Br. Poult. Sci. 40(5):644–652. https://doi.org/10.1080/00071669987034.

Villar-Patiño, G., Díaz-Cruz, A., Ávila-González, E., Guinzberg, R., Pablos, J.L. and Piña, E. (2002) Effects of dietary supplementation with vitamin C or vitamin E on cardiac lipid peroxidation and growth performance in broilers at risk of developing ascites syndrome. Am. J. Vet. Res. 63(5):673–676. https://doi.org/10.2460/ajvr.2002.63.673.

Villaverde, C., Baucells, M.D., Bou, R. and Barroeta, A.C. (2004a) Use of oxidized sunflower oil: effect on vitamin E deposition in different tissues in poultry. Proc. 22nd World's Poult. Congr., Istanbul, Turkey.

Villaverde, C., Cortinas, L., Barroeta, A.C., Martín-Orúe, S.M. and Baucells, M.D. (2004b) Relationship between dietary unsaturation and vitamin E in poultry. J. Anim. Physiol. Anim. Nutr. (Berl) 88(3–4):143–149. https://doi.org/10.1111/j.1439-0396.2003.00471.x.

Villaverde, C., Baucells, M.D., Manzanilla, E.G. and Barroeta, A.C. (2008) High levels of dietary unsaturated fat decrease α-tocopherol content of whole body, liver and plasma of chickens without variations in intestinal apparent absorption. Poult. Sci. 87(3):497–505. https://doi.org/10.3382/ps.2007-00292.

Vink-van Wijngaarden, T., Birkenhäger, J.C., Kleinekoort, W.M., van den Bemd, G.J., Pols, H.A. and van Leeuwen, J.P. (1995) Antiestrogens inhibit in vitro bone resorption stimulated by 1, 25-dihydroxyvitamin D_3 and the vitamin D_3 analogs EB1089 and KH1060. Endocrinology 136(2):812–815. https://doi.org/10.1210/endo.136.2.7835315.

Virtanen, E., Remus, J., Rosi, L., McNaughton, J. and Augustine, P. (1996) The effect of betaine and salinomycin during coccidiosis in broilers. Poult. Sci. 75(1):149.

Vo, K.V., Bashaw, A.J., Adefope, N.A., Catlin, C. and Wakefield, T. (1996) Effect of ascorbic acid and sucrose supplementation to broiler chicks subjected to delayed placement on early mortality, hemo-stress response, and growth performance. Poult. Sci. 75(suppl. 1):150.

Vo, K.V., Adefope, N.A., Fenderson, C.L. and Kolison, S.H. (1999) Effect of vitamin and trace mineral withdrawal on performance of broilers reared under high density stress. Poult. Sci. 78(suppl. 1):58.

Vogt, H. and Harnisch, S. (1991) Choline in layer diets. Archiv. Geflügelk 55:236–240.

Völker, L. and Fenster, R. (1991) Supplementation with ascorbic acid for increasing carcass yield in broiler chickens and turkeys prior to slaughter. Proc. 8th Eur. Symp. Poult. Nutr., Venice, Italy. (pp. 274–276).

Wagner, C. (2001) Biochemical role of folate in cellular metabolism. Clin. Res. Regul. Aff. 18(3):161–180. https://doi.org/10.1081/CRP-100108171.

Wagner, C., Briggs, W.T. and Cook, R.J. (1984) Covalent binding of folic acid to dimethylglycine dehydrogenase. Arch. Biochem. Biophys. 233(2):457–461. https://doi.org/10.1016/0003-9861(84)90467-3.

Wagstaff, R.K. (1978) Two hidden vitamins worth 0.137 lb 0.024 FC. Broiler Ind. 41(8):93.

Wahle, K.W.J., Hoppe, P.P. and McLntosha, G. (1993) Effects of storage and various intrinsic vitamin E concentrations on lipid oxidation in dried egg powders. J. Sci. Food Agric. 61(4):463–469. https://doi.org/10.1002/jsfa.2740610414.

Waldenstedt, L. (2006) Nutritional factors of importance for optimal leg health in broilers: a review. Anim. Feed Sci. Technol. 126(3–4):291–307. https://doi.org/10.1016/j.anifeedsci.2005.08.008.
Waldroup, P.W., Hellwig, H.M., Spencer, G.K., Smith, N.K., Fancher, B.I., Jackson, M.E., Johnson, Z.B. and Goodwin, T.L. (1985) The effects of increased levels of niacin supplementation on growth rate and carcass composition of broiler chickens. Poult. Sci. 64(9):1777–1784. https://doi.org/10.3382/ps.0641777.
Waldroup, P.W. and Fritts, C.A. (2005) Evaluation of separate and combined effects of choline and betaine in diets for male broilers. Int. J. Poult. Sci. 4(7):442–448. https://doi.org/10.3923/ijps.2005.442.448.
Waldroup, P.W., Motl, M.A., Yan, F. and Fritts, C.A. (2006) Effects of betaine and choline on response to methionine supplementation to broiler diets formulated to industry standards. J. Appl. Poult. Res. 15(1):58–71. https://doi.org/10.1093/japr/15.1.58.
Walsh, M.M., Kerry, J.F., Buckley, D.J., Arendt, E.K. and Morrissey, P.A. (1998) Effect of dietary supplementation with α-tocopheryl acetate on the stability of reformed and restructured low nitrite cured turkey products. Meat Sci. 50(2):191–201. https://doi.org/10.1016/s0309-1740(98)00030-8.
Walter, E.D. and Jensen, L.S. (1963) Effectiveness of selenium and non-effectiveness of sulfur amino acids in preventing muscular dystrophy in the turkey poult. J. Nutr. 80(3):327–331. https://doi.org/10.1093/jn/80.3.327.
Walters, B.S., Wu, W. and Maurer, A.J. (1991) Effect of flat peas (*Lathyrus silvestris*) on broiler chicks. Poult. Sci. 70(1):127.
Walton, J.P., Julian, R.J. and Squires, E.J. (2001) The effects of dietary flax oil and antioxidants on ascites and pulmonary hypertension in broilers using a low temperature model. Br. Poult. Sci. 42(1):123–129.
Wang, H., Zhang, H.J., Wang, X.C., Wu, S.G., Wang, J., Xu, L. and Qi, G.H. (2017) Dietary choline and phospholipid supplementation enhanced docosahexaenoic acid enrichment in egg yolk of laying hens fed a 2% Schizochytrium powder-added diet. Poult. Sci. 96(8):2786–2794. https://doi.org/10.3382/ps/pex095.
Wang, J., Clark, D.L., Jacobi, S.K. and Velleman, S.G. (2020a) Effect of vitamin E and omega-3 fatty acids early post hatch supplementation on reducing the severity of wooden breast myopathy in broilers. Poult. Sci. 99(4):2108–2119. https://doi.org/10.1016/j.psj.2019.12.033.
Wang, J., Clark, D.L., Jacobi, S.K. and Velleman, S.G. (2020b) Effect of early post hatch supplementation of vitamin E and omega-3 fatty acids on the severity of wooden breast, breast muscle morphological structure and gene expression in the broiler breast muscle. Poult. Sci. 99(11):5925–5935. https://doi.org/10.1016/j.psj.2020.08.043.
Wang, J., Qiu, L., Gong, H., Celi, P., Yan, L., Ding, X., Bai, S., Zeng, Q., Mao, X., Xu, S., Wu, C. and Zhang, K. (2020c) Effect of dietary 25-hydroxycholecalciferol supplementation and high stocking density on performance, egg quality, and tibia quality in laying hens. Poult. Sci. 99(5):2608–2615. https://doi.org/10.1016/j.psj.2019.12.054.
Wang, J., Clark, D.L., Jacobi, S.K. and Velleman, S.G. (2021a) Effect of vitamin E and alpha lipoic acid on intestinal development associated with wooden breast myopathy in broilers. Poult. Sci. 100(3):100952. https://doi.org/10.1016/j.psj.2020.12.049.
Wang, J., Zhang, C., Zhang, T., Yan, L., Qiu, L., Yin, H., Ding, X., Bai, S., Zeng, Q., Mao, X., Zhang, K., Wu, C., Xuan, Y. and Shan, Z. (2021b) Dietary 25-hydroxyvitamin D improves intestinal health and microbiota of laying hens under high stocking density. Poult. Sci. 100(7):101132. https://doi.org/10.1016/j.psj.2021.101132.
Wang, J.S., Rogers, S.R. and Pesti, G.M. (1987) Influence of choline and sulphate on copper and toxicity and substitution of and antagonism between methionine and copper supplements to chick diets. Poult. Sci. 66(9):1500–1507. https://doi.org/10.3382/ps.0661500.
Wang, Y., Li, L., Gou, Z., Chen, F., Fan, Q., Lin, X., Ye, J., Zhang, C. and Jiang, S. (2020) Effects of maternal and dietary vitamin A on growth performance, meat quality, antioxidant status, and immune function of offspring broilers. Poult. Sci. 99(8):3930–3940. https://doi.org/10.1016/j.psj.2020.03.044.
Ward, N.E. (1993) Vitamin supplementation rates for U.S. commercial broilers, turkeys and layers. J. Appl. Poult. Res. 2(3):286–296. https://doi.org/10.1093/japr/2.3.286.
Ward, N.E. (1995) Research examine use of 25-OH vitamin D_3 in broiler chicks. Feedstuffs 67:12–15.
Ward N. E. (2014) U.S. Commercial broiler vitamin survey DSM Nutritional Products https://www.dsm.com/content/dam/dsm/anh/en_na/documents/2014-US-Commercial-Broiler-Survey.pdf.

Ward, N.E. (2017) Vitamins in eggs. In "Egg innovations and strategies for improvements" Hester, Y. (ed.). Elsevier. (pp. 207–220). https://doi.org/10.1016/B978-0-12-800879-9.00020-2.

Ward, N. E. (2022) Vitamin requirements for broilers Proceedings Arkansas Nutrition Conference, September 13-15, 2022 – Rogers Convention Centre, Rogers, AR.

Ward, N.E., Jones, J.E. and Maurice, D.V. (1985) Inefficacy of propionic-acid for depleting laying hens and their progeny of vitamin-B_{12}. Nutr. Rep. Int. 32:1325–1332.

Warren, M.F., Vu, T.C., Toomer, O.T., Fernandez, J.D. and Livingston, K.A. (2020) Efficacy of 1-α-hydroxycholecalciferol supplementation in young broiler feed suggests reducing calcium levels at grower phase front. Vet. Sci. 10. https://doi.org/10.3389/fvets.2020.00245.

Wasserman, R.H. (1981) Intestinal absorption of calcium and phosphorus. Fed. Proc. 40(1):68–72. PMID:7192650.

Watkins, B.A. (1989a) Influence of biotin deficiency and dietary trans-fatty acids on tissue lipids in chickens. Br. J. Nutr. 61(1):99–111. https://doi.org/10.1079/BJN19890096.

Watkins, B.A. (1989b) Levels of dihomo-γ-linoleate are depressed in heart phosphatidylcholine and phosphatidylethanolamine in the biotin-deficient chick. Poult. Sci. 68(5):698–705. https://doi.org/10.3382/ps.0680698.

Watkins, B.A. (1993) Diet and leg weakness. In. In poultry "Recent advances in animal nutrition" Garnsworthy, P.C. and Cole, D.J.A. (ed.). Nottingham University Press. (pp. 131–141).

Watkins, B.A. and Kratzer, F.H. (1987a) Dietary biotin effects on polyunsaturated fatty acids in chick tissue lipids and prostaglandin E_2 levels in freeze-clamped hearts. Poult. Sci. 66(11):1818–1828. https://doi.org/10.3382/ps.0661818.

Watkins, B.A. and Kratzer, F.H. (1987b) Effects of dietary biotin and linoleate on polyunsaturated fatty acids in tissue phospholipids. Poult. Sci. 66(12):2024–2031. https://doi.org/10.3382/ps.0662024.

Watkins, B.A. and Kratzer, F.H. (1987c) Tissue lipid fatty acid composition of biotin- adequate and biotin-deficient chicks. Poult. Sci. 66(2):306–313. https://doi.org/10.3382/ps.0660306.

Weber, G. (2001) Nutritional effects on poultry meat quality, stability and flavor. Proc. 13th Eur. Symp. Poult. Nutr., Blankenberge, Belgium. (pp. 9–16).

Weber, G.M. (2009) Improvement of flock productivity through supply of vitamins for higher laying performance and better egg quality. Poult. Sci. 65(3):443–458. https://doi.org/10.1017/S0043933909000312.

Wei, I.L. and Young, T.K. (1994) Vitamin B_6 metabolism is altered in chronic renal failure rats. Nutr. Res. 14(2):271–278. https://doi.org/10.1016/S0271-5317(05)80385-9.

Weiser, H. and Vecchi, M. (1982) Stereoisomers of α-tocopheryl acetate. II. Biopotencies of all eight stereoisomers, individually or in mixtures, as determined by rat resorption-gestation tests. Int. J. Vitam. Nutr. Res. 52(3):351–370. PMID:7174231.

Weiser, H., Schlachter, M., Probst, H.P. and Kormann, A.W. (1990) The relevance of ascorbic acid for bone metabolism. Proc. 2nd symp. ascorbic acid domest. anim., Kartause, Ittingen, Switzerland. ETH Zürich. (pp. 73–95).

Weiser, H., Schlachter, M., Probst, H.P., Flachowsky, G. and Schone, F. (1991) Importance of vitamins D_3, C and B_6 for bone metabolism. Friedrich Schiller Univ. Jena Germany:(26–27).

Weiss, F.G. and Scott, M.L. (1979) Influence of vitamin B_6 upon reproduction and upon plasma and egg cholesterol in chickens. J. Nutr. 109(6):1010–1017. https://doi.org/10.1093/jn/109.6.1010.

Wen, J., Morrissey, P.A., Buckley, D.J. and Sheehy, P.J.A. (1996) Oxidative stability and α-tocopherol retention in turkey burgers during refrigerated and frozen storage as influenced by dietary α-tocopheryl acetate. Br. Poult. Sci. 37(4):787–795. https://doi.org/10.1080/00071669608417908.

Wen, J., Lin, J. and Wang, H.M. (1997) Effect of dietary vitamin E and ascorbic acid on the growth and immune function of chicks. Chin. Agric. Sci. (145–149) https://www.cabdirect.org/cabdirect/abstract/19981410004.

Wen, J., McCarthy, S.N., Higgins, F.M.J., Morrissey, P.A., Buckley, D.J. and Sheehy, P.J.A. (1997b) Effect of dietary α-tocopheryl acetate on the uptake and distribution of α-tocopherol in turkey tissue and lipid stability. Ir. J. Agric. Food Res. 36(1):65–74.

Wen, J., Livingston, K.A. and Persia, M.E. (2019) Effect of high concentrations of dietary vitamin D_3 on pullet and laying hen performance, skeleton health, eggshell quality, and yolk vitamin D_3 content when fed to W36 laying hens from day of hatch until 68 wk of age. Poult. Sci. 98(12):6713–6720. https://doi.org/10.3382/ps/pez386.

West, C.E., Sijtsma, S.R., Kouwenhoven, B., Rombout, J.H.W.M. and van der Zijpp, A.J. (1992a) Epithelia-damaging virus infections affect vitamin A status in chickens. J. Nutr. 122(2):333–339. https://doi.org/10.1093/jn/122.2.333.

West, C.E., Sijtsma, S.R., Peters, H.P.E., Rombout, J.H. and van der Zijpp, A.J. (1992b) Production of chickens with marginal vitamin A deficiency. Br. J. Nutr. 68(1):283–291. https://doi.org/10.1079/BJN19920085.

Whanger, P.D. (1981) Selenium and heavy metal toxicity. In "Selenium in biology and medicine" Spallholz, J.E., Martin, J.L. and Ganther, H.E. (ed.) AVI Publishing Co., Westport, Connecticut, USA.

White, H.B. (1996) Sudden death of chicken embryos with hereditary riboflavin deficiency. J. Nutr. 126(4)(suppl.):1303S–1307S. https://doi.org/10.1093/jn/126.suppl_4.1303S.

White, W.S., Peck, K.M., Ulman, E.A. and Erdman, J.W. (1993) The ferret as a model for evaluation of the bio-availabilities of all-trans-beta-carotene and its isomers. J. Nutr. 123(6):1129–1139.

Whitehead, C.C. (1977) The use of biotin in poultry nutrition. Worlds Poult. Sci. J. 33(3):140–154. https://doi.org/10.1079/WPS19770012.

Whitehead, C.C. (1978) Effect of nutrient deficiencies in animals: Biotin. In "Handbook series in nutrition and food: nutrition disorders" Rechcigl Jr., M. (ed.). CRC Press Inc.

Whitehead, C.C. (1984) Biotin intake and transfer to the egg and chick in broiler breeder hens housed on litter or in cages. Br. Poult. Sci. 25(2):287–292. https://doi.org/10.1080/00071668408454868.

Whitehead, C.C. (1985) Assessment of biotin deficiency in animals. Ann. N. Y. Acad. Sci. 447(1):86–96. https://doi.org/10.1111/j.1749-6632.1985.tb18427.x.

Whitehead, C.C. (1987) Requirements for vitamins. In "Nutrient requirements of poultry and nutritional research" Fisher, C. and Boorman, K.N. (ed.). Butterworths. (pp. 173–190).

Whitehead, C.C. (1988a) Vitamin nutrition update. Broiler Ind. 51(9):60.

Whitehead, C.C. (1988b) Nutrition of breeding stock: recent advances in turkey science. Proc. 21st World Poultr. Congr., Montréal, Canada. (pp. 91–117).

Whitehead, C.C. (1991a) Effects of vitamins on leg weakness in poultry. Proc. 7th Eur. Symp. Poult. Nutr. Venezia, Mestre. (pp. 157–166).

Whitehead, C.C. (1991b) Relationships between tissue and dietary levels of vitamins A and E in lines of genetically lean and fat broilers. Proc. 8th Eur. Symp. Poult. Nutr., Venice, Italy. (pp. 295–297).

Whitehead, C.C. (1993) Vitamin supplementation of cereal diets for poultry. Anim. Feed Sci. Technol. 45(1):81–95. https://doi.org/10.1016/0377-8401(93)90073-S.

Whitehead, C.C. (1995a) Nutrition and skeletal disorders in broilers and layers. Poult. Int.12(40–48).

Whitehead, C.C. (1995b) The role of vitamin D metabolites in the prevention of tibial dyschondroplasia. Anim. Feed Sci. Technol. 53(2):205–210. https://doi.org/10.1016/0377-8401(95)02013-P.

Whitehead, C.C. (1996) Nutrition issues: changing standard requirements. Poult. Int. 9:24–26.

Whitehead, C.C. (1998) The influence of vitamins on the performance and health status of laying hens and turkeys. Multi-State Poult. Meeting.

Whitehead, C.C. (1999) The impact of vitamins on health and performance in fowls. Proc. 12th Eur. Symp. Poult. Nutr., Veldhoven, The Netherlands. (pp. 73–82).

Whitehead, C.C. (2000a) Recent developments on the effects of nutrition on skeletal disease. Proc. 21st World's Poult. Congr., Montreal, Canada.

Whitehead, C.C. (2000b) Update on vitamin and trace mineral requirements for poultry. Proc. Md Nutr. Conf.

Whitehead, C.C. (2001) Nicotinic acid in poultry nutrition. Feed Mix 1:32–34.

Whitehead, C.C. (2002a) Vitamins in feedstuffs. In "Poultry feedstuffs, supply, composition and nutritive value" McNab, M. and Boorman, K.N. (ed.), CABI Pub. (pp. 181–190).

Whitehead, C.C. (2002b) Influence of vitamins and minerals on bone formation and quality. Proc. 11th Eur. Poultr. Conf., Bremen, Germany.

Whitehead, C.C. (2002c) Nutrition and poultry welfare. Poult. Sci. 58(3):349–356. https://doi.org/10.1079/WPS20020027.

Whitehead, C.C. (2003) Papel de la nutrición para mejorar el bienestar y la calidad de vida de las aves. Proc. 40th Symp., WPSA's Spanish Branch, Girona, Spain.

Whitehead, C.C. (2004a) Nutritional and metabolic disorders in meat poultry. Proc. 21st World Poultr. Congr., Montréal, Canada.

Whitehead, C.C. (2004b) Overview of bone biology in the egg-laying hen. Poult. Sci. 83(2):193–199.

Whitehead, C.C. (2005) Mechanisms and nutritional influences in skeletal development: influence of macro- and microelements on bone formation. Proc. 15th Eur. Symp. Poult. Nutr., Balatonfured, Hungary. (pp. 142–150).

Whitehead, C.C. and Bannister, D.W. (1980) Biotin status, blood pyruvate carboxylase EC 6.4.1.1 activity and performance in broilers under different conditions of bird husbandry and diet processing. Br. J. Nutr. 43(3):541–549. https://doi.org/10.1079/bjn19800121.

Whitehead, C.C. and Blair, R.B. (1974) The involvement of biotin in the fatty liver and kidney syndrome in broiler chickens. Worlds Poult. Sci. J. 30:231.

Whitehead, C.C. and Keller, T. (2003) An update on ascorbic acid in poultry. Worlds Poult. Sci. J. 59(2):161–184. https://doi.org/10.1079/WPS20030010.

Whitehead, C.C. and Portsmouth, J.I. (1989) Vitamin requirements and allowances for poultry. In "Recent advances in animal nutrition" Haresign, W. and Cole, D.G.A. (ed.). Butterworths, London, UK.

Whitehead, C.C. and Randall, C.J. (1982) Interrelationships between biotin, choline and other B-vitamins and the occurrence of fatty liver and kidney syndrome and sudden death syndrome in broiler chickens. Br. J. Nutr. 48(1):177–184. https://doi.org/10.1079/bjn19820099.

Whitehead, C.C. and Siller, W.G. (1983) Experimentally induced fatty liver and kidney syndrome in the young turkey. Res. Vet. Sci. 34(1):73–76.

Whitehead, C.C., Bannister, D.W., Evans, A.J., Siller, W.G. and Wight, P.A.L. (1976a) Biotin deficiency and fatty liver and kidney syndrome in chicks given purified diets containing different fat and protein levels. Br. J. Nutr. 35(1):115–125. https://doi.org/10.1079/BJN19760015.

Whitehead, C.C., Blair, R., Bannister, D.W., Evans, A.J. and Jones, R.M. (1976b) The involvement of biotin in preventing the fatty liver and kidney syndrome in chicks. Res. Vet. Sci. 20(2):180–184. https://doi.org/10.1016/S0034-5288(18)33453-2.

Whitehead, C.C., Armstrong, J.A. and Waddington, D. (1982) The determination of the availability to chicks of biotin in feed ingredients by a bioassay based on the response of blood pyruvate carboxylase (EC 6.4.1.1) activity. Br. J. Nutr. 48(1):81–88. https://doi.org/10.1079/bjn19820090.

Whitehead, C.C., Pearson, R.A. and Herron, K.M. (1985) Biotin requirements of broiler breeders fed diets of different protein content and effect of insufficient biotin on the viability of progeny. Br. Poult. Sci. 26(1):73–82. https://doi.org/10.1080/00071668508416789.

Whitehead, C.C., McCormack, H.A. and Webster, C. (1992) A quantitative estimate of the replaceability of methionine by choline in broiler diets. Proc. 19th World's Poult. Congr., Amsterdam, The Netherlands. (pp. 639–640).

Whitehead, C.C., Rennie, J.S., Farquharson, C. and Fleming, R.H. (1993a) Recent findings on tibial dyschondroplasia in broilers and osteoporosis in caged layers. Proc. Br. Soc. Anim. Prod. (1972) 1993:70–70. https://doi.org/10.1017/S0308229600023965.

Whitehead, C.C., Rennie, J.S., McCormack, H.A. and Hocking, P.M. (1993b) Defective down syndrome in chicks is not caused by riboflavin deficiency in breeders. Br. Poult. Sci. 34(3):619–623. https://doi.org/10.1080/00071669308417618.

Whitehead, C.C., Farquharson, C., Rennie, J.S. and McCormack, H.A. (1994) Nutrition and cellular factors affecting tibial dyschondroplasia in broilers. Proc. Aust. Poultr. Sci. Symp., Sydney. (pp. 13–19).

Whitehead, C.C., McCormack, H.A., Rennie, J.S. and Frigg, M. (1995) Folic acid requirements of broilers. Br. Poult. Sci. 36(1):113–121. https://doi.org/10.1080/00071669508417757.

Whitehead, C.C., McCormack, H.A., McTeir, L. and Fleming, R.H. (2004a) High vitamin D_3 requirements in broilers for bone quality and prevention of tibial dyschondroplasia and interactions with dietary calcium, available phosphorus and vitamin A. Br. Poult. Sci. 45(3):425–436. https://doi.org/10.1080/00071660410001730941.

Whitehead, C.C., McCormack, H.A., Mcteir, L. and Fleming, R.H. (2004b) The maximum legal limit for vitamin D_3 in broiler diets may need to be increased. Br. Poult. Sci. 45(1)(suppl. 1):S24-S26. https://doi.org/10.1080/00071660410001698074.

Whitfield, G.K., Hsieh, J.C., Jurutka, P.W., Selznick, S.H., Haussler, C.A., MacDonald, P.N. and Haussler, M.R. (1995) Genomic actions of 1,25-dihydroxyvitamin D_3. J. Nutr. 125(6)(suppl.):1690S-1694S.

Wiedermann, U., Hanson, L.A., Kahu, H. and Dahlgren, U.I. (1993) Aberrant T-cell function in vitro and impaired T-cell dependent antibody response *in vivo* in vitamin A-deficient rats. Immunology 80(4):581–586.

Williams, B., Solomon, S., Waddington, D., Thorp, B. and Farquharson, C. (2000a) Skeletal development in the meat-type chicken. Br. Poult. Sci. 41(2):141–149. https://doi.org/10.1080/713654918.

Williams, B., Waddington, D., Solomon, S. and Farquharson, C. (2000b) Dietary effects on bone quality and turnover, and Ca and P metabolism in chickens. Res. Vet. Sci. 69(1):81–87. https://doi.org/10.1053/rvsc.2000.0392.

Williams, C.J. and Zedek, A.S. (2010) Comparative field evaluations of *in ovo* applied technology. Poult. Sci. 89(1):189–193. https://doi.org/10.3382/ps.2009-00093.

Wilson, H.R. (1997) Effects of maternal nutrition on hatchability. Poult. Sci. 76(1):134–143. https://doi.org/10.1093/ps/76.1.134.

Wiseman, E.M., Bar-El, D.S. and Reifen, R. (2017) The vicious cycle of vitamin A deficiency. Crit. Rev. Food Sci. Nutr. 57(17):3703–3714. https://doi.org/10.1080/10408398.2016.1160362.

Witkowska, D., Sedrowicz, L. and Oledzka, R. (1992) Effect of a diet with an increased content of vitamin B_6 on the absorption of amino acids in the intestine of rats intoxicated with carbaryl propoxur and thiuram. Methionine. Bromatol. Chem. Toksykoleziczna 25:25.

Witztum, J.L. (1989) Current approaches to drug therapy for the hypercholesterolemic patient. Circulation 80(5):1101–1114.

Wolf, G. (1991) The intracellular vitamin A-binding proteins: an overview of their functions. Nutr. Rev. 49(1):1–12. https://doi.org/10.1111/j.1753-4887.1991.tb07349.x.

Wolf, G. (1993) The newly discovered retinoic acid-X receptors (RXRs). Nutr. Rev. 51(3):81–84. https://doi.org/10.1111/j.1753-4887.1993.tb03075.x.

Wolf, G. (1995) The enzymatic cleavage of beta-carotene: still controversial. Nutr. Rev. 53(5):134–137. https://doi.org/10.1111/j.1753-4887.1995.tb01537.x.

Wolf, G. (2006) How an increased intake of α-tocopherol can suppress the bioavailability of gamma-tocopherol. Nutr. Rev. 64(6):295–299. https://doi.org/10.1111/j.1753-4887.2006.tb00213.x.

Wolf, G. (2007) Identification of a membrane receptor for retinol-binding protein functioning in the cellular uptake of retinol. Nutr. Rev. 65(8 Pt 1):385–388. https://doi.org/10.1111/j.1753-4887.2007.tb00316.x.

Wolf, G. and Carpenter, K.J. (1997) Early Research into the vitamins: the work of Wilhelm Stepp. J. Nutr. 127(7):1255–1259. https://doi.org/10.1093/jn/127.7.1255.

Workel, H., Keller, T., Reeve, A. and Lauwaerts, A. (1998) Choline the rediscovered vitamin: world poultry magazine on production processing and marketing 14:22–25.

Workel, H.A., Keller, T.H., Reeve, A. and Lauwaerts, A. (1999) Choline – the rediscovered vitamin. Poult. Int.:4(44–47).

World Poultry (2001) Vitamins. World poultry magazine on production processing and marketing special, Elsevier (ed).

Wu, C.C., Dorairajan, T. and Lin, T.L. (2000) Effect of ascorbic acid supplementation on the immune response of chickens vaccinated and challenged with infectious bursal disease virus. Vet. Immunol. Immunopathol. 74(1–2):145–152. https://doi.org/10.1016/s0165-2427(00)00161-6.

Wyatt, C.L. (1991) Effect of high levels of vitamin A supplementation on skin pigmentation and growth performance in broiler chicks. Poult. Sci. J. 68(1):161.

Xiang, R.P., Sun, W.D., Wang, J.Y. and Wang, X.L. (2002) Effect of vitamin C on pulmonary hypertension and muscularization of pulmonary arterioles in broilers. Br. Poult. Sci. 43(5)(suppl.):705–712. https://doi.org/10.1080/0007166021000025064.

Xie, J., Tang, L., Lu, L., Zhang, L., Lin, X., Liu, H.C., Odle, J. and Luo, X. (2015) Effects of acute and chronic heat stress on plasma metabolites, hormones and oxidant status in restrictedly fed broiler breeders. Poult. Sci. 94(7):1635–1644. https://doi.org/10.3382/ps/pev105.

Xu, T., Leach, R.M., Hollis, B. and Soares, J.H. (1997) Evidence of increased cholecalciferol requirement in chicks with tibial dyschondroplasia. Poult. Sci. 76(1):47–53. https://doi.org/10.1093/ps/76.1.47.

Xu, Y., Chen, J., Yu, X., Tao, W., Jiang, F., Yin, Z. and Liu, C. (2010) Protective effects of chlorogenic acid on acute hepatotoxicity induced by lipopolysaccharide in mice. Inflamm. Res. 59(10):871–877. https://doi.org/10.1007/s00011-010-0199-z.

Yair, R., Shahar, R. and Uni, Z. (2015) *In ovo* feeding with minerals and vitamin D_3 improves bone properties in hatchlings and mature broilers. Poult. Sci. 94(11):2695–2707. https://doi.org/10.3382/ps/pev252.

Yan, H.J., Lee, E.J., Nam, K.C., Min, B.R. and Ahn, D.U. (2006) Dietary functional ingredients: performance of animals and quality and storage stability of irradiated raw turkey breast. Poult. Sci. 85(10):1829–1837.

Yang, C.P. and Jeng, S.L. (1989) Pyridoxine deficiency and requirements in mule duckling. J. Chin. Agric. Chem. Soc. 27:450.

Yang, H., Qazi, I.H., Pan, B., Angel, C., Guo, S., Yang, J., Zhang, Y., Ming, Z., Zeng, C., Meng, Q., Han, H. and Zhou, G. (2019) Dietary selenium supplementation ameliorates female reproductive efficiency in aging mice. Antioxidants (Basel) 8(12):634. https://doi.org/10.3390/antiox8120634.

Yang, H.S., Waibel, P.E. and Brenes, J. (1973) Evaluation of vitamin D_3 supplements by biological assays using the turkey. J. Nutr. 103(8):1187–1194. https://doi.org/10.1093/jn/103.8.1187.

Yang, J., Ding, X., Bai, S., Wang, J., Zeng, Q., Peng, H., Su, Z., Xuan, Y., Scott Fraley, G.S. and Zhang, K. (2020a) Effects of maternal dietary vitamin E on the egg characteristics, hatchability, and offspring quality of prolonged storage eggs of broiler breeder hens. J. Anim. Physiol. Anim. Nutr. (Berl) 104(5):1384–1391. https://doi.org/10.1111/jpn.13371.

Yang, J., Ding, X., Bai, S., Wang, J., Zeng, Q., Peng, H., Xuan, Y., Su, Z. and Zhang, K. (2020b) The effects of broiler breeder dietary vitamin E and egg storage time on the quality of eggs and newly hatched chicks. Animals (Basel) 10(8):1409. https://doi.org/10.3390/ani10081409.

Yang, L. and Wang, H. (1996a) Effect of dietary riboflavin level on performance and nutritional status of broilers. 20th World's Poult. Congr., New Delhi, India. (pp. 148–150).

Yang, L. and Wang, H. (1996b) Effect of riboflavin on the utilization of methionine and metabolism of protein of liver. 20th World´s Poult. Congr., New Delhi, India. (pp. 212–213).

Yang, M. and Wu, W. (1997) Dietary supplementation of thiamine in excess of NRC recommendation can prevent immunosuppression caused by toxic *Fusarium proliferatum*. Poult. Sci. 78(suppl. 1):125.

Yang, N., Larsen, C.T., Dunnington, T.E., Geraert, P.A., Picard, P.M. and Siegel, P.B. (2000) Immune competence of chicks from two lines divergently selected for antibody response to sheep red blood cells as affected by supplemental vitamin E. Poult. Sci. 79(6):799–803. https://doi.org/10.1093/ps/79.6.799.

Yang, P., Wang, H., Zhu, M. and Ma, Y. (2019) Effects of choline chloride, copper sulfate and zinc oxide on long-term stabilization of microencapsulated vitamins in premixes for weanling piglets. Animals (Basel) 9(12):1154. https://doi.org/10.3390/ani9121154.

Yang, P., Wang, H., Zhu, M. and Ma, Y. (2020) Evaluation of extrusion temperatures, pelleting parameters and vitamin forms on vitamin stability in feed. Animals 10(5):894. https://doi.org/10.3390/ani10050894.

Yao, L., Wang, T., Persia, M., Horst, R.L. and Higgins, M. (2013) Effects of vitamin D_3-enriched diet on egg yolk vitamin D_3 content and yolk quality. J. Food Sci. 78(2):C178–C183. https://doi.org/10.1111/1750-3841.12032.

Yarger, J.G., Quarles, C.L., Hollis, B.W. and Gray, R.W. (1995a) Safety of 25-hydroxycholecalciferol as a source of cholecalciferol in poultry rations. Poult. Sci. 74(9):1437–1446. https://doi.org/10.3382/ps.0741437.

Yarger, J.G., Saunders, C.A., McNaughton, J.L., Quarles, C.L., Hollis, B.W. and Gray, R.W. (1995b) Comparison of dietary 25-hydroxycholecalciferol and cholecalciferol in broiler chickens. Poult. Sci. 74(7):1159–1167. https://doi.org/10.3382/ps.0741159.

Yaripour, M., Seidavi, A., Dadashbeiki, M., Laudadio, V., Tufarelli, V., Ragni, M. and Payan-Carreira, R. (2018) Impact of dietary supra-nutritional levels of vitamins A and E on fertility traits of broiler breeder hens in late production phase. Agriculture 8(10):149. https://doi.org/10.3390/agriculture8100149.

Yaroshenko, F.A., Ionov, I.A. and Surai, P.F. (1995) Vitamin E and quality of newly hatched chicks. Proc. Ukr. Conf. Physiol. Biochem. Farm Anim.

Yegani, M.D., Miles, R.H., Nilipour, A.D. and Butcher, G. (2001) Vitamin C – practical applications in modern poultry production. World Poult. 17:10.

Yeh, Y.L., Chou, P.C., Chen, Y.H., Lai, L.S., Chung, T.K., Walzem, R.L., Huang, S.Y. and Chen, S.E. (2020) Dietary supplementation of 25-hydroxycholecalciferol improves cardiac function and livability in broiler breeder hens-amelioration of blood pressure and vascular remodeling. Poult. Sci. 99(7):3363–3373. https://doi.org/10.1016/j.psj.2020.03.015 .

Yen, J.T., Jensen, A.H. and Baker, D.H. (1977) Assessment of the availability of niacin in corn, soybeans and soybean meal. J. Anim. Sci. 45(2):269–278.

Yersin, A.G., Edens, F.W. and Simmons, D.G. (1989) The effects of *Bordetella avium* on tracheal cilia of turkey poults receiving exogenous niacin. Poult. Sci. 70(suppl. 1):162 (abstract).

Yin, M.C., Faustman, C., Riesen, J.W. and Williams, S.N. (1993) α-tocopherol and ascorbate delay oxymyoglobin and phospholipid oxidation *in vitro*. J. Food Sci. 58(6):1273–1276. https://doi.org/10.1111/j.1365-2621.1993.tb06164.x.

Yin, M.C. and Cheng, W.S. (1997) Oxymyoglobin and lipid oxidation in phosphatidylcholine liposomes retarded by α-tocopherol and β-carotene. J. Food Sci. 62(6):1095–1097. https://doi.org/10.1111/j.1365-2621.1997.tb12220.x.

Yonke, J.A. and Cherian, G. (2019) Choline supplementation alters egg production performance and hepatic oxidative status of laying hens fed high-docosahexaenoic acid microalgae. Poult. Sci. 98(11):5661–5668. https://doi.org/10.3382/ps/pez339.

Yoshida, H. and Takagi, S. (1999) Antioxidative effects of sesamol and tocopherols at various concentrations in oils during microwave heating. J. Sci. Food Agric. 79(2):220–226. https://doi.org/10.1002/(SICI)1097-0010(199902)79:2<220::AID-JSFA173>3.0.CO;2-8.

Yoshida, M. and Hoshii, H. (1976) Effect of dilauryl succinate on reproduction of the cock and hen and preventive effect of vitamin E. J. Nutr. 106(8):1184–1191. https://doi.org/10.1093/jn/106.8.1184.

Yotova, I., Yotsov, S., Pashov, D., Afanasov, K., Sotirov, L. and Stoyanccev, E. (1990) Effect of vitamin C on some factors of immune reactivity of broiler chicks infected with Marek's disease virus. Vet. Bull. 12:1200.

Young, J.F., Stagsted, J., Jensen, S.K., Karlsson, A.H. and Henckel, P. (2003) Ascorbic acid, α-tocopherol and oregano supplements reduce stress-induced deterioration of chicken meat quality. Poult. Sci. 82(8):1343–1351. https://doi.org/10.1093/ps/82.8.1343.

Young, L.G., Lun, A., Pos, J., Forshaw, R.P. and Edmeades, D.E. (1975) Vitamin E stability in corn and mixed feed. J. Anim. Sci. 40(3):495–499. https://doi.org/10.2527/jas1975.403495x.

Young, R.J., Norris, L.C. and Heuser, G.F. (1955) The chick's requirement for folic acid in the utilization of choline and its precursors betaine and methylamino ethanol. J. Nutr. 55(3):353–362. https://doi.org/10.1093/jn/55.3.353.

Youssef, D.A., Miller, C.W., El-Abbassi, A.M., Cutchins, D.C., Cutchins, C., Grant, W.B. and Peiris, A.N. (2011) Antimicrobial implications of vitamin D. Derm. Endocrinol. 3(4):220–229. https://doi.org/10.4161/derm.3.4.15027.

Youssef, I.M.I., Beineke, A., Rohn, K. and Kamphues, J. (2012) Influences of increased levels of biotin, zinc or mannan-oligosaccharides in the diet on foot pad dermatitis in growing turkeys housed on dry and wet litter. J. Anim. Physiol. Anim. Nutr. (Berl) 96(5):747–761. https://doi.org/10.1111/j.1439-0396.2010.01115.x.

Yu, D.G., Namgung, N., Kim, J.H., Won, S.Y., Choi, W.J. and Kil, D.Y. (2021) Effects of stocking density and dietary vitamin C on performance, meat quality, intestinal permeability, and stress indicators in broiler chickens. J. Anim. Sci. Technol. 63(4):815–826. https://doi.org/10.5187/jast.2021.e77.

Yu, M., Guan, K. and Zhang, C. (2011) The promoting effect of retinoic acid on proliferation of chicken primordial germ cells by increased expression of cadherin and catenins. Amino Acids 40(3):933–941. https://doi.org/10.1007/s00726-010-0717-x.

Yuan, J., Roshdy, A.R., Guo, Y., Wang, Y. and Guo, S. (2014) Effect of dietary vitamin A on reproductive performance and immune response of broiler breeders. PLOS ONE 9(8):e105677. https://doi.org/10.1371/journal.pone.0105677.

Yunis, R., Ben-David, A., Heller, E.D. and Cahaner, A. (2000) Immunocompetence and viability under commercial conditions of broiler groups differing in growth rate and in antibody response to *Escherichia coli* vaccine. Poult. Sci. 79(6):810–816. https://doi.org/10.1093/ps/79.6.810.

Zaghari, M., Sedaghat, V. and Shivazad, M. (2013) Effect of vitamin E on reproductive performance of heavy broiler breeder hens. J. Appl. Poult. Res. 22(4):808–813. https://doi.org/10.3382/japr.2012-00718.

Zakaria, A.H. and Al-Anezi, M.A. (1996) Effect of ascorbic acid and cooling during egg incubation on hatchability, culling, mortality, and the body weights of broiler chickens. Poult. Sci. 75(10):1204–1209. https://doi.org/10.3382/ps.0751204.

Zang, H., Zhang, K., Ding, X., Bai, S., Hernández, J.M. and Yao, B. (2011) Effects of different dietary vitamin combinations on the egg quality and vitamin deposition in the whole egg of laying hens. Rev. Bras. Cienc Avic 13(3):189–196. https://doi.org/10.1590/S1516-635X2011000300005.

Zaniboni, L. and Cerolini, S. (2006) Lipid changes in chicken sperm during ageing and α-tocopherol dietary supplementation. Worlds Poult. Sci. J. 62:415–415.

Zaniboni, L. and Cerolini, S. (2009) Liquid storage of turkey semen: changes in quality parameters, lipid composition and susceptibility to induced in vitro peroxidation in control, n-3 fatty acids and α-tocopherol rich spermatozoa. Anim. Reprod. Sci. 112(1–2):51–65. https://doi.org/10.1016/j.anireprosci.2008.04.002.

Zanini, S.F., Torres, C.A.A., Bragagnolo, N., Turatti, J.M., Silva, M.G. and Zanini, M.S. (2003a) Oil sources and vitamin E levels in the diet on the composition of fatty acid in rooster's meat. Proc. XVI16th Symp. Qual. Poult. Meat, St.-Brieuc, France. (pp. 199–210).

Zanini, S.F., Torres, C.A.A., Bragagnolo, N., Turatti, J.M., Silva, M.N. and Zanini, M.S. (2003b) Evaluation of the ratio of omega-6, omega-3 fatty acids and vitamin E levels in the diet on the reproductive performance of cockerels. Arch. Anim. Nutr. 57(6):429–442. https://doi.org/10.1080/0003942032000161072.

Zapata, L.F. and Gernat, A.G. (1995) The effect of four levels of ascorbic acid and two levels of calcium on eggshell quality of forced-molted White Leghorn hens. Poult. Sci. 74(6):1049–1052. https://doi.org/10.3382/ps.0741049.

Zdanowska-Sąsiadek, Z., Michalczuk, M., Damaziak, K. and Niemiec, J. (2016a) Dietary vitamin E supplementation on cholesterol, vitamin E content and fatty acid profile in chicken muscles. Can. J. Anim. Sci. 120(2):114–120. https://doi.org/10.1139/cjas-2015-0103.

Zdanowska-Sąsiadek, Ż., Michalczuk, M., Damaziak, K., Niemiec, J., Poławska, E., Gozdowski, D. and Różańska, E. (2016b) Effect of vitamin E supplementation on growth performance and chicken meat quality. Eur. Poult. Sci. 80(2):1–14. https://doi.org/10.1399/eps.2016.152.

Zduńczyk, Z., Jankowski, J. and Koncicki, A. (2002) Growth performance and physiological state of turkeys fed diets with higher content of lipid oxidation products, selenium, vitamin E and vitamin A. Poult. Sci. 58(3):357–364. https://doi.org/10.1079/WPS20020028.

Zee, J.A., Carmichael, L., Codère, D., Poirier, D. and Fournier, M. (1991) Effect of storage conditions on the stability of vitamin C in various fruits and vegetables produced and consumed in Quebec. Journal of Food Composition and Analysis 4(1):77–86. https://doi.org/10.1016/0889-1575(91)90050-G.

Zeisel, S.H. (1981) Dietary choline: biochemistry, physiology, and pharmacology. Annu. Rev. Nutr. 1:95–121. https://doi.org/10.1146/annurev.nu.01.070181.000523.

Zeisel, S.H. (1990) Choline deficiency. J. Nutr. Biochem. 1(7):332–349. https://doi.org/10.1016/0955-2863(90)90001-2.

Zeisel, S.H. (2006) Choline: critical role during fetal development and dietary requirements in adults. Annu. Rev. Nutr. 26:229–250. https://doi.org/10.1146/annurev.nutr.26.061505.111156.

Zeisel, S.H. and Niculescu, M.D. (2006) Perinatal choline influences brain structure and function. Nutr. Rev. 64(4):197–203. https://doi.org/10.1111/j.1753-4887.2006.tb00202.x.

Zempleni, J., Green, G.M., Spannagel, A.W. and Mock, D.M. (1997) Biliary excretion of biotin and biotin metabolites is quantitatively minor in rats and pigs. J. Nutr. 127(8):1496–1500. https://doi.org/10.1093/jn/127.8.1496.

Zhai, Q.H., Dong, X.F., Tong, J.M., Guo, Y.M. and Bao, Y.E. (2013) Long-term effects of choline on productive performance and egg quality of brown-egg laying hens. Poult. Sci. 92(7):1824–1829. https://doi.org/10.3382/ps.2012-02854.

Zhang, C., Li, D., Wang, F. and Dong, T. (2003) Effects of dietary vitamin K levels on bone quality in broilers. Arch. Tierernahr. 57(3):197–206. https://doi.org/10.1080/0003942031000136620.

Zhang, H., Elliott, K.E.C., Durojaye, O.A., Fatemi, S.A., Schilling, M.W. and Peebles, E.D. (2019) Effects of *in ovo* injection of l-ascorbic acid on growth performance, carcass composition, plasma antioxidant capacity, and meat quality in broiler chickens. Poult. Sci. 98(9):3617–3625. https://doi.org/10.3382/ps/pez173.

Zhang, J.Z., Henning, S.M. and Swendseid, M.E. (1993) Poly(ADP-ribose) polymerase activity and DNA strand breaks are affected in tissues of niacin-deficient rats. J. Nutr. 123(8):1349–1355.

Zhang, M.Y., Jia, J.S., Qin, J.H. and Zhao, Y.L. (1994) Improvement of hatchability by treatment of hatching eggs with vitamin B_{12} during incubation. Poult. Husb. Dis. Control 5:21.

Zhang, X., Liu, G., McDaniel, G.R. and Roland, D.A. (1997) Responses of broiler lines selected for tibial dyschondroplasia incidence to supplementary 25-hydroxycholecalciferol. J. Appl. Poult. Res. 6(4):410–416. https://doi.org/10.1093/japr/6.4.410.

Zhang, Y., Zhang, N., Liu, L., Wang, Y., Xing, J. and Li, X. (2021) Transcriptome analysis of effects of folic acid supplement on gene expression in liver of broiler chickens. Front. Vet. Sci. 8:686609. https://doi.org/10.3389/fvets.2021.686609.

Zhao, H., Chen, Y., Wang, S., Wen, C. and Zhou, Y. (2021) Effects of dietary natural vitamin E supplementation on laying performance, egg quality, serum biochemical indices, tocopherol deposition and antioxidant capacity of laying hens. Ital. J. Anim. Sci. 20(1):2254–2262. https://doi.org/10.1080/1828051X.2021.2002733.

Zhao, P., Yan, L., Zhang, T., Yin, H., Liu, J. and Wang, J. (2021) Effect of 25-hydroxyvitamin D and essential oil complex on productive performance, egg quality, and uterus antioxidant capacity of laying hens. Poult. Sci. 100(11):101410. https://doi.org/10.1016/j.psj.2021.101410.

Zhao, Z. and Ross, A.C. (1995) Retinoic acid repletion restores the number of leukocytes and their subsets and stimulates natural cytotoxicity in vitamin A deficient rats. J. Nutr. 125(8):2064–2073. https://doi.org/10.1093/jn/125.8.2064.

Zheng, W. and Teegarden, D. (2013) Vitamin D. In "Handbook of vitamins" 5th ed. Zempleni, J., Suttie, J., Gregory, J. and Stover P. J. (ed.). CRC Press, Taylor & Francis Group, LLC. (pp. 51–88).

Zhu, M., Wesley, I.V., Nannapaneni, R., Cox, M., Mendonca, A., Johnson, M.G. and Ahn, D.U. (2003) The role of dietary vitamin E in experimental Listeria monocytogenes infections in turkeys. Poult. Sci. 82(10):1559–1564. https://doi.org/10.1093/ps/82.10.1559.

Zhu, Y., Li, S., Duan, Y., Ren, Z., Yang, X. and Yang, X. (2020) Effects of *in ovo* feeding of vitamin C on post-hatch performance, immune status and DNA methylation-related gene expression in broiler chickens. Br. J. Nutr. 124(9):903–911. https://doi.org/10.1017/S000711452000210X.

Zhu, Y., Zhao, J., Wang, C., Zhang, F., Huang, X., Ren, Z., Yang, X., Liu, Y. and Yang, X. (2021) Exploring the effectiveness of *in ovo* feeding of vitamin C based on the embryonic vitamin C synthesis and absorption in broiler chickens. J. Anim. Sci. Biotechnol. 12(1):86. https://doi.org/10.1186/s40104-021-00607-w.

Zhu, Y.F., Li, S.Z., Sun, Q.Z. and Yang, X.J. (2019) Effect of in ovo feeding of vitamin C on antioxidation and immune function of broiler chickens. Animal 13(9):1927–1933. https://doi.org/10.1017/S1751731118003531.

Zimmermann, N.G., Twining, P., Harter-Dennis, J. and FitzCoy, S. (1996) Betaine as a methionine substitute and coccidial deterrent in broilers. Poult. Sci. 75(1):154.

Zuidhof, M.J., Schneider, B.L., Carney, V.L., Korver, D.R. and Robinson, F.E. (2014) Growth, efficiency, and yield of commercial broilers from 1957, 1978, and 2005. Poult. Sci. 93(12):2970–2982. https://doi.org/10.3382/ps.2014-04291.

Zulkifli, I., Norma, M.T.C., Chong, C.H. and Loh, T.C. (2001) The effects of crating and road transportation on stress and fear responses of broiler chickens treated with ascorbic acid. Arch. Geflügelk 65:33–37.

Zwaan, J. and Lam, K.W. (1992) Comparison of ascorbic-acid levels in the eye and remainder of the chicken-embryo during development. Exp. Eye Res. 54(3):411–413. https://doi.org/10.1016/0014-4835(92)90053-u.

Index

A
acetylcholine 31, 93, 123, 146–8
African swine fever 11
Agriculture Research Council (ARC) 3, 6, 9
amino acids 29, 33, 75, 80, 92–3, 99, 106, 123, 280, 318
antimicrobial drugs 47
antioxidants 11, 16, 42, 72–5, 107, 141–2, 170–2, 177–8, 182, 244–5
appetite 30, 31, 45, 67, 94, 108–9, 119, 258
ascites 82, 144, 203, 244–5
ascorbic acid *see* vitamin C

B
B complex vitamins 6, 11, 31–2, 183–5, 305–14
  optimum supplementation 254–69
  productivity 17
  sensitivity 41
  stability 13
  see also individual B vitamins by name
bedding 111, 203, 236–7, 255, 264, 266–7
benzoic acid 41
beriberi 21–3, 25, 91, 94
bioavailability 9–10, 38
biotin (vitamin B_8) 6, 10, 14, 31, 41
  biochemical functions 128–9
  and breeding 191–4
  chemical structure and properties 125
  commercial forms 127
  deficiency signs 129–32
  laying hens 311–13
  metabolism 127–8
  natural sources 125–7
  nutritional assessment 129
  optimum supplementation 265–8
  toxicity 132
black tongue 26, 119
blood clotting 30, 76–7, 85–7, 88–9, 183, 303
body temperature 95, 202, 240, 272, 315
bone development 29, 54, 57, 63–4, 66–7, 85–6, 130, 173, 192, 222, 228, 254, 257, 273, 279, 292, 294–5, 304
breeding
  optimum supplementation 151–98
  see also reproduction
brewer's yeast 91
broilers
  body composition 199–200
  growth rates 199
  optimum supplementation 205–78
  product quality 203

C
carbon emissions 1, 2
carbon footprint 2
carbon tax savings 2–3
cardiovascular function 107
carotenoids 12, 41, 43, 48, 51–2, 170–2
  see also vitamin A
cholecalciferol 59
  see also vitamin D
choline 29, 32, 318–22
  biochemical functions 147–9
  and breeding 197–8
  chemical structure and properties 145
  commercial forms 146
  deficiency signs 149–50
  metabolism 146–7
  natural sources 145–6
  nutritional assessment 149
  optimum supplementation 276
  toxicity 150
citric acid cycle *see* Krebs cycle
cobalamin 6, 110–11, 113, 136, 308
  see also vitamin B_{12}
coccidiosis vaccine 6–9, 44
cod liver oil 23, 60, 61
collagen 64, 100, 107, 141–4, 257, 260, 273, 315
confinement, of poultry 41, 131
crazy chick disease *see* encephalomalacia 78
curled-toe paralysis 31, 101–2, 114
cyanocobalamin *see* vitamin B_{12}

D
deficiency signs and symptoms 21–3, 30–2
  biotin (vitamin B_8) 129–32
  choline 149–50
  folic acid (vitamin B_9) 136–8
  niacin (vitamin B_3) 119–20
  pantothenic acid (vitamin B_5) 123–5
  vitamin A 54–8, 168
  vitamin B_1 94–6
  vitamin B_2 100–3
  vitamin B_3 107–9
  vitamin B_{12} 113–15
  vitamin C 144–5
  vitamin D 66–7
  vitamin E 74, 78–82
  vitamin K 88–9
dermal lesions 129–30
dermatitis 17, 25, 31, 102, 107, 119, 120, 193, 203, 225, 266–7
Dietary Supplement Ingredient Database (DSID) 33

E
egg production 30–1, 39, 45, 55, 82, 102, 109, 114, 119, 120, 124, 131, 132, 137, 144, 150, 152, 168, 171–4, 177, 183, 185, 189, 191–5, 224, 279–80, 287–8, 290–3, 295–7, 299–301, 303, 305–13, 315–22
eggs
  fortification of 323–8
  nutritional composition 322–6
  shell quality 45, 307, 309, 311, 313, 315, 317–18
  storage 179, 181, 185, 301–3
  vitamin transfer to yolks 324–6
  yolk colour 52, 171, 281, 290, 301, 320
encephalomalacia 30, 45, 46, 78–80, 108, 239, 245
energy efficiency 1
epithelial tissue disorders 56
essential oils 249
ethoxyquin 10, 12
exudative diathesis 78–9

F
fat-soluble vitamins 10, 11, 29–30, 47, 162–3, 222
  see also individual vitamins by name
feed conversion ratio (FCR) 3–5, 39, 172, 174, 189–90, 199–200, 206, 224, 230, 269–71, 277, 286, 289, 295–6
feedstuffs
  biotin content 126–7
  cost-benefit relationship 204
  ingredients 203–4
  storage 9–12, 38, 49–50, 69, 121, 127, 132, 139
  variations in 203–4
  vitamin concentrations in 40
  vitamins in 33–47
  see also optimum supplementation
fertility 30, 31, 57, 73, 76, 81, 132, 143, 151, 153–4, 168–9, 171, 175–7, 180–1, 184, 193, 196
  see also reproduction
folic acid (vitamin B_9) 6, 14, 32, 41, 114
  biochemical functions 134–6
  and breeding 194–5
  chemical structure and properties 132–3
  commercial forms 133
  deficiency signs 136–8
  laying hens 313–14
  metabolism 134
  natural sources 133
  nutritional assessment 136
  optimum supplementation 268–9
  toxicity 138
Food and Drug Administration (FDA) 33
fowl typhoid 43, 45, 144
free radicals 42, 73–4, 141–2, 176, 180
free-range systems 39, 281

G
greenhouse gases 1–2
growth retardation 102, 137, 149

H
hatchability 102, 109, 114, 119, 124, 131, 137, 169, 172–85, 188–95, 189, 243, 308, 311–13
heat stress 43–6, 82, 101, 142, 152, 169, 170, 181, 196–7, 203, 240–1, 249, 255, 258
Hippocrates 21

I
immune impairment 56–7
immunity 16, 42, 53, 64, 76, 107, 141–2, 169–70, 182, 221–2, 229, 235–6, 241–4, 272–3
Institut National de Recherche Agronomique et l'Environnement (INRAE) 3

K
kidneys 52, 55, 61, 64, 67, 77, 114, 131, 149, 305
Krebs cycle 5, 93, 113, 118, 123

L
laying hens, optimum supplementation 280–322
lesions 55, 58, 81, 96, 123–4, 129–30, 137, 193, 222, 236, 244, 264, 266–7

M
meat quality 30, 46, 75, 206, 210, 222, 237, 239–40, 245–7, 251, 262, 274
menadione salts 84
metabolic functions 5, 6, 85, 147, 183, 199, 279
metabolism 93, 141, 147–8
micronutrients 5
muscular dystrophy 78, 80–1
mycotoxins 10, 45, 46, 55, 89, 242, 255, 300, 309

N
National Research Council (NRC) 3, 6, 9
National Research Institute for Agriculture, Food and Environment 3
nervous disorders 108–9, 113
net-zero 1
niacin (vitamin B_3) 6, 13, 29, 31
  biochemical functions 118–19
  and breeding 190–1
  chemical structure and properties 115
  commercial forms 116
  deficiency signs 119–20
  laying hens 309–11
  metabolism 116–18
  natural sources 115–16
  nutritional assessment 119
  optimum supplementation 261–4
  toxicity 120
night blindness 21, 25, 30
nobel prize winners 27

O
optimum supplementation 3, 5–9, 14–20
  B complex vitamins 254–69
  breeding 151–98
  broilers and turkeys 205–78
  choline 276–8
  laying hens 280–322
  vitamin A 221–3
  vitamin C 269–76
  vitamin D 223–9
  vitamin E 239–54
  vitamin K 254–5
osteomalacia 30, 63, 66
outdoor grazing 39
oxidation 12, 69, 72–5, 98–100, 108, 113, 118–19, 123, 125, 138, 143, 178, 203, 246–50
  see also antioxidants

P
pantothenic acid (vitamin B_5) 6, 14, 20, 32, 41
  biochemical functions 122–3
  and breeding 191
  chemical structure and properties 120–1
  commercial forms 121–2
  deficiency signs 123–5
  laying hens 311
  metabolism 122
  natural sources 121
  nutritional assessment 123
  optimum supplementation 264–5
  stability 121
  toxicity 125
Paris Climate Agreement (COP 21) 2015 1
pellagra 22, 24–6
pelleted feed *see* feedstuffs
pernicious anemia 26, 113
perosis 31, 32, 102, 108, 113–14, 119–20, 124, 130–1, 136–8, 149, 257, 267
polyneuritis 22, 31, 94–6, 185, 257, 306
productivity 5, 14–15, 17, 20, 174, 210, 258
pyridoxine *see* vitamin B_3

R
Recommended Daily Allowances (RDA) 33, 302
reproduction 16, 57–8, 65, 76, 81–2, 151
  see also breeding; fertility
retinol 48, 50–2, 53–4
  see also vitamin A
riboflavin *see* vitamin B_2
rickets 25, 66, 222, 223–4, 227–8
  see also bone development

S
Science Based Targets initiative (SBTi) 1
scurvy 21–5, 142, 143
selenium 42, 44, 46–7, 74–82, 141, 178, 181, 239, 244, 245, 247, 253, 274, 288, 301, 324
spiking syndrome 45
stress 6–9, 44–5, 82, 142, 176, 240, 270–1
  see also heat stress
supplementation *see* optimum supplementation
sustainability 1
Sustainable Development Goals 1

T
temperature (body) 95, 202, 240, 271, 315
thiamine *see* vitamin B_1
tryptophan 29, 31, 33, 106, 116–20, 138, 190, 261, 309
turkeys
  body composition 202
  body weights 199, 201
  optimum supplementation 205–78
  product quality 203

twisted feet 245, 266
see also curled-toe paralysis
twisted leg 130, 238

U
ultraviolet (UV) light stimulation 29
ultraviolet (UV) radiation 59–60, 125, 133
United Nations, Sustainable Development Goals 1

V
value-added tax (VAT) 2
vision 27, 30, 53, 55
vitamin A 30
bioavailability 10
biochemical functions 52–3
and breeding 163, 168–72
chemical structure and properties 48–9
commercial forms 49–50
deficiency signs 54–8, 168
and immunity 42–3, 53, 56–7, 169–70, 221–2
laying hens 287–90
metabolism 50–1
natural sources 49
nutritional assessment 54
optimum supplementation 221–3
sensitivity 41
stability 11–12, 50
toxicity 58–9
vitamin B_1 6, 13, 31
biochemical functions 92–4
and breeding 185
chemical structure and properties 90–1
commercial sources 91
deficiency signs 94–6
laying hens 306
metabolism 91–2
natural sources 91
nutritional assessment 94
optimum supplementation 257–8
toxicity 96
vitamin B_2 6, 13, 31
biochemical functions 98–100
and breeding 188
chemical structure and properties 96–7
commercial forms 97
deficiency signs 100–3
laying hens 306–7
metabolism 97–8
natural sources 96–7
nutritional assessment 100
optimum supplementation 258–9
toxicity 103
vitamin B_3 *see* niacin (vitamin B_3)
vitamin B_6 6, 13, 31
biochemical functions 106–7
and breeding 188–9
chemical structure and properties 103–4
commercial forms 105
deficiency signs 107–9
and immunity 107
laying hens 307–8
metabolism 105
natural sources 103–5
nutritional assessment 107
optimum supplementation 259–60
toxicity 109
vitamin B_{12} 13, 31
biochemical functions 112–13
and breeding 189–90
chemical structure and properties 110
commercial forms 111
deficiency signs 113–15
laying hens 308–9
metabolism 111
natural sources 110
nutritional assessment 113
optimum supplementation 261
toxicity 115
vitamin C 16–17, 21, 29, 32
absorption of minerals 143
biochemical functions 140–4
and breeding 195–7
chemical structure and properties 138–9
commercial forms 139–40
conversion of vitamin D3 143, 230, 273
deficiency signs 144–5
and immunity 42, 45–6, 141–2, 272–3
laying hens 314–18
metabolism 140
natural sources 139
nutritional assessment 144
optimum supplementation 269–76
sensitivity 41
stability 14
toxicity 145
vitamin D 29, 30
biochemical functions 62–5
and breeding 172–6
chemical structure and properties 59–60
commercial forms 60
deficiency signs 66–7
and immunity 64, 229, 235–6
laying hens 290–9
metabolism 60–2

natural sources 60
nutritional assessment 65–6
optimum supplementation 223–9, 324–5
sensitivity 41
stability 12
toxicity 67–8
vitamin E 16, 30
biochemical functions 72–7
and breeding 176–82
chemical structure and properties 68–9
commercial forms 70
deficiency signs 74, 78–82
and immunity 42–4, 76, 182, 241–4
laying hens 299–303
metabolism 70–2
natural sources 69–70
nutritional assessment 78
optimum supplementation 239–54, 324–5
sensitivity 41
stability 12, 69–70
toxicity 82–3
vitamin K 30
biochemical functions 85–7
and breeding 183
chemical structure and properties 83
commercial sources 84
deficiency signs 88–9
laying hens 303–5
metabolism 84–5
natural sources 83–4
nutritional assessment 87–8
optimum supplementation 254–5
sensitivity 41
stability 13
toxicity 90
vitamins
absorption 47
antagonists 46
bioavailability 9–10, 38
conversion factors 36–9
definition 29
as essential micronutrients 5
fat-soluble 10, 11, 29–30, 47, 162–3, 222
and food quality 17–18
history of 21–8
production 27–8
requirements and utilization 38
reserves 47
role of 3–5
sensitivity of 41
solubility 34–5
stability 69–70
stability and volatility 11–14, 50
synthesis 29
water-soluble 29, 90, 183–5, 254–7, 305–6
see also optimum supplementation; *individual vitamins by name*

W
water-soluble vitamins 29, 90, 183–5, 254–7, 305–6
welfare 16–17, 203

X
xerophthalmia 21, 23, 25, 30, 55